REFERENCE

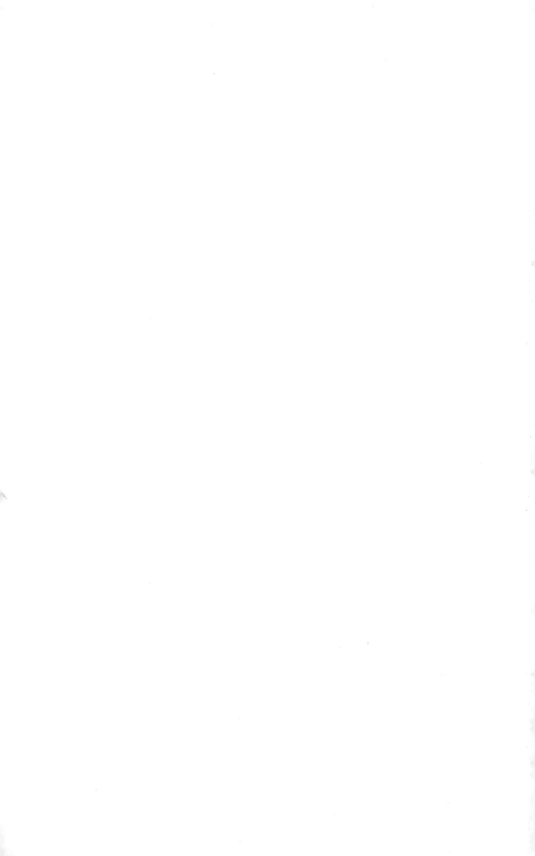

Chemical Exposure and Human Health

This book is dedicated to Ray Phillips.
He helped me define the person
I wanted to be and would eventually become.
He taught me that only by pursuing my dreams
could I make them become realities.

Chemical Exposure and Human Health

*A Reference to 314 Chemicals
with a Guide to Symptoms
and a Directory of Organizations*

by
CYNTHIA WILSON

McFarland & Company, Inc., Publishers
Jefferson, North Carolina, and London

British Library Cataloguing-in-Publication data are available

Library of Congress Cataloguing-in-Publication Data

Wilson, Cynthia, 1953–
    Chemical exposure and human health : a reference to 314 chemicals
with a guide to symptoms and a directory of organizations / by
Cynthia Wilson.
        p.   cm.
    Includes bibliographical references and index.
    ISBN 0-89950-810-3 (library binding : 50# alk. paper) ∞
    1. Environmentally induced diseases.   2. Environmental health.
3. Toxicology   4. Chemicals — Health aspects.   5. Environmental
health — Directories.   I. Title.
    [DNLM: 1. Environmental Exposure.   2. Hazardous Substances —
directories.   3. Hazardous Substances — toxicity.   QV 600 W747
1993]
RB152.W49   1993
615.9′02 — dc20
DNLM/DLC
for Library of Congress   92-51010
                                                            CIP

Manufactured in the United States of America

McFarland & Company, Inc., Publishers
  Box 611, Jefferson, North Carolina 28640

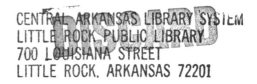
Table of Contents

Acknowledgments

I truly must thank my neglected husband, John, for his constant support and belief in this project—though I think he may be sorry he ever suggested I turn my research into this book.

A special thank you goes to Cindy Duehring for being there when I needed advice, help with tracking down sources, or just someone to talk to—even if it was at three in the morning.

I'd also like to thank Connie Davis. Without her help and support much of what I've accomplished simply wouldn't have been possible.

Last, I would like to thank Bonnye Matthews, Claire Baiz, and Eileen Smith for their efforts in gathering materials that I wouldn't have been able to obtain on my own.

Introduction

Whether by design or default, there is a cloud of ignorance that obscures general knowledge and acceptance of chemically induced health problems. This is particularly true for people who suffer from multiple chemical sensitivities (MCS).

In my own case, it took three years and seven doctors before one was finally able to diagnose me with formaldehyde poisoning. I'm one of the lucky ones.

According to the Institute of Medicine (IOM), there is a shortage of doctors able to respond adequately to the consequences of toxic occupational and environmental exposures which makes it unlikely that a person who may be suffering from chemically related health problems will be able to find responsive, knowledgeable medical help (27, 28).

In 1988, the IOM published *The Role of the Primary Care Physician in Occupational and Environmental Medicine,* which stated, "There is widespread agreement that, with few exceptions, physicians are inadequately trained in occupational and environmental medicine. Lacking a solid foundation in occupational and environmental medicine as well as in the related disciplines of epidemiology and toxicology, most primary care physicians are hard-pressed to keep up with developments in the field. Indeed, the general medical literature contains relatively little about occupational and environmental medicine" (27).

In a survey of medical schools, the IOM found that only 66 percent provided any instruction in occupational and environmental medicine, and only four curriculum hours were required in this field over four years. A 1987 survey conducted by the American Medical Colleges found only 1.4 percent of all students took elective courses in occupational medicine, and 50 percent of the students considered their instruction time in public health and community medicine inadequate (27).

In 1991, the IOM published *Addressing the Physician Shortage in Occupational and Environmental Medicine,* which gave the following as factors contributing to the shortage of doctors willing to become involved in toxic health issues:

1. A shortage of specially trained physicians to serve as teachers, researchers, and consultants to physicians;
2. A lack of readily accessible information on toxic substances in the workplace and the general environment; and
3. Barriers in medical education and clinical practice that limit physician involvement, including the perception that occupational and environmental health conditions are infrequent, difficult, and time- consuming to diagnose and treat; the existence of significant economic disincentives such as the fragmented and often adversarial worker's compensation insurance system; and the pervasive presence of complex ethical and legal issues [28].

In addition, intense infighting among medical disciplines has left most chemical victims without ready access to medical help. Those doctors who practice conventional medicine but recognize chemically induced illnesses are routinely ostracized by their peers or at the very least are referred to as controversial. And the differences between conventional doctors and doctors who practice environmental medicine (also known as clinical ecology) are so great that the American Academy of Medicine and other medical associations have issued position papers condemning this emerging field of medicine. In large part, environmental medicine is growing because of the increasing number of people suffering from MCS. For these victims, diagnosis and treatment is almost nonexistent in orthodox medicine (5, 6).

The main difference, however, between conventional physicians and those doctors who diagnose chemically related health problems appears to be a matter of perception.

For the most part, conventional doctors believe if a person has suffered for years from chronic bronchitis, the illness is a medically established condition and must therefore bear no relation to the patient's environment. They prescribe medication knowing the patient will recover, but also knowing the problem will recur. Sometimes the condition will even reappear on a regular, predictable schedule (7, 298).

These doctors fail to recognize that it often takes years for the results of chemical exposures to become manifest in illnesses but that once these effects are established, re-exposure will reintroduce the illness. Unless the condition progresses to the point where the patient develops chemical sensitivities, the patient is as unlikely as the doctor to recognize the connection. If the patient does make the connection and raises the issue, conventional doctors will generally refer the patient for psychiatric treatment (5, 7, 280, 298, 300).

Chemically aware doctors instead ask why the patient has had chronic bronchitis for years, and they acknowledge that chemicals can and do cause medically established illnesses and diseases. These doctors look for a pattern between the patient's medical condition and chemical exposures. If they find a connection, they usually treat the patient by recommending avoidance of the inciting chemical or protective equipment to minimize the exposure (5, 6, 280, 298).

Short of an acute chemical exposure from a massive spill or widespread community health complaints linked to a toxic waste site, most doctors are reluctant even to consider the possibility that chemical exposures may be at the root of a health problem. While much of their reluctance may be attributed to their lack of training, it is a common misperception that chemicals adversely impact only a small subpopulation of people who are particularly susceptible to the effects of toxic chemicals (27, 291).

This belief is fostered by the American Conference of Government Industrial Hygienists (ACGIH), which consistently maintains that "because of wide variation in individual susceptibility, ... a small percentage of workers may experience discomfort from some substances at concentrations at or below the threshold limit values (TLVs); a smaller percentage may be affected more seriously by aggravation of a pre-existing condition or by development of an occupational illness." This dogma is almost universally repeated by government agencies, industry, and the medical community (291).

Yet a review of the available supporting documentation used by the ACGIH for the 1976 TLVs uncovered only 11 studies that showed no adverse effects at or below the TLV. Most of the studies reported adverse health effects in substantial numbers of the exposed workers. Eight studies even showed 100 percent of the workers were adversely affected at or below the TLVs. On average the documentation showed 17 percent of workers suffered adverse health effects at or below TLVs (291).

In 1988, the ACGIH lowered many of the TLVs and subsequently lowered the average for adverse health effects to 14 percent; however, most of the available supporting documentation still showed TLVs at which substantial numbers, even up to 100 percent, of the workers were at risk. These 1988 TLVs were adopted by the Occupational Safety and Health Administration (291).

To compound the myth of chemical safety, all products must now have Material Safety Data Sheets (MSDS), and physicians are encouraged to obtain copies of these when confronted with a patient claiming chemical injury. While an MSDS is a good place for a physician to start, it shouldn't be relied on to tell the whole story. The law requires that only the active ingredients and major health effects be listed (7, 301).

The story of a woman on the West Coast is a good illustration of how incomplete MSDS information is. This woman was given an adhesive by her dentist which she used over a six-month period to fix a partial plate that kept breaking. The MSDS listed 2-butanone and toluene as the ingredients, which helps explain her subsequent brain damage but does nothing to explain why her jaw bone died. Her attorney discovered that beta-chloroprene was an inactive ingredient not required to be listed on the MSDS. Beta-chloroprene causes necrosis (bone and tissue death) when absorbed (304).

The MSDS, however, only described the health hazards (acute and chronic) as follows:

1. Inhalation may cause irritation of the respiratory tract, excessive exposure causes dizziness up to unconsciousness.
2. Contact with eyes causes irritation.
3. Contact with skin may cause irritation.
4. May be absorbed by skin.
5. Ingestion may cause stomach-ache, nausea and vomiting.
6. Excessive exposure during a long period may cause liver and kidney damage as well as disturbances of the central nervous system [18].

The woman's brain damage was diagnosed as severe and irreversible, and she is facing major reconstructive surgery to replace her jaw but it has yet to be established in court that the product was responsible.

There is hope. Progress is being made, in spite of the general ignorance, misconceptions, and reluctance in the medical community to address chemically related health issues. The technology to prove chemical injuries is finally beginning to catch up to the technology that created them, but it is still in its infancy. As new testing procedures are discovered and existing procedures are refined to measure smaller and smaller changes in body functions, more evidence of chemical damage is being observed. Often, though, the significance of what is found is not fully understood because of the inadequacy of our knowledge of body systems and cellular interaction (1, 2, 4, 5, 6, 32, 33, 280, 300, 451, 454, 455).

Two major areas of concern are emerging as going hand in hand with both acute and chronic chemical exposures. They are nervous system and immune system damage (33, 300).

Most, but certainly not all, victims of chemical exposure have some form of brain damage impairing higher cognitive functions such as memory, reasoning, or the ability to acquire or process new information. This central nervous system damage is often accompanied by damage to the peripheral nervous system as well (33, 301, 302, 304).

Changes in the immune system are also found in the majority of victims. Such changes may include immune system activation and or suppression, formation of antibodies to chemicals, and the formation of two or more types of autoimmune antibodies (32, 280, 300).

Most often, these autoimmune antibodies are to the liver, thyroid, kidneys, intestines, stomach, and myelin sheathing; but they may not be organ-specific as in the case of antibodies associated with certain forms of lupus. Whether these autoimmune antibodies will eventually develop into the associated autoimmune diseases has not been clearly established. Much research is still needed in this area (280, 300).

The etiology of how chemicals are creating this damage is also unknown, especially in the area of MCS. As of October 1991, the Environmental Protection Agency, the National Institutes of Health, and the National Institute of Environmental Health Sciences were not funding research into MCS issues even though the National Academy of Sciences, the National Research Council, and other agencies have been calling for basic MCS research since the early 1980s (5, 6, 10, 32, 280).

Coming to terms with the fact that personal hygiene products, laundry detergents, or the photocopier at work may be adversely affecting one's health or emotional stability is not easy, and the medical community doesn't make it any easier. There are, however, qualified doctors who can help. Chapter 6 lists organizations that deal with these health issues; many of them make doctor referrals.

Because of the medical profession's inconsistency in diagnosing chemical injuries, a list of the tests that are most often used either to find or to rule out chemically related health problems has been provided. These tests need, however, to be ordered and interpreted by qualified doctors experienced in chemical injuries. This is especially true for the neuropsychological testing (1, 2, 4, 5, 6, 33, 454, 455).

Chemicals, their metabolites, or heavy metals in the body: 1) blood tests; 2) urine tests; 3) fat biopsies.

Immune system testing: 1) antibody assay testing for chemical antibody formation; 2) activated lymphocyte profiles; 3) autoimmune disease profiles; 4) autoimmune profiles for nervous system disorders; 5) allergy testing for foods, molds, pollens, and chemicals.

Neuropsychological testing: 1) complete neurological examination; 2) neurobehavioral testing (Halstead-Reitan or Pittsburgh Occupational Exposure Tests); 3) Positron Emission Tomography (PET) scans; 4) Magnetic Resonance Imaging (MRI) scans; 5) Quantitive Electroencephalogram (EEG); 6) Single Photon Emission Computed Tomography (SPECT) scans.

Other testing considerations: 1) enzyme testing for cholinesterase levels, antioxidant levels, liver enzymes, etc. (see Chapter 2); 2) amino acids profiles (Standard Panel or Neuropsychiatric Panel); 3) conditions and disorders associated with specific chemical exposures such as aplastic anemia, pulmonary function tests, etc. (see Chapter 2); 4) challenge testing to chemicals in an environmental unit. The latter may be needed for individuals suffering from multiple chemical sensitivities because sensitivities may develop before otherwise detectable chemical damage has occurred.

A Note on Alphabetization

The alphabetization of chemical names is a confusing matter for the reader with a nonscientific background.

The alphabetization used in this book generally follows the same rules as *The Register of Toxic Effects of Chemical Substances* published by the National Institute of Occupational Safety and Health.

The many prefixes used in organic chemistry are disregarded in alphabetizing; these include: ortho-, meta-, para-, alpha-, beta-, gamma-, see-, tert-, sym-, as-, uns-, cis-, trans-, endo-, exo-, d-, l-, dl-, n-, N-, O-, as well as all numbers that involve structure. Hyphens are ignored within a word, as are numbers and many of the prefixes listed above when used in an inter word position. So "1, 8-p-Methadiene" will be found in the m's. And "1-Chloro-2, 3-epoxypropane" is alphabetized as if it were spelled "Chloroepoxypropane." Punctuation is ignored no matter where it appears.

A strict letter-by-letter alphabetization is thus required for Chapter 5, the chemical directory. Methylcarbinol will appear before methyl cellosolve, for example.

In chapters 2, 3 and 4, the far more common word-by-word form of alphabetization is used. While letter-by-letter alphabetization is the more correct method of alphabetizing chemical names (and, given the elements that one disregarded, the only truly practical one), the word-by-word method is much easier to use in the three chapters dealing with the symptoms, targets and sources of chemical exposure, permitting, as it does, like elements to stay grouped. Nervous system damage will appear before nervousness, for example.

The index permits access to prefixed chemical names in two ways — either ignoring the prefixes listed above or considering them part of the name. The chemicals are listed both ways to improve usability for readers unfamiliar with the conventions of chemical nomenclature.

1

The Chemical Gauntlet

Whatever befalls the Earth, befalls the sons of the Earth.
Man did not weave the web of life, he is merely a strand
in it. Whatever he does to the web, he does to himself.

— Chief Sealth, 1854

Every minute of every day we are inundated by chemicals. While some of these exposures may be harmless, many are not. Between 1965 and 1982 over 4 million distinct chemical compounds were formulated, with as many as 6,000 new formulations being created each week since then. The National Institute for Occupational Safety and Health (NIOSH) maintains files on over 100,000 chemicals. The Environmental Protection Agency (EPA) regulates approximately 65,000 toxic chemicals and receives about 1,500 requests per year to register new compounds (296, 414, 447).

Approximately 3,000 chemicals are deliberately added to our food, 700 have been found in drinking water, 400 have been identified in human tissue, over 500 can be found under the kitchen sink or in the laundry room in the average home, and approximately 100 pounds of hazardous waste have been tucked away in such storage places as the basement or garage (25, 296).

With over 70,000 of these chemicals in daily use, many people are becoming increasingly concerned about health and safety issues. Recently a man on a television talk show asked why the government, or anyone for that matter, should be concerned about a chemical estimated to harm only 300 to 400 people. The answer can be found in simple arithmetic (296).

The Food and Drug Administration (FDA) allows pesticide residue on food if it is estimated to pose a cancer risk to only 1 person in 1 million. So if we use the same risk/safety ratio of 1:1,000,000 for all known health hazards associated with the EPA's 65,000 chemicals, we could assume given the United States' population, at least 16,250,000 chemical injury victims

1

immediately with 375,000 new victims each year. Figures in the NIOSH's files suggest as many as 25 million victims (448).

Some chemicals, however, are known or suspected to adversely affect considerably more people than one in a million. Formaldehyde has been estimated by various institutions and government agencies to adversely influence the health of between 10 and 20 percent of the population at any exposure level. Formaldehyde is such a ubiquitous chemical, found in everything from food to plywood, that it has the statistical capability to harm the health of 25 to 50 million people (129, 278, 279).

Approximately 80 million people, or 3 out of every 10, in the United States can expect to contract some form of cancer during their lifetime. The National Cancer Institute has estimated in at least one communiqué that as many as 98 percent of all cancers may be linked to chemical exposures, according to Lynn Montandon, founder of the Response Team for the Chemically Injured (303).

Until recently, the federal government has concentrated most of its resources on researching cancer and the effects of acute chemical exposures, paying very little attention to the effects of long-term, low-level chemical exposures or to the neurological, reproductive, developmental, or immunological effects that chemicals may cause. The government is just beginning to look at these non-cancer health risks, and the existing research into these other health effects is, on the whole, inadequate to nonexistent. According to the National Research Council, no toxicity data are available for over 39,000 commercially used chemicals (301, 302, 449, 453).

Along with more accepted non-cancer health concerns such as birth defects, a "new" and controversial illness is sweeping the country and has been getting more and more attention. It has been given many names, such as Environmental Illness and Total Allergy Syndrome, but Multiple Chemical Sensitivities (MCS) seems to be one of the more popular and accurate names (5, 6, 457).

People are becoming so sensitized by either acute or chronic low-level chemical exposures that they can no longer tolerate exposure levels that most governmental agencies and the medical and scientific communities consider too low to pose any significant health risk. The condition's symptoms range in severity from sneezing and mild headaches to seizures, violent headaches and other reactions so overwhelming the victims must totally withdraw from society to control their environments (5, 6).

Multiple Chemical Sensitivities has also been called the "Twentieth Century Disease" by some professionals. That was even the title of a 1970s PBS documentary dealing with this highly complex, little-understood illness. There is, however, evidence that MCS was first observed as early as the 1800s. Alfred B. Nobel (1833–1896), the inventor of dynamite, suffered from dynamite-induced headaches, as did many of his factory workers.

The French author Marcel Proust (1871–1922) isolated himself in a cork-lined room. His biographer noted a number of instances in which perfumes made Proust ill, and he had to set visitors' chairs outside to air because they became contaminated by the scents of the occasional guest (6, 24).

While MCS appears to have existed for some time, the energy conservation effort in the 1970s sharply exacerbated the problem. While reducing the volume of outside air allowed into homes and workplaces to conserve energy, no consideration was given to the health effects on people being exposed to the resulting higher levels of volatile organic compounds and other biological contaminants trapped inside. The health problems created by this energy conservation are being called the "Sick Building Syndrome" (428).

The extent to which chemicals are damaging health is unknown because injuries of this nature are hard to spot. For example, when a woman has a miscarriage, a test to check for solvents known to induce spontaneous abortions is not routinely done and in most cases is not even considered. A person suffering from depression is given counseling and medication, but rarely does anyone think to see if that person is being exposed to one of the 40 chemicals known to cause depression. There are headache clinics all over the country, but it is doubtful that many, if any, routinely take the trouble to rule out chemicals as a potential cause (7, 27, 293, 413).

An important question is how many people have been classified as hypochondriacs or as being mentally ill because chemical injuries have not been detected through routine medical tests. How many continue to suffer from the medical community's general reluctance to consider chemical causes (5, 298)?

The National Academy of Sciences (NAS) estimates that "up to 15 percent of the population may have heightened sensitivity to chemicals...." According to Zane Gard, M.D., the NAS has further reported that by 1993, 30 percent of the population may be adversely affected, and in the next generation the percentage could double again to 60 percent (21, 281).

In spite of increasing evidence of chemically related health problems, the United States as a nation remains chemically ignorant. Citizens rely on government agencies like the FDA, EPA, or the Occupational Safety and Health Administration (OSHA) for protection, but by law these agencies are limited in their powers to protect (286, 301, 302, 447).

The NIOSH found 884 neurotoxic chemical compounds used in the cosmetic and perfume industries. Yet no regulations exist to prohibit the use of those chemicals, nor does the Federal Food, Drug, and Cosmetic Act require cosmetic ingredients to undergo pre-market toxicity testing. The consumer cannot even make an informed decision about whether to use these products because these industries are exempt from ingredient labeling laws (201, 302).

Pesticides, insecticides, and herbicides (collectively referred to as "pesticides") represent another class of substances from which the American people falsely believe they are being protected. A pesticide registered by the EPA is not guaranteed to be safe for three major reasons (10, 447).

First, the EPA registers pesticides not on safety but on a cost-benefit basis, balancing health and environmental concerns against the economic gain to the manufacturer and the end user of the product (447). In fact, out of the 600 active ingredients under its control, the EPA can provide safety assurances for only six (467).

It is illegal to make or imply safety claims for pesticide products. Such claims as "EPA registered," "safe when used as directed," and "containing all natural ingredients" are among the most common safety claims that are unlawfully made to dispel public apprehension about their use. Unfortunately, while laws barring these statements are on the books, they are rarely enforced (447).

Second, the law is flawed by a major loophole regarding inert ingredients used in these products. Inert ingredients are those that are not directly active in the product's stated function. Other than that restriction, an inert ingredient can be anything. Inerts are important to the public because they make up from 50 percent to 99 percent of a product and are not required to be EPA registered or even listed on the product label. Many of these so-called inert ingredients, when not used as inerts in pesticide products, are regulated by as many as 22 different federal agencies, including the EPA (11, 286).

The Northwest Coalition for Alternatives to Pesticides (NCAP), in a Freedom of Information Act lawsuit, obtained from the EPA a list of 1,400 of the 2,000 substances being used as inert ingredients. From that list, the NCAP learned that substances such as hazardous waste, Chicago sludge, asbestos, and some banned chemicals such as DDT are being used as inert ingredients. The EPA banned DDT as an active ingredient because of its potential toxicity to humans and the environment (23).

Congress has made the de facto decision that the Trade Secrets Act, which protects manufacturers from having to fully disclose ingredients, supersedes the public's right to know what it's being exposed to and the health hazards resulting from those exposures. Some states are seriously considering legislation to require full ingredient disclosures, but no state has yet enacted such a law (11, 23, 286).

Third, only the active ingredient in the product is required to undergo toxicity testing. No studies of any kind are required on the inert ingredients or the possible potentiation, synergistic, additive, or cumulative effects of the total chemical composition of the product that is actually sold to the public. That means there would be no way to evaluate effectively the potential health hazards associated with the use of these products even if all the ingredients were listed (11, 286).

In addition, the EPA defines disinfectants as one of several types of antimicrobial pesticides and requires only the active ingredients to be registered. In some instances, one may be exposed to potentially harmful disinfectants that are not even known to work (450).

Loopholes in the laws are not the only problems. Some decisions by regulating agencies have the potential to create as many problems as they were intended to solve.

For instance, in spite of a significant correlation between birth defects and outdoor air pollution, the EPA is promoting the burning of hazardous waste as a method of disposal. Substances that the agency deems too hazardous to put into landfills are now being put into the air. An incinerator that is 99.9999 percent efficient is still capable of dumping approximately 300,000 pounds of toxins into the air; one that is only 91 percent efficient may generate as much as 270 million pounds (294, 458).

James Walsh, a scientist employed by the U.S. National Bureau of Standards, studied the EPA emissions monitoring process and concluded that the same numbers the EPA uses to obtain a 99.99 percent efficiency rating could with equal validity represent a destruction capability of only 79.23 percent. In addition, the EPA acknowledges that the technology needed to accurately monitor emissions from these smoke stacks does not exist. Yet we are led to believe that burning these hazardous materials is based on environmental concerns and adequate technology (286a, 458).

In 1988, the EPA removed new carpet from its Washington, D.C., headquarters after 122 staff members complained of adverse reactions. However, beyond removing the carpeting, the EPA did not respond to general concerns that carpeting may be a health threat. Because of this lack of response, the National Federation of Federal Employees (NFFE) petitioned the EPA on January 11, 1990, to investigate the toxicity of carpeting and promulgate rules for conducting research on the mechanism of causation and the extent of adverse health effects (31a, 461).

On April 16, 1990, the EPA denied the NFFE petition, but two days later it announced a "dialogue" program to encourage the carpet industry to voluntarily reduce carpet emissions. Upon completing the "dialogue," the EPA in March of 1992 published a brochure stating that "limited research to date has found no link between adverse health effects and the levels of chemicals emitted by new carpet" (31a, 461)

In 1991, 26 state attorneys general petitioned the Consumer Product Safety Commission (CPSC) to require health warnings on new carpet and installation materials. The warnings were to list the possible reactions and advise consumers to take such precautions as fully ventilating newly carpeted rooms. The CPSC refused (31a).

Then, in August 1992, Rosalind Anderson, Ph.D., a physiologist, announced the results of her experiments with specific carpets that people had claimed made them ill. Using standard testing methods, she exposed mice to air blown over these carpet samples. The fumes from the nine carpet samples she tested killed the majority of the mice. The carpet fumes worked like a nerve gas, causing the mice to gasp for air, turn blue, lose their balance, and suffer paralysis and lung hemorrhaging. Within four hours many of the mice were dead. In one experiment, Anderson found that not only a carpet sample but simply an air sample from the room in which the carpet was installed caused the mice to die (31a).

It is too early to tell whether Anderson's finding will significantly influence the EPA's position on carpet toxicity.

The FDA and EPA are not the only governmental agencies failing to protect the public interest. Created to protect workers, OSHA establishes and regulates permissible exposure levels (PELs) for toxic chemicals found in the workplace. In 1988, OSHA PELs were taken directly from the threshold limit values (TLVs) established by the American Conference of Governmental Industrial Hygienists (ACGIH), a voluntary organization with no official government ties. Industry interests have played a major role in establishing these exposure levels. In some instances TLVs have been established and the supporting worker safety documentation has consisted of nothing more than a telephone call from an industry representative to the ACGIH. In addition, the ACGIH refused to release the minutes of the meetings where the TLVs were established to researchers trying to verify the safety data used to determine exposure levels. The available supporting documentation strongly suggests that an industry's ability to meet a particular exposure level played as large a role in determining TLVs as did the health risks to workers (12, 291; see Introduction for more information on TLVs).

In addition, OSHA PELs are often based on a dose-response measurement and do not take into account the potential of many chemicals to accumulate in human tissue, blood, and body fat until a toxic level has been reached (1, 296, 305, 306).

In acknowledging and regulating potentially hazardous chemicals, OSHA frequently lags far behind other federal agencies. Asbestos has long been accepted in the medical and scientific communities, the EPA, the NIOSH, and other federal agencies as a carcinogen. It is not, however, regulated by OSHA as one. In his testimony on the Indoor Air Quality Act of 1991 (HR 1006, S 455), John Moran, director of occupational safety and health for the Laborers' Health and Safety Fund of North America, stressed that Congress should mandate that interim regulations be drafted within six months of the bill's enactment because of government agencies' traditional resistance to regulating indoor contaminants. Moran went on to explain that the need for a time frame was "particularly important regarding the workplaces under OSHA jurisdiction, for which OSHA must continue to bear responsibility, as OSHA continues to evidence a complete lack of will or ability to establish required standards within a time frame considered reasonable by nearly anyone" (12, 18, 304, 322).

To make matters worse, on July 7, 1992, the 11th Circuit Court of Appeals ruled that OSHA's standards for 428 toxic substances were invalid due to inadequate research on exposure levels and effects. If the court's ruling is allowed to stand, it will eliminate the newly adopted workplace exposure limits for 164 toxic substances and return PEL limits for 212 previously regulated air contaminants to higher, outdated, and less protective PELs established more than 20 years earlier (416a, 416b).

At the time of this writing, OSHA had requested a rehearing, claiming that in vacating the entire standard, the court went far beyond its judicial function and exceeded the remedies that any petitioner could properly seek, with the result that workers could face serious health risks while OSHA's hands were tied (416b).

While significant problems exist within the federal agencies charged with protecting the public, these agencies are also understaffed and grossly underfunded to carry out the tasks set for them by Congress. As one doctor put it, chemical compounds are being thrown at researchers faster than they have the capacity to test them. There are also countless instances in which Congress has given an agency the responsibility for solving a problem without giving it the authority to effect change. For example, the EPA lists indoor air pollution as fourth out of 31 environmental concerns; however, in 1991 less that 4 percent of the EPA's overall air program budget was spent on the problem because Congress prioritizes the way the EPA spends its funds, and indoor air pollution is not a priority concern (446).

Perhaps it should be. According to the American Lung Association of Washington, "a recent survey of office workers nationwide showed that 24 percent of office workers were aware of air quality problems in their offices. Twenty percent felt that their work performance was adversely affected by air quality problems" (3).

Protecting the public from all known health hazards was the original mandate for many U.S. government agencies, but over the years that goal has been proven virtually unattainable. Since the 1950s, when little was known about the full range of health effects chemicals can cause, the government has slowly developed a policy of risk assessment. As the number of chemical related injuries has grown, the General Accounting Office has questioned the validity of these risk assessment models, stating that these models underestimate the potential risks to all minority groups, women, children, infants, fetuses, and minority groups in general (301, 448).

Because of the federal government's lack of leadership in protecting its citizens, many states are now starting to take their own measures. For example, the EPA will allow drinking water to be contaminated with arsenic at 50 parts per billion, a level which poses a cancer risk to 1 person in every 100. The California EPA wants to lower its state's arsenic level standard to 2 parts per trillion and thus reduce the cancer risk to approximately one person in a million (289).

In many instances dangerous chemical substances have entered the market because the best available chemical structure, technical review, and risk assessment models at the time indicated they were safe. Only later, at the expense of human health and in some cases lives were these models proved wrong (301).

No one debates that every day toxic chemicals cause adverse health effects. The battle lines are drawn on the dosage at which damage may occur, the extent of the damage, the route of exposure (inhalation, ingestion, or skin absorption) needed to cause damage, and chronic low-level exposures versus acute exposures.

This book will not settle the debate. In fact, it is intended to add fuel to the fire. California Senator Nicolas C. Petris said it best when he wrote, "Pesticides are still better categorized in terms of what we do not know than what is known about them." However, Senator Petris' statement could equally apply to most chemicals currently in use (11, 453).

While the chemicals in this book represent only a small sampling of the chemicals in daily use, none has been tested for the full range of its toxic potential—making the public the experimental test animals.

While much more research in this area is needed, it appears that effects on a person's health depend not only on the chemical but on a person's genetic makeup and the level and duration of the exposure. Generally, no person will get all the symptoms listed for any chemical, nor will everyone who is exposed become ill. Science still has not determined how two people can work side by side with only one becoming ill (5, 6, 32).

Chapter 2 lists those symptoms that have been associated with a particular chemical exposure. The following criteria were used in selecting what health effects were to be included.

Health effects are stated as fact if a federal or state governmental publication printed the adverse health effect as a fact without using a qualifier, if human epidemiological studies were confirmed by supporting animal research, or if medical case reports established a dose related cause and effect relationship and the reports underwent peer review.

Health effects are stated as suspected if a variety of animal studies showed consistent results across species but no human evidence was available, or if epidemiological human studies were insufficient or inadequate and no animal studies existed.

Health effects were not included if insufficient or inadequate animal and or human studies existed, if medical case reports did not establish a clear cause and effect relationship, or if medical or scientific reports were not peer reviewed.

Many chemicals are known to target specific organs, systems, or body parts (end-point targets) for damage. While these chemicals may cause damage in other areas of the body, end-point targets are where the primary damage can be expected to take place. Chapter 3 deals with these end-point targets.

Chemicals were chosen based on where a person might expect to be exposed to them. As labeling laws don't require complete disclosure, chemical usage was the hardest part to research and many non-technical sources were used. Chapter 4 lists usages, but because of the Trade Secrets Act it is impossible to know how complete this information is. Where possible major categories such as cleaning products were split into subcategories such as household cleaning products. It is in these subcategories, however, where limited information was available.

Chapter 5 provides a profile for each chemical. These profiles contain trade names and synonyms which have also been cross-referenced to their chemical names.

The OSHA permissible exposure levels (PELs) are given. The exposure standards of the NIOSH and the American Conference of Governmental Industrial Hygienists have also been included where available and when they are lower than OSHA standards. These standards may be used to establish relative toxicity: a higher exposure standard generally means a lower risk. These standards are not intended, however, to protect all workers (12, 291)

Methylene chloride, for example, currently has an OSHA PEL of 500 parts per million (ppm), but OSHA is considering lowering the standard to 50 ppm in order to save approximately 600 lives. The higher PEL is based on the exposure level at which methylene chloride's irritating effects can be observed (419).

The following is provided to give a frame of reference for the quantity at which chemicals are measured and regulated: 1 part per million (ppm) equates to 1 minute in 2 years; 1 part per billion (ppb) equates to 1 second in 32 years; and 1 part per trillion (ppt) equates to 1 second in 320 centuries (293).

Chapter 5 also restates the potential and suspected health effects, end-point targets, and usages for each chemical from chapters 2, 3, and 4. In addition, where available, other pertinent information has been included.

Chapter 6 is a resource guide. Over 400 organizations were contacted, but only those responding are included. Some of these organizations work for a reduction in the use of toxic chemicals while others are support groups for people whose health has been adversely affected.

Making the world a safer place in which to live starts with the general public, not the government. Modern society's dependence on chemicals has forced its members to run a chemical gauntlet in which not only the environment but millions of people are at risk. We are left to choose whether protecting our carpet from our children is more important that protecting our children from potentially toxic carpet fumes. Chemicals, even toxic chemicals, are often the substances of life, and doing away with them is not the solution nor is it practical. We do need, however, to look for less toxic substitutes and demand complete product toxicity testing and full ingredient label disclosure in order to minimize health risks. Most important, we need to start treating these substances with the respect they deserve.

2
Symptoms, Diseases, and Health Conditions: Potential Chemical Causatives

Abdominal cramps Azinphos-methyl; Benzyl chloride; Carbaryl; Chlorpyrifos; Demeton; EPN; Ethyl chloride; Hydroquinone; Lead; Malathion; Methyl bromide; Methyl parathion; Naled; Nickel; N-Nitrosodimethylamine; Phosdrin; n-Propyl alcohol; TEDP.

Abdominal discomfort 2-Aminopyridine; Chlorine dioxide; 1,3-Dichloropropene.

Abdominal distention Hydrogen peroxide.

Abdominal pain Acetylene tetrabromide; Arsine; Boron; Bromine; 2-Butoxyethanol; Cadmium; Carbon tetrachloride; Chromium; 2,4-D; Diethylamine; Epichlorohydrin; 2-Ethoxyethyl acetate; Ethylene glycol dinitrate; Fluorides; Hydrazine; Iodine; Isopropyl alcohol; Lead; Limonene; Methyl cellosolve acetate; Naphthalene; Nicotine; Nitric oxide; Nitrophenols; Pentachlorophenol; Phenol; Phosphine; Phosphorus; Picric acid; Pindone; Propylene dichloride; Stibine; Sulfur dioxide; 1,1,2,2-Tetrachloroethane; Tetraethyl lead; Tetramethyl lead; Thallium; Tin; Toluene; Toluene-2,4-diisocyanate;

Turpentine; Vinyl chloride; Warfarin; Xylenes; Zinc chloride.

Abdominal pain, upper Methyl alcohol.

Abdominal soreness Demeton.

Abdominal spasms Cyanides; Hydrogen cyanide.

Abdominal spasms, tonic Pentaborane.

Abortions, spontaneous Antimony; Arsenic; Benzene; beta-Chloroprene; Dinitrotoluenes; Ethylene oxide; Lead; Mercury; Phenol; Vinyl chloride.

Abortions, suspected of causing spontaneous Acrolein; Copper; Dibutylphthalate; 2,4-Dichlorophenol; Styrene; Tetrachloroethylene; Xylenes.

Acidosis 2-Aminopyridine; 2-Butoxyethanol; Cobalt; Dinitro-o-cresol; 2,4-D; Formaldehyde; Formic acid; Methyl alcohol; Paraldehyde.

Acidosis metabolic Ethyl ether; Isopropyl ether; Pentaborane; Sulfur dioxide.

Acroosteolysis, occupational (spontaneous dissolution of the finger tips.) Vanadium pentoxide; Vinyl chloride.

Adrenal damage, suspected of causing 2,3-Benzofuran.

Adrenal gland cellular vacuolization Beryllium.

Adrenal gland congestion Beryllium.

Adrenal lesions, suspected of causing 2,3-Benzofuran.

Adrenal tissue death Ethylene dichloride; Pentachloronaphthalene; Tetrachloronaphthalene.

Aggressiveness Tin.

Agitation Chlorinated camphene; Nicotine; Sulfur dioxide.

Alcohol intolerance Dimethylformamide; Thiram.

Allergic sensitization Pyrethrum; Titanium dioxide; Trichloroethylene.

Allergic-like reactions *also see* Chemical sensitivity Methylene bisphenyl isocyanate; Toluene-2,4-diisocyanate.

Alveolar congestion Chloropicrin.

Alveolar septal distension, suspected of causing 1,2-Dichloroethylene.

Alveolar swelling Chloropicrin; Phosgene.

Alzheimer's Disease, suspected of causing Aluminum.

Amino acids, excessive Lead.

Anemia Aniline; Arsenic; Benzene; Benzidine; n-Butyl acetate; sec-Butyl acetate; tert-Butyl acetate; Cadmium; Chlorinated diphenyl; Chloropicrin; Chromium; Decaborane; Diborane; o-Dichlorobenzene; p-Dichlorobenzene; Dinitrobenzenes; Dinitrotoluenes; Ethylene dichloride; Formaldehyde; Isobutyl acetate; Lead; Molybdenum; p-Nitroaniline; Nitrobenzene; p-Nitrochlorobenzene; Pentaborane; p-Phenylene diamine; Phosphorus; Propylene dichloride; Tetraethyl lead; Tetramethyl lead; Toluene; o-Toluidine; 2,4,6-Trinitrotoluene.

Anemia, agranulocytic Picric acid.

Anemia, aplastic Benzene; Chlorinated camphene; Dinitrobenzenes; Lindane; Pentachlorophenol; 2,4,6-Trinitrotoluene.

Anemia, hemolytic Chromium; Cresols; p-Dichlorobenzene; Dinitrobenzenes; Formaldehyde; Hydroquinone; Isopropyl alcohol; Methyl mercaptan; Naphthalene; Nitrophenols; Phenol; Phenylhydrazine; Propylene dichloride; Stibine; Trimellitic anhydride.

Anemia, hypochromic normocytic Lead.

Anemia, low grade Acrylonitrile.

Anemia, suspected of causing Copper; 1,1-Dimethylhydrazine; Ethyl silicate; Ethylene glycol dinitrate; Fluorides; Methyl cellosolve; Polychlorinated biphenyls; Selenium; Tin.

Anemia, suspected of causing hemolytic 1,1-Dimethylhydrazine.

Anemia, suspected of causing macrocytic Beryllium.

Angina Carbon monoxide; Ethylene glycol dinitrate.

Ankle drops or dangles Arsenic.

Ankle reflex, absence of Phosphine.

Ankles, numbness/tingling/prickling sensation of the Dinitrobenzenes.

Ankles, paralysis of Lead.

Antibodies, decreased Benzene.

Antibodies to the chemical, formation of Benzene; Chlorinated diphenyl; Cobalt; Formaldehyde; alpha-Methyl styrene; Trimellitic anhydride.

Anxiety Acetonitrile; Acrylamide; Arsenic; Chlorine; Chlorpyrifos; Dinitro-o-cresol; Lead; Malathion; Manganese; Methyl parathion; Naled; Nitric oxide; Picric acid; Styrene;

Tetraethyl lead; Tetramethyl lead; Trichloroethylene.

Apathy Azinphos-methyl; Chlorpyrifos; Demeton; Dinitrobenzenes; Formaldehyde; Methyl alcohol; Naled.

Appetite, loss of Acetonitrile; Acetylene tetrabromide; Aniline; Antimony; Azinphos-methyl; Benzene; Benzyl chloride; Beryllium; Bromine; Carbaryl; Carbon disulfide; Chlorinated diphenyl; Cobalt; 2,4-D; Decaborane; Demeton; Diborane; p-Dichlorobenzene; Dichlorvos; Dimethyl sulfate; 1,1-Dimethylhydrazine; EPN; Ethyl ether; Ferbam; n-Heptane; Hexone; Isopropyl ether; Lead; Malathion; Mercury; Methyl alcohol; Methyl bromide; Methyl parathion; Naled; Naphtha; 1-Nitropropane; 2-Nitropropane; Paraldehyde; Pentaborane; Pentachloronaphthalene; Pentachlorophenol; n-Pentane; Phenol; Phenylhydrazine; Phosdrin; Phosphine; Pindone; Polychlorinated biphenyls; Pyridine; TEDP; Tellurium; TEPP; 1,1,2,2-Tetrachloroethane; Tetrachloroethylene; Tetrachloronaphthalene; Tetraethyl lead; Tetramethyl lead; Thiram; o-Toluidine; Trichloroethylene; 2,4,6-Trinitrotoluene; Triorthocresyl phosphate; Vanadium pentoxide; Warfarin; Xylenes.

Appetite, suspected of causing loss of Molybdenum; Silver.

Apprehension Acrylonitrile; Dichlorodifluoromethane; Sodium fluoroacetate.

Arteries, abnormal tension of Cumene; Manganese.

Arteriosclerosis 1,3-Butadiene.

Asbestosis Asbestos.

Asphyxia Acetic anhydride; Acetonitrile; Acrolein; Acrylonitrile; Azinphos-methyl; Benzene; Carbaryl; Carbon dioxide; Chlorpyrifos; Cyanides; Dichloromonofluoromethane; Dichlorotetrafluoroethane; EPN; Hydrogen cyanide; Sulfur dioxide.

Astheno-autonomic syndrome (weakness in self regulating body functions.) Vanadium pentoxide.

Asthma Bromine; Chloropicrin; Chromium; Cobalt; Ethylenediamine; Methylene bisphenyl isocyanate; Pyrethrum; Toluene-2,4-diisocyanate; Trimellitic anhydride.

Asthma, allergic Nickel carbonyl; p-Phenylene diamine.

Asthma, bronchial Maleic anhydride; p-Phenylene diamine; Phthalic anhydride; Sulfur dioxide.

Asthma, intrinsic (adult onset) Formaldehyde.

Asthma, occupational Maleic anhydride; Phthalic anhydride.

Asthmatic bronchitis Chlorine dioxide; Epichlorohydrin.

Atherosclerosis Polycyclic aromatic hydrocarbons.

Attention, impaired capacity to attain Formaldehyde.

Attention span, short Formaldehyde.

Autoimmune diseases Cadmium; Hydrazine; Mercury; Polychlorinated biphenyls; Silica; Vanadium pentoxide; Vinyl chloride.

Autonomic dysfunction (self-controlling body functions) Ethyl acrylate.

Back aches, lower Ethylene glycol.

Back pain Arsine; Methyl alcohol; Pindone; Warfarin.

Back pain (lumbar) 2-Butoxyethanol; 2-Ethoxyethyl acetate; Methyl cellosolve acetate; Stibine.

Back pain, lower Manganese; Zinc oxide.

Balance, loss of or impaired Benzene; Chromium; Ethylene dichloride; Hexone; Methyl chloride; Nitrobenzene; Styrene; 1,1,2,2-Tetrachloroethane; 1,1,1-Trichloroethane; 1,1,2-Trichloroethane; Xylenes.

Behavior/Emotions *see* specific headings under Aggressiveness; Agitation; Anxiety; Apathy; Apprehension; Behavioral; Belligerence; Boastfulness; Delirium; Delusions; Depression; Disorientation; Emotional; Euphoria; Excitement; Exhilaration; Feeling of being spacey; Feeling of oppression; Giddiness; Hallucinations; Hyperactivity; Hysteria; Incoherence; Indecision; Irrational; Irritability; Judgment; Lethargy; Listlessness; Mania; Mental disorders; Nervousness; Neurobehavioral; Neurosis; Perceptual distortions; Peripheral-vegetative disorders; Personality changes; Psychological; Psychomotor; Psychoneurological; Psychosis; Restlessness; Schizophrenic; Sense of well being; Uneasiness; Vegetative disorders; Violent behavior.

Behavioral changes, suspected of causing Cyanides; Hydrogen cyanide.

Behavioral effects/problems/changes n-Butyl acetate; Cadmium; Carbon disulfide; Chlorinated camphene; Ethanol; Isoamyl alcohol; Lead; Methylene chloride; Pentaborane; Trichloroethylene.

Belching Phosphorus.

Belligerence Acetone; Ethyl acetate.

Birth defects Arsenic; beta-Chloroprene; 2,4-D; Dinitrobenzenes; Ethanol; Isoamyl alcohol; Manganese; Mercury; Toluene; Warfarin.

Birth defects, suspected of causing Acrolein; Acrylonitrile; Benzene; 1,3-Butadiene; Cadmium; Calcium arsenate; Carbon disulfide; Chloroform; Chromium; Copper; Cumene; Cyanides; Cyclohexanone; Dinitrotoluenes; Dimethylaniline; 1,1-Dimethylhydrazine; Di-sec octyl phthalate; Endosulfan; Epichlorohydrin; Ethylene oxide; Hydrogen cyanide; Limonene; Methyl bromide; Methyl cellosolve; Methyl chloride; Methyl iodide; Methyl

parathion; Nicotine; Nitrobenzene; Nitrophenols; Polycyclic aromatic hydrocarbons; Thallium; Tin; 1,1,1-Trichloroethane; Turpentine; Vanadium pentoxide; Vinyl chloride; Xylenes.

Birth weight, low Arsenic; Chlorinated diphenyl; Polychlorinated biphenyls.

Birth weight, suspected of causing low Acetone; Cadmium; Chloroform; Chromium; Ethylene oxide; Methylene chloride; Nickel; Nicotine; Nitrobenzene; Polycyclic aromatic hydrocarbons; Styrene; Tetrachloroethylene; Tin; 1,1,1-Trichloroethane; Vanadium pentoxide.

Births, premature Benzene; Chlorinated diphenyl; Polychlorinated biphenyls.

Births, suspected of causing premature Chlorine dioxide.

Bladder cancer Benzidine; Chloroform.

Bladder cancer, suspected of causing Aniline; o-Toluidine.

Bladder inflammation Benzidine; Ethyl ether; Isopropyl ether; Naphthalene; Turpentine.

Bladder tissue death Aniline.

Bladder wall ulceration Aniline.

Blood, abnormal amounts of uric acid in the Lead.

Blood, abnormal increase in granulocytes in the 2-Butoxyethanol.

Blood, chocolate colored Aniline.

Blood, decreased bilirubin in the Naphthalene; Pentachloronaphthalene.

Blood, decreased erythrocytes in Benzene; 1,3-Butadiene; Chloroform; Methyl parathion.

Blood, decreased hematocrit in the 1,3-Butadiene.

Blood, decreased hemoglobin in the 1,3-Butadiene; Chloroform; Chromium; Lead; Phenylhydrazine.

Blood, decreased leukocytes in Benzene; Benzyl chloride; Stibine.

Blood, decreased neutrophils in the 1,3-Butadiene.

Blood, decreased platelets in Benzene; 1,3-Butadiene; Chromium; N-Nitrosodimethylamine; Polycyclic aromatic hydrocarbons; Vanadium pentoxide; Vinyl chloride.

Blood, decreased polymorphonuclear leukocytes in the Crotonaldehyde.

Blood, decreased potassium levels in Barium.

Blood, decreased surface sulfydryls in the Crotonaldehyde.

Blood, deficiency of lymphocytes in the Pentaborane.

Blood, delayed hemoglobin oxidizing into ferric form Dimethylaniline.

Blood, denatured erythrocytes in the Isopropyl alcohol.

Blood, depression of plasma in the Methyl parathion.

Blood, destruction of erythrocytes in the Lead; Picric acid.

Blood, excessive calcium in the Ethylene dichloride.

Blood, excessive eosinophils in the Chromic acid; Ethyleneimine; Pyrethrum.

Blood, excessive gamma globin in Chloroform.

Blood, excessive monocytes in the Acetylene tetrabromide; Chromic acid; 1,1,2,2-Tetrachloroethane.

Blood, excessive potassium in the Allyl chloride; Barium.

Blood, excessive protein in the Allyl chloride.

Blood, excessive sodium in the Allyl chloride.

Blood, hemoglobin oxidizes to

ferric form in the n-Amyl acetate; o-Dichlorobenzene; Dinitrobenzenes; Dinitrotoluenes; Ethylene glycol dinitrate; Hydroquinone; Methyl mercaptan; Monomethyl aniline; p-Ni-troaniline; p-Nitrochlorobenzene; Nitrophenols; 1-Nitropropane; Phenol; Phenylhydrazine; Tetramethyl succinonitrile; o-Toluidine; 2,4,6-Trinitrotoluene; Xylidine.

Blood, increased bilirubin in the Benzyl chloride; Hexachloronaphthalene; Methylene chloride; Nickel; Nitrophenols; Pentachloronaphthalene; Phenol; Phenylhydrazine; 2,4,6-Trinitrotoluene.

Blood, increased erythrocytes in the Stibine.

Blood, increased hemoglobin in the Cyanides; Hydrogen cyanide.

Blood, increased leukocytes in the 2-Butoxyethanol; o-Chlorobenzylidene malononitrile; Chromic acid; Chromium; Cyanides; Ethylene glycol; Ethyleneimine; Hydrogen cyanide; Hydrazine; Magnesium oxide; Nickel; Nickel carbonyl; p-Nitroaniline; Paraldehyde; Pentaborane; Phenylhydrazine; Phosgene; 2,4,6-Trinitrotoluene; Zinc oxide.

Blood, increased nitrogenous bodies in 2,4-D; Lead; Paraldehyde.

Blood, increased reticulocytes in the 2-Butoxyethanol; Lead; Naphthalene; Nickel; 2,4,6-Trinitrotoluene.

Blood; increased uric acid in Molybdenum.

Blood, insufficient oxygenation of Chlorine; Propane.

Blood, reduction of cellular elements in the Methyl cellosolve.

Blood, suspected of causing changes in the Diacetone alcohol.

Blood, suspected of causing decreased erythrocytes in the Styrene.

Blood, suspected of causing

decreased hematocrit in the Cresols; 1,1-Dimethylhydrazine.

Blood, suspected of causing decreased hemoglobin in the Cresols; 1,1-Dimethylhydrazine; Styrene.

Blood, suspected of causing increased erythrocytes in the Chlorinated diphenyl; Polychlorinated biphenyls.

Blood, suspected of causing increased hemoglobin in the Chlorinated diphenyl; Polychlorinated biphenyls; Vanadium pentoxide.

Blood calcium, abnormally low Fluorides; Hydrogen fluoride; Zinc chloride.

Blood cancers *also see* **Blood malignancies** Vinyl chloride.

Blood cell damage Endosulfan.

Blood cells, decrease in or depression of red Arsenic; Arsine; 1,3-Butadiene; 2-Butoxyethanol; Cresols; 1,1-Dimethylhydrazine.

Blood cells, decrease in or depression of white Arsenic; Arsine; Benzene; 1,3-Butadiene; Calcium arsenate; Chromic acid; Chromium; 1,1,2,2-Tetrachloroethane.

Blood cells, destruction of red Acetic acid; Aniline; Arsenic; Arsine; Benzidine; 2-Butoxyethanol; 1,1-Dimethylhydrazine; Isopropyl alcohol; Methyl hydrazine; n-Propyl alcohol; Stibine.

Blood cells, affects the production; development of 1,3-Butadiene.

Blood cells, excessive of red Cobalt; Ethyl ether; Ethyleneimine; Isopropyl ether.

Blood cells, granules in red Aniline; p-Dichlorobenzene; Methyl hydrazine; Naphthalene; p-Nitroaniline; p-Nitrochlorobenzene; Nitrophenols; Phenol; Phenylhydrazine.

Blood cells, increased sedimentation rate of red Chromium.

Blood cells, intravascular destruction of red Bromine; Chromium; Iodine.

Blood cells, suspected of causing decrease in or depression of white Diglycidyl ether.

Blood cells, suspected of causing granules in red Styrene.

Blood cells, suspected of causing intravascular destruction of red 2-Ethoxyethyl acetate.

Blood cells, suspected of causing the destruction of red Tin.

Blood cells, suspected of affecting the production; development of Diglycidyl ether; Ethylene dibromide.

Blood cells, toxic production; development of Polycyclic aromatic hydrocarbons.

Blood clotting, changes in 1,1,2, 2-Tetrachloroethane; 1,1,1-Trichloroethane.

Blood clotting, inhibits Acetic anhydride; Chromium; Ethylene dichloride; Nitric acid; Phosphoric acid; Phosphorus; Pindone; Sulfur monochloride; Vinyl chloride.

Blood clotting in the blood vessels Phenylhydrazine.

Blood damage, suspected of causing 1,2,3-Trichloropropane.

Blood diseases/disorders Benzene; p-Dichlorobenzene; Ethyl chloride; Lindane; Trichloroethylene; 2,4,6-Trichlorophenol.

Blood disorders (indices), abnormal Warfarin.

Blood malignancies *also see* **Blood cancer** 1,3-Dichloropropene; Polychlorinated biphenyls.

Blood plasma, a relative increase in red blood cells caused by a decrease in the volume of (hemoconcentration) Phosgene.

Blood poisoning Acetone.

Blood pressure, high or increased
Acetonitrile; 2-Aminopyridine; Antimony; Azinphos-methyl; Barium; Cadmium; Carbaryl; Carbon dioxide; Carbon disulfide; Chlorinated diphenyl; Chlorpyrifos; Dimethylformamide; Endosulfan; EPN; Nicotine; Polychlorinated biphenyls; TEDP; Vanadium pentoxide.

Blood pressure, low or decreased
Acetic acid; Acetone; Acetonitrile; Azinphos-methyl; Bromine; 1,3-Butadiene; 2-Butoxyethanol; Chloroform; Chloropicrin; Cyanides; 2,4-D; Demeton; Diacetone alcohol; Dichlorvos; 1,1-Dimethylhydrazine; Dimethylphthalate; EPN; Ethyl acetate; Ethyl methacrylate; Ethylene dichloride; Ethylene glycol dinitrate; Ferbam; Hydrogen cyanide; Iodine; Isopropyl alcohol; Lead; Linalyl alcohol; Magnesium oxide; Methyl chloride; Methyl methacrylate; Methyl parathion; Naled; Nicotine; Nitrophenols; Oxalic acid; Paraldehyde; Pentachlorophenol; Phenol; Phenylhydrazine; Phosdrin; Phthalic anhydride; n-Propyl alcohol; TEPP; 1,1,2,2-Tetrachloroethane; Tetraethyl lead; Tetramethyl lead; 1,1,1-Trichloroethane.

Blood sugar, abnormal amounts of Lead.

Blood sugar, high: (hyperglycemia) 2,4-D; Ethyl ether; Isopropyl ether.

Blood sugar, low: (hypoglycemia) Ethyl acetate; Ethylene dichloride.

Blood sugar, suspected of causing high: (hyperglycemia) Nickel.

Blood sugar, suspected of causing low: (hypoglycemia) Dimethyl sulfate.

Blood vessel, dilatation of 2,4-D; Linalyl alcohol.

Blood vessel blockage Vinyl chloride.

Blood vessel collapse; peripheral Acetone; Ethyl acetate.

Blood vessel congestion Boron; Methyl parathion.

Blood vessel endothelial damage Methyl parathion.

Blood vessel hemorrhaging Methyl parathion.

Blood vessel lesions Arsenic.

Blood vessel walls, thickening of Vinyl chloride.

Blood vessels, hemorrhaging around (perivascular) Boron.

Blood vessels, swelling around (perivascular) Ethylene glycol.

Blood vessels, widespread injury to the small Phosphine.

Boastfulness Acetone; Ethyl acetate.

Body, retarded growth of the Lead.

Body aches Formaldehyde; Zinc oxide.

Body temperature, depressed *also see* hypothermia 2,4-D; Formaldehyde; Furfuryl alcohol; Nickel; Nitrophenols.

Boils Zinc oxide.

Bone death *also see* Tissue/Bone death Phosphorus.

Bone degeneration, suspected of causing 2,3-Benzofuran.

Bone diseases Aluminum.

Bone fractures, spontaneous Phosphorus.

Bone marrow, suspected of causing excessive proliferation of normal cells in 2,4,6-Trichlorophenol.

Bone marrow atrophy, suspected of causing 2,4-Dichlorophenol.

Bone marrow cytotoxicity, suspected of causing Diglycidyl ether.

Bone marrow damage 2-Butoxyethanol.

Bone marrow depression Benzene; Methyl cellosolve; Polycyclic aromatic hydrocarbons.

Bone marrow depression, suspected of causing 2-Ethoxyethyl acetate.

Bones, increases softness in Aluminum; Cadmium.

Brain *also see* **headings under Electroencephalogram.**

Brain *also see* **headings under Meninges.**

Brain *also see* **headings under Nervous system, central.**

Brain, cerebellar atrophy of the Ethanol; Isoamyl alcohol.

Brain, cerebellar dysfunction of the n-Hexane; Sodium fluoroacetate.

Brain, cerebellar neurologic symptoms in the Methyl iodide.

Brain, cerebral difficulties in the Phosphine.

Brain, cerebral embolisms in the Hydrogen peroxide.

Brain, cerebral hemorrhaging in the Pindone; Warfarin.

Brain, cerebral swelling of the Benzene; Chromium; Ethylene glycol; Nickel carbonyl.

Brain, enlarged Chromium.

Brain, neurofibrillary tangles in the Aluminum.

Brain, organic affective syndrome of the Tetrachloroethylene; Toluene.

Brain, petechial hemorrhaging on the surface of the Phosphine.

Brain, suspected of causing cerebellum damage Nitrobenzene.

Brain, suspected of causing cerebral dysfunction in the Benzyl acetate; Benzyl alcohol; Benzyl chloride; Cresols; Dinitro-o-cresol; Dinitrotoluenes; Toluene-2,4-diisocyanate; o-Toluidine; 2,4,6-Trinitrotoluene; Vinyl toluene; Xylenes.

Brain atrophy Sodium fluoroacetate.

Brain cancer Vanadium pentoxide.

Brain catecholamines, adversely effects Benzene.

Brain congestion Barium.

Brain damage Boron; Carbon monoxide; Mercury; Methyl bromide; Methyl cellosolve acetate; Sodium fluoroacetate.

Brain damage, suspected of causing Cadmium; Methylene chloride.

Brain degeneration Boron; Pentaborane.

Brain dysfunction Acrylamide; Aluminum; Arsenic; Carbon disulfide; Hydrogen sulfide; Lead; Methyl cellosolve; Methyl methacrylate; Pentaborane; Tetraethyl lead; Tetramethyl lead.

Brain dysfunction, nonspecific Ammonia.

Brain dysfunction, toxic Tetrachloroethylene; Toluene; Triorthocresyl phosphate.

Brain function depression Carbon monoxide.

Brain hemorrhaging Chlorinated camphene; Nickel carbonyl; Xylenes.

Brain hemorrhaging, suspected of causing Chloroform.

Brain inflammation Ethylene glycol.

Brain irritation Octane.

Brain lesions Carbon monoxide; 2-Ethoxyethyl acetate; Methyl cellosolve acetate.

Brain swelling Barium; Dinitro-o-cresol; Endosulfan.

Brain tumors Acrylonitrile.

Brain waves, marker delay in certain p-Dichlorobenzene.

Brainstem damage, suspected of causing Nitrobenzene.

Breath, bitter almond Acetonitrile.

Breath, chemical smell on Nitrophenols; Phenol.

Breath, garlic Arsenic; Calcium arsenate; Phosphorus; Selenium; Tellurium.

Breath, shortness of Beryllium; Carbon monoxide; Cyanides; Diborane; Dinitrobenzenes; Dinitro-o-cresol; Ethyleneimine; Formaldehyde; Hydrogen cyanide; Propane; Propylene imine; Pyrethrum; Trimellitic anhydride.

Breath, turpentine odor on Turpentine.

Bronchi, complete inflammatory destruction of Nitrogen dioxide.

Bronchi, diphtheria-like mutations of the Propylene imine.

Bronchi degeneration Phosgene.

Bronchial constriction Azinphosmethyl; Carbaryl; Chlorine; Chlorpyrifos; Fluorotrichloromethane; Malathion; Methyl parathion; Naled; TEDP.

Bronchial constriction, reflex Sulfur dioxide.

Bronchial dilation Ethyl ether; Isopropyl ether.

Bronchial irritation n-Hexane; Selenium.

Bronchial mucous destruction 1,1-Dimethylhydrazine.

Bronchial secretions Chloromethyl methyl ether; Ethyl ether; Isopropyl ether; Malathion.

Bronchial spasms Ammonia; Antimony; Chlorine dioxide; Chromium; Formaldehyde; Sulfur dioxide; Toluene-2,4-diisocyanate.

Bronchioles inflammation Chloropicrin.

Bronchitis Acetaldehyde; Acetic anhydride; Acetone; Arsenic; Benzene; Chlorinated camphene; Chlorine; Chlo-rine dioxide; Chloromethyl methyl ether; Chromium; 2,4-D; Ethylene oxide; Ethyleneimine; Formaldehyde; Formic acid; Furfuryl alcohol; Hydrazine; Hydrogen fluoride; Iodine; Maleic anhydride; Manganese; Nickel; Nitric acid; Phosphine; Phthalic anhydride; Propylene imine; Selenium; Sulfur dioxide; Sulfuric acid; Titanium dioxide; Vanadium pentoxide.

Bronchitis, allergic Methylamine.

Bronchitis, chemical Methylamine.

Bronchitis, chronic Acetic acid; Epichlorohydrin; Portland cement.

Bronchitis, suspected of causing 2-Diethylaminoethanol.

Bruising, intravascular Boron.

Bruising, massive Pindone.

Calves, cramps in Triorthocresyl phosphate.

Cancer Arsenic; Arsine; Asbestos; Benzene; Benzidine; Cadmium; Chlorinated camphene; Chlorinated diphenyl; Chloroform; Chloromethyl methyl ether; Chromium; Creosotes; Ethylene oxide; Ethyleneimine; Hydrazine; Nickel; Nickel carbonyl; 2-Nitropropane; N-Nitrosodimethylamine; Polychlorinated biphenyls; Polycyclic aromatic hydrocarbons; beta-Propiolactone; Styrene; 1,1,2,2-Tetrachloroethane; Vanadium pentoxide; Vinyl chloride.

Cancer, suspected of causing Acetaldehyde; Acrolein; Acrylamide; Acrylonitrile; Aniline; 2,3-Benzofuran; Benzyl chloride; Beryllium; 1,3-Butadiene; Calcium arsenate; Carbon tetrachloride; beta-Chloroprene; Chromic acid; 2,4-D; o-Dichlorobenzene; p-Dichlorobenzene; 1,1-Dichloroethane; Dichloroethyl ether; 1,3-Dichloropropene; Diglycidyl ether; Dimethyl sulfate; Dimethylformamide; 1,1-Dimethylhydrazine; Dinitrotoluenes; Di-sec octyl phthalate; Epichlorohydrin; Ethyl acrylate; Ethyl chloride; Ethylene dibromide; Ethylene dichloride; Ethylenediamine; Formaldehyde; Hexachloroethane; Hydrazine; Hydrogen fluoride; Isobutyl alcohol; Isophorone; Lead; Limonene; Methyl bromide; Methyl cellosolve; Methyl chloride; Methyl hydrazine; Methyl iodide; Methylene bisphenyl isocyanate; Methylene chloride; Nitrobenzene; p-Nitrochlorobenzene; Pentachlorophenol; Phenyl glycidyl ether; Phenylhydrazine; Propylene dichloride; Propylene imine; Propylene oxide; Silica; Sodium hydroxide; Styrene; Tetrachloroethylene; Titanium dioxide; Toluene-2,4-diisocyanate; o-Toluidine; 1,1,2-Trichloroethane; Trichloroethylene; 2,4,6-Trichlorophenol; Turpentine.

Capillary congestion (engorgement) Stibine.

Capillary leakage Phosgene.

Cardiac *also see* **Heart.**

Cardiac dilation Phosphorus pentasulfide.

Cardiopulmonary arrest Chromium; Ethylene dibromide.

Cardiopulmonary collapse Arsenic.

Cardiovascular collapse Aniline; Monomethyl aniline; p-Nitroaniline; Phenol; Phosphorus; o-Toluidine.

Cardiovascular constriction Nicotine.

Cardiovascular disorders tert-Butyl acetate.

Cardiovascular failure Methyl parathion.

Cardiovascular paralysis Magnesium oxide.

Cartilage, dark pigmentation of the Phenol.

Cataracts o-Dichlorobenzene; Dinitro-o-cresol; Ethylene oxide; Naphthalene; Nitrophenols; Picric acid; 2,4,6-Trinitrotoluene.

Cataracts, suspected of causing Cumene.

Catatonia *also see* **Vegetative disorders** Thiram.

Cell division, decreases Aluminum.

Cell division, effects Dimethyl acetamide.

Cell membranes, destruction of Cadmium.

Cells, granular cytoplasmic degeneration in Hydrazine.

Cells, poisonous condition caused by insufficient oxygen to Cyanides; Hydrogen cyanide.

Cells, suspected of causing excessive proliferation of normal 2,3-Benzofuran; Creosotes.

Cellular damage 1,1,2,2-Tetrachloroethane; 1,1,1-Trichloroethane.

Cellular respiration, inhibits Cyanides.

Cerebrospinal fluid, albumin in Acetonitrile.

Cerebrospinal system, distal axoneuropathy of the Dichlorodifluoromethane.

Chemical poisoning *also see* **Chemical sensitivity** Hydrogen sulfide.

Chemical sensitivity or hypersensitivity Benzidine; n-Butyl alcohol; sec-Butyl alcohol; Chloropicrin; Crotonaldehyde; Diborane; 1,3-Dichloropropene; Epichlorohydrin; Ethyl acrylate; Ethylenediamine; Formaldehyde; Formic acid; Hexachloronaphthalene; Hydrazine; Isobutyl alcohol; Isopropyl alcohol; Maleic anhydride; Methyl acrylate; Methyl methacrylate; p-Phenylene diamine; Phthalic anhydride; Picric acid; Pindone; n-Propyl alcohol; Pyrethrum; Sulfur dioxide; Trichloroethylene; Turpentine.

Chemical sensitivity or hypersensitivity, suspected of causing Ferbam.

Chest, burning sensation in the Diborane.

Chest cavity, fluid in Hydrazine.

Chest constriction o-Chlorobenzylidene malononitrile; Ethyl benzene; Isopropyl acetate; Methyl acetate; Phosgene; n-Propyl acetate; Sulfur dioxide; Zinc chloride.

Chest heaviness Diborane; Ethylenediamine.

Chest oppressions Dimethyl sulfate; Methyl formate.

Chest pains Acetonitrile; Ammonia; Butylamine; Chlorobenzene; beta-Chloroprene; 1,3-Dichloropropene; Dimethyl sulfate; 1,1-Dimethylhydrazine; Formaldehyde; Furfuryl alcohol; Magnesium oxide; Mercury; Methylene bisphenyl isocyanate; Nitrogen dioxide; Pentachlorophenol; Phosgene; Pyrethrum; Sulfur dioxide; Thallium; Thiram; Toluene-2,4-diisocyanate; Turpentine; Zinc chloride.

Chest pressure Phosphine.

Chest tightness Azinphos-methyl; Benzene; Cadmium; Carbaryl; Chlorinated diphenyl; Demeton; Diborane; Dichlorvos; EPN; Formaldehyde; Iodine; Malathion; Manganese; Methyl parathion; Naled; Nickel carbonyl; Phosdrin; Phosphine; Polychlorinated biphenyls; TEDP; TEPP; Zinc oxide.

Chest x-rays, abnormal Vinyl chloride.

Chills Cadmium; Chloromethyl methyl ether; Diborane; Phosphine; Propane; Selenium; Trimellitic anhydride; Zinc oxide.

Chloracne *also see* **Dermatitis.** Chlorinated diphenyl; 2,4-D; 2,4-Dichlorophenol; Hexachloronaphthalene; Pentachloronaphthalene; Polychlorinated biphenyls.

Choking Bromine; Chlorine; 1,1-Dimethylhydrazine; Hydrogen chloride; Nitric oxide; Phosgene; Propylene dichloride; Sulfur dioxide; Toluene-2,4-diisocyanate; Turpentine.

Cholera Calcium arsenate.

Chromosomal aberrations Acetaldehyde; Antimony; Arsenic; Chlorinated camphene; beta-Chloroprene; Chromium; Dinitro-o-cresol; Epichlorohydrin; Ethylene oxide; Hydrogen fluoride; Nickel; Phenol; Propylene oxide; Vanadium pentoxide; Vinyl toluene; Zinc chloride.

Chromosomal aberrations, suspected of causing Cadmium; Cobalt; Copper; Cyclohexanol; Ethylene dibromide; Fluorides; Lead; Malathion; Methyl bromide; Methylene chloride; Phosphine; Styrene; 1,1,1-Trichloroethane.

Chromosomal aberrations of leukocytes Benzene.

Chromosomal abnormalities Trichloroethylene.

Chromosomal breaks o-Dichlorobenzene.

Chromosomal breaks, suspected of causing Antimony.

Chromosomal damage Benzene; Phenol.

Chromosomal damage, suspected of causing Formaldehyde.

Circulation in fingers; toes, loss of Arsenic.

Circulatory collapse Acetic anhydride; Bromine; Dinitro-o-cresol; Ethanol; Formic acid; Iodine; Isoamyl alcohol; Isopropyl alcohol; Methyl alcohol; Nitric acid; Phosphoric acid; n-Propyl alcohol; Sulfur monochloride.

Circulatory collapse, peripheral Tetramethyl lead.

Circulatory failure Acetone; Dimethyl sulfate; Ethylene dichloride; Nitrophenols; Phosgene.

Circulatory shock Acetic acid; Phosphoric acid; Sulfur monochloride.

Cirrhosis Calcium arsenate; p-Dichlorobenzene; Ethanol; Isoamyl alcohol; Methyl chloride; N-Nitrosodithylamine; 1,1,2,2-Tetraloroethane.

Clumsiness Ethanol; Isoamyl alcohol.

Cognitive functions, changes in higher Formaldehyde.

Cold, sensitivity to Vinyl chloride.

Cold-like symptoms Benzyl chloride; Formaldehyde.

Colic Chloropicrin; Dimethylformamide; Lead; Propane; Tetraethyl lead; Tetramethyl lead.

Colitis Hexone.

Colitis, ulcerative Hydrogen peroxide.

Collapse Acetone; Acrylonitrile; Bromine; Calcium oxide; Dichloromonofluoromethane; Dichlorotetrafluoroethane; Diethylamine; Dimethylaniline; Ethyl bromide; Ethylene dibromide; Fluorotrichloromethane; Hydrogen peroxide; Hydrogen sulfide; Hydroquinone; Iodine; Nicotine; Oxalic acid; Paraldehyde; Pentachlorophenol; Phenol; Phosphorus pentasulfide; Pyrethrum; Sodium hydroxide; Tetrachloroethylene.

Colon, ruptured Hydrogen peroxide.

Colon cancer Chloroform.

Colon cancer, suspected of causing Ethyl acrylate.

Coma Acetone; Acetonitrile; 2-Aminopyridine; n-Amyl acetate; Aniline; Arsenic; Azinphos-methyl; n-Butyl acetate; n-Butyl alcohol; sec-Butyl alcohol; Calcium arsenate; Camphor; Carbaryl; Carbon dioxide; Carbon monoxide; Carbon tetrachloride; Chloroacetaldehyde; Chloroform; Chlorpyrifos; Cresols; Cumene; Cyanides; Cyclohexane; Cyclohexanone; 2,4-D; Demeton; Dichlorodifluoromethane; Dichloromonofluoromethane; Dichlorotetrafluoroethane; Dimethyl sulfate; Dimethylaniline; Dimethylphthalate; Dinitro-o-cresol; EPN;

Ethanol; Ethyl acetate; Ethyl benzene; Ethyl butyl ketone; Ethyl methacrylate; Ethylene dichloride; Ethylene glycol; Ferbam; Fluorotrichloromethane; Formaldehyde; Hexachloronaphthalene; Hexone; Hydrogen cyanide; Hydrogen sulfide; Isoamyl alcohol; Isobutyl alcohol; Isopropyl alcohol; Lindane; Limonene; Malathion; Mesityl oxide; Methyl n-amyl ketone; Methyl alcohol; Methyl bromide; Methyl cellosolve acetate; Methyl chloride; 5-Methyl-3-heptanone; Methyl iodide; Methyl mercaptan; Monomethyl aniline; Naled; Nitrobenzene; Oxalic acid; Paraldehyde; Pentachloronaphthalene; 2-Pentanone; Phenol; p-Phenylene diamine; Phosphorus; Phosphorus pentasulfide; Picric acid; n-Propyl alcohol; Propylene dichloride; Sodium fluoroacetate; 1,1,2,2-Tetrachloroethane; Tetrachloroethylene; Tetrachloronaphthalene; Tetraethyl lead; Tetramethyl lead; Tetramethyl succinonitrile; Thiram; Toluene; 1,1,2-Trichloroethane; Trifluorobromomethane; 2,4,6-Trinitrotoluene; Turpentine.

Coma, suspected of causing 2,4-Dichlorophenol.

Concentrate, inability to Chloroform; Pentaborane; Styrene; Tin.

Concentration, difficult or impaired Formaldehyde; Methyl parathion.

Confusion Acetonitrile; n-Amyl acetate; Aniline; Arsenic; Azinphosmethyl; n-Butyl acetate; n-Butyl alcohol; sec-Butyl alcohol; Camphor; Carbon dioxide; Carbon monoxide; Chlorinated camphene; Chlorpyrifos; Cresols; Cumene; Cyanides; Demeton; Dichlorodifluoromethane; Dichloromonofluoromethane; Dichlorotetrafluoroethane; Dimethyl acetamide; Dimethylaniline; EPN; Ethylene dichloride; Ferbam; Fluorotrichloromethane; Hexachloronaphthalene; Hydrogen cyanide; Isobutyl alcohol; Isopropyl alcohol; Malathion; Manganese; Methyl parathion; Monomethyl aniline; Naled; Naphthalene; Nicotine; Nitric oxide; p-Nitroaniline; Nitrobenzene; n-Pentane; Phenol; Phosphorus pentasulfide; n-Propyl alcohol; TEDP; Thiram; Toluene; o-Toluidine; Trichloroethylene; Trifluorobromomethane; Xylenes.

Conjunctiva congestion Chromium; Cobalt; Ethyl bromide; Ethylene dichloride; Isoamyl acetate; Turpentine.

Conjunctiva congestion, suspected of causing Phosgene.

Conjunctiva hemorrhaging Ethyl bromide; Propylene dichloride.

Conjunctiva irritation Cyclohexanol; Isopropyl acetate.

Conjunctiva pain Phosphorus pentasulfide.

Conjunctiva redness Hexachloroethane.

Conjunctiva swelling Acetic anhydride; Dimethyl sulfate.

Conjunctivitis Acetaldehyde; Acetic acid; Acetic anhydride; Acetone; Acetonitrile; Allyl chloride; Benzyl chloride; Beryllium; Boron; Calcium arsenate; Chlorine; o-Chlorobenzylidene malononitrile; Chloropicrin; beta-Chloroprene; Chromic acid; Creosotes; Crotonaldehyde; Dibutylphthalate; Dimethyl sulfate; Dimethylamine; 1,1-Dimethylhydrazine; Epichlorohydrin; Ethyleneimine; Formaldehyde; Formic acid; Hexachloroethane; Hydrazine; Hydrogen sulfide; Hydroquinone; Iodine; Maleic anhydride; Methyl alcohol; Methylamine; Pentaborane; Phosphorus pentasulfide; Phthalic anhydride; Propylene imine; Pyrethrum; Stibine; Sulfuric acid; Sulfuryl fluoride; Toluene-2,4-diisocyanate; Zinc chloride; Zinc oxide.

Conjunctivitis, suspected of causing 2-Butoxyethanol.

Consciousness, decreased level of Dichlorodifluoromethane; Pentaborane.

Constipation Acetic acid; Calcium arsenate; Dimethylformamide; Ethyl ether; Formaldehyde; Isopropyl ether; Lead; Mercury; 1,1,2,2-Tetrachloroethane; Tetraethyl lead; Tetramethyl lead.

Convulsions Acetone; Acrylonitrile; 2-Aminopyridine; Aniline; Arsenic; Azinphos-methyl; Barium; Benzene; Benzyl alcohol; Butylamine; Calcium arsenate; Camphor; Carbaryl; Carbon dioxide; Carbon monoxide; Chlorinated camphene; Chloroform; Chlorpyrifos; Chromium; Creosotes; Cyanides; 2,4-D; Decaborane; Demeton; Diborane; Dichlorvos; Dimethyl sulfate; Dimethylaniline; 1,1-Dimethylhydrazine; Endosulfan; EPN; Ethyl acetate; Ethyl acrylate; Ethyl ether; Ethyl methacrylate; Ethylene glycol; Formaldehyde; Hydrazine; Hydrogen cyanide; Hydrogen sulfide; Hydroquinone; Isopropyl ether; Lead; Limonene; Malathion; Methyl acrylate; Methyl alcohol; Methyl bromide; Methyl chloride; Methyl hydrazine; Methyl iodide; Methyl mercaptan; Monomethyl aniline; Naled; Nickel; Nicotine; p-Nitroaniline; Nitrophenols; Octane; Oxalic acid; Pentaborane; Pentachlorophenol; Phenol; p-Phenylene diamine; Phosdrin; Phosphorus; Phosphorus pentasulfide; Picric acid; Sodium fluoroacetate; Sulfur dioxide; TEDP; TEPP; Tetramethyl lead; Tetramethyl lead; Tetramethyl succinonitrile; Thallium; Tin; o-Toluidine; Tributyl phosphate; 1,1,2-Trichloroethane; Turpentine.

Convulsions, asphyxial Hydrogen sulfide; Phosphorus pentasulfide.

Convulsions, clonic Endosulfan; Hydrogen peroxide; Lindane; Methyl bromide; Pyrethrum.

Convulsions, epileptiform Acetonitrile; Camphor; Xylenes.

Convulsions, grand mal Lindane.

Convulsions, opisthotono Acetonitrile.

Convulsions, suspected of causing Cresols; Ethylene oxide; Sulfuryl fluoride.

Convulsions, suspected of causing clonic 2,4-Dichlorophenol.

Convulsions, tonic Acetonitrile; Endosulfan; Hydrogen peroxide; Phosphine.

Coordination, impaired hand/eye Ethylene oxide.

Coordination, loss of Acetone; Acrylamide; n-Amyl acetate; Aniline; Azinphos-methyl; Benzene; 2-Butanone; n-Butyl acetate; n-Butyl alcohol; sec-Butyl alcohol; Carbon monoxide; Carbon tetrachloride; Chlorobenzene; Chlorpyrifos; Copper; Cumene; Cyanides; Decaborane; Demeton; p-Dichlorobenzene; Dichlorvos; 2,4-Dichlorophenol; Dimethylaniline; Dinitrobenzenes; Dinitrotoluenes; EPN; Ethanol; Ethyl acetate; Ethyl chloride; Ferbam; Fluorotrichloromethane; Hexone; Hydrazine; Hydrogen cyanide; Isoamyl alcohol; Isobutyl alcohol; Isopropyl alcohol; Limonene; Malathion; Mercury; Methyl bromide; Methyl cellosolve; Methyl hydrazine; Methyl iodide; Methyl parathion; Methylene chloride; Monomethyl aniline; Naled; Nickel; Nicotine; p-Nitroaniline; Pentaborane; Phosdrin; Phosphine; n-Propyl alcohol; Propylene oxide; Pyrethrum; Sodium fluoroacetate; Styrene; TEDP; 1,1,2,2-Tetrachloroethane; Tetrachloroethylene; Tetraethyl lead; Thallium; Thiram; Toluene; o-Toluidine; 1,1,1-Trichloroethane; 1,1,2-Trichloroethane; Trichloroethylene; Turpentine; Xylenes.

Coordination, suspected of causing loss of Cresols; Cyclohexanone; 1,1-Dimethylhydrazine; Ethyl mercaptan; Linalyl alcohol; Molybdenum.

Cornea, calcium deposits in the superficial layer of the Benzyl alcohol.

Cornea overgrowths Acetic acid.

Corneal abnormalities Ethyl acetate.

Corneal abrasions Ethylene dichloride.

Corneal blistering Chromium.

Corneal burns Acetic anhydride; Allyl chloride; Ethylene oxide; Phenyl ether-biphenyl mixture; Propylene oxide.

Corneal clouding Epichlorohydrin.

Corneal damage/injury Aniline; Crotonaldehyde; Sulfur dioxide.

Corneal damage/injury, suspected of causing Ethylene dibromide.

Corneal erosion Formaldehyde.

Corneal inflammation n-Butyl acetate; n-Butyl alcohol; Calcium arsenate; Chlorine; Ethyleneimine; Formic acid; Hydroquinone; Maleic anhydride; Propylene imine; Quinone; Stibine; Triethylamine.

Corneal numbness Pentachlorophenol.

Corneal opaque areas or blind spots (opacity): *also see* **Vision, loss of and Vision, dimness of.** Acetic anhydride; 2-Diethylaminoethanol; Epichlorohydrin; Ethylene dichloride; Pentaborane; Pentachlorophenol; Phosphorus; Phosphorus pentasulfide; beta-Propiolactone; Sodium hydroxide.

Corneal opaque areas or blind spots (opacity), suspected of causing Nitrophenols.

Corneal reflexes, loss of Bromine.

Corneal swelling Acetic anhydride; Benzyl alcohol; Diethylamine; Dimethylamine; Ethylamine; Morpholine; Sodium hydroxide; Triethylamine.

Corneal tissue death Allyl alcohol; beta-Chloroprene; Diacetone alcohol; Epichlorohydrin.

Corneal ulcers Hydrogen peroxide;

Hydroquinone; Pentaborane; Quinone; Sodium hydroxide.

Corneal vacuolization Xylenes.

Corneal vesiculation Hydrogen sulfide; Phosphorus pentasulfide.

Costervertebral angle tenderness 2-Ethoxyethyl acetate.

Cough Acetaldehyde; Acetic acid; Acetic anhydride; Aluminum; Ammonium sulfamate; n-Amyl acetate; Antimony; Benzyl chloride; Beryllium; Bromine; 1,3-Butadiene; n-Butyl acetate; n-Butyl alcohol; sec-Butyl alcohol; Butylamine; Cadmium; Calcium oxide; Chlorine; Chlorine dioxide; o-Chlorobenzylidene malononitrile; Chloromethyl methyl ether; Chloropicrin; Chromium; Cobalt; Cumene; Cyanides; 2,4-D; Diborane; Dichloroethyl ether; 1,3-Dichloropropene; Dimethyl sulfate; Dimethylamine; Dinitro-o-cresol; Epichlorohydrin; Ethyl acrylate; Ethyl ether; Ethyleneimine; Formaldehyde; Formic acid; Furfuryl alcohol; Hydrogen chloride; Hydrogen cyanide; Hydrogen sulfide; Iodine; Isoamyl acetate; Isobutyl alcohol; Isopropyl acetate; Isopropyl ether; Magnesium oxide; Maleic anhydride; Manganese; Mercury; Methylamine; Methylene bisphenyl isocyanate; Mica; Morpholine; Naled; Nickel; Nickel carbonyl; Nitric acid; Nitric oxide; Nitroethane; Nitrogen dioxide; Pentachlorophenol; Phosgene; Phosphine; Phosphorus; Phosphoric acid; Phosphorus pentasulfide; Portland cement; n-Propyl acetate; Propylene dichloride; Pyrethrum; Selenium; Silica; Sodium hydroxide; Sulfur dioxide; Sulfur monochloride; Thiram; Tin; Toluene-2,4-diisocyanate; Trimellitic anhydride; 2,4,6-Trinitrotoluene; Turpentine; Vanadium pentoxide; Zinc chloride; Zinc oxide.

Cranial *also see* **headings under Nervous system, peripheral.**

Cranial neuropathy Arsenic;

Trichloroethylene.

Cyanosis Acrylonitrile; Aniline; Arsenic; Azinphos-methyl; Bromine; Calcium arsenate; Carbaryl; Carbon monoxide; Chlorpyrifos; Creosotes; 2,4-D; Demeton; Dichlorvos; Dimethyl sulfate; Dimethylaniline; Dinitro-o-cresol; Dinitrobenzenes; Dinitrotoluenes; Endosulfan; Epichlorohydrin; EPN; Ethyl bromide; Ethylene glycol; Ethylene oxide; Hydroquinone; Iodine; Lindane; Limonene; Malathion; Methyl cellosolve acetate; Methyl hydrazine; Methyl mercaptan; Monomethyl aniline; Naled; Nickel; Nicotine; Nitric oxide; p-Nitroaniline; p-Nitrochlorobenzene; Nitrogen dioxide; Nitrophenols; 1-Nitropropane; Oxalic acid; Paraldehyde; Phenol; Phenylhydrazine; Phosdrin; Phosgene; Picric acid; Sulfur dioxide; TEDP; TEPP; o-Toluidine; 2,4,6-Trinitrotoluene; Turpentine; Xylidine; Zinc chloride.

Cyanosis, suspected of causing Ethyl mercaptan.

Cytochrome P-450, decrease in: (A protein important in catalyzing the metabolism of steroid hormones, fatty acids,; detoxification of a variety of chemical substances.) Lead.

Death Acetaldehyde; Acetic acid; Acetone; Acetonitrile; Acrolein; Acrylonitrile; Allyl alcohol; Allyl chloride; 2-Aminopyridine; Ammonia; n-Amyl acetate; Aniline; Arsenic; Azinphos-methyl; Barium; Benzene; Benzyl acetate; Boron; Bromine; 1,3-Butadiene; n-Butyl acetate; n-Butyl alcohol; sec-Butyl alcohol; Butylamine; Cadmium; Calcium arsenate; Calcium oxide; Camphor; Carbaryl; Carbon dioxide; Carbon monoxide; Carbon tetrachloride; Chlorinated camphene; Chlorinated diphenyl; Chlorine; Chlorine dioxide; Chloroform; Chlorpyrifos; Chromium; Cobalt; Copper; Creosotes; Cresols; Cumene; Cyanides; 2,4-D; Diacetone alcohol; p-Dichlorobenzene; Dichlorodifluoromethane;

Dichloroethyl ether; Dichloromonofluoromethane; Dichlorotetrafluoroethane; Diethylamine; Dimethyl sulfate; 1,1-Dimethylhydrazine; Dinitro-o-cresol; Dinitrotoluenes; Endosulfan; Epichlorohydrin; EPN; Ethanol; Ethyl acetate; Ethyl acrylate; Ethyl bromide; Ethyl chloride; Ethyl ether; Ethyl methacrylate; Ethylene dibromide; Ethylene dichloride; Ethylene glycol; Ferbam; Fluorides; Fluorotrichloromethane; Formaldehyde; Formic acid; n-Hexane; Hydrogen cyanide; Hydrogen fluoride; Hydrogen sulfide; Iodine; Isoamyl alcohol; Isobutyl alcohol; Isopropyl alcohol; Isopropyl ether; Lead; Lindane; Limonene; Malathion; Methyl alcohol; Methyl bromide; Methyl cellosolve; Methyl cellosolve acetate; Methyl chloride; Methyl iodide; Methyl methacrylate; Methyl parathion; Methylene chloride; Monomethyl aniline; Naled; Naphthalene; Nickel; Nickel carbonyl; Nicotine; Nitric acid; p-Nitroaniline; Nitrobenzene; Nitrophenols; 2-Nitropropane; N-Nitrosodimethylamine; Oxalic acid; Pentachlorophenol; n-Pentane; Petroleum distillates; p-Phenylene diamine; Phosgene; Phosphine; Phosphoric acid; Phosphorus; Phosphorus pentasulfide; Picric acid; Pindone; Propane; n-Propyl alcohol; Pyrethrum; Sodium fluoroacetate; Sodium hydroxide; Stibine; Sulfur dioxide; Sulfur monochloride; TEDP; 1,1,2,2-Tetrachloroethane; Tetrachloroethylene; Tetraethyl lead; Tetramethyl lead; Thallium; Thiram; Tin; Toluene; o-Toluidine; Tributyl phosphate; 1,1,1-Trichloroethane; 1,1,2-Trichloroethane; Triethylamine; Trifluorobromomethane; 2,4,6-Trinitrotoluene; Triorthocresyl phosphate; Turpentine; Vanadium pentoxide; Vinyl chloride; Warfarin; Xylenes; Zinc chloride.

Death, suspected of causing Ethyl acetate; Methyl acetate; Vinyl acetate.

Dehydration Arsenic.

Delirium n-Amyl acetate; Benzene; Benzyl alcohol; Bromine; n-Butyl acetate; n-Butyl alcohol; sec-Butyl alcohol; Calcium arsenate; Camphor; Dimethyl sulfate; Ethylene glycol dinitrate; Hydroquinone; Iodine; Isobutyl alcohol; Limonene; Methyl alcohol; Nickel; Nitrophenols; Paraldehyde; Phosphorus; Tetraethyl lead; Tetramethyl lead; Thallium; Thiram; Toluene; Turpentine.

Delirium, toxic Lead.

Delusions Dimethyl acetamide; Lead; Paraldehyde; Tetraethyl lead.

Depression Acrrylamide; Arsenic; Butylamine; Camphor; Chlorinated diphenyl; Chloroform; Cresols; Cyanides; Demeton; Dimethyl acetamide; Dinitro-o-cresol; Ethyl ether; Ethylene dibromide; Formaldehyde; Hydrogen cyanide; Isopropyl ether; Lead; Magnesium oxide; Manganese; Methyl formate; Methyl parathion; Naled; Polychlorinated biphenyls; Propylene oxide; Styrene; Tetraethyl lead; Tetramethyl lead.

Depression, suspected of causing 1,1-Dimethylhydrazine.

Dermatitis *also see* listings for Skin. Acetaldehyde; Acetonitrile; Allyl alcohol; n-Amyl acetate; sec-Amyl acetate; Aniline; Arsenic; Arsine; Benzene; Benzidine; 1,3-Butadiene; sec-Butyl acetate; tert-Butyl acetate; sec-Butyl alcohol; Calcium arsenate; Calcium oxide; Carbon disulfide; Chlorine; o-Chlorobenzylidene malononitrile; Chloromethyl methyl ether; beta-Chloroprene; Chromium; Cobalt; Copper; Cresols; Cumene; Cyclohexane; Cyclohexanone; 2,4-D; Diacetone alcohol; Diisobutyl ketone; Diisopropylamine; Dimethylamine; Dimethylformamide; Epichlorohydrin; Ethyl acetate; Ethyl benzene; Ethyl butyl ketone; Ethylamine; Ethylene dichloride; Ferbam; Fluorides; Fluorotrichloromethane; Formaldehyde; Formic acid; Furfural; n-Heptane;

n-Hexane; Hexone; Hydrazine; Hydrogen chloride; Hydroquinone; Isoamyl acetate; Isobutyl acetate; Isobutyl alcohol; Isophorone; Isopropyl acetate; Isopropyl ether; Isopropylamine; Lindane; Maleic anhydride; Mesityl oxide; Methyl acrylate; Methyl n-amyl ketone; 5-Methyl-3-heptanone; Methyl iodide; Methyl isobutyl carbinol; Methyl methacrylate; alpha-Methyl styrene; Methylamine; Methylene bisphenyl isocyanate; Naphtha; Naphthalene; Nitrobenzene; Nitroethane; Nitromethane; Octane; Paraquat; n-Pentane; 2-Pentanone; Phenol; Phosphoric acid; Phthalic anhydride; Portland cement; n-Propyl acetate; Propylene dichloride; Propylene imine; Pyrethrum; Pyridine; Quinone; Selenium; Stibine; Stoddard solvent; Sulfuric acid; Tellurium; 1,1,2,2-Tetrachloroethane; Thiram; Tin; Toluene; Toluene-2,4-diisocyanate; o-Toluidine; Trichloroethylene; 2,4,6-Trinitrotoluene; Xylenes; Zinc oxide.

Dermatitis, acne-form Chlorinated diphenyl; Hexachloronaphthalene; Octachloronaphthalene; Pentachloronaphthalene; Polychlorinated biphenyls; Tetrachloronaphthalene.

Dermatitis, allergic Creosotes; Methyl parathion; p-Nitrochlorobenzene; Thiram; Vanadium pentoxide.

Dermatitis, allergic contact Nickel.

Dermatitis, contact Arsenic; Benzoyl peroxide; Beryllium; n-Butyl alcohol; Cadmium; Chromium; 2,4-D; Dimethyl acetamide; Ethyl methacrylate; Ethylenediamine; Hydrazine; Isopropyl alcohol; Linalyl alcohol; Limonene; Methyl acrylate; Nickel carbonyl; Pentachlorophenol; Phenylhydrazine; Picric acid; Propylene oxide; Pyrethrum; Silver; Titanium dioxide; Turpentine.

Dermatitis, defatting Acetone; Diacetone alcohol; Dichlorodifluoromethane; Dichloromonofluoromethane; Dichlorotetrafluoroethane; Ethylene dichloride; Fluorotrichloromethane; Isopropyl acetate; n-Pentane; n-Propyl acetate; Propylene dichloride; Styrene; Trifluorobromomethane.

Dermatitis, delayed contact 1,3-Dichloropropene.

Dermatitis, exfoliative Boron.

Dermatitis, scaling Acrylonitrile.

Dermatitis, sensitive Acetic acid; Acetic anhydride; Chloroacetaldehyde; Chromic acid; p-Phenylene diamine; Phenyl glycidyl ether; Turpentine.

Dermatitis with vesiculation Ethylene dibromide.

Dermatosis (non-inflammatory skin diseases) Antimony, Arsenic; Zinc chloride.

Developmental effects Aluminum.

Developmental effects, suspected of causing 2-Butanone; Cyclohexanone; Hydroquinone; 2,4,6-Trichlorophenol.

Diabetes 1,3-Butadiene.

Diarrhea Acetaldehyde; Acetic acid; n-Amyl acetate; Antimony; Arsenic; Arsine; Azinphos-methyl; Barium; Benzyl acetate; Benzyl alcohol; Benzyl chloride; Boron; Bromine; 2-Butoxyethanol; n-Butyl acetate; n-Butyl alcohol; sec-Butyl alcohol; Cadmium; Calcium arsenate; Camphor; Carbaryl; Carbon tetrachloride; Chloropicrin; Chlorpyrifos; Chromium; Cobalt; Copper; 2,4-D; Decaborane; Demeton; Diborane; o-Dichlorobenzene; Dichlorvos; Diethylamine; Dimethyl sulfate; EPN; 2-Ethoxyethyl acetate; Ethylene dibromide; Ethylene dichloride; Ethylene oxide; Ferbam; Fluorides; Formaldehyde; Formic acid; Furfuryl alcohol; Hexone; Hydrazine; Hydroquinone; Iodine; Isoamyl alcohol; Isobutyl alcohol; Lead; Malathion; Mercury; Methyl alcohol; Methyl cellosolve acetate; Methyl hydrazine;

Methyl iodide; Methyl parathion; Naled; Naphthalene; Nickel; Nicotine; p-Nitroaniline; 1-Nitropropane; 2-Nitropropane; N-Nitrosodimethylamine; Pentaborane; Phenol; Phenylhydrazine; Phosdrin; Phosphine; Phosphorus; Phosphorus pentasulfide; Picric acid; Pindone; Polycyclic aromatic hydrocarbons; n-Propyl alcohol; Pyrethrum; Stibine; Sulfur dioxide; Sulfur monochloride; TEDP; TEPP; 1,1,2,2-Tetrachloroethane; Tetraethyl lead; Tetramethyl lead; Thallium; Thiram; 1,1,1-Trichloroethane; Trichloroethylene; Turpentine; Warfarin; Zinc chloride.

Diarrhea, bloody Nitrophenols.

Diarrhea, suspected of causing 2,4-Dichlorophenol; 1,1-Dimethylhydrazine; Molybdenum.

Disorientation Aniline; Azinphosmethyl; Carbon dioxide; Chloroform; Chlorpyrifos; Dimethyl acetamide; Dimethylaniline; EPN; Ethylene dibromide; Formaldehyde; Monomethyl aniline; Naled; p-Nitroaniline; Pentaborane; Propane; Propylene dichloride; TEDP; Tetrachloroethylene; Tetraethyl lead; Tin; o-Toluidine.

Dizziness Acetone; Acetonitrile; 2-Aminopyridine; Aniline; Antimony; Arsine; Benzene; Benzyl chloride; Bromine; 2-Butanone; n-Butyl acetate; n-Butyl alcohol; sec-Butyl alcohol; Butylamine; Camphor; Carbon dioxide; Carbon disulfide; Carbon monoxide; Carbon tetrachloride; Chlorinated diphenyl; Chlorine; Chlorobenzene; Chloroform; beta-Chloroprene; Chromium; Copper; Cumene; Cyanides; 2,4-D; Decaborane; Demeton; Diborane; Dibutylphthalate; p-Dichlorobenzene; Dichlorodifluoromethane; 1,1-Dichloroethane; 1,2-Dichloroethylene; Diisobutyl ketone; Dimethyl acetamide; Dimethylaniline; Dimethylformamide; Dimethylphthalate; Dinitrotoluenes; Ethanol; Ethyl benzene; Ethyl chloride; Ethyl ether; Ethyl methacrylate; Ethylene glycol dinitrate; Ethyleneimine; Ferbam; Formaldehyde; Formic acid; Furfuryl alcohol; n-Hexane; Hexone; sec-Hexyl acetate; Hydrazine; Hydrogen cyanide; Hydrogen sulfide; Hydroquinone; Iodine; Isoamyl alcohol; Isobutyl acetate; Isophorone; Isopropyl alcohol; Isopropyl ether; Limonene; Malathion; Mercury; Methyl bromide; Methyl chloride; Methyl formate; Methyl iodide; Methyl parathion; Methylene chloride; Monomethyl aniline; Naphtha; Nicotine; Nitrophenols; Paraldehyde; Pentaborane; Pentachlorophenol; n-Pentane; Petroleum distillates; Phenol; Phosphine; Phosphorus pentasulfide; Polychlorinated biphenyls; Propane; n-Propyl acetate; n-Propyl alcohol; Propylene dichloride; Propylene imine; Pyridine; Stoddard solvent; Tetrachloroethylene; Tetrahydrofuran; Thiram; Toluene; o-Toluidine; 1,1,1-Trichloroethane; 1,1,2-Trichloroethane; Trichloroethylene; 1,2,3-Trichloropropane; 2,4,6-Trinitrotoluene; Turpentine; Vanadium pentoxide; Vinyl chloride; Xylenes; Xylidine.

DNA, binds to Ethylene dibromide; Polycyclic aromatic hydrocarbons.

DNA, interferes with Aluminum; Nickel.

DNA, suspected of causing methylated Methyl bromide.

DNA damage Acetaldehyde; Benzene; Chloromethyl methyl ether; 2,4-D; Ethyleneimine; Formaldehyde; Propylene oxide; Vanadium pentoxide.

DNA damage, suspected of causing Antimony; 1,1-Dimethylhydrazine; Lead; Methyl chloride; Methylene chloride; N-Nitrosodimethylamine; Thallium; Tin.

DNA synthesis, inhibits Thiram.

DNA synthesis, unscheduled Demeton.

Dreaming, excessive Azinphos-methyl; Chlorpyrifos; Naled.

Drooping or dropping body parts Thallium.

Drowsiness Acetaldehyde; Acetone; Aniline; Azinphos-methyl; Benzene; 1,3-Butadiene; 2-Butoxyethanol; n-Butyl acetate; sec-Butyl acetate; tert-Butyl acetate; n-Butyl alcohol; sec-Butyl alcohol; Chlorobenzene; Chlorpyrifos; Cumene; Cyclohexane; Decaborane; Diborane; o-Dichlorobenzene; 1,2-Dichloroethylene; Dinitrotoluenes; EPN; 2-Ethoxyethyl acetate; Ethyl acetate; Ethyl acrylate; Ethyl ether; Ethylene glycol; N-Ethylmorpholine; Ferbam; Formaldehyde; Hexachloro-naphthalene; Hexone; Isoamyl acetate; Isobutyl acetate; Isobutyl alcohol; Isopropyl acetate; Isopropyl alcohol; Isopropyl ether; Malathion; Methyl acetate; Methyl alcohol; Methyl cellosolve; Methyl cellosolve acetate; Methyl iodide; Methyl isobutyl carbinol; alpha-Methyl styrene; Monomethyl aniline; Naled; Naphtha; Nitric oxide; p-Nitroaniline; Octane; Paraldehyde; Pentaborane; Pentachloronaphthalene; n-Pentane; Petroleum distillates; n-Propyl alcohol; Propylene dichloride; Styrene; TEDP; 1,1,2,2-Tetrachloroethane; Tetrachloroethylene; Tetrachloronaphthalene; Thiram; Toluene; o-Toluidine; 1,1,1-Trichloroethane; 1,1,2-Trichloroethane; Trichloroethylene; Vanadium pentoxide; Vinyl chloride; Vinyl toluene; Xylenes.

Drowsiness, suspected of causing Furfuryl alcohol.

Duodenal ulcers Chromium.

Duodenum inflammation Acetone.

Duodenum tissue death Phosphoric acid.

Ear, humming in Dichlorodifluoromethane.

Ear aches Formaldehyde.

Ears, noise in Camphor.

Ears, ringing or tingling sound in Aniline; Benzene; Cumene; Cyanides; Dimethylaniline; Formaldehyde; Hydrogen cyanide; Hydroquinone; Monomethyl aniline; p-Nitroaniline; Nitrophenols; Phenol; Pyrethrum; 1,1,2, 2-Tetrachloroethane; o-Toluidine; 1,1, 1-Trichloroethane.

Eczema *also see* **headings under Dermatitis.** Chromium; Formaldehyde; Hydrazine; Vanadium pentoxide

Electroencephalogram, abnormal Nickel carbonyl; Styrene.

Electroencephalogram, suspected of causing abnormal Benzyl acetate; Benzyl alcohol; Benzyl chloride; Cresols; Dinitro-o-cresol; Dinitrotoluenes; Toluene; Toluene-2,4-diisocyanate; o-Toluidine; 2,4,6-Trinitrotoluene; Vinyl toluene.

Embryo death, suspected of causing Methyl cellosolve; Thallium.

Emotional detachment Dimethyl acetamide.

Emotional disturbances Mercury.

Emotional liability/instability/ upset Acetone; Arsenic; Azinphos-methyl; Carbon disulfide; Carbon monoxide; Chlorpyrifos; Ethyl acetate; Ferbam; Formaldehyde; Manganese; Naled; Tetraethyl lead; Thiram; Toluene.

Emphysema Acrolein; Beryllium; 1,3-Butadiene; Cadmium; Chlorine; Chlorine dioxide; 2,4-D; Ethylene oxide; Nickel; Phthalic anhydride; Propylene dichloride; Sulfur dioxide; Sulfuric acid; Vinyl chloride.

Enzyme activities, altered beta-Chloroprene; Lead; Triphenyl phosphate.

Enzyme function, inhibits superoxide production from normal Crotonaldehyde.

Enzyme levels, elevated serum Arsenic; 2,4-Dichlorophenol; 2,4,6-Trinitrotoluene.

Enzyme poisoning, cholinesterase Carbaryl.

Enzymes, deficiency of thrombin Ethylene dichloride.

Enzymes, elevated lactic dehydrogenase Phosphoric acid.

Enzymes, increased blood amylase Zinc chloride.

Enzymes, inhibits cholinesterase Azinphos-methyl; Chlorpyrifos; Demeton; Dichlorvos; EPN; Malathion; Methyl parathion; Naled; TEDP; Triorthocresyl phosphate; Triphenyl phosphate.

Enzymes, inhibits production of Cyanides; Hydrogen cyanide.

Enzymes, suspected of inhibiting chloinesterase Tributyl phosphate.

Epigastric cramps Dimethylformamide.

Epigastric distress Chlorinated diphenyl; Polychlorinated biphenyls.

Epigastric pain Acetic anhydride; Chlorinated diphenyl; Formic acid; Nickel; Nickel carbonyl; Phosphine; Phosphoric acid; Polychlorinated biphenyls; Sulfur monochloride; Vanadium pentoxide; Zinc chloride.

Esophageal, necrotic lesions in Nitrophenols.

Esophageal burns 2,4-D.

Esophageal corrosion Nitric acid.

Esophageal hemorrhaging Dimethylphthalate.

Esophageal inflammation Dimethylphthalate; Hydrogen peroxide.

Esophageal pain Nitric acid; Oxalic acid.

Esophageal perforation Acetic acid; Calcium oxide; Sodium hydroxide.

Esophageal perforation, delayed Diethylamine.

Esophageal strictures Acetic acid; Acetic anhydride; Calcium oxide; Formic acid; Iodine; Nitric acid; Phosphoric acid; Sodium hydroxide; Sulfur monochloride; Zinc chloride.

Esophageal swelling Calcium oxide; Sodium hydroxide.

Euphoria Benzene; Cumene; Ethanol; Isoamyl alcohol; Methyl formate; Toluene; Trifluorobromomethane; Vanadium pentoxide; Vinyl chloride.

Excitement 2-Aminopyridine; Camphor; Diacetone alcohol; Ethyl ether; Fluorotrichloromethane; Hydrogen sulfide; Isopropyl ether; Limonene; Methyl alcohol; Naphthalene; Nitrophenols; Paraldehyde; Phenol; Picric acid; Propane; Pyrethrum; Turpentine; Xylenes.

Exhaustion Chloroform; Ethyl ether; Isopropyl ether.

Exhaustion, absolute Dimethyl sulfate; Nicotine; Pyrethrum.

Exhilaration Acetone; Ethyl acetate; n-Pentane.

Expectoration, bloody Chlorine; Cyanides; Hydrogen cyanide; Trimellitic anhydride.

Expectoration, excessive Portland cement.

Expectoration, frothy Nitric oxide.

Extremities, bruising of Warfarin.

Extremities, burning sensation in 1,1,2,2-Tetrachloroethane; 1,1,1-Trichloroethane.

Extremities, cold/clammy Calcium arsenate; Methyl alcohol.

Extremities, cyanosis of Vinyl chloride.

Extremities, numbness/tingling/prickling sensation in Acrylamide; 2-Butanone; Calcium arsenate; Cyanides; Hydrogen cyanide; n-Hexane; Methylene chloride; 1,1,2,2-Tetrachloroethane; 1,1,1-Trichloroethane.

Extremities, pain in Methyl methacrylate.

Extremities, tonic spasms of the Pentaborane.

Extremities, weakness in Acrylonitrile.

Eye, impaired choroidal perfusion of the Cobalt.

Eye aches/pains Allyl chloride; Azinphos-methyl; Carbaryl; o-Chlorobenzylidene malononitrile; 2,4-D; Demeton; Dichlorvos; EPN; Ethyl methacrylate; Malathion; Naled; TEDP; TEPP.

Eye burns Acetaldehyde; Acetic acid; Ammonia; Boron trifluoride; Bromine; Carbon disulfide; Chlorine; Chlorobenzene; Dimethyl sulfate; Ethylene oxide; Ethyleneimine; Hydrazine; Hydrogen chloride; Hydrogen fluoride; Isopropylamine; Limonene; Methyl acetate; Methyl acrylate; Methyl hydrazine; Oxalic acid; Phosphoric acid; Phosphorus; Propylene imine; Selenium; Sodium hydroxide; Sulfur dioxide; Sulfur monochloride; Sulfuric acid; o-Toluidine; Turpentine.

Eye damage/injury Benzene; Benzyl chloride; Boron; Chloroacetaldehyde; Chromic acid; 2-Diethylaminoethanol.

Eye disorder where both eyes don't focus of the same object Thallium.

Eye irritation Acetaldehyde; Acetic anhydride; Acetone; Acetonitrile; Acetylene tetrabromide; Acrolein; Acrylamide; Acrylonitrile; Allyl alcohol; Allyl chloride; Ammonia; Ammonium sulfamate; n-Amyl acetate; sec-Amyl acetate; Aniline; Antimony; Barium; Benzene; Benzoyl peroxide; Benzyl acetate; Benzyl chloride; Boron; 1,3-Butadiene; 2-Butanone; 2-Butoxyethanol; n-Butyl acetate; sec-Butyl acetate; tert-Butyl acetate; n-Butyl alcohol; sec-Butyl alcohol; Butylamine; Calcium oxide; Camphor; Carbon tetrachloride; Chlorinated diphenyl; Chlorine dioxide; Chloroacetaldehyde; alpha-Chloroacetophe-

none; Chlorobenzene; o-Chlorobenzylidene malononitrile; Chloroform; Chloromethyl methyl ether; Chloropicrin; beta-Chloroprene; Copper; Creosotes; Cresols; Crotonaldehyde; Cumene; Cyanides; Cyclohexane; Cyclohexanol; Cyclohexanone; 2,4-D; Demeton; Diacetone alcohol; Dibutylphthalate; o-Dichlorobenzene; p-Dichlorobenzene; 1,3-Dichloro-5,5-dimethylhydantoin; Dichloroethyl ether; 1,2-Dichloroethylene; Dichlorvos; Diethylamine; 2-Diethylaminoethanol; Diglycidyl ether; Diisobutyl ketone; Diisopropylamine; Dimethyl sulfate; Dimethylamine; 1,1-Dimethylhydrazine; Di-sec octyl phthalate; Epichlorohydrin; EPN; Ethanol; Ethanolamine; 2-Ethoxyethyl acetate; Ethyl acetate; Ethyl acrylate; Ethyl benzene; Ethyl bromide; Ethyl butyl ketone; Ethyl chloride; Ethyl ether; Ethyl formate; Ethyl methacrylate; Ethyl silicate; Ethylamine; Ethylene dibromide; Ethylene dichloride; Ethylene oxide; N-Ethylmorpholine; Ferbam; Fluorides; Formaldehyde; Formic acid; Furfural; Furfuryl alcohol; Glycidol; Hexachloroethane; n-Hexane; Hexone; Hydrazine; Hydrogen cyanide; Hydrogen fluoride; Hydrogen peroxide; Hydrogen sulfide; Hydroquinone; Iodine; Isoamyl acetate; Isoamyl alcohol; Isobutyl acetate; Isobutyl alcohol; Isophorone; Isopropyl acetate; Isopropyl alcohol; Isopropyl ether; Isopropylamine; Ketene; Lead; Lindane; Limonene; Magnesium oxide; Malathion; Maleic anhydride; Mercury; Mesityl oxide; Methyl n-amyl ketone; Methyl acetate; Methyl acrylate; Methyl alcohol; Methyl bromide; Methyl cellosolve; Methyl cellosolve acetate; Methyl formate; 5-Methyl-3-heptanone; Methyl hydrazine; Methyl iodide; Methyl isobutyl carbinol; Methyl methacrylate; alpha-Methyl styrene; Methylal; Methylamine; Methylene bisphenyl isocyanate; Methylene chloride; Morpholine; Naled; Naphtha; Naphthalene; Nitric acid; Nitric oxide;

Nitrobenzene; Nitroethane; Nitrogen dioxide; 1-Nitropropane; Octane; Oxalic acid; Paraquat; Pentaborane; Pentachlorophenol; n-Pentane; 2-Pentanone; Petroleum distillates; Phenol; Phenyl ether; Phenyl ether-biphenyl mixture; Phenyl glycidyl ether; Phosdrin; Phosgene; Phosphoric acid; Phosphorus; Phosphorus pentasulfide; Phthalic anhydride; Picric acid; Polychlorinated biphenyls; Portland cement; n-Propyl acetate; n-Propyl alcohol; Propylene dichloride; Propylene imine; Propylene oxide; Pyridine; Quinone; Selenium; Sodium hydroxide; Stoddard solvent; Styrene; Sulfur dioxide; Sulfur monochloride; Sulfuric acid; TEDP; 1,1,2,2-Tetrachloroethane; Tetrachloroethylene; Tetraethyl lead; Tetrahydrofuran; Tetramethyl succinonitrile; Thiram; Tin; Toluene; Tributyl phosphate; 1,1,1-Trichloroethane; 1,1,2-Trichloroethane; Trichloroethylene; 1,2,3-Trichloropropane; Triethylamine; Trimellitic anhydride; 2,4,6-Trinitrotoluene; Turpentine; Vanadium pentoxide; Vinyl acetate; Vinyl toluene; Xylenes; Zinc chloride.

Eye irritation, suspected of causing sec-Hexyl acetate; Molybdenum.

Eye member inflammation *see* **Conjunctivitis.**

Eye movement, involuntary Ethanol; Ethylene dichloride; Ethylene glycol; Hydrazine; Isoamyl alcohol; Naled; Sodium fluoroacetate.

Eye movement, suspected of causing involuntary Benzyl acetate; Benzyl alcohol; Benzyl chloride; Cresols; Dinitro-o-cresol; Dinitrotoluenes; Toluene; Toluene-2,4-diisocyanate; o-Toluidine; 2,4,6-Trinitrotoluene; Vinyl toluene; Xylenes.

Eye swelling 2,4-D; p-Dichlorobenzene; Ethyl methacrylate.

Eye twitching Hexachloroethane.

Eyelid swelling Acetic acid; Chloropicrin.

Eyelid tremors/spasms Benzyl chloride; Bromine; o-Chlorobenzylidene malononitrile; Dimethyl sulfate; Phosgene; Phosphorus; Turpentine.

Eyelids, inability to close Hexachloroethane.

Eyelids, red Allyl chloride; o-Chlorobenzylidene malononitrile.

Eyes, blue-gray Silver.

Eyes, burning sensation in o-Chlorobenzylidene malononitrile.

Eyes, changes in Carbon disulfide.

Eyes, difficult focusing Diborane.

Eyes, dry n-Butyl acetate.

Eyes, dry; red Chlorinated camphene.

Eyes, itching; burning Calcium arsenate.

Eyes, itchy; inflamed tert-Butyl acetate.

Eyes, nerve inflammation behind the 2-Butanone.

Eyes, numbness/tingling/prickling sensation around 2-Aminopyridine.

Eyes, pain behind the Allyl alcohol.

Eyes, pale Lead.

Eyes, red Selenium.

Eyes, sensitive to light Acetaldehyde; Acetic anhydride; Allyl alcohol; Aniline; Bromine; n-Butyl alcohol; Calcium arsenate; 2,4-D; Dibutylphthalate; Diethylamine; Dimethyl sulfate; Dimethylamine; Ethyl mercaptan; Ethylene dichloride; Hexachloroethane; Hydrogen sulfide; Hydroquinone; Maleic anhydride; alpha-Methyl styrene; Phosphorus; Phosphorus pentasulfide; Sodium hydroxide; Tin.

Eyes, swelling around the Dimethyl sulfate.

Eyes, yellowing Dinitrobenzenes.

Face, flushed Acetone; Dimethylformamide; Ethyl acetate; Picric acid; Tetrachloroethylene.

Facial angioedema Chromium.

Facial congestion Dimethylformamide.

Facial numbness/tingling/prickling sensation Ethylenediamine; n-Hexane; Sodium fluoroacetate.

Facial paralysis Cresols.

Facial redness Ethyl bromide.

Facial spasms, tonic Pentaborane.

Facial swelling 1,1-Dimethylhydrazine; Ethyleneimine; Pyrethrum.

Facial twitching Demeton.

Faintness Butylamine; Isophorone; Nicotine; Phenol; Phosphine.

Fatigue Acrylamide; Arsenic; Benzene; Beryllium; 1,3-Butadiene; 2-Butanone; Carbon disulfide; Carbon monoxide; Chlorinated diphenyl; Chlorine; Chloroform; Chloropicrin; beta-Chloroprene; Cyanides; 2,4-D; Decaborane; Diborane; 1,1-Dichloroethane; 1,2-Dichloroethylene; Dinitro-o-cresol; Dinitrobenzenes; Epichlorohydrin; Ethyl ether; Formaldehyde; n-Hexane; Hexone; Hydrogen cyanide; Hydrogen sulfide; Isoamyl acetate; Isopropyl ether; Lead; Manganese; Mercury; Methyl alcohol; Methyl bromide; Methyl cellosolve; Methyl chloride; Methylene chloride; Nickel; Nitric oxide; Nitrogen dioxide; Pentachloronaphthalene; n-Pentane; Phenylhydrazine; Phosphine; Phosphorus pentasulfide; Picric acid; Polychlorinated biphenyls; Pyrethrum; Selenium; Styrene; Sulfur dioxide; 1,1,2,2-Tetrachloroethane; Tetrachloronaphthalene; Tetraethyl lead; Tetramethyl succinonitrile; Toluene; 1,1,1-Trichloroethane; 1,1,2-Trichloroethane; 1,2,3-Trichloropropane; 2,4,6-Trinitrotoluene; Xylenes; Zinc oxide.

Fatigue, excessive Trichloroethylene.

Fecal bleeding Bromine; Calcium arsenate; Formaldehyde; Iodine; Pindone; Tetramethyl lead; Warfarin.

Feces, black tarry Pindone.

Feeling of being spacey Formaldehyde.

Feeling of oppression Bromine; Phosgene.

Feet, numbness/tingling/prickling sensation of the Arsenic; Dinitrobenzenes; Triorthocresyl phosphate.

Feet, swelling of p-Dichlorobenzene.

Feet, weak Triorthocresyl phosphate.

Feet become sensitive to touch Arsenic.

Feet phenomenon, burning Thallium.

Fertility, decreased Chlorinated diphenyl; Polychlorinated biphenyls.

Fertility, suspected of causing decreased Copper; Di-sec octyl phthalate; Methyl chloride; Polycyclic aromatic hydrocarbons; Thallium.

Fertility, suspected of reducing male p-Dichlorobenzene.

Fetal alcohol syndrome Ethanol.

Fetal anomalies; developmental delays *also see* **Birth defects.** Toluene.

Fetal asphyxiation Formaldehyde.

Fetal brain damage Carbon monoxide; Mercury.

Fetal brain death Carbon monoxide.

Fetal central nervous system dysfunction Toluene.

Fetal growth retardation, suspected of causing Thallium.

Fetal lungs unexpanded at birth Camphor; Chlorine; Cyclohexanone; Propylene dichloride.

Fetal neurobehavioral deficits Chlorinated diphenyl; Polychlorinated biphenyls.

Fetal toxicity, suspected of causing 2-Butoxyethanol; Endosulfan.

Fetuses, suspected of causing effects or impairs neurological development of Cadmium; Methyl parathion.

Fetuses, suspected of causing structural alterations in the brains of Thallium.

Fever Calcium oxide; Chloromethyl methyl ether; 2,4-D; Diborane; Dimethyl sulfate; Dinitro-o-cresol; Hydrazine; Isopropyl alcohol; Limonene; Nickel carbonyl; N-Nitrosodimethylamine; Pentachlorophenol; Picric acid; Pyrethrum; Selenium; Sulfur dioxide; Trimellitic anhydride; Turpentine; Zinc chloride; Zinc oxide.

Fever, delayed Decaborane.

Fever, flu-like Magnesium oxide; Manganese.

Fever above 106 degrees Carbon monoxide; Dinitro-o-cresol; Pentachlorophenol; Picric acid.

Fibrosis, interstitial Asbestos; Lead.

Fibrosis, nodular diffused Cobalt.

Fibrosis, progressive massive Silica.

Finger clubbing Asbestos.

Finger tips, numbness/tingling of the Formaldehyde.

Finger tremors Benzyl chloride.

Fingernail changes Selenium.

Fingernail changes caused by defective nutrition or metabolism (dystrophy) Ethyl methacrylate.

Fingernail damage Paraquat.

Fingers, numbness of Thallium.

Flu, TMA Trimellitic anhydride.

Flu-like symptoms Formaldehyde; Trimellitic anhydride.

Food intolerance, fatty Chlorinated diphenyl; Polychlorinated biphenyls.

Forearms, numbness/tingling/prickling sensation of the Dinitrobenzenes; Formaldehyde.

Frostbite 1,3-Butadiene; Carbon dioxide; Ethyl chloride; Ethylene oxide; Fluorotrichloromethane; Methyl chloride; Propane.

Gag reflexes, loss of 1,1,2,2-Tetrachloroethane.

Gait, disturbed/staggering/unsteady Acrylamide; Benzene; 2-Butoxyethanol; Copper; Ethanol; 2-Ethoxyethyl acetate; n-Hexane; Hydrogen sulfide; Isoamyl alcohol; Malathion; Manganese; Methyl cellosolve; Methyl chloride; Methyl iodide; Paraldehyde; Styrene; 1,1,2,2-Tetrachloroethane; 1,1,2-Trichloroethane; Vanadium pentoxide; Xylenes.

Gait, suspected of causing staggering Benzyl acetate; Benzyl alcohol; Benzyl chloride; Cresols; Dinitro-o-cresol; Dinitrotoluenes; Toluene; Toluene-2,4-diisocyanate; o-Toluidine; 2,4,6-Trinitrotoluene; Vinyl toluene.

Gastric disorders *see* **Stomach.**

Gastroduoenum inflammation Acetone.

Gastrointestinal cancer Chlorinated diphenyl; Chloroform; Polychlorinated biphenyls.

Gastrointestinal congestion 1,1,2-Trichloroethane.

Gastrointestinal cramps Calcium arsenate.

Gastrointestinal damage Benzyl chloride.

Gastrointestinal damage, upper Ammonia.

Gastrointestinal disorders/diseases Boron; sec-Butyl acetate; tert-Butyl acetate; beta-Chloroprene;

Hydrogen sulfide; Hydroquinone; Isobutyl acetate.

Gastrointestinal distress Calcium arsenate; Ferbam; Hydrogen sulfide; 1-Nitropropane; Phosphorus pentasulfide; Selenium; Silver; Triorthocresyl phosphate.

Gastrointestinal disturbances Ammonium sulfamate; Arsenic; Mercury; Zinc oxide.

Gastrointestinal hemorrhaging n-Amyl acetate; Barium; n-Butyl alcohol; sec-Butyl alcohol; Chromium; Ethylene dichloride; Isobutyl alcohol; Vinyl chloride.

Gastrointestinal hemorrhaging, suspected of causing 1,3-Dichloro-5,5-dimethylhydantoin.

Gastrointestinal hemorrhaging, upper Ammonia.

Gastrointestinal inflammation Barium; Chloropicrin; Formaldehyde; Isopropyl alcohol; Lindane; Picric acid; n-Propyl alcohol; 1,1,2-Trichloroethane; Zinc oxide.

Gastrointestinal inflammation, corrosive Bromine.

Gastrointestinal irritation Arsenic; Benzyl acetate; Cadmium; Chlorine dioxide; Chloroform; Cresols; Dimethylphthalate; Ethyl acrylate; Paraquat; Phosphine; Phosphorus.

Gastrointestinal irritation, upper Methyl parathion.

Gastrointestinal lesions Creosotes.

Gastrointestinal pain n-Propyl alcohol.

Gastrointestinal spasms Cyanides; Hydrogen cyanide.

Genetic mutation, suspected of causing dominant lethal Methyl chloride.

Genetic mutation, suspected of causing sex-linked recessive lethal 1,3-Dichloro-5,5-dimethylhydantoin.

Genetic mutations Chloroform; p-Dichlorobenzene; Epichlorohydrin; Phenol; Polycyclic aromatic hydrocarbons.

Genetic mutations, suspected of causing Benzyl chloride; 1,3-Butadiene; Cadmium; Copper; 1,1-Dichloroethane; 1,3-Dichloropropene; Dinitro-o-cresol; Ethylene dibromide; Ethylene dichloride; Ethyleneimine; Formaldehyde; Methyl bromide; Methyl chloride; Methyl iodide; Methylene bisphenyl isocyanate; Methylene chloride; Tin; Toluene-2,4-diisocyanate; o-Toluidine; 1,2,3-Trichloropropane.

Genetic mutations in males, suspected of causing dominant lethal Thallium.

Genital organs, prolapsed Vinyl chloride.

Giddiness Acetonitrile; n-Amyl acetate; Azinphos-methyl; Benzene; n-Butyl acetate; n-Butyl alcohol; sec-Butyl alcohol; Chlorpyrifos; Cumene; Demeton; Dichlorvos; Dimethyl sulfate; EPN; n-Heptane; n-Hexane; Isobutyl alcohol; Malathion; Methyl alcohol; Naled; Nickel; Nickel carbonyl; Octane; Phenylhydrazine; Phosphine; Phosphorus pentasulfide; Pyridine; TEDP.

Gingival *see* Gums.

Glands, swollen Formaldehyde.

Glaucoma Dinitro-o-cresol.

Glottis corrosion Formic acid.

Glottis edema Acetic acid; Acetic anhydride; Bromine; Calcium oxide; Dimethyl sulfate; Formic acid; Iodine; Nitric acid; Phosphorus; Sodium hydroxide; Sulfur monochloride.

Goiters, endemic Cyanides; Hydrogen cyanide.

Gout-like symptoms Molybdenum.

Gum disorders Sulfur dioxide.

Gum inflammation beta-Chloroprene.

Gums, bleeding Chlorine; Pindone; Warfarin.

Gums, lead line Lead.

Gums, swollen Limonene; Turpentine.

Hair, bleached Hydrogen peroxide.

Hair, yellow stained Dinitro-o-cresol; Dinitrobenzenes; Picric acid.

Hair growth, excessive or in unusual places 2,4-Dichlorophenol.

Hair loss beta-Chloroprene; Decaborane; Diborane; Pentaborane; Stibine; Thallium.

Hair loss, temporary Sodium hydroxide.

Hallucinations Acrylamide; Arsenic; n-Butyl acetate; Camphor; Carbon monoxide; Chloroform; Manganese; Tetraethyl lead; Tetramethyl lead; Thiram; Toluene.

Hallucinations, auditory Dimethyl acetamide; Paraldehyde; Sodium fluoroacetate.

Hallucinations, visual Dimethyl acetamide; Paraldehyde.

Hand tremors Methyl bromide; 1,1,2,2-Tetrachloroethane.

Hands, numbness/tingling/prickling sensation of the Arsenic; Dinitrobenzenes; Trichloroethylene; Triorthocresyl phosphate.

Hands, stiff Vinyl chloride.

Hands, swelling of p-Dichlorobenzene.

Hands, weakness in Triphenyl phosphate.

Head; congenitally abnormally small Ethanol.

Headaches Acetone; Acetonitrile; Acetylene tetrabromide; Acrylamide; Acrylonitrile; 2-Aminopyridine; n-Amyl acetate; Aniline; Antimony; Arsenic; Arsine; Azinphos-methyl; Benzene; Benzyl chloride; Bromine; 1,3-Butadiene; 2-Butanone; 2-Butoxyethanol; n-Butyl acetate; sec-Butyl acetate; tert-Butyl acetate; n-Butyl alcohol; sec-Butyl alcohol; Butylamine; Cadmium; Calcium arsenate; Camphor; Carbaryl; Carbon dioxide; Carbon disulfide; Carbon monoxide; Carbon tetrachloride; Chlorinated diphenyl; Chlorine; Chlorine dioxide; Chlorobenzene; o-Chlorobenzylidene malononitrile; Chloroform; Chloropicrin; beta-Chloroprene; Chlorpyrifos; Chromium; Creosotes; Cumene; Cyanides; Cyclohexanol; Cyclohexanone; 2,4-D; Decaborane; Demeton; Diborane; Dibutylphthalate; o-Dichlorobenzene; p-Dichlorobenzene; 1,1-Dichloroethane; 1,2-Dichloroethylene; 1,3-Dichloropropene; Dichlorvos; Diisobutyl ketone; Diisopropylamine; Dimethyl sulfate; Dimethylformamide; Dinitro-o-cresol; Dinitrobenzenes; Dinitrotoluenes; EPN; 2-Ethoxyethyl acetate; Ethyl acetate; Ethyl acrylate; Ethyl benzene; Ethyl butyl ketone; Ethyl ether; Ethyl methacrylate; Ethyl mercaptan; Ethylene dibromide; Ethylene dichloride; Ethylene glycol; Ethylene glycol dinitrate; Ethylene oxide; Ethyleneimine; Ferbam; Fluorides; Formaldehyde; Furfural; n-Hexane; Hexone; sec-Hexyl acetate; Hydrogen cyanide; Hydrogen fluoride; Hydrogen sulfide; Hydroquinone; Iodine; Isoamyl acetate; Isoamyl alcohol; Isobutyl acetate; Isobutyl alcohol; Isophorone; Isopropyl alcohol; Isopropyl ether; Lead; Lindane; Malathion; Maleic anhydride; Manganese; Mercury; Methyl n-amyl ketone; Methyl acetate; Methyl alcohol; Methyl bromide; Methyl cellosolve; Methyl cellosolve acetate; Methyl formate; 5-Methyl-3-heptanone; Methyl isobutyl carbinol; Methyl parathion; Monomethyl aniline; Naled; Naphtha; Naphthalene; Nickel; Nickel carbonyl; Nicotine; Nitric oxide; p-Nitroaniline; Nitrobenzene; p-Nitrochlorobenzene; Nitrophenols; 1-Nitropropane; 2-Nitropropane;

N-Nitrosodimethylamine; Octane; Oxalic acid; Pentaborane; Pentachloronaphthalene; Pentachlorophenol; n-Pentane; 2-Pentanone; Petroleum distillates; Phenol; Phosdrin; Phosgene; Phosphine; Phosphorus pentasulfide; Picric acid; Polychlorinated biphenyls; Propane; n-Propyl alcohol; Propylene dichloride; Propylene imine; Pyrethrum; Pyridine; Selenium; Stibine; Styrene; TEDP; TEPP; 1,1,2,2-Tetrachloroethane; Tetrachloroethylene; Tetrachloronaphthalene; Tetraethyl lead; Tetrahydrofuran; Tetramethyl succinonitrile; Thiram; Tin; Toluene; o-Toluidine; Tributyl phosphate; 1,1,1-Trichloroethane; 1,1,2-Trichloroethane; Trichloroethylene; 1,2,3-Trichloropropane; Trimellitic anhydride; Triorthocresyl phosphate; Turpentine; Vanadium pentoxide; Vinyl chloride; Xylenes; Xylidine; Zinc oxide.

Healing, slow Acrylonitrile.

Hearing, loss of Acetone; Cobalt; Lead.

Hearing disturbances Cyanides; Hydrogen cyanide; Mercury.

Hearing sensitivity Acetaldehyde; Formaldehyde.

Heart, abnormal/altered electrocardiogram of the Antimony; Arsenic; Arsine; Chlorobenzene; Dichlorodifluoromethane; Ethylene oxide; Lead; Methyl chloride; Thallium; Xylenes.

Heart, acute myocardial lesions of the Ethylene dibromide.

Heart; arterial hypoxemia of the Beryllium.

Heart, changes in the myocardium of the Chromium.

Heart, depressed S-T segment of electrocardiogram of the Carbon monoxide.

Heart, electrocardiogram T-wave abnormalities of the Cyanides; Fluorotrichloromethane; Hydrogen cyanide.

Heart, enlarged Beryllium; Hydrazine.

Heart, insufficient oxygen supply to the myocardial of the Methyl parathion.

Heart, left ventricle muscle hemorrhaging of the Chromium.

Heart, myocardial damage/injury of the Barium; Phosphine; Thallium.

Heart, myocardial degeneration of the Bromine; Methyl parathion.

Heart, myocardial depression of the Ethyl ether; Isopropyl ether.

Heart, myocardial fragmentation of the Tetramethyl lead.

Heart, myocardial hemorrhaging of the Calcium arsenate.

Heart, myocardial infarction of the Carbon monoxide; Nickel carbonyl.

Heart, myocardial swelling of the Stibine.

Heart, myocardium diseases of the Cobalt.

Heart, myocardium dystrophy of the beta-Chloroprene.

Heart, pericardial pain in the Diborane.

Heart, premature or excessive constriction of the Barium; 1,1-Dichloroethane.

Heart, premature ventricular contraction of the Arsenic.

Heart, right atrial; ventricular hypertrophy of the Beryllium; Zinc chloride.

Heart, suspected of causing coronary constriction of the Nickel.

Heart, suspected of causing myocardial depression of the Nickel.

Heart, suspected of causing myocardium effect of the Methyl acetate.

Heart, suspected of causing myocardium fibrous swelling of the 1,2-Dichloroethylene.

Heart, suspected of causing pericardial swelling of the Chlorinated diphenyl; Polychlorinated biphenyls.

Heart, ventricular fibrillation of the Cumene; Sodium fluoroacetate; Xylenes.

Heart arrest/failure Acetonitrile; Barium; n-Butyl alcohol; sec-Butyl alcohol; Carbon tetrachloride; Chlorine; o-Chlorobenzylidene malononitrile; Chloroform; Cobalt; Dichlorodifluoromethane; Dichloromonofluoromethane; Dichlorotetrafluoroethane; Ethyl bromide; Ethyl chloride; Fluorotrichloromethane; Isobutyl alcohol; Magnesium oxide; Methyl methacrylate; Nickel; Nitrophenols; Paraldehyde; Pentachlorophenol; Phenol; Phosgene; Sodium fluoroacetate; Thallium; Trichloroethylene.

Heart arrhythmias Acetic acid; Arsenic; Azinphos-methyl; Barium; n-Butyl acetate; n-Butyl alcohol; sec-Butyl alcohol; Chloroform; Chlorpyrifos; Cyanides; 2,4-D; Dichlorodifluoromethane; 1,1-Dichloroethane; Dichloromonofluoromethane; Dichlorotetrafluoroethane; Ethyl bromide; Ethyl chloride; Ethyl ether; Fluorides; Fluorotrichloromethane; Formaldehyde; Hydrazine; Hydrogen cyanide; Hydrogen fluoride; Isobutyl alcohol; Isopropyl ether; Malathion; Monomethyl aniline; p-Nitroaniline; Phenol; Phosphorus pentasulfide; 1,1,2,2-Tetrachloroethane; Trichloroethylene; Trifluorobromomethane; o-Toluidine; 1,1,1-Trichloroethane.

Heart beat, abnormal Sodium fluoroacetate.

Heart beat, weak/irregular Chloropicrin; Dinitro-o-cresol.

Heart collapse Benzene.

Heart damage/impairment Arsine; Dimethyl sulfate; Ethanol; Ethyl acetate; Formaldehyde; Malathion; Paraquat; Phenol; Stibine.

Heart degeneration Ethyl bromide.

Heart depression Antimony; 1,1-Dimethylhydrazine.

Heart disease, chronic rheumatic 1,3-Butadiene.

Heart disease, coronary Carbon disulfide.

Heart disorders/diseases/effects 1,3-Butadiene; p-Nitrochlorobenzene; Trifluorobromomethane.

Heart failure, congestive Carbon monoxide; Pentachloronaphthalene; Tetrachloronaphthalene.

Heart irregularities Azinphosmethyl; Cyanides; Demeton; Dichlorvos; EPN; Hydrogen cyanide; Naled; Phosdrin; TEDP; TEPP; 2,4,6-Trinitrotoluene.

Heart lesions Cadmium; Carbonmonoxide; 2-Ethoxyethyl acetate; Lead; Methyl cellosolve acetate.

Heart lesions, ischemic Acetic anhydride; Phosphoric acid.

Heart lesions, suspected of causing 1,2-Dichloroethylene.

Heart muscle, changes in Methyl hydrazine.

Heart muscle degeneration Tetramethyl lead.

Heart muscle swelling Tetramethyl lead.

Heart palpitations sec-Butyl acetate; tert-Butyl acetate; beta-Chloroprene; Cyanides; Dichlorodifluoromethane; Dichloromonofluoromethane; Dichlorotetrafluoroethane; Dinitrobenzenes; Ethylene glycol dinitrate; Formaldehyde; Hydrogen cyanide; Isoamyl acetate; Isobutyl acetate; Methyl acetate; Phosphorus pentasulfide; Xylenes.

Heart physiology, changes in Barium.

Heart rate, increased Carbon dioxide; Ethyl ether; Isopropyl ether.

Heart rate, decreased or slow Chlorobenzene; Malathion; n-Propyl alcohol; 1,1,2,2-Tetrachloroethane; 1,1,1-Trichloroethane; Trichloroethylene.

Heart rate over 100 beats per minute Acetone; Aniline; Arsenic; Azinphos-methyl; Bromine; Calcium arsenate; Carbon monoxide; Chlorine; Chlorpyrifos; 2,4-D; Dinitro-o-cresol; Endosulfan; Ethyl acetate; Ethylene dichloride; Iodine; Isopropyl alcohol; Limonene; Methyl alcohol; Methyl chloride; Naled; Nicotine; p-Nitroaniline; Nitrogen dioxide; Pentachlorophenol; Picric acid; Propylene dichloride; Pyrethrum; Sodium fluoroacetate; TEDP; Thiram; Turpentine.

Heart rate under 60 beats per minute Acetonitrile; Chlorpyrifos; Cyanides; Demeton; Fluorotrichloromethane; Hydrogen cyanide; Isopropyl alcohol; Methyl alcohol; Methyl parathion; Naled; TEDP; Tetraethyl lead.

Heart shock (cardiogenic) Cobalt.

Heartburn Acetic acid; Hexone; Trimellitic anhydride.

Hemorrhaging Camphor; Diborane; p-Dichlorobenzene; Endosulfan; Ethylene dichloride; N-Nitrosodimethylamine; Octane; Phosphorus; 2,4,6-Trinitrotoluene.

Hepatitis Chloroform; Ferbam; Picric acid; Thiram.

Hepatitis, occupational alpha-Methyl styrene.

Hepatitis; toxic beta-Chloroprene; Dinitro-o-cresol; Hexachloronaphthalene; Paraldehyde; Pentachloronaphthalene; 1,1,2,2-Tetrachloroethane; 2,4,6-Trinitrotoluene.

Hives *also see* **Dermatitis.** Phthalic anhydride.

Hodgkin's disease (cancer) Ethylene oxide.

Hodgkin's disease (cancer), suspected of causing Pentachlorophenol.

Hyperactivity p-Dichlorobenzene; Endosulfan; Formaldehyde; Lindane.

Hyperventilation *also see* **Respiration, rapid** 2,4-D.

Hypothalamic disorders Triorthocresyl phosphate.

Hypothermia *also see* **Body temperature, reduced.** Acetone; Azinphos-methyl; Chlorpyrifos; Creosotes; Ethanol; Ethyl acetate; Isoamyl alcohol; Isopropyl alcohol; Limonene; Naled; Phenol; n-Propyl alcohol; Tetraethyl lead; Turpentine.

Hypothermia, suspected of causing Cyclohexanone; TEDP.

Hysteria Dichloroethyl ether.

IgG protein, chemical binds to Vinyl chloride.

Immune complex glomerulonephritis Cadmium; Mercury.

Immune system, autoimmune responses similar to sclerosis in the Vinyl chloride.

Immune system abnormalities Trichloroethylene.

Immune system activation Chlorpyrifos.

Immune system activation, suspected of causing Cadmium; Manganese.

Immune system damage Benzene; Copper.

Immune system damage, suspected of causing Chlorinated camphene; Chlorobenzene; Chloroform; p-Dichlorobenzene; 2,4-Dichlorophenol; Endosulfan; Lead; Methyl chloride; Tin.

Immune system depression Asbestos.

Immune system disorders 1,1,2-Trichloroethane.

Immune system response, cell-mediated Beryllium.

Immune system sensitization *also see* **Chemical sensitivity.** Chromium, Cobalt, Formaldehyde, Styrene, Trimellitic anhydride.

Immune system suppression, suspected of causing Cadmium; Chlorinated diphenyl; 1,1-Dimethylhydrazine; Methyl parathion; Polychlorinated biphenyls; Vinyl acetate.

Impotence beta-Chloroprene; Manganese; Vinyl chloride.

Impotence, suspected of causing Ethanol.

Incoherence Hydrazine.

Incontinence Acetone; Acetonitrile; Azinphos-methyl; Carbaryl; Carbon monoxide; Chlorpyrifos; EPN; Ethyl acetate; Methyl parathion; Naled; TEDP.

Indecision Mercury.

Indigestion Bromine; Hexachloronaphthalene; Isoamyl acetate; Naphtha; Pentachloronaphthalene; Tetrachloronaphthalene.

Inebriation n-Butyl acetate; Ethanol; Ethyl chloride; Isophorone; Propylene oxide; 1,1,2,2-Tetrachloroethane; 1,1,1-Trichloroethane; Vanadium pentoxide.

Infection, increased susceptibility to Acetone.

Intelligence, impaired Carbon disulfide; Paraldehyde.

Intelligence Quotient (IQ), lowered Ethanol; Lead.

Intelligence Quotient (IQ) profile, inconsistent Formaldehyde.

Intestinal cancer, suspected of causing Acrylonitrile.

Intestinal congestion Ethyl bromide.

Intestinal congestion, suspected of causing Cyclohexanone.

Intestinal hemorrhaging Dinitro-o-cresol; Ethyl bromide.

Intestinal irritation n-Hexane; Hydroquinone; Tin.

Intestinal pain Formaldehyde; Hexone.

Intestinal swelling Malathion.

Intracellular swelling Sodium hydroxide.

Intracranial pressure 1,2-Dichloroethylene; Tetraethyl lead.

Iris inflammation Sulfur dioxide.

Irrational behavior Camphor.

Irritability Acrylamide; Acrylonitrile; Aniline; Arsenic; Benzyl chloride; Bromine; Carbon monoxide; Chloroform; beta-Chloroprene; Dinitrotoluenes; Ethyl methacrylate; Formaldehyde; Hydrogen sulfide; Isophorone; Lindane; Lead; Manganese; Mercury; Methyl iodide; Methyl methacrylate; Methylamine; p-Nitroaniline; Phosphorus pentasulfide; Selenium; Styrene; 1,1,2,2-Tetrachloroethane; Tetraethyl lead.

Itching, severe Dimethyl sulfate; Pentachloronaphthalene; Phosphorus; Picric acid; Pyrethrum; Tin.

Jaundice Acetylene tetrabromide; Acrylonitrile; Arsine; Calcium arsenate; Chloroform; o-Dichlorobenzene; p-Dichlorobenzene; Dimethyl acetamide; Dimethyl sulfate; Dinitrobenzenes; Dinitrotoluenes; Ethylene dichloride; Formaldehyde; Hexachloronaphthalene; Methyl chloride; Naphthalene; p-Nitroaniline; Nitrobenzene; N-Nitrosodimethylamine; Octachloronaphthalene; Pentachloronaphthalene; Phenylhydrazine; Phosphine; Phosphorus; Picric acid; Stibine; 1,1,2,2-Tetrachloroethane; Tetrachloronaphthalene; 2,4,6-Trinitrotoluene.

Jaw, stiffness in lower Acetonitrile.

Jaw, swollen Phosphorus.

Jaw bones, inflammation (osteo-

myelitis) of the Phosphine; Phosphorus; Phosphorus pentasulfide.

Jaw pain Phosphorus.

Jejunum tissue death Phosphoric acid.

Joint aches Formaldehyde.

Joint pain Bromine; Chlorinated diphenyl; Formaldehyde; Lead; Polychlorinated biphenyls; Trimellitic anhydride; Vinyl chloride.

Joint swelling Formaldehyde.

Judgment, impaired Acrylonitrile; Benzene; Carbon monoxide; Pentaborane.

Kidney, fatty degeneration of Chloroform; Tetramethyl succinonitrile.

Kidney congestion Benzene; Beryllium; Cobalt.

Kidney congestion, suspected of causing Chlorinated camphene.

Kidney damage/injury Acetylene tetrabromide; Allyl chloride; n-Amyl acetate; Aniline; 2,3-Benzofuran; Boron; 2-Butoxyethanol; n-Butyl acetate; n-Butyl alcohol; sec-Butyl alcohol; Cadmium; Carbon disulfide; Carbon tetrachloride; Chlorobenzene; Chloroform; beta-Chloroprene; Chromic acid; Chromium; Copper; Creosotes; Cresols; Diacetone alcohol; Diborane; o-Dichlorobenzene; p-Dichlorobenzene; 1,1-Dichloroethane; 2,4-Dichlorophenol; Dimethyl acetamide; Dimethyl sulfate; Dimethylformamide; 1,1-Dimethylhydrazine; Dinitro-o-cresol; Epichlorohydrin; 2-Ethoxyethyl acetate; Ethyl acetate; Ethyl chloride; Ethyl ether; Ethylene dibromide; Ethylene dichloride; Ethylene glycol; Ethylenediamine; Formic acid; Hexachloroethane; Hexone; Hydrazine; Isobutyl alcohol; Isophorone; Isopropyl ether; Limonene; Mesityl oxide; Methyl cellosolve acetate; Methyl chloride; Methyl hydrazine; Methylene chloride; Mono-methyl aniline; Morpholine; Nitric acid; 1-Nitropropane; Oxalic acid; Paraquat; Pentachlorophenol; Phenol; Phenylhydrazine; Phosphorus; Propylene dichloride; Pyridine; Stibine; Styrene; 1,1,2,2-Tetrachloroethane; Tetrachloroethylene; Thallium; Tin; 1,1,2-Trichloroethane; 2,4,6-Trinitrotoluene; Turpentine; Xylenes; Xylidine.

Kidney damage/injury, suspected of causing Boron trifluoride; Chlorinated diphenyl; Chlorobenzene; Decaborane; Diacetone alcohol; 2,4-Dichlorophenol; Diglycidyl ether; Di-sec octyl phthalate; Endosulfan; Ethyl benzene; Ethyl mercaptan; Ethyl silicate; Ethylene glycol dinitrate; Ethylene oxide; Ferbam; Methyl cellosolve; Molybdenum; Nickel; Nitroethane; Pentaborane; Polychlorinated biphenyls; Selenium; Sulfuryl fluoride; 1,2,3-Trichloropropane.

Kidney degeneration Ethyl bromide; Methyl parathion; Paraldehyde.

Kidney degeneration, suspected of causing Chlorinated camphene; Creosotes.

Kidney degenerative lesions Phenyl ether; Phenyl ether-biphenyl mixture.

Kidney diseases Ethyl bromide; Formic acid; Lead.

Kidney diseases, immune complex Malathion.

Kidney diseases, suspected of causing Propylene dichloride.

Kidney dysfunction Cadmium; Isopropyl alcohol; Malathion; n-Propyl alcohol; Sodium fluoroacetate.

Kidney effects, suspected of causing Methyl acetate.

Kidney enlargement, suspected of causing Chlorinated camphene.

Kidney failure Acetic anhydride; Ammonia; Barium; Chromium; Cresols; 2-Ethoxyethyl acetate; Ethylene dibromide; Ethylene dichloride; Ethylene glycol; Methyl bromide; Methyl cellosolve acetate; Methyl iodide; Naphthalene; Nitric acid; Phosphoric acid; Propylene dichloride; Sodium fluoroacetate; Sulfur monochloride; Trichloroethylene.

Kidney function, reduced N-Nitrosodimethylamine.

Kidney function, suspected of causing reduced Endosulfan.

Kidney hemorrhaging Ethylene dichloride.

Kidney impairment Chromium; Cresols; Isopropyl alcohol; n-Propyl alcohol.

Kidney inflammation Allyl alcohol; Arsenic; Chromium; Diacetone alcohol; Ethyl ether; Isopropyl ether; 1,1,2,2-Tetrachloroethane.

Kidney inflammation, glomerular Stibine.

Kidney inflammation, hemorrhagic Bromine; Iodine; Picric acid.

Kidney insufficiency Barium; Dinitro-o-cresol; Monomethyl aniline; Methyl cellosolve acetate; p-Nitroaniline; Nitrophenols; Pentachlorophenol; Phenol; Phosphorus; o-Toluidine.

Kidney irritation Vinyl chloride.

Kidney ischemic lesions Nitric acid.

Kidney lesions Acetone; Cadmium; Camphor; Chlorinated camphene; Cresols; Diacetone alcohol; Limonene; Methyl methacrylate; Picric acid; Tetraethyl lead; Turpentine.

Kidney pain Formaldehyde.

Kidney swelling Pentachloronaphthalene; Tetrachloronaphthalene.

Kidney swelling, suspected of causing Chlorinated camphene.

Kidney tissue death Cadmium; Lindane; Thallium.

Kidney tissue death, hemorrhagic Ethylene glycol.

Kidney tissue death, suspected of causing Chlorinated camphene.

Laryngeal irritation p-Phenylene diamine.

Laryngeal paralysis; partial Formaldehyde.

Laryngeal spasms Azinphosmethyl; Dichloromonofluoromethane; Dichlorotetrafluoroethane; Dichlorvos; EPN; Ethyl ether; Formaldehyde; Isopropyl ether; Malathion; Naled; Phosdrin.

Laryngeal spasms, suspected of causing Hydrogen chloride.

Laryngeal swelling Ammonia; Dichloromonofluoromethane; Dichlorotetrafluoroethane; Dimethyl sulfate; Ethyleneimine; Propylene imine; Sulfur dioxide.

Laryngitis Benzene; Hydrogen chloride; Iodine.

Lassitude Arsenic; Benzene; Carbaryl; Diborane; Dinitro-o-cresol; Manganese; Lead; Styrene; Tetraethyl lead; Zinc oxide.

Learning disability Lead.

Leg aches Triorthocresyl phosphate.

Leg cramps; pain Methyl alcohol.

Leg weakness Arsenic; Chlorpyrifos.

Legs, paralysis of Thallium.

Lethargy Acrylamide; Aniline; 2,4-D; Dimethyl acetamide; Dimethyl sulfate; Dimethylaniline; 1,1-Dimethylhydrazine; Ethanolamine; Ethyl acrylate; Ferbam; Hydrazine; Manganese; Methyl acrylate; Monomethyl aniline; Naphthalene; Nickel; Nitric oxide; p-Nitroaniline; Phosphine; Thiram; o-Toluidine.

Lethargy, suspected of causing Cresols; Cyclohexanone; 2,4-Dichlorophenol; Methyl mercaptan.

Leukemia Benzene; Ethylene oxide.

Leukemia, non-lymphocytic Benzene.

Leukemia, suspected of causing o-Dichlorobenzene; 1,3-Dichloropropene; Pentachlorophenol; Styrene; 2,4,6-Trichlorophenol.

Libido, altered Carbon disulfide; Mercury.

Libido, decreased Manganese; Vinyl chloride.

Libido, loss of beta-Chloroprene; 2,4-D.

Libido, suspected of causing a decline in Vanadium pentoxide.

Libido, suspected of causing altered Cadmium.

Ligaments, dark pigmentation of the Phenol.

Ligaments of ribs; pelvis, calcification of Fluorides.

Lightheadedness Acrylonitrile; Benzene; 1,3-Butadiene; 2-Butanone; Chlorine dioxide; Decaborane; Demeton; Diborane; Dichlorodifluoromethane; Dichloromonofluoromethane; Dichlorotetrafluoroethane; Ethylene dichloride; n-Heptane; n-Hexane; Hexone; Methyl alcohol; Methylene chloride; Naphtha; Pentaborane; Propylene dichloride; 1,1,2,2-Tetrachloroethane; Tetrachloroethylene; 1,1,1-Trichloroethane; 1,1,2-Trichloroethane; Trifluorobromomethane; Xylenes.

Lips, bleeding Warfarin.

Lips, blue Ethyl acrylate.

Lips, navy blue to black Aniline; p-Nitroaniline; o-Toluidine.

Lips, numbness/tingling/prickling sensation of the Pyrethrum.

Lips, swollen Dimethyl sulfate; Limonene; Turpentine.

Listlessness Naphthalene; Styrene.

Listlessness, suspected of causing Molybdenum; Silver.

Liver, accumulation of serous fluid (ascites) in the N-Nitrosodimethylamine.

Liver, altered serum chemistry of the Nitrobenzene; Thallium.

Liver, insufficient blood supply to the Cobalt.

Liver, petechial hemorrhaging on the surface of the Phosphine.

Liver, suspected of causing fatty degeneration of the 1,2-Dichloroethylene.

Liver, swollen or enlarged Arsenic; Carbon monoxide; Chloroform; beta-Chloroprene; Dimethyl sulfate; Dimethylformamide; Hexachloronaphthalene; Hexone; Hydrazine; Nitrobenzene; N-Nitrosodimethylamine; Pentachloronaphthalene; Phenylhydrazine; Phosphorus; 1,1,2,2-Tetrachloroethane; Tetrachloronaphthalene; Toluene; Vanadium pentoxide; Vinyl chloride.

Liver, tender Arsenic; Dimethyl sulfate; Hydrazine; Nitrobenzene; Phosphorus; Picric acid; 1,1,2,2-Tetrachloroethane.

Liver atrophy p-Dichlorobenzene.

Liver atrophy, suspected of causing Nickel.

Liver cancer Chlorinated diphenyl; 2-Nitropropane; Polychlorinated biphenyls; Vanadium pentoxide.

Liver cancer, suspected of causing p-Dichlorobenzene; Dinitrotoluenes; Di-sec octyl phthalate; 2,4,6-Trichlorophenol.

Liver cells, destruction of parenchymal 2-Nitropropane.

Liver congestion Allyl alcohol; Boron; Cobalt; Methyl bromide.

Liver damage, suspected of causing Chlorobenzene.

Liver damage/injury Acetone; Acrylonitrile; Allyl chloride; Ammonia; n-Amyl acetate; Aniline; Arsine; 2,3-Benzofuran; Boron; n-Butyl acetate; n-Butyl alcohol; sec-Butyl alcohol; Calcium arsenate; Carbon disulfide; Carbon tetrachloride; Chlorinated diphenyl; Chlorobenzene; o-Chlorobenzylidene malononitrile; Chloroform; beta-Chloroprene; Chromic acid; Chromium; Cobalt; Copper; Cresols; 2,4-D; Diacetone alcohol; o-Dichlorobenzene; 1,1-Dichloroethane; 2,4-Dichlorophenol; Dimethyl acetamide; Dimethyl sulfate; Dimethylformamide; 1,1-Dimethylhydrazine; Dimethylphthalate; Dinitrobenzenes; Epichlorohydrin; Ethanol; Ethyl acetate; Ethyl chloride; Ethylene dibromide; Ethylene dichloride; Ethylenediamine; Ethyleneimine; Hexachloroethane; Hydrazine; Isoamyl alcohol; Isobutyl alcohol; Isophorone; Mesityl oxide; Methyl cellosolve; Methyl chloride; Methyl hydrazine; Methylene chloride; Monomethyl aniline; Morpholine; p-Nitroaniline; 1-Nitropropane; 2-Nitropropane; Octachloronaphthalene; Paraquat; Pentachlorophenol; Phenol; Phenylhydrazine; Phosphine; Polychlorinated biphenyls; Propylene dichloride; Pyridine; Stibine; Tellurium; Tetrachloroethylene; Tetrachloronaphthalene; Tetramethyl succinonitrile; Thallium; Toluene; 1,1,1-Trichloroethane; 1,1,2-Trichloroethane; Trichloroethylene; 1,2,3-Trichloropropane; 2,4,6-Trinitrotoluene; Vanadium pentoxide; Vinyl chloride; Xylenes; Xylidine.

Liver damage/injury, delayed Acetylene tetrabromide.

Liver damage/injury, suspected of causing Cadmium; Decaborane; Diacetone alcohol; Diborane; Dichloroethyl ether; Diglycidyl ether; Di-sec octyl phthalate; Ethyl benzene; Ethyl mercaptan; Ethyl silicate; Ethylene glycol dinitrate; Ethylene oxide; Lindane; Molybdenum; Nitroethane; Pentaborane; Selenium; 2,4,6-Trichlorophenol.

Liver destruction/degeneration Barium; Boron; Cadmium; Ethyl bromide; Methyl parathion.

Liver diseases, suspected of causing Propylene dichloride.

Liver dysfunction/disorders/diseases/effects Benzidine; sec-Butyl acetate; tert-Butyl acetate; p-Dichlorobenzene; Ethyl bromide; Ethylene dibromide; Isobutyl acetate; Isopropyl alcohol; n-Propyl alcohol; Sodium fluoroacetate; 1,1,2,2-Tetrachloroethane; Thiram; Toluene; 2,4,6-Trinitrotoluene; Zinc oxide.

Liver effects, suspected of causing 1,3-Dichloropropene; Methyl acetate.

Liver failure Creosotes; Dimethyl sulfate; Ethylene dibromide; Ethylene dichloride; Phosphorus; Trichloroethylene; 2,4,6-Trinitrotoluene; Vanadium pentoxide.

Liver fatty changes Thallium.

Liver fatty degeneration Chloroform; Tetramethyl succinonitrile; Tin.

Liver focal hemorrhaging Methyl bromide.

Liver function, abnormal Lead.

Liver function, impaired Chloroform.

Liver function, reduced beta-Chloroprene; N-Nitrosodimethylamine.

Liver granulomas Mica.

Liver inflammation, suspected of causing Cresols.

Liver irritation Hexachloroethane.

Liver lesions Cresols; 2-Ethoxyethyl acetate; Methyl cellosolve acetate; Methyl methacrylate; Phenyl ether; Phenyl ether-biphenyl mixture.

Liver lesions, ischemic Acetic anhydride; Phosphoric acid.

Liver lesions, suspected of causing 1,2-Dichloroethylene.

Liver pain 2,4-D; Ethylene dichloride.

Liver tissue death Beryllium; Calcium arsenate; 2,4-D; Dinitrobenzenes; Ethylene dibromide; Ethylene dichloride; Hexachloronaphthalene; N-Nitrosodimethylamine; Pentachloronaphthalene; Thallium; 2,4,6-Trinitrotoluene.

Liver tissue death, suspected of causing 2-Butoxyethanol; 2,4-Dichlorophenol; Tin.

Lockjaw Acetonitrile.

Lung blood vessel damage Chlorine.

Lung burns Bromine.

Lung cancer Acrylonitrile; Arsenic; Cadmium; Chloromethyl methyl ether; Chromium; Nickel; Polycyclic aromatic hydrocarbons; Vanadium pentoxide.

Lung cancer, suspected of causing Acrylonitrile; Beryllium; Calcium arsenate; Dimethyl sulfate; Methylene chloride; Silica.

Lung congestion Acrolein; Chlorinated camphene; Chloroform; Chloromethyl methyl ether; p-Dichlorobenzene; Isophorone; Nickel carbonyl; Phosgene; Vinyl acetate; Xylenes.

Lung damage/injury Acetylene tetrabromide; 2,3-Benzofuran; Benzyl chloride; Chlorobenzene; beta-Chloroprene; Cresols; p-Dichlorobenzene; Ethyl acetate; Manganese; Mesityl oxide; Mica; Pentachlorophenol; Pyrethrum; Xylenes; Xylidine.

Lung damage/injury, suspected of causing Chlorobenzene; Cyclohexanone; Diglycidyl ether; Methyl cellosolve.

Lung degeneration Isophorone.

Lung diseases, suspected of causing fatal Chloropicrin.

Lung edema Acetic acid; Allyl alcohol; Allyl chloride; Ammonia; Arsenic; Benzyl chloride; Bromine; n-Butyl acetate; n-Butyl alcohol; sec-Butyl alcohol; Cadmium; Carbon monoxide; Chlorinated camphene; Chlorine; Chlorine dioxide; Chloroacetaldehyde; alpha-Chloroacetophenone; o-Chlorobenzylidene malononitrile; Chloromethyl methyl ether; Chloropicrin; Chromium; Cobalt; 2,4-D; Diborane; Dimethyl sulfate; Dimethylamine; 1,1-Dimethylhydrazine; Dinitro-o-cresol; Ethyl acrylate; Ethyl bromide; Ethylene dibromide; Ethylene oxide; Ethyleneimine; Fluorides; Formaldehyde; Hydrazine; Hydrogen fluoride; Hydrogen sulfide; Iodine; Isobutyl alcohol; Isopropylamine; Ketene; Limonene; Methyl bromide; Methyl cellosolve acetate; Methyl methacrylate; Methyl parathion; Monomethyl aniline; Nickel carbonyl; Nitric oxide; Nitrogen dioxide; Nitrophenols; Octane; Paraldehyde; Phenol; Phosgene; Phosphine; Phosphorus pentasulfide; Propylene imine; Sodium fluoroacetate; Sulfur dioxide; Sulfur monochloride; Sulfuric acid; Tetramethyl succinonitrile; Thallium; Toluene-2,4-diisocyanate; Tributyl phosphate; Trimellitic anhydride; Turpentine; Vinyl acetate; Xylenes; Zinc chloride.

Lung edema, delayed Acetaldehyde; Acrolein; Dichloroethyl ether; Nitric acid.

Lung edema, hemorrhagic Isopropyl alcohol.

Lung edema, suspected of causing Crotonaldehyde; Cyclohexanone; 2-Ethoxyethyl acetate; Hydrogen chloride; Lead; Methyl acetate; Methyl formate; Nitroethane; Sulfuryl fluoride.

Lung fibrosis Aluminum; Beryllium; Cadmium; p-Dichlorobenzene; Titanium dioxide; Vinyl chloride; Zinc chloride.

Lung function, abnormal Acrolein.

Lung function, reduced/restricted/impaired Asbestos; Chlorinated diphenyl; Chromium; Cobalt; Manganese; N-Nitrosodimethylamine;

Phosphoric acid; Polychlorinated biphenyls; Silica; Sulfur dioxide; Xylenes; Zinc oxide.

Lung granulomas Beryllium; p-Dichlorobenzene.

Lung hemorrhagic lesions Arsenic.

Lung hemorrhaging Benzene; Chloroform; Octane; Paraldehyde; Phosgene; Trichloroethylene; Vinyl acetate; Xylenes.

Lung hemorrhaging, suspected of causing Cyclohexanone; 2,4-Dichlorophenol; 1,1-Dimethylhydrazine; Lead.

Lung infections, increased Manganese.

Lung inflammation Epichlorohydrin; Manganese; Nitrogen dioxide; Paraquat.

Lung inflammation, suspected of causing Ethyl benzene.

Lung irritation Arsenic; Cadmium; Diborane; Dichlorodifluoromethane; Dichloromonofluoromethane; Diisopropylamine; Fluorotrichloromethane; Formaldehyde; Ketene; Methyl bromide; Methyl iodide; Methyl mercaptan; Phosphine; Propylene oxide; Stibine; Titanium dioxide; Trifluorobromomethane; Vinyl chloride.

Lung irritation, suspected of causing Ethyl mercaptan; Lead.

Lung lesions Cresols; Methyl cellosolve acetate; Titanium dioxide.

Lung lesions, suspected of causing 1,2-Dichloroethylene.

Lung rales Azinphos-methyl; Carbaryl; Chlorpyrifos; Cobalt; Naled; Nitroethane; TEDP.

Lung secretions Methylene bisphenyl isocyanate.

Lung sensitization *also see* **Chemical sensitivity.** Methylene bisphenyl isocyanate; Toluene-2,4-diisocyanate.

Lung tissue death Nickel carbonyl.

Lungs, dry-land drowning from accumulating blood in the Phosgene.

Lupus erythematous, systemic Hydrazine; Polychlorinated biphenyls; Silica; Vinyl chloride.

Lymph node hypertrophy Acetic acid.

Lymphatic cancer Vinyl chloride.

Lymphatic tissue lesions, suspected to causing 2,3-Benzofuran.

Lymphocyctic neuropathy Chlorpyrifos.

Lymphoma (cancer), suspected of causing Styrene.

Malaise (a general feeling of being unwell) Arsine; Carbon dioxide; 2,4-D; 1,3-Dichloropropene; Dimethyl sulfate; Dinitro-o-cresol; Formaldehyde; Magnesium oxide; Manganese; Methyl bromide; Methyl hydrazine; Naphthalene; N-Nitrosodimethylamine; Phosgene; Styrene; 1,1,2,2-Tetrachloroethane; Trimellitic anhydride; Zinc oxide.

Malaise, suspected of causing Silver.

Malnutrition Lead; Phosphorus.

Mania Calcium arsenate; Ethyl ether; Isopropyl ether; Methyl alcohol; Tetraethyl lead; Tetramethyl lead.

Manual dexterity, impaired 1,1,2,2-Tetrachloroethane; 1,1,1-Trichloroethane.

Mediastinum tissue inflammation Calcium oxide.

Membrane, tissue ulceration Acetic acid; Acetic anhydride; Formic acid.

Memory, changes in Styrene.

Memory, impaired/defective Arsenic; Carbon disulfide; Carbon monoxide; Lead; Manganese; Methyl parathion; Paraldehyde; Tin.

Memory, inability to recall words; names from Formaldehyde.

Memory, loss of recent Pentaborane.

Memory disorders Ethylene dichloride.

Memory loss Carbaryl; Dichlorodifluoromethane; Ethanol; Ethylene oxide; Formaldehyde; n-Hexane; Hydrogen sulfide; Isoamyl alcohol; Methyl methacrylate; Methyl parathion; Paraldehyde; Phosphorus pentasulfide; Tin; Vanadium pentoxide; Xylenes.

Memory loss, retrograde Propane.

Memory loss, short term Formaldehyde; Xylenes.

Memory loss, suspected of causing Silver.

Meninges (brain/spinal cord membranes) inflammation Ethylene glycol.

Meninges (brain/spinal cord membranes) lesions 2-Ethoxyethyl acetate; Methyl cellosolve acetate.

Menstrual cycles, altered Carbon disulfide; Polychlorinated biphenyls.

Menstrual disorders/irregularities Benzene; Formaldehyde; Lead; Mercury; Sulfur dioxide.

Menstrual disorders/irregularities, suspected of causing Tetrachloroethylene.

Menstrual disturbances Antimony; Vinyl chloride.

Menstrual flow, deficient amount of Formaldehyde.

Menstrual pain Benzene; Formaldehyde.

Mental activity, impaired Ethanol; Isoamyl alcohol; 1,1,2,2-Tetrachloroethane.

Mental disorders/illness Ethyl ether; Isopropyl ether; Methyl parathion.

Mental disturbances Formic acid.

Mental dullness Chloroform; De-

caborane; Isoamyl alcohol; Methyl cellosolve; Propylene imine; 1,1,1-Trichloroethane; Trifluorobromomethane.

Mental retardation in children Lindane.

Mesothelioma Asbestos.

Metabolic pigment disorders Polycyclic aromatic hydrocarbons.

Metabolic stress Carbon dioxide.

Metabolism, changes in Barium.

Metabolism, suspected of altering Boron.

Metabolism defect causing myocardial disorders of the heart Thiram.

Metal fume fever (resembles the flu) Antimony; Arsenic; Cadmium; Cobalt; Copper; Diborane; Lead; Magnesium oxide; Manganese; Mercury; Nickel; Tin; Zinc oxide.

Mitochondria degeneration Thallium.

Mitochondrial changes Lead.

Mood swings Ethanol; Isoamyl alcohol.

Motor control impairment, suspected of causing n-Butyl alcohol.

Motor dysfunction Methyl alcohol.

Motor polyneuropathy n-Hexane.

Motor restlessness Cumene; Methyl alcohol.

Motor skill retardation in children Lindane.

Motor skills, impaired Ethyl acetate; n-Pentane; Toluene; Triphenyl phosphate.

Mouth, bad taste in Dinitrobenzenes, 2-Aminopyridine, p-Nitrochlorobenzene.

Mouth, bitter taste in Acetonitrile; Ethyl mercaptan; Picric acid.

Mouth, burning pain in Limonene.

Mouth, burning sensation in

Chlorine; Dinitrobenzenes; Nicotine; Nitrophenols; Turpentine.

Mouth, dry 1,3-Butadiene; Tellurium.

Mouth, foamy bloodstained Acetonitrile.

Mouth, frothing from Carbaryl; Nitrophenols; Phenol.

Mouth, gasoline taste in n-Pentane.

Mouth, metallic taste in Antimony; Arsenic; Calcium arsenate; Copper; Ethylene dichloride; Formaldehyde; Lead; Selenium; Tellurium; Tetraethyl lead; Tetramethyl lead; Vanadium pentoxide; Zinc oxide.

Mouth, necrotic lesions in Nitrophenols.

Mouth, numbness/tingling of Barium.

Mouth, peculiar taste in Ethylene oxide.

Mouth, sweet taste in Calcium arsenate; Ethyl mercaptan; Zinc oxide.

Mouth burns 2,4-D.

Mouth corrosion Nitric acid.

Mouth hemorrhaging Creosotes.

Mouth irritation Antimony; Cresols.

Mouth pain Nitric acid.

Mouth redness Sulfur dioxide.

Mucous membrane, navy blue to black Aniline; p-Nitro aniline; o-Toluidine.

Mucous membrane burns Chromium; Dimethylamine; 1,1-Dimethylhydrazine; Methylamine.

Mucous membrane congestion Hydrogen peroxide.

Mucous membrane corrosion Acetic anhydride; Phosphoric acid; Sulfur monochloride.

Mucous membrane hemorrhaging Cumene.

Mucous membrane irritation Acrolein; Benzoyl peroxide; Butylamine; Calcium arsenate; Camphor; Chloroacetaldehyde; Chloropicrin; beta-Chloroprene; Chloromethyl methyl ether; Chromium; Copper; Cumene; Cyclohexane; Cyclohexanone; 1,3-Dichloro-5,5-dimethylhydantoin; Dichloroethyl ether; 1,3-Dichloropropene; Dimethylamine; 1,1-Dimethylhydrazine; Dimethylphthalate; Di-sec octyl phthalate; Ethyl acrylate; Ethyl benzene; Ethyl butyl ketone; Ethyl chloride; Ethyl formate; Ethyl mercaptan; Ethyl methacrylate; Ethyl silicate; Ethylamine; Ferbam; Furfuryl alcohol; Hexachloroethane; Isophorone; Isopropyl ether; Mesityl oxide; Methyl n-amyl ketone; 5-Methyl-3-heptanone; Nitroethane; Nitromethane; Oxalic acid; Pentaborane; 2-Pentanone; Phthalic anhydride; n-Propyl acetate; Propylene dichloride; Selenium; Thiram; Tributyl phosphate.

Mucous membrane lesions Cumene.

Mucous membrane pain Phosphoric acid; Sulfur monochloride.

Mucous membrane secretions Ammonia.

Mucous membrane tissue death Sodium hydroxide; Sulfur monochloride.

Mucous membrane ulcers Chromium.

Multiple sclerosis–like symptoms Carbon monoxide.

Mumps Iodine.

Muscle aches/pain Cadmium; 2,4-D; Methyl bromide; Nickel; Pentaborane; Phenol; Phosphine; Picric acid; Tetraethyl lead; Tetraethyl lead; Tetramethyl lead; Trimellitic anhydride; 2,4,6-Trinitrotoluene; Vinyl chloride; Zinc oxide.

Muscle contractions, involuntary Azinphos-methyl; Carbaryl; Chlorpyrifos; Cumene; Demeton; Diborane; Dichlorvos; EPN; Malathion; Methyl parathion; Naled; TEDP.

Muscle cramps Calcium arsenate; Carbaryl; Formaldehyde; Lead; n-Hexane; Pentaborane; Phosphorus pentasulfide; Picric acid; Tetraethyl lead; Tetramethyl lead; Thallium; Zinc oxide.

Muscle damage 2,4-D.

Muscle failure n-Pentane.

Muscle fatigue Diborane; Toluene.

Muscle fiber death Thallium.

Muscle fiber degeneration Hydrazine.

Muscle fiber splitting Thallium.

Muscle hemorrhaging, skeletal 1,3-Dichloropropene.

Muscle irritation Paraldehyde.

Muscle membrane hemorrhaging Warfarin.

Muscle movements, jerky or spastic Camphor; Carbaryl; Cyanides; n-Hexane; Mercury; Tetraethyl lead.

Muscle nerve supply (denervation) atrophy; degeneration n-Hexane.

Muscle rigidity Copper; Cyanides; 2,4-D; Hydrogen cyanide; Manganese.

Muscle spasms Barium; Carbaryl; Chlorinated camphene; Chlorobenzene; 2,4-D; Decaborane; EPN; Formaldehyde; Lindane; Naled.

Muscle spasms, ciliary TEDP.

Muscle tenderness 2,4-D; Isopropyl alcohol; Picric acid; n-Propyl alcohol.

Muscle tension Naled.

Muscle tissue, hardening of Isopropyl alcohol; n-Propyl alcohol.

Muscle tissue death Lindane.

Muscle tone, autonomic impaired Methyl methacrylate.

Muscle tone, loss of Ferbam; Thiram.

Muscle twitching Azinphos-methyl; Carbaryl; Chlorpyrifos; Creosotes; 2,4-D; Demeton; EPN; Hydroquinone; Malathion; Naled; Nickel carbonyl; Phenol; Sodium fluoroacetate; TEDP; TEPP; Thallium; Tributyl phosphate.

Muscle weakness Acrylamide; n-Amyl acetate; Barium; 2-Butanone; n-Butyl acetate; n-Butyl alcohol; sec-Butyl alcohol; 2,4-D; Diborane; 2,4-Dichlorophenol; n-Hexane; Isobutyl alcohol; Lead; Pentachlorophenol; Tetraethyl lead; Tetramethyl lead.

Muscle weakness, proximal Carbaryl.

Muscle weakness, suspected of causing Triphenyl phosphate.

Muscles, abnormal tension of Cumene; Manganese.

Muscular excitement Camphor.

Muscular fibrillation Pyrethrum.

Muscular swelling n-Hexane; Isopropyl alcohol; n-Propyl alcohol.

Myasthenia gravis Chlorine.

Mycosis fungoides (cancer), suspected of causing Ethylenediamine.

Nasal atrophy Chromium.

Nasal bleeding, ulcerative Phthalic anhydride.

Nasal burns Acetic acid; Formaldehyde.

Nasal cancer Nickel.

Nasal congestion Cyanides; Formaldehyde; Hydrazine; Hydrogen cyanide; Hydrogen fluoride; Pyrethrum.

Nasal crusting Formaldehyde.

Nasal discharge Azinphos-methyl; Carbaryl; Chlorine; Chromium; Demeton; Dichlorvos; EPN; Formic acid; Malathion; Naled; Phosdrin; Phthalic anhydride; Propylene imine; Pyrethrum; Sulfur dioxide; Sulfuryl fluoride; TEDP; TEPP; Trimellitic anhydride.

Nasal drip, post Formaldehyde.

Nasal inflammation Acetaldehyde; Arsenic; Calcium arsenate; p-Dichlorobenzene; Formaldehyde; Formic acid; Hydrogen chloride; Phosphorus pentasulfide; Pyrethrum; Trimellitic anhydride.

Nasal inflammation, allergic Benzyl chloride.

Nasal inflammation, suspected of causing Ethylene oxide.

Nasal inflammation with profuse discharge Epichlorohydrin; Ethylenediamine; Iodine.

Nasal irritation Acetaldehyde; Acetic acid; Acetic anhydride; Acetone; Acetylene tetrabromide; Acrylonitrile; Allyl chloride; Ammonia; Ammonium sulfamate; n-Amyl acetate; sec-Amyl acetate; Antimony; Arsenic; Benzene; Benzyl chloride; Boron; Boron trifluoride; 1,3-Butadiene; 2-Butanone; 2-Butoxyethanol; sec-Butyl acetate; tert-Butyl acetate; n-Butyl alcohol; Butylamine; Carbon tetrachloride; Chlorine dioxide; Chloroacetaldehyde; Chlorobenzene; o-Chlorobenzylidene malononitrile; Chromium; Copper; Cresols; Crotonaldehyde; Cyclohexanol; 2,4-D; Diacetone alcohol; o-Dichlorobenzene; Dichloroethyl ether; Diisobutyl ketone; Dimethyl sulfate; Dimethylamine; 2-Ethoxyethyl acetate; Ethyl acetate; Ethyl benzene; Ethyl ether; Ethyl formate; Ethyl silicate; Ethylene oxide; Ethylenediamine; Ethyleneimine; N-Ethylmorpholine; Ferbam; Formaldehyde; Glycidol; n-Hexane; Hexone; Hydrazine; Hydrogen fluoride; Hydrogen peroxide; Iodine; Isoamyl alcohol; Isobutyl acetate; Isobutyl alcohol; Isophorone; Isopropyl acetate; Isopropyl alcohol; Isoamyl acetate; Isopropyl ether; Isopropylamine; Ketene; Lindane; Magnesium oxide; Maleic anhydride; Methyl acetate; Methyl cellosolve; Methyl formate; Methyl methacrylate; alpha-Methyl styrene; Methylamine; Methylene bisphenyl isocyanate; Methylene chloride; Morpholine; Naphtha; Nitric oxide; Nitroethane; Octane; Paraquat; Pentachlorophenol; Petroleum distillates; Phenol; Phenyl ether; Phenyl ether-biphenyl mixture; Portland cement; n-Propyl acetate; n-Propyl alcohol; Selenium; Sodium hydroxide; Stoddard solvent; Styrene; Sulfur dioxide; Sulfur monochloride; Sulfuric acid; Tetrachloroethylene; Tetramethyl succinonitrile; Toluene-2,4-diisocyanate; 1,1,2-Trichloroethane; Trichloroethylene; Triethylamine; Trimellitic anhydride; Turpentine; Vinyl acetate; Xylenes; Zinc chloride.

Nasal irritation, suspected of causing sec-Hexyl acetate; Molybdenum.

Nasal itching Chromium.

Nasal passages, burning sensation in Acetic anhydride; Chlorine.

Nasal passages, dry 1,3-Butadiene.

Nasal passages; frothing from the Carbaryl; Nitrophenols; Phenol.

Nasal septum, blue-gray Silver.

Nasal septum perforation Calcium oxide; Chromic acid; Chromium; Copper.

Nasal septum ulcers Arsenic; Calcium oxide; Chlorine; Chromium; Ethyleneimine; Propylene imine; Sodium hydroxide; Stibine; Sulfur dioxide; Zinc chloride.

Nasal soreness Chromium.

Nausea Acetaldehyde; Acetic anhydride; Acetone; Acetonitrile; Acetylene tetrabromide; Acrylonitrile; 2-Aminopyridine; n-Amyl acetate; Aniline; Antimony; Arsenic; Arsine; Azinphosmethyl; Benzene; Benzyl chloride; 1,3-Butadiene; 2-Butanone; 2-Butoxyethanol; n-Butyl acetate; n-Butyl alcohol; sec-Butyl alcohol; Butylamine; Cadmium; Camphor; Carbaryl; Carbon monoxide; Carbon tetrachloride;

Chlorinated camphene; Chlorinated diphenyl; Chlorine; Chlorine dioxide; Chlorobenzene; Chloroform; Chloropicrin; Chlorpyrifos; Chromium; Cobalt; Copper; Cumene; Cyanides; Cyclohexanol; Decaborane; Demeton; Diborane; Dibutylphthalate; o-Dichlorobenzene; o-Dichlorobenzene; p-Dichlorobenzene; 1,1-Dichloroethane; Dichloroethyl ether; 1,2-Dichloroethylene; 1,3-Dichloropropene; Dichlorvos; 2-Diethylaminoethanol; Diisopropylamine; Dimethyl sulfate; Dimethylformamide; 1,1-Dimethylhydrazine; Dinitro-o-cresol; Dinitrotoluenes; Epichlorohydrin; EPN; Ethanol; 2-Ethoxyethyl acetate; Ethyl acetate; Ethyl acrylate; Ethyl benzene; Ethyl chloride; Ethyl ether; Ethyl mercaptan; Ethylene dibromide; Ethylene dichloride; Ethylene glycol; Ethylene glycol dinitrate; Ethylene oxide; Ethyleneimine; Ferbam; Fluorides; Formaldehyde; Formic acid; Furfuryl alcohol; n-Heptane; Hexachloronaphthalene; n-Hexane; Hexone; sec-Hexyl acetate; Hydrazine; Hydrogen cyanide; Hydrogen fluoride; Hydroquinone; Isoamyl alcohol; Isobutyl acetate; Isobutyl alcohol; Isophorone; Isopropyl alcohol; Isopropyl ether; Lead; Lindane; Limonene; Magnesium oxide; Malathion; Maleic anhydride; Mercury; Methyl alcohol; Methyl bromide; Methyl cellosolve acetate; Methyl chloride; Methyl formate; Methyl hydrazine; Methyl iodide; Methyl parathion; Methylene chloride; Monomethyl aniline; Naled; Naphtha; Naphthalene; Nickel; Nicotine; Nitric acid; Nitric oxide; p-Nitroaniline; Nitrobenzene; Nitroethane; Nitrogen dioxide; 1-Nitropropane; 2-Nitropropane; N-Nitrosodimethylamine; Pentaborane; Pentachloronaphthalene; Pentachlorophenol; n-Pentane; Petroleum distillates; Phenol; Phenyl ether; Phenyl ether-biphenyl mixture; Phenylhydrazine; Phosdrin; Phosgene; Phosphine; Phosphoric acid; Phosphorus; Phosphorus pentasulfide; Picric acid; Pindone; Polychlorinated biphenyls; n-Propyl acetate; n-Propyl alcohol; Propylene dichloride; Propylene imine; Propylene oxide; Pyrethrum; Pyridine; Selenium; Stibine; Styrene; Sulfur dioxide; Sulfur monochloride; TEDP; Tellurium; TEPP; 1,1,2,2-Tetrachloroethane; Tetrachloroethylene; Tetrachloronaphthalene; Tetraethyl lead; Tetrahydrofuran; Tetramethyl lead; Tetramethyl succinonitrile; Thallium; Thiram; Toluene; Toluene-2, 4-diisocyanate; o-Toluidine; Tributyl phosphate; 1,1,1-Trichloroethane; 1,1,2-Trichloroethane; Trichloroethylene; 1,2,3-Trichloropropane; Trimellitic anhydride; 2,4,6-Trinitrotoluene; Triorthocresyl phosphate; Turpentine; Vinyl chloride; Warfarin; Xylenes; Zinc chloride; Zinc oxide.

Neck, flushed Tetrachloroethylene.

Neck, numbness/tingling of the Barium.

Neck spasms, tonic Pentaborane.

Neonate hemolytic anemia Naphthalene.

Neonate jaundice Naphthalene.

Neonate lethality, suspected of causing Acetone; Cyclohexanone; Dibutylphthalate; 2,4-Dichlorophenol; Ethylene oxide; Lead; Polycyclic aromatic hydrocarbons.

Nerve cell damage, suspected of causing Cadmium.

Nerve cells, destruction of Pentaborane.

Nerve damage, peripheral Trichloroethylene.

Nerve degeneration of axons; myelin sheaths; peripheral Allyl chloride; Thallium.

Nerve disturbances, peripheral Dinitrobenzenes.

Nerve inflammation Hydrogen sulfide.

Nerve inflammation, peripheral Picric acid; Sulfur dioxide; Thallium.

Nerve inflammation Hydrogen sulfide.

Nerve system, multi-nerve inflammation of the Triorthocresyl phosphate.

Nerves, removes myelin sheath from Arsenic; Thallium; Triorthocresyl phosphate.

Nerves controlling muscular blood vessels (vasomotor), disorders of the Vanadium pentoxide.

Nervous excitement Pentaborane.

Nervous system, central neuronal tissue death of the Camphor.

Nervous system, central neuropathy of the Arsenic.

Nervous system, distal axon degeneration of the Arsenic.

Nervous system, neural degenerative lesions of the Cyanides; Hydrogen cyanide.

Nervous system, peripheral neuropathy of the Arsenic; Arsine; Calcium arsenate; Carbaryl; Carbon disulfide; Chlorpyrifos; Dichlorodifluoromethane; Dichloromonofluoromethane; Ethylene oxide; n-Hexane; Hydrogen sulfide; Phosphorus pentasulfide; Thiram; Trichloroethylene; 2,4,6-Trinitrotoluene; Triorthocresyl phosphate; Vinyl chloride.

Nervous system, polyneuropathy of the Acrylamide; Allyl chloride; Carbon disulfide; 2,4-D; Lead; Mercury; Methyl bromide; n-Pentane; Thallium.

Nervous system, silver deposits in neuron of the central Silver.

Nervous system, swelling in the white matter of the central Tin.

Nervous system, topical neuropathy of the Cyanides; Hydrogen cyanide.

Nervous system cancer, central Vinyl chloride.

Nervous system damage/injury Hydrogen sulfide; Trichloroethylene.

Nervous system damage/injury, central Carbon dioxide; Decaborane; Methyl bromide; Phosphorus; Propylene dichloride.

Nervous system degeneration, central Copper.

Nervous system depression, central Acetaldehyde; Acetylene tetrabromide; sec-Amyl acetate; Benzene; Benzyl alcohol; Benzyl chloride; 2-Butoxyethanol; n-Butyl acetate; sec-Butyl acetate; tert-Butyl acetate; Camphor; Carbon tetrachloride; Chlorobenzene; Chloroform; beta-Chloroprene; Cumene; Cyclohexane; Diacetone alcohol; 1,1-Dichloroethane; 1,2-Dichloroethylene; Dichloromonofluoromethane; 2,4-Dichlorophenol; Dichlorotetrafluoroethane; Dimethylaniline; Dinitrotoluenes; 2-Ethoxyethyl acetate; Ethyl benzene; Ethyl bromide; Ethyl chloride; Ethyl ether; Ethyl formate; Ethyl mercaptan; Ethyl silicate; Ethylene dichloride; Ethylene glycol; Ethylene glycol dinitrate; Formaldehyde; Formic acid; Glycidol; Hexachloroethane; n-Hexane; Hexone; Hydrazine; Isoamyl acetate; Isobutyl alcohol; Isophorone; Isopropyl acetate; Isopropyl alcohol; Isopropyl ether; Linalyl alcohol; Mesityl oxide; Methyl n-amyl ketone; Methyl alcohol; Methylchloride; Methyl formate; Methyl iodide; Methyl methacrylate; alpha-Methyl styrene; Methylal; Nicotine; Nitromethane; Octane; n-Pentane; Propane; n-Propyl alcohol; Propylene oxide; Pyridine; Styrene; Sulfuryl fluoride; 1,1,2,2-Tetrachloroethane; Toluene; 1,1,1-Trichloroethane; 1,1,2-Trichloroethane; Trichloroethylene; 1,2,3-Trichloropropane.

Nervous system depression, suspected of causing central Diisobutyl ketone; Ethyl acetate; Fluorotrichloromethane.

Nervous system disorders/effects tert-Butyl acetate; Paraquat; Pentachlorophenol; Sulfur dioxide; Trifluorobromomethane.

Nervous system disorders/effects, central Carbon disulfide; Cresols; Ethyl methacrylate.

Nervous system dysfunction Ethyl chloride.

Nervous system dysfunction, central beta-Chloroprene; Ethanol; Picric acid; Toluene.

Nervous system dysfunction, peripheral beta-Chloroprene.

Nervous system excitement, central Glycidol; Hydroquinone; Lindane; Nicotine; Phthalic anhydride.

Nervous system impairment, central Hexone.

Nervous system lesions, suspected of causing 2,3-Benzofuran.

Nervous system neuropathy Ethylene oxide.

Nervous system paralysis, central Magnesium oxide.

Nervous system pathology; central Lead.

Nervousness Acrylamide; Arsenic; Benzene; Carbon disulfide; Decaborane; Dimethylformamide; Ethylene dichloride; Lead; Manganese; Methyl acetate; Pyridine; Selenium; Styrene; 1,1,2,2-Tetrachloroethane; Toluene; Vanadium pentoxide.

Neurobehavioral changes Toluene.

Neurobehavioral impairment Lead.

Neurochemistry changes Lead.

Neurologic disturbances 1,1,2, 2-Tetrachloroethane.

Neurologic impairment/dysfunction Sodium fluoroacetate.

Neurosis Azinphos-methyl; Chlorpyrifos; Naled.

Neurotic symptoms sec-Amyl acetate; Ethyl acrylate; Sulfur dioxide; 2,4,6-Trinitrotoluene.

Nightmares Azinphos-methyl; Chlorpyrifos; Naled; Tetraethyl lead; Tetramethyl lead.

Nosebleeds Boron trifluoride; Bromine; Chlorine; Chromium; Cyanides; Formaldehyde; Hydrogen cyanide; Maleic anhydride; Paraquat; Pindone; Propylene dichloride; Selenium; Thiram; Trimellitic anhydride; Warfarin.

Numb/tingling/prickling sensation Arsenic; Ethylene oxide.

Numbers, impaired ability to work with Xylenes.

Numbness, general Chlorobenzene; Dibutylphthalate; p-Dichlorobenzene; Phosphine; Propane; Vinyl chloride.

Nutritional malabsorbtion Zinc chloride.

Olfactory fatigue Acetonitrile; N-Ethylmorpholine; Methylamine; Sulfur dioxide.

Olfactory nerve paralysis *also see* **Smell, loss of.** Hydrogen sulfide.

Optic atrophy, Leber's hereditary Cyanides; Hydrogen cyanide.

Optic congestion Methyl alcohol.

Optic nerve atrophy Cobalt; Methyl acetate.

Optic neuropathy n-Hexane.

Organ congestion, suspected of causing 1,2-Dichloroethylene.

Organs, dropping or drooping of Thallium.

Organs or body, underdevelopment of Benzene.

Osteoporosis Cadmium.

Osteoporosis, suspected of causing Beryllium.

Ovarian atrophy Benzene.

Ovarian dysfunction Vinyl chloride.

Ovarian dysfunction, suspected of causing Vanadium pentoxide.

Ovaries, suspected of causing non-functioning Dinitrotoluenes.

Oxygen, inability to utilize Chloroform; Dimethylaniline; Dinitro-o-cresol; Dinitrobenzenes; 1,1-Dimethylhydrazine; Dinitrotoluenes; Ethylene glycol; Hydroquinone; Methyl hydrazine; Nitric oxide; Nitrobenzene; p-Nitrochlorobenzene; Phosgene; o-Toluidine; Xylidine.

Oxygen deprivation Dichloromonofluoromethane; Magnesium oxide.

Pain; absence of normal sense of *also see* Sensation loss of. Dimethyl sulfate; Ethyl chloride.

Pain, localized Oxalic acid.

Pallor Benzene; Ethyl ether; Isopropyl ether; Lead; Methyl cellosolve; Phenol; Pindone; Pyrethrum; Selenium; Tetraethyl lead; Vinyl chloride; Warfarin.

Palmar planter hyperkeratoses Calcium arsenate.

Pancreas damage, suspected of causing Di-sec octyl phthalate.

Pancreas inflammation Cresols; Zinc chloride.

Pancreas lesions Cresols.

Pancreas tissue death Phosphoric acid.

Pancreatic cancer Ethylene oxide.

Pancreatic disorders Ethanol; Isoamyl alcohol.

Paralysis Acetonitrile; 2-Aminopyridine; Arsenic; Azinphos-methyl; Barium; Benzene; Demeton; Dichlorvos; Dimethyl sulfate; EPN; 2-Ethoxyethyl acetate; Hexachloroethane; n-Hexane; Malathion; Naled; Nitrobenzene; Phosdrin; Pindone; Pyrethrum; TEDP; TEPP; 1,1,2,2-Tetrachloroethane; Tributyl phosphate; Trichloroethylene; Triorthocresyl phosphate.

Paralysis, flaccid 2,4-D; Ferbam; Thiram.

Paralysis, partial Tin.

Paralysis, suspected of causing Methyl bromide; Triphenyl phosphate.

Paralysis of lower limbs, partial Cyanides; Hydrogen cyanide.

Paralysis on one side of the body Cyanides; Hydrogen cyanide; Hydrogen peroxide.

Parkinson-like symptoms Carbon disulfide; Carbon monoxide; Cyanides; Hydrogen cyanide; Manganese; Methyl iodide.

Paroxysmal atrial fibrosis Nicotine.

Patience, loss of Xylenes.

Perception, impaired 1,1,2,2-Tetrachloroethane; 1,1,1-Trichloroethane.

Perceptual distortions Dimethyl acetamide; Toluene.

Performance impairment (mental and/or physical) n-Butyl acetate, Decaborane, Dichlorodifluoromethane, Isobutyl alcohol, Methylene chloride,; Trifluorobromomethane.

Peribronchial swelling Phosgene.

Peripheral-vegetative syndrome Vanadium pentoxide.

Personality changes 2-Butoxyethanol; Ethanol; 2-Ethoxyethyl acetate; Isoamyl alcohol; Mercury; Methyl cellosolve; Methyl chloride

Pharyngeal hemorrhaging Creosotes.

Pharyngeal inflammation Acetone; Bromine; Chlorine.

Pharyngeal irritation Acetic anhydride; p-Phenylene diamine.

Pharyngeal itching Chromium.

Pharyngeal redness Sulfur dioxide.

Pharyngeal swelling Acetic acid; Calcium oxide; Sodium hydroxide.

Pharyngeal ulcers Ethylene dibromide.

Physical strength, decrease in *also see* **Weakness.** Vanadium pentoxide.

Pleural disease Asbestos.

Pneumonconiosis Amorphous silica; Antimony; Barium; Chromium; Mica; Molybdenum; Stibine.

Pneumonia Acetone; Bromine; Cadmium; Calcium oxide; Chlorine; o-Chlorobenzylidene malononitrile; Chloromethyl methyl ether; Chloropicrin; Chromium; Cobalt; Cresols; 2,4-D; Diborane; Ethanol; Ethyl acetate; Formaldehyde; Iodine; Isoamyl alcohol; Limonene; Manganese; Nickel; Nickel carbonyl; Nitric acid; Nitric oxide; Phosgene; n-Propyl alcohol; Pyrethrum; Sodium hydroxide; Tetramethyl succinonitrile; Turpentine; Zinc oxide.

Pneumonia, aspirative Isopropyl alcohol.

Pneumonia, bronchial Acetic acid; Ammonia; Carbon monoxide; Chlorinated camphene; Chlorine; Chloropicrin; Dichlorodifluoromethane; Ethyleneimine; Hydrogen sulfide; Isopropyl alcohol; Mercury; Methyl bromide; Phosphorus pentasulfide; Propylene dichloride; Propylene imine; Zinc chloride.

Pneumonia, chemical Beryllium; n-Heptane; n-Hexane; Nickel carbonyl; Octane; n-Pentane.

Pneumonia, chemical bronchial Sulfur dioxide.

Pneumonia, hemorrhagic Cumene.

Pneumonia, suspected of causing Boron trifluoride.

Polyps, ethmoid Formaldehyde.

Porphyria cutanea tarda 2,4-Dichlorophenol.

Pregnant toxemia Vinyl chloride.

Prostate cancer Cadmium.

Prostate cancer, suspected of causing Acrylonitrile.

Psoriasis *also see* **dermatitis** Linalyl alcohol.

Psychological impairment Copper; Dichlorodifluoromethane.

Psychomotor agitation/deficits/ impairment Carbon disulfide; Lead; Sodium fluoroacetate.

Psychoneurological disturbances Tetrachloroethylene; Tin.

Psychosis Carbon disulfide; Lead; Manganese; Tetraethyl lead; Thallium; Toluene.

Psychosis, alcoholic Acetone.

Psychotic episodes/disturbances Chloroform; Ethyl ether; Isopropyl ether; Hydrogen sulfide; Methyl iodide; Phosphorus pentasulfide; Tin.

Psychotic-like behavior 2-Aminopyridine.

Pulmonary *see* **Lung.**

Pulse, alternating weak/strong Sodium fluoroacetate.

Pulse, increased Isoamyl acetate; Methyl chloride; Pyridine.

Pulse, irregular Acetonitrile; Nitrophenols; Phenol; Stibine.

Pulse, rapid Acetic acid; Acetic anhydride; Acetone; Acetonitrile; Calcium oxide; Camphor; Ethyl acetate; Ethyl bromide; Formic acid; Nitric acid; Phosphoric acid; Sulfur monochloride; Zinc chloride.

Pulse, slow Acetonitrile; Barium; 1,3-Butadiene; Methyl alcohol; n-Propyl alcohol.

Pulse, thready Creosotes.

Pulse, weak Acetic acid; Acetic anhydride; Acetonitrile; Calcium arsenate; Camphor; Carbon monoxide; Chromium; Cresols; Formic acid; Nitric acid; Nitrophenols; Phenol; Phosphoric acid; Stibine; Sulfur monochloride.

Pulse pressure, increased Carbon dioxide.

Pupillary reflexes, loss of Creosotes.

Pupils, constricted Azinphos-methyl; Carbaryl; Demeton; Dichlorvos; EPN; Malathion; Naled; Paraldehyde; Phosdrin; TEDP.

Pupils, dilated Acetone; Acetonitrile; Azinphos-methyl; Carbaryl; Chlorpyrifos; EPN; Ethyl acetate; Ethyl bromide; Isopropyl alcohol; Naled; Paraldehyde; Pentachlorophenol; Toluene.

Pyloric strictures Acetic acid; Acetic anhydride; Benzene; Formic acid; Iodine; Nitric acid; Phosphoric acid; Sulfur monochloride; Zinc chloride.

Rales Manganese; Vanadium pentoxide; Zinc oxide.

Rales, bilateral diffused Phosphine.

Rales, mucous Nitrophenols.

Raynaud's Disease Arsenic; Vanadium pentoxide; Vinyl chloride.

Reaction time, slowed/impaired Acetone; Ethyl acetate; 1,1,2,2-Tetrachloroethane; Toluene; 1,1,1-Trichloroethane; Xylenes.

Rectal cancer, suspected of causing Ethyl acrylate.

Rectum/anus inflammation (proctitis) Hydrogen peroxide.

Reflexes, absense/loss of Arsenic; Carbon monoxide; 2,4-D; Ethylene glycol; Isopropyl alcohol; Malathion; n-Propyl alcohol; 1,1,2,2-Tetrachloroethane.

Reflexes, depressed Carbon monoxide; 2,4-D.

Reflexes, hyperexcitable/hyperactive Chlorinated camphene; Cumene; Cyanides; Hydrogen cyanide; Tetraethyl lead.

Reflexes, slowed/diminished Pyridine.

Remorse Acetone; Ethyl acetate.

Renal *see* **Kidney.**

Reproductive damage, suspected of causing male Fluorides; Hydrogen fluoride.

Reproductive effects, suspected of causing Acrylonitrile; 2,3-Benzofuran; 1,3-Butadiene; Cyclohexanone; Hydroquinone; 2,4,6-Trichlorophenol.

Reproductive organs, inflammatory diseases of the Formaldehyde.

Respiration, Cheyne-Stokes TEDP; TEPP.

Respiration, decreased Endosulfan.

Respiration, gasping Cyanides; Hydrogen cyanide; Vinyl acetate.

Respiration, heavy Ethanol; Isoamyl alcohol.

Respiration, increased rate/depth of Acetonitrile; Cyanides; Dinitro-o-cresol; Hydrogen cyanide; Nickel; Nitric oxide; Picric acid; Pyridine.

Respiration, irregular Acrylonitrile; Cresols; Ethyl ether; Isopropyl ether; Nickel.

Respiration, labored/difficult Acetic anhydride; Acetonitrile; 2-Aminopyridine; Ammonia; Ammonium sulfamate; n-Amyl acetate; Aniline; Arsine; Asbestos; Azinphos-methyl; n-Butyl acetate; n-Butyl alcohol; sec-Butyl alcohol; Cadmium; Carbaryl; Carbon dioxide; Chlorine; Chlorine dioxide; Chloromethyl methyl ether; Chlorpyrifos; Cobalt; Cresols; Cyanides; 2,4-D; p-Dichlorobenzene; Dimethyl sulfate; Dimethylamine; 1,1-Dimethylhydrazine; Dinitrotoluenes; Endosulfan; EPN; Ethyl benzene; Ethylene dichloride; Ethylene oxide; Formic acid; Hydrogen cyanide; Hydrogen sulfide; Hydroquinone; Isoamyl acetate; Isoamyl alcohol; Isobutyl alcohol; Manganese; Mercury; Methyl acetate; Methyl alcohol Methyl bromide; Methyl formate;

Methylene bisphenyl isocyanate; Mica; Monomethyl aniline; Naled; Nickel carbonyl; Nicotine; Nitric acid; Nitric oxide; p-Nitroaniline; Nitroethane; Nitrogen dioxide; Paraldehyde; Pentachlorophenol; Phenylhydrazine; Phosgene; Phosphine; Phosphoric acid; Phosphorus pentasulfide; Picric acid; Pyrethrum; Selenium; Silica; Stibine; Sulfur dioxide; TEDP; Toluene-2,4-diisocyanate; Trimellitic anhydride; 2,4,6-Trinitrotoluene; Turpentine; Vanadium pentoxide; Vinyl acetate; Xylenes; Zinc chloride; Zinc oxide.

Respiration, painful Phosgene.

Respiration, rapid *also see* **Hyperventilation.** Carbon monoxide; Cresols; Cyanides; Dinitro-o-cresol; Ethyl acrylate; Hydrogen cyanide; Hydroquinone; Isoamyl acetate; Methyl acrylate; Nitric oxide; p-Nitroaniline; Nitrogen dioxide; Pentachlorophenol; Phosphorus pentasulfide; Zinc chloride.

Respiration, shallow Acetic anhydride; Demeton; Nitric acid; Nitric oxide; Nitrophenols; Phenol; Phosphoric acid.

Respiration, slow Cyanides; Ethyl acetate; Hydrogen cyanide.

Respiration, suspected of causing labored/difficult Crotonaldehyde; Decaborane; 2,4-Dichlorophenol; Ethyl silicate; Molybdenum; 2,4,6-Trichlorophenol.

Respiration labored/difficult on exertion Portland cement.

Respiration that provokes a snoring sound, laborious Nitrophenols.

Respiratory arrest/failure Acetaldehyde; Acetone; Acetonitrile; Ammonia; 2-Aminopyridine; n-Amyl acetate; Azinphos-methyl; Barium; Benzene Boron; n-Butyl acetate; n-Butyl alcohol; sec-Butyl alcohol; Camphor; Carbaryl; Carbon monoxide; Chlorinated camphene; Chloroform;

Chromium; Cresols; Cumene; Cyanides; Diacetone alcohol; 2,4-Dichlorophenol; Endosulfan; EPN; Ethylene dichloride; Ethylene glycol; Hydrogen cyanide; Hydroquinone; Isoamyl alcohol; Isobutyl alcohol; Isopropyl alcohol; Limonene; Methyl alcohol; Methyl bromide; Naled; Nickel carbonyl; p-Nitroaniline; Nitrophenols; Picric acid; n-Propyl alcohol; Pyrethrum; Sulfur dioxide; TEDP; 1,1,2,2-Tetrachloroethane; Tetraethyl lead; Thallium; 1,1,1-Trichloroethane; Turpentine; Xylenes.

Respiratory arrest/failure, suspected of causing 2,4-Dichlorophenol.

Respiratory blockage Acrolein, Ammonia, Antimony.

Respiratory burns Ammonia.

Respiratory collapse Dinitro-o-cresol.

Respiratory congestion, upper Acrolein; Acrylonitrile.

Respiratory depression Acetonitrile; 2,4-D; o-Dichlorobenzene; Dinitrotoluenes; Furfuryl alcohol; Isopropyl alcohol; Linalyl alcohol; Methylal; Paraldehyde; n-Propyl alcohol; Tin.

Respiratory depression, suspected of causing Ethyl methacrylate.

Respiratory difficulty beta-Chloroprene; Lindane.

Respiratory discomfort Isopropyl ether.

Respiratory disease, chronic Acrolein.

Respiratory diseases/disorders/effects Beryllium; 1,3-Butadiene; bromide; 2-Butanone; Ethyl bromide; Vanadium pentoxide.

Respiratory distress 2-Aminopyridine; Arsenic; Creosotes; Diborane; 1,1-Dimethylhydrazine; Epichlorohydrin; p-Nitroaniline; Tetramethyl succinonitrile.

Respiratory dryness, upper sec-Butyl acetate.

Respiratory function, impaired/decreased Arsenic; Cadmium; Fluorides; Hydrogen fluoride; Methyl bromide; Vinyl chloride.

Respiratory inflammation Acetic acid; Acetone; Calcium oxide; Chloropicrin.

Respiratory insufficiency Zinc chloride.

Respiratory irritation Allyl chloride; Ammonia; Antimony; Arsenic; Benzene; Benzyl acetate; Chlorine dioxide; alpha-Chloroacetophenone; beta-Chloroprene; Chromic acid; Cobalt; Crotonaldehyde; Cyclohexane; 2,4-D; p-Dichlorobenzene; 1,3-Dichloro-5,5-dimethylhydantoin; Dichloroethyl ether; 1,2-Dichloroethylene; Dichlorotetrafluoroethane; Diethylamine; 2-Diethylaminoethanol; Diglycidyl ether; Ethanolamine; Ethyl acetate; Ethyl acrylate; Ethyl bromide; Ethylamine; Ethylene dibromide; Ethylenediamine; Ferbam; Fluorides; sec-Hexyl acetate; Hydrazine; Hydrogen peroxide; Hydrogen sulfide; Isophorone; Methyl hydrazine; Methylamine; Mica; Morpholine; Nitroethane; 1-Nitropropane; 2-Nitropropane; Octane; Phenyl ether; Phosgene; Phosphorus; Phosphorus pentasulfide; Sulfur monochloride; Sulfuryl fluoride; Tetramethyl succinonitrile; Toluene; Tributyl phosphate; Triethylamine; Trimellitic anhydride; Vinyl acetate; Xylenes.

Respiratory irritation, upper Acrolein; Allyl alcohol; sec-Amyl acetate; Barium; Benzyl chloride; Boron; 2-Butanone; n-Butyl acetate; tert-Butyl acetate; Calcium oxide; Chloropicrin; Cyanides; Dibutylphthalate; Dimethylphthalate; Ethyl benzene; Ethyl ether; Ethyl formate; Fluorotrichloromethane; Furfural; Hydrogen cyanide; Isoamyl acetate; Isobutyl acetate; Isopropyl acetate; Isopropyl ether; Maleic anhydride; Methyl acetate; Methyl acrylate; Methylal; Pentachlorophenol; Phenyl glycidyl ether; Phosphoric acid; Phthalic anhydride; Propylene imine; Propylene oxide; Silver; Sodium hydroxide; Tetrachloroethylene; Tetrahydrofuran; Tin; Vinyl toluene.

Respiratory lesions, suspected of causing Ethylene dibromide; Ethylene oxide.

Respiratory oppression, upper Acrylonitrile.

Respiratory paralysis Acetaldehyde; Aniline; Benzyl alcohol; 1,3-Butadiene; Carbaryl; Chloroform; Epichlorohydrin; Ethyl bromide; Ethyl ether; Ferbam; Hydrogen sulfide; Isopropyl ether; Magnesium oxide; Methyl parathion; Monomethyl aniline; Nicotine; Phosphorus pentasulfide; Pyrethrum; Sulfur dioxide; Thiram; o-Toluidine; Triorthocresyl phosphate.

Respiratory passage disease, hyperactive Formaldehyde.

Respiratory sensitivity/hypersensitivity *also see* **Chemical sensitivity.** Chloroacetaldehyde; Cobalt.

Respiratory soft tissue, freezing of Trifluorobromomethane.

Respiratory tract, inability to utilize oxygen in the upper Octane.

Respiratory tract cancer Vinyl chloride.

Restlessness Acetone; Azinphosmethyl; Camphor; Carbon dioxide; Chlorpyrifos; Dinitro-o-cresol; Malathion; Methyl alcohol; Naled; Nitric oxide; Picric acid; Pyrethrum; Tetraethyl lead; Tetramethyl lead.

Retching Propylene imine.

Retina hemorrhaging Warfarin.

Retrosternal pain Zinc chloride.

Retrosternal soreness Toluene-2,4-diisocyanate.

Retrosternal tightness Thallium.

Rhabdomyolysis (a disease characterized by the destruction of skeletal muscles.) 2,4-D; Pentaborane.

Rickets, suspected of causing Beryllium.

Salivation, excessive Acetonitrile; Azinphos-methyl; Calcium arsenate; Calcium oxide; Carbaryl; Chlorinated camphene; Creosotes; Cumene; Demeton; Dichlorvos; 1,1-Dimethylhydrazine; Endosulfan; EPN; Ethyl ether; Fluorides; Formic acid; Furfuryl alcohol; Iodine; Isopropyl ether; Limonene; Malathion; Mercury; Methyl parathion; Naled; Nickel; Nicotine; Phosdrin; Phosphorus; Phosphorus pentasulfide; Propane; Sodium fluoroacetate; Sodium hydroxide; TEDP; Turpentine.

Schizophrenic-type symptoms Formaldehyde; Methyl parathion.

Scleroderma *also see* **Skin diseases.** Silica; Vanadium pentoxide; Vinyl chloride.

Scleroderma-like skin changes Vinyl chloride.

Scrotal cancer Polycyclic aromatic hydrocarbons.

Seizures *see* **Convulsions.**

Sensation, numbness/tingling/prickling Acrylamide; Carbon dioxide; Chlorpyrifos; 2,4-D; Fluorides; Hydrogen fluoride; Mercury; Methyl alcohol; n-Pentane; Sulfuryl fluoride; Tetraethyl lead; Tetramethyl lead; Trichloroethylene; Toluene; Trifluorobromomethane; Vanadium pentoxide.

Sensation, painful "pins, needles" Arsenic.

Sensation, partial or complete loss of Ethyl acetate; Ethyl bromide; Methyl chloride; Methyl iodide; Methylene chloride; Paraldehyde; Phosphine.

Sensation due to anesthetic effects, loss of Acetaldehyde; Acetone; Benzyl alcohol; Camphor; Chloroform; Cyclohexane; 2,4-D; o-Dichlorobenzene; 1,1-Dichloroethane; Ethanol; Ethyl ether; n-Hexane; Isoamyl alcohol; Isobutyl acetate; Isopropyl ether; Magnesium oxide; Methyl bromide; Methylal; Tin; 1,1,1-Trichloroethane; Trichloroethylene; Vanadium pentoxide; Vinyl tolune.

Sensation of being hot/warm Benzyl chloride; Camphor; Dinitro-o-cresol; Isoamyl acetate.

Sensation of tingling Dichlorodifluoromethane.

Sense of well being Dinitro-o-cresol.

Sensory disturbances/impairments Acetone; Ethanol; Isoamyl alcohol; Tin.

Sensory polyneuropathy n-Hexane.

Sexual disorders Acrylamide; Arsenic; Lead; Manganese; Styrene.

Shaking Methyl iodide.

Shivering Diborane.

Shock Acetic anhydride; Acetone; Arsenic; Bromine; Butylamine; Calcium arsenate; Calcium oxide; Ethyl acetate; Formaldehyde; Formic acid; Iodine; Monomethyl aniline; p-Nitroaniline; Nitrophenols; Oxalic acid; Phenol; Phosphorus; Sodium hydroxide; Stibine; o-Toluidine.

Shock, hemorrhagic Pindone; Warfarin.

Shock-like symptoms Nitrophenols.

Silicosis Silica; Stibine.

Silo-fillers disease Nitrogen dioxide.

Skin, black Acetic acid.

Skin, blood vessel dilation of the Magnesium oxide.

Skin, blue-gray Silver.

Skin, bronze Arsine.

Skin, burning sensation on p-Dichlorobenzene.

Skin, clammy Acetic acid; Acetic anhydride; Camphor; Formic acid; Nitric acid; Phosphoric acid; Sulfur monochloride.

Skin, cold; clammy Calcium oxide; Ethanol; Isoamyl alcohol; Sodium hydroxide.

Skin, cold; painful Ethyl acetate.

Skin, dry; peeling/cracking Benzoyl peroxide; n-Butyl alcohol; sec-Butyl alcohol; Ethyl ether; Isopropyl alcohol; Isopropyl ether; Octane; Petroleum distillates; n-Propyl alcohol.

Skin, flushed Butylamine; Dinitro-o-cresol; Ethylene glycol dinitrate; Pentaborane.

Skin, hemorrhaging beneath the 1,3-Dichloropropene.

Skin, hyperpigmentation with interspersed spots of hypopigmentation on the Arsenic.

Skin, multi-colored p-Dichlorobenzene.

Skin, painful; tender Chlorine.

Skin, pale; clammy Formaldehyde.

Skin, pale; cold Acetone.

Skin, sensitivity to light Creosotes; Hexachloronaphthalene; Pyrethrum.

Skin, slate gray Aniline; p-Nitroaniline; o-Toluidine.

Skin, thickens Arsine; Vinyl chloride.

Skin, yellow stained Dinitro-o-cresol; Dinitrobenzenes; Picric acid.

Skin blisters Acetylene tetrabromide; Carbon dioxide; Carbon disulfide; Chlorine; Cumene; o-Dichlorobenzene; Ethyl benzene; Ethylene dibromide; Methyl bromide; Methyl iodide; beta-Propiolactone; Propylene oxide; Vinyl acetate.

Skin burns Acetaldehyde; Acetic anhydride; Allyl alcohol; Ammonia; Barium; Benzyl chloride; Boron trifluoride; Bromine; Butylamine; Carbon disulfide; Chloroacetaldehyde; Chlorobenzene; Chloromethyl methyl ether; Chromium; Creosotes; Diglycidyl ether; Dimethyl sulfate; Dimethylamine; 1,1-Dimethylhydrazine; Epichlorohydrin; Ethyl benzene; Ethylamine; Ethylene oxide; Ethyleneimine; Formic acid; Hydrazine; Hydrogen chloride; Hydrogen fluoride; Iodine; Isophorone; Isopropylamine; Limonene; Mercury; Methyl hydrazine; Methylamine; Phenol; Phosgene; Phosphoric acid; Phosphorus; Propane; beta-Propiolactone; Propylene imine; Propylene oxide; Selenium; Sodium hydroxide; Sulfur dioxide; Sulfur monochloride; Sulfuric acid; Tetrachloroethylene; Tin; Trichloroethylene; Turpentine; Zinc chloride.

Skin cancer Arsenic; Arsine; Chlorinated diphenyl; Creosotes; Polychlorinated biphenyls; Polycyclic aromatic hydrocarbons.

Skin cancer, suspected of causing Carbon tetrachloride; p-Nitrochlorobenzene.

Skin cells, excessive proliferation of normal Dimethyl acetamide.

Skin cracking Isoamyl alcohol; Isobutyl alcohol; Isopropyl acetate; 1,1,2,2-Tetrachloroethane; 1,1,1-Trichloroethane.

Skin damage/injury Benzene; Boron.

Skin desquamation Acrylonitrile.

Skin discoloration, blotchy p-Dichlorobenzene.

Skin dryness sec-Butyl acetate; n-Pentane; 1,1,2,2-Tetrachloroethane; Toluene; 1,1,1-Trichloroethane.

Skin eruptions Benzyl chloride; Bromine; Picric acid.

Skin erythema Acrylonitrile; Boron; Butylamine.

Skin granulomas Beryllium.

Skin hemorrhaging *also see* **bruising** Creosotes; p-Dichlorobenzene.

Skin hyperpigmentation Calcium arsenate; 2,4-Dichlorophenol.

Skin hypersensitivity *also see* **Chemical sensitivity** Iodine; Methylene bisphenyl isocyanate.

Skin inflammation Chlorine; Chlorobenzene; Cresols; Ethyl benzene; Ethylene dibromide; Propylene imine; 1,1,2,2-Tetrachloroethane.

Skin irritation Acetic anhydride; Acrolein; Acrylamide; Allyl alcohol; Allyl chloride; n-Amyl acetate; Antimony; Arsenic; Barium; Benzoyl peroxide; Benzyl acetate; Benzyl chloride; 1,3-Butadiene; n-Butyl acetate; sec-Butyl acetate; sec-Butyl alcohol; Calcium oxide; Camphor; Carbaryl; Carbon tetrachloride; Chlorinated camphene; Chlorinated diphenyl; Chloroacetaldehyde; alpha-Chloroacetophenone; Chlorobenzene; Chloroform; Chloromethyl methyl ether; Chloropicrin; beta-Chloroprene; Chromium; Creosotes; Cresols; Crotonaldehyde; Cyanides; Cyclohexane; Cyclohexanol; 2,4-D; Demeton; o-Dichlorobenzene; p-Dichlorobenzene; 1,1-Dichloroethane; Dichlorvos; Diethylamine; 2-Diethylaminoethanol; Dimethylamine; Dimethyl acetamide; Dimethylamine; EPN; Ethanol; Ethanolamine; Ethyl acrylate; Ethyl benzene; Ethyl bromide; Ethyl ether; Ethyl formate; Ethylene dichloride; Ethylene glycol dinitrate; Ferbam; Glycidol; Hexachloroethane; Hydrogen cyanide; Isobutyl acetate; Isobutyl alcohol; Isopropyl acetate; Isopropyl alcohol; Isopropyl ether; Ketene; Linalyl alcohol; Lindane; Limonene; Malathion; Maleic anhydride; Mercury; Mesityl oxide; Methyl n-amyl ketone; Methyl acrylate; Methyl bromide; Methyl iodide; Methylal; Methylamine; Methylene chloride; Morpholine; Naled; Naphtha; Nitric acid; Nitromethane; Oxalic acid;

Pentaborane; n-Pentane; Phenyl ether; Phenyl ether-biphenyl mixture; Phenyl glycidyl ether; Phosdrin; Phosphoric acid; Polychlorinated biphenyls; beta-Propiolactone; n-Propyl acetate; Propylene dichloride; Propylene imine; Propylene oxide; Pyridine; Quinone; Silver; Sodium hydroxide; Sulfur dioxide; TEDP; Tin; Toluene; Tributyl phosphate; 1,1,1-Trichloroethane; 1,2,3-Trichloropropane; Triethylamine; Trimellitic anhydride; Turpentine; Vinyl toluene; Zinc chloride.

Skin irritation with deep pain Epichlorohydrin.

Skin itching Acrylonitrile; Ethyl acrylate; Methyl bromide; Nitrophenols.

Skin lesions Arsenic; Beryllium; Boron; sec-Butyl acetate; tert-Butyl acetate; Carbon monoxide; Creosotes; o-Dichlorobenzene; Formaldehyde; Isobutyl acetate; Methyl bromide; Polycyclic aromatic hydrocarbons; Sulfur dioxide; Tellurium; Thiram; o-Toluidine; Warfarin.

Skin overgrowths Arsenic.

Skin pain Hydrogen sulfide.

Skin rash, petechial Pindone; Warfarin.

Skin rashes Cyanides; Decaborane; Diborane; Hydrogen cyanide; Iodine; Pentaborane; Picric acid; Trichloroethylene.

Skin redness o-Chlorobenzylidene malononitrile; Creosotes; Cumene; 1,3-Dichloropropene; Diethylamine; Ethylene dibromide; Hydrogen peroxide; Hydrogen sulfide; Methyl bromide; Methyl methacrylate; Nitrophenols; Pyrethrum; Quinone; Tetrachloroethylene; 1,1,1-Trichloroethane.

Skin redness; pain on contact Phosphorus pentasulfide.

Skin scaling 1,1,2,2-Tetrachloroethane; 1,1,1-Trichloroethane.

Skin sensitivity/hypersensitivity, delayed Beryllium.

Skin sensitization/sensitivity Aluminum; Ethyleneimine; Limonene; Toluene-2,4-diisocyanate.

Skin swelling Benzene; 1,3-Dichloropropene; 1,1,1-Trichloroethane.

Skin tissue death Acrolein; Chromium; Dimethyl sulfate; Dinitro-o-cresol; Propylene imine; Propylene oxide; Quinone; Warfarin.

Skin tissue death, suspected of causing Ethylene oxide.

Skin ulcers Chromic acid; Chromium; Quinone; Silver.

Skin vesiculations Acetic anhydride; Acrylonitrile; Ammonia; o-Chlorobenzylidene malononitrile; Diethylamine; Hydrogen peroxide; Methyl bromide.

Sleep, inability to (insomnia) Acrylamide; Antimony; Arsenic; Azinphosmethyl; Benzyl chloride; beta-Chloroprene; Chlorpyrifos; Ethylene dichloride; Formaldehyde; Hexone; Hydrogen sulfide; Lead; Manganese; Mercury; Methyl alcohol; Naled; Naphtha; Phosphorus pentasulfide; Pyridine; Styrene; 1,1,2,2-Tetrachloroethane; Tetraethyl lead; Tetramethyl lead; Toluene; Trichloroethylene.

Sleep, poor Carbon disulfide.

Sleep, temporary cessation of breathing during Carbaryl; Cyanides; Hydrogen cyanide; Hydrogen sulfide; Methyl alcohol; Phosphorus pentasulfide.

Sleepiness (somnolence) Chlorobenzene; Demeton; Diacetone alcohol; Dimethyl acetamide; Ethyl benzene; Ethyl ether; Hexone; Hydrazine; Isopropyl ether; Limonene; Methyl cellosolve; Methylene chloride; p-Nitroaniline; Pyridine; Tellurium; Tetrachloroethylene; 1,1,1-Trichloroethane; Trichloroethylene; Turpentine; Vanadium pentoxide.

Sleeping difficulty/disturbances Dimethylformamide; Vanadium pentoxide.

Smell, acute sense of Formaldehyde.

Smell, altered sense of Cyanides; Hydrogen cyanide; Sulfur dioxide.

Smell, decreased sense of 2,4-D; Ethanol; Isoamyl alcohol.

Smell, loss of Cadmium; Formaldehyde; Phosphorus pentasulfide; Selenium; Sulfur dioxide.

Smell properly, inability to Antimony.

Sneezing Acrylonitrile; Chlorine; Dimethylamine; Formaldehyde; Iodine; Pentachlorophenol; Pyrethrum; Selenium; Sulfur dioxide; Trimellitic anhydride; 2,4,6-Trinitrotoluene.

Speech, loss of Dimethyl sulfate; Ethanol; Isoamyl alcohol; Sodium fluoroacetate.

Speech, monotone Demeton.

Speech, recrudescent stuttering 2-Ethoxyethyl acetate.

Speech, slurred Acetone; Azinphos-methyl; 2-Butoxyethanol; Carbaryl; Chlorpyrifos; EPN; 2-Ethoxyethyl acetate; Ethyl acetate; Malathion; Methyl chloride; Methyl iodide; Methyl parathion; Naled; Pyridine; TEDP.

Speech changes Dichlorodifluoromethane.

Speech difficulties p-Dichlorobenzene; Dimethyl sulfate; Formaldehyde; Manganese.

Speech impairment, spastic Hydrogen cyanide.

Speech impairments Cyanides; n-Hexane; Isopropyl alcohol; Mercury; Paraldehyde.

Speech impairments, suspected of causing Benzyl acetate; Benzyl alcohol; Benzyl chloride.

Speech pattern, retarded Formaldehyde.

Sperm abnormalities Carbon disulfide.

Sperm abnormalities, suspected of causing Acetone; Chloroform; Copper; Ethanol; Ethylene dibromide; Nickel; Vinyl acetate.

Sperm count, low Dibutylphthalate; Ethylene oxide.

Sperm count, suspected of causing low Dinitrotoluenes; Ethylene dibromide; Manganese; Methylene chloride; Nitrobenzene.

Sperm damage Lead.

Sperm death, suspected of causing 2,4,6-Trichlorophenol.

Sperm heads, suspected of causing abnormal p-Dichlorobenzene.

Sperm production, suspected of causing altered Mercury.

Spermatogenous disturbances beta-Chloroprene.

Spinal cord *see* **headings under Meninges.**

Spinal cord *see* **headings under Nervous system, central.**

Spine stiffness Fluorides.

Spleen, enlarged Vanadium pentoxide.

Spleen, excessive proliferation of normal cells in the Stibine.

Spleen damage Aniline.

Spleen damage, suspected of causing 2,4-Dichlorophenol; 2,4,6-Trichlorophenol.

Spleen infarction Benzene.

Sputum, bloody Chloromethyl methyl ether; Phosgene; Phthalic anhydride.

Sputum, copious amounts of Zinc chloride.

Sputum, fluorescent green Phosphine.

Sputum, foamy Acetonitrile; Phosgene.

Sputum, mucoid frothy Nitrogen dioxide.

Sputum, pink frothy Ammonia.

Stannosis (a benign form of pneumoconiosis.) Tin.

Sterility Formaldehyde.

Sterility, female Lead.

Sterility, suspected of causing Cadmium; Epichlorohydrin; Pentaborane; Polycyclic aromatic hydrocarbons.

Stillbirths Warfarin.

Stomach burns 2,4-D.

Stomach cramps Antimony; Copper.

Stomach cysts, suspected of causing Chlorinated diphenyl; Polychlorinated biphenyls.

Stomach discomfort/distress/disturbances Acetonitrile; Camphor; Chloroform; Fluorides; Hydrogen fluoride; Methyl alcohol; Xylenes.

Stomach distention, suspected of causing Creosotes.

Stomach hemorrhaging Acetic acid; Acetic anhydride; Dimethylphthalate; Fluorides; Nitric acid; Phosphoric acid; Sulfur monochloride.

Stomach hemorrhaging, suspected of causing Chlorinated diphenyl; Polychlorinated biphenyls.

Stomach inflammation Acetone; Benzene; 2,3-Benzofuran; Calcium arsenate; Carbon disulfide; Chlorinated diphenyl; Chromium; Ethyl acetate; Formaldehyde; Hydrogen peroxide; Iodine; Mercury; p-Phenylene diamine; Polychlorinated biphenyls; Sulfuric acid; Triorthocresyl phosphate.

Stomach inflammation, congestive Benzene.

Stomach inflammation; hemorrhaging Paraldehyde.

Stomach inflammation, ulcerative Formic acid.

Stomach irritation Calcium oxide; Dibutylphthalate; Limonene; Tin; Turpentine.

Stomach mucosa congestion Chromium.

Stomach necrotic lesions Nitrophenols.

Stomach pain Chloroform; Chromium; o-Dichlorobenzene; Dimethylformamide; Dimethylphthalate; Hexone; Oxalic acid.

Stomach perforation Calcium oxide.

Stomach perforation, delayed Diethylamine.

Stomach strictures Acetic acid; Acetic anhydride; Formic acid; Nitric acid; Phosphoric acid; Sulfur monochloride.

Stomach tissue death Cyanides; Hydrogen cyanide; Phosphoric acid.

Stomach ulcers Chromium.

Stomach ulcers, suspected of causing Chlorinated diphenyl; Polychlorinated biphenyls.

Stomach upsets Dinitro-o-cresol.

Strokes Nickel carbonyl.

Stupor Acetone; Acetonitrile; 2-Aminopyridine; Bromine; Calcium arsenate; Cumene; Cyanides; 2,4-D; Ethanol; Ethyl acetate; Ethyl chloride; Ethylene dichloride; n-Heptane; Hydrogen cyanide; Iodine; Isoamyl alcohol; Isopropyl alcohol; Limonene; Octane; Oxalic acid; Phosphine; Picric acid; Propane; n-Propyl alcohol; Pyrethrum; Pyridine; 1,1,2-Trichloroethane; Turpentine.

Substernal burning Beryllium; Phosphine.

Substernal pain Cadmium; Calcium oxide; Chlorine; Cumene; Nickel; Phosphine.

Sudden infant death syndrome, suspected of causing Lead.

Suffocation, feeling of Acetic acid; Acetic anhydride; Bromine; Calcium oxide; Dimethyl sulfate; Ethyl methacrylate; Formic acid; Hydroquinone; Iodine; Isophorone; Limonene; Nitric acid; Phosphorus; Sodium hydroxide; Sulfur monochloride; Turpentine.

Swallowing, inability/difficulty Acetic acid; Acetic anhydride; Calcium arsenate; Dimethyl sulfate; Formaldehyde; Formic acid; Nitric acid; Phenol; Phosphoric acid; Sulfur dioxide; Sulfur monochloride.

Sweat, inability to Tellurium.

Sweating, localized Acrylamide; Demeton; TEDP; TEPP.

Sweating, profuse/intense Acetone; Acetonitrile; 2-Aminopyridine; Antimony; Azinphos-methyl; Calcium arsenate; Carbaryl; Carbon dioxide; Carbon monoxide; Chlorpyrifos; 2,4-D; Dichlorvos; Dinitro-o-cresol; Ethyl acetate; Ethyl ether; Fluorides; Isopropyl ether; Malathion; Methyl parathion; Naled; Naphthalene; Nickel carbonyl; Nicotine; Nitrophenols; Pentaborane; Pentachlorophenol; Phenol; Phosphorus pentasulfide; Picric acid; Pyrethrum; Tellurium; 1,1,2,2-Tetrachloroethane.

Sweats, cold Nicotine; Phenol.

Sweats, night Formaldehyde; Propylene dichloride.

Sympathoadrenal discharge Carbaryl.

Talkativeness Acetone; Ethyl acetate.

Taste, altered sense of Sulfur dioxide.

Taste, decreased sense of 2,4-D; Ethanol; Isoamyl alcohol.

Taste, loss of sense of Formaldehyde.

Tearing Acetaldehyde; Acetic acid; Acetic anhydride; Acrolein; Allyl alcohol; Azinphos-methyl; Bromine; n-Butyl alcohol; Calcium arsenate; Carbaryl; Chlorine; o-Chlorobenzylidene malononitrile; Chloropicrin; 2,4-D; Demeton; Dichloroethyl ether; Diisobutyl ketone; Dimethyl sulfate; Epichlorohydrin; EPN; Ethyl acrylate; Ethyl methacrylate; Ethyl silicate; Formaldehyde; Formic acid; Hexachloroethane; Hydrogen sulfide; Hydroquinone; Iodine; Malathion; Mercury; Methyl acetate; Methyl formate; Methyl parathion; Naled; Phosgene; Phosphoric acid; Phosphorus; Phosphorus pentasulfide; Phthalic anhydride; Sulfur dioxide; Sulfur monochloride; TEDP; TEPP; Toluene; Toluene-2,4-diisocyanate.

Tearing, suspected of causing Cyclohexanone; Nitroethane.

Teeth, decay of (dental caries) Sulfur dioxide.

Teeth, disease around (periodontum) beta-Chloroprene.

Teeth, disorders of the tissue (periodontal) surrounding the Sulfur dioxide.

Teeth, inflammation of the tissue (periodontal) surrounding the beta-Chloroprene.

Teeth, painful (dental) Phosphorus.

Teeth, sensitivity to temperature changes in Sulfur dioxide.

Teeth erosion/corrosion (dental) Acetic acid; Chlorine; beta-Chloroprene; Nitric acid; Nitric oxide; Sulfuric acid.

Temple pain *also see* **Headaches.** Propylene imine.

Tendon reflex, absent/decreased deep Acrylamide; Ammonia; Barium; Triphenyl phosphate.

Tendon reflex suppression Ferbam; Thiram.

Tendon reflexes, absent/impaired Acetone; Ethyl acetate; Isopropyl alcohol.

Testicular atrophy Chloroform.

Testicular atrophy, suspected of causing Cobalt; Dinitrotoluenes; Methyl bromide; Methyl cellosolve.

Testicular cancer, suspected of causing Dimethylformamide.

Testicular damage Lead.

Testicular damage, suspected of causing Boron; Cadmium; Di-sec octyl phthalate; Manganese; Vinyl chloride.

Testicular degeneration, suspected of causing Cobalt; Dibutylphthalate; Dinitrotoluenes; Ethylene oxide; Methyl bromide; Nickel; Nitrobenzene.

Testicular lesions, suspected of causing Methyl chloride.

Testicular pain Formaldehyde.

Testicular tissue death; suspected of causing Diglycidyl ether.

Testosterone, suspected of causing decreased levels of n-Butyl alcohol.

Thirst Acetic acid; Acetic anhydride; 2-Aminopyridine; Calcium arsenate; Dinitro-o-cresol; Dinitrobenzenes; Fluorides; Formaldehyde; Formic acid; Lead; Nitric acid; Phosphine; Phosphoric acid; Picric acid; Sulfur monochloride; Tetramethyl lead.

Throat, blue-gray Silver.

Throat, burning pain in Limonene; Nitrophenols; Turpentine.

Throat, burning sensation in Acetic anhydride; 2-Aminopyridine; Nicotine.

Throat, dry Aniline; Dinitrobenzenes; Isoamyl acetate; Manganese; Monomethyl aniline; p-Nitroaniline; Tetramethyl lead; o-Toluidine; Trichloroethylene; Zinc oxide.

Throat, dry burning Phosgene.

Throat, sore Calcium arsenate; Chloromethyl methyl ether; Formaldehyde; Hexone; 2,4,6-Trinitrotoluene.

Throat burns Formaldehyde; Hydrogen chloride.

Throat constriction Acetonitrile; Calcium arsenate.

Throat corrosion Nitric acid.

Throat inflammation Hydrogen chloride.

Throat irritation Acetaldehyde; Acetic acid; Acetone; Acrolein; Ammonia; Ammonium sulfamate; n-Amyl acetate; Antimony; Arsenic; Boron; 1,3-Butadiene; 2-Butanone; 2-Butoxyethanol; n-Butyl acetate; sec-Butyl acetate; tert-Butyl acetate; n-Butyl alcohol; sec-Butyl alcohol; Butylamine; Carbon tetrachloride; Chlorine dioxide; Chloroacetaldehyde; o-Chlorobenzylidene malononitrile; Copper; Cresols; Cyclohexanol; 2,4-D; Diacetone alcohol; Dibutylphthalate; Dichloroethyl ether; Diisobutyl ketone; Dimethylamine; Ethyl acetate; Ethyl benzene; Ethylene glycol; Ethylene oxide; Ethyleneimine; N-Ethylmorpholine; Ferbam; Formaldehyde; Formic acid; Glycidol; n-Hexane; Hexone; Hydrazine; Hydrogen fluoride; Hydrogen peroxide; Isoamyl acetate; Isoamyl alcohol; Isobutyl acetate; Isobutyl alcohol; Isophorone; Isopropyl alcohol; Isopropylamine; Ketene; Lindane; Maleic anhydride; Methyl acetate; Methyl cellosolve; Methyl methacrylate; alpha-Methyl styrene; Methylamine; Methylene bisphenyl isocyanate; Methylene chloride; Naphtha; Nitric oxide; Nitroethane; Pentachlorophenol; Petroleum distillates; Phenol; Phosgene; Phosphoric acid; n-Propyl acetate; n-Propyl alcohol; Selenium; Stoddard solvent; Styrene; Sulfur dioxide; Sulfur monochloride; Sulfuric acid; Tetrachloroethylene; Tetramethyl succinonitrile; Toluene-2, 4-diisocyanate; Tributyl phosphate; Trichloroethylene; 1,2,3-Trichloropropane; Triethylamine; Trimellitic anhydride; Turpentine; Vanadium pentoxide; Vinyl acetate; Xylenes; Zinc chloride.

Throat irritation, suspected of causing Molybdenum.

Throat malaise Formic acid.

Throat numbness Acetonitrile.

Throat pain Nitric acid; Oxalic acid.

Thyroid, decreased iodine uptake by the Cobalt.

Thyroid, enlarged Cyanides; Hydrogen cyanide; Thiram.

Thyroid, excessive proliferation of normal cells in the Bromine; Cobalt.

Thyroid damage/injury, suspected of causing 2,3-Benzofuran; Chlorinated camphene; Di-sec octyl phthalate.

Thyroid disease, autoimmune Polychlorinated biphenyls.

Thyroid disorders/dysfunction/ effects Bromine; Cyanides; Hydrogen cyanide; Iodine; Sodium fluoroacetate.

Thyroid function, inhibits Sulfur dioxide.

Thyroid function, suspected of causing inhibited Lead.

Thyroid lesions, suspected of causing 2,3-Benzofuran.

Tissue, dark pigmentation of fibrous Phenol.

Tissue/Bone death Allyl alcohol; Benzyl alcohol; Carbon disulfide; Chlorine; Chloromethyl methyl ether; Chloropicrin; beta-Chloroprene; Creosotes; 1,3-Dichloro-5,5-dimethylhydantoin; Ethylene dibromide; Hydrazine.

Tissue corrosion Sodium hydroxide.

Tissue damage Acrolein; Allyl alcohol; Arsenic; Benzyl acetate.

Tissue proteins, altered Formaldehyde.

Tissues, insufficient oxygen supply to Iodine.

Toes, numbness of Pyrethrum; Thallium.

Tongue, coated Selenium.

Tongue, green Vanadium pentoxide.

Tongue, navy blue to black Aniline; p-Nitroaniline; o-Toluidine.

Tongue, swollen Dimethyl sulfate; Limonene; Turpentine.

Touch, dulled sensitivity to 2,4-D.

Trachea, diphtheria-like mutations of the Propylene imine.

Trachea degeneration Phosgene.

Trachea inflammation (tracheitis) Formaldehyde; Hydrazine; Sulfur dioxide.

Trachea inflammation, granular Benzene.

Tracheobronchial inflammation Cadmium; Formaldehyde; Phosphorus pentasulfide; Sulfuric acid.

Tracheobronchial inflammation, hemorrhagic Isopropyl alcohol.

Tremors Acrylamide; 2-Aminopyridine; Benzene; 2-Butoxyethanol; Camphor; Carbaryl; Carbon disulfide; Carbon dioxide; Chlorinated camphene; Chlorpyrifos; Copper; Cumene; Cyanides; Cyclohexanol; Decaborane; Diborane; Dichlorodifluoromethane; Dichloromonofluoromethane; Dichlorotetrafluoroethane; Dinitrobenzenes; Endosulfan; 2-Ethoxyethyl acetate; Ethyl silicate; Ethylene dichloride; Ethylene glycol; Fluorotrichloromethane; Hydrazine; Hydrogen cyanide; Lead; Malathion; Manganese; Mercury; Methyl cellosolve; Methyl chloride; Methyl hydrazine; Methyl parathion; Nickel carbonyl; Nicotine; Nitrobenzene; Paraldehyde; Pentaborane; Phenol; p-Phenylene diamine; Phosphine; Sulfur dioxide; 1,1,2,2-Tetrachloroethane; Tetrachloroethylene; Tetraethyl lead; Thallium; Thiram; Tin; Toluene-2, 4-diisocyanate; Trichloroethylene; Trifluorobromomethane; Xylenes.

Tremors, suspected of causing Benzyl acetate; Benzyl alcohol; Cresols; Cyclohexanone; 2,4-Dichlorophenol; 2-Diethylaminoethanol; Dinitro-o-cresol; Dinitrotoluenes; Sulfuryl fluoride; Toluene; o-Toluidine; 2,4,6-Trinitrotoluene; Vinyl toluene.

Tuberculosis, predisposition to Chlorine.

Unconsciousness Acetonitrile; Allyl chloride; Ammonia; Benzene; 2-Butanone; n-Butyl acetate; sec-Butyl acetate; Carbon dioxide; Carbon tetrachloride; Chlorinated camphene; Chlorobenzene; Chloromethyl methyl ether; Chromium; 2,4-D; Dichlorodifluoromethane; Dimethylaniline; Dimethylphthalate; Dinitrotoluenes; Ethylene glycol; n-Heptane; Hydrazine; Hydrogen sulfide; Isobutyl acetate; Methyl acetate; Methyl parathion; Methylene chloride; Nitric oxide; Nitric oxide; Nitrophenols; n-Pentane; Phenol; Phosphorus pentasulfide; Picric acid; Propane; 1,1,2,2-Tetrachloroethane; Tetrachloroethylene; 1,1,1-Trichloroethane; Trichloroethylene; Vinyl chloride; Xylenes.

Unconsciousness due to inadequate blood flow to the brain Calcium arsenate; Carbon monoxide; Chlorine; Cyanides; Hydrogen cyanide; Phosphine; Tin.

Unconsciousness due to narcotic effects n-Amyl acetate; 1,3-Butadiene; tert-Butyl acetate; sec-Butyl alcohol; Butylamine; Chloroacetaldehyde; Chloroform; Cumene; Cyclohexane; Cyclohexanol; Cyclohexanone; Diacetone alcohol; Ethyl acetate; Ethyl benzene; Ethyl butyl ketone; Ethyl chloride; Ethyl ether; Ethyl formate; Ethyl silicate; Glycidol; Hexone; Isoamyl acetate; Isoamyl alcohol; Isophorone; Isopropyl acetate; Isopropyl ether; Mesityl oxide; Methyl n-amyl ketone; 5-Methyl-3-heptanone; Methyl mercaptan; 2-Pentanone; Phenyl glycidyl ether; n-Propyl acetate; Styrene; Vanadium pentoxide; Xylenes.

Unconsciousness due to narcotic effects, suspected of causing sec-Hexyl acetate; Linalyl alcohol; Methyl acetate; Nitroethane; Sulfuryl fluoride.

Uneasiness Nitric oxide.

Uremia (a toxic condition associated with renal insufficiency.) Ethylene glycol.

Urinary tract effects, suspected of causing 1,3-Dichloropropene.

Urinate, inability to Arsine.

Urination, difficulty in Dimethyl sulfate; Ethyl ether; Isopropyl ether; beta-Propiolactone.

Urination, frequent Methyl cellosolve acetate; Picric acid; beta-Propiolactone; Pyridine.

Urination, irregular Benzidine.

Urination, painful Aniline; Benzidine; Dimethyl sulfate; Ethyl ether; Isopropyl ether; Limonene; Monomethyl aniline; p-Nitroaniline; beta-Propiolactone; o-Toluidine; Turpentine.

Urination with pain, frequent Formaldehyde.

Urine, albumin in Acetaldehyde; Acetonitrile; 2-Butoxyethanol; Calcium arsenate; Camphor; Carbon monoxide; Chloroform; 2,4-D; Dimethyl sulfate; Dinitro-o-cresol; 2-Ethoxyethyl acetate; Ethyl ether; Ethylene glycol; Ethyleneimine; Formic acid; Hydrogen sulfide; Isopropyl ether; Limonene; Methyl chloride; Oxalic acid; Paraldehyde; Phosphorus; Phosphorus pentasulfide; Picric acid; Stibine; Tetraethyl lead; Tetramethyl lead; Turpentine.

Urine, bilirubin in Acetylene tetrabromide.

Urine, blood in Allyl alcohol; Aniline; Arsine; Benzidine; 2-Butoxyethanol; Calcium arsenate; Dimethyl sulfate; Dinitro-o-cresol; 2-Ethoxyethyl acetate; Ethylene glycol; Ethyleneimine; Formaldehyde; Formic acid; Limonene; Methyl hydrazine; Monomethyl aniline; Naphthalene; p-Nitroaniline; Oxalic acid; Pentachlorophenol; Phosphorus; Picric acid; Pindone; beta-Propiolactone; Propylene dichloride; Stibine; o-Toluidine; Turpentine; Warfarin.

Urine, cylindroids in Tetraethyl lead; Tetramethyl lead.

Urine, dark Dimethyl sulfate; Phenol; Nitrophenols; Phenylhydrazine; Picric acid.

Urine, decrease in phosphorus in the Lead.

Urine, diminished/reduced amount of Aniline; Bromine; Carbon monoxide; 2,4-D; 2-Ethoxyethyl acetate; Ethylene dichloride; Iodine; Isopropyl alcohol; Methyl cellosolve acetate; Monomethyl aniline; Oxalic acid; Paraldehyde; Phosphorus; Picric acid; n-Propyl alcohol; Propylene dichloride; Tetraethyl lead; Tetramethyl lead.

Urine, excessive phosphorus in the Lead.

Urine, excessive urobilin in Acetylene tetrabromide; Isoamyl acetate; Phenylhydrazine.

Urine, glucose in n-Amyl acetate; n-Butyl acetate; n-Butyl alcohol; sec-Butyl alcohol; Calcium arsenate; Isobutyl alcohol.

Urine, green or green-brown Hydroquinone.

Urine, hemoglobin in Acetic acid; Aniline; 2-Butoxyethanol; Monomethyl aniline; Naphthalene; p-Nitroaniline; Stibine; Tetraethyl lead; Tetramethyl lead; o-Toluidine.

Urine, methemoglobin in p-Dichlorobenzene; Methyl hydrazine; Nitrobenzene; Nitrogen dioxide.

Urine, myoglobin in 2,4-D; Isopropyl alcohol.

Urine, protein in Cadmium; Calcium arsenate; 2,4-D; Lead; Malathion; Mercury; Methyl bromide; Methyl chloride; Naphthalene.

Urine, pus in Dinitro-o-cresol.

Urine, smokey Pindone.

Urine, suspected of causing blood in p-Nitrochlorobenzene.

Urine, suspected of causing hemoglobin in p-Nitrochlorobenzene.

Urine, suspected of causing protein in Nitrophenols.

Urine, transient excessive discharge of 2-Ethoxyethyl acetate.

Urine formation, absence of Acetic acid; Bromine; 2-Butoxyethanol; Calcium arsenate; Camphor; Cresols; 2-Ethoxyethyl acetate; Ethylene glycol; Iodine; Methyl bromide; Methyl cellosolve acetate; Methyl chloride; Phosphorus; Picric acid; Stibine.

Urine formation, excessive Furfuryl alcohol; Isopropyl alcohol; Methyl cellosolve acetate; Picric acid; n-Propyl alcohol.

Urine retention Acetonitrile; Camphor; Tin.

Uterine growths, benign Vinyl chloride.

Vaginal inflammation, chronic Formaldehyde.

Vascular *see* **Blood vessel.**

Vegetative disorders Bromine.

Vein inflammation in conjunction with the formation of a blood clot Paraldehyde.

Vertigo Acetone; Acetonitrile; Aniline; Azinphos-methyl; Benzene; sec-Butyl acetate; tert-Butyl acetate; n-Butyl alcohol; Calcium arsenate; Camphor; Chloropicrin; Chlorpyrifos; Creosotes; Cumene; 2,4-D; Diborane; 1,2-Dichloroethylene; Dimethylaniline; Dinitrotoluenes; EPN; Ethyl acetate; Ethyl benzene; Ethylene dichloride; Fluorides; Formaldehyde; Formic acid; n-Hexane; Hydrogen fluoride; Isobutyl acetate; Isobutyl alcohol; Methyl acetate; Methyl alcohol; Methyl bromide; Methyl chloride; Methyl iodide; Monomethyl aniline; Naled; Naphthalene; Nickel; Nickel carbonyl; p-Nitroaniline; Nitrobenzene; p-Nitrochlorobenzene; Octane; Pentachloronaphthalene; p-Phenylene diamine; Phosphine; Phosphorus pentasulfide; Picric acid; Propylene dichloride; Sulfur dioxide; TEDP; 1,1,2,2-Tetrachloroethane; Tetrachloroethylene; Tetrachloronaphthalene; Tin; Toluene; o-Toluidine; Trichloroethylene; Triorthocresyl phosphate; Turpentine.

Violent behavior, sporadic Hydrazine.

Vision, blurred Allyl alcohol; Ammonia; Azinphos-methyl; Benzene; Benzyl acetate; Benzyl alcohol; Benzyl chloride; 2-Butoxyethanol; n-Butyl alcohol; Carbaryl; Diethylamine; Dimethylamine; 2-EPN; Ethoxyethyl acetate; Formaldehyde; n-Hexane; Malathion; Methyl alcohol; Methyl bromide; Methyl parathion; Naled; Sodium fluoroacetate; TEDP; TEPP; Triethylamine; Zinc oxide.

Vision, central blind spots in Dinitrobenzenes; Methyl alcohol.

Vision, changes in Carbon disulfide.

Vision, constricted or narrowed field of Dinitrobenzenes; alpha-Methyl styrene.

Vision, dimness of Azinphos-methyl; Carbaryl; Carbon dioxide; Carbon monoxide; Chlorpyrifos; Cyanides; EPN; Methyl alcohol; Naled.

Vision, double Acetone; Diborane; Ethanol; Ethyl acetate; Isoamyl alcohol; Maleic anhydride; Methyl bromide; Methyl iodide; Phosphine.

Vision, foggy Morpholine.

Vision, hazy blue Ethylamine.

Vision, loss of (blindness) Butylamine; Cresols; Ethyl acrylate; Ethyl bromide; Formaldehyde; Lead; Methyl acetate; Methyl alcohol; Nickel; Sulfur dioxide; Trichloroethylene.

Vision, impaired field of Mercury.

Vision, misty; halos Dimethylamine.

Vision, suspected of causing blurred Cresols; Dinitro-o-cresol; Dinitrotoluenes; Toluene; Toluene-2, 4-diisocyanate; o-Toluidine; 2,4,6-Trinitrotoluene; Vinyl toluene; Xylenes.

Vision, temporary loss of Allyl alcohol; 2-Butanone; Carbon dioxide; Hydrazine; Methyl formate.

Vision disorders/impairment Demeton; Tin.

Vision disturbances n-Amyl acetate; Benzyl alcohol; Camphor; Carbon disulfide; Carbon monoxide; Cobalt; Cyanides; Diethylamine; Diisopropylamine; Dimethylamine; Dimethylaniline; Dinitrobenzenes; N-Ethylmorpholine; Formic acid; Hydrogen cyanide; Isopropylamine; Mercury; Methyl acetate; Methyl alcohol; Methyl bromide; Methyl chloride; Methyl formate; Methyl iodide; Morpholine; Nicotine; Pentaborane; Quinone; Selenium; Tetraethyl lead; Tetramethyl lead; Toluene; Trichloroethylene; Triethylamine; Turpentine; Vanadium pentoxide.

Vision loss in half the field involving one or both eyes Cyanides; Hydrogen cyanide.

Vision weakness Aniline.

Visual acuity, reduced Ethanol; Isoamyl alcohol; Methyl alcohol.

Vocal cord ulceration Propylene imine.

Voice, hoarseness of Arsenic; Cumene; Dimethyl sulfate; Formaldehyde.

Voice, huskiness of Chlorine.

Voice, loss of Acetic acid; Acetic anhydride; Bromine; Calcium oxide; Chlorine; Dimethyl sulfate; Formic acid; Iodine; Nitric acid; Phosphorus; Sodium hydroxide; Sulfur monochloride.

Vomiting Acetaldehyde; Acetic acid; Acetic anhydride; Acetone; Acetonitrile; Acetylene tetrabromide; Acrylonitrile; n-Amyl acetate; Aniline; Antimony; Arsenic; Arsine; Azinphos-methyl; Barium; Benzene; Benzyl acetate; Benzyl alcohol; Benzyl chloride; Boron; Bromine; 2-Butanone; 2-Butoxyethanol; n-Butyl acetate; n-Butyl alcohol; sec-Butyl alcohol; Butylamine; Cadmium; Calcium arsenate; Calcium oxide; Camphor; Carbaryl; Carbon dioxide; Carbon monoxide; Carbon tetrachloride; Chlorinated camphene; Chlorine; Chlorobenzene; Chloroform; Chloropicrin; Chlorpyrifos; Chromium; Cobalt; Copper; Creosotes; Cresols; Cumene; Cyanides; 2,4-D; Decaborane; Demeton; Diborane; o-Dichlorobenzene; p-Dichlorobenzene; Dichloroethyl ether; 1,3-Dichloropropene; Dichlorvos; Diethylamine; 2-Diethylaminoethanol; Diisopropylamine; Dimethyl sulfate; Dimethylformamide; 1,1-Dimethylhydrazine; Dinitro-o-cresol; Dinitrotoluenes; Epichlorohydrin; EPN; Ethanol; 2-Ethoxyethyl acetate; Ethyl acetate; Ethyl benzene; Ethyl chloride; Ethyl ether; Ethyl methacrylate; Ethylene dibromide; Ethylene dichloride; Ethylene glycol; Ethylene glycol dinitrate; Ethyleneoxide; Ethyleneimine; Ferbam; Fluorides; Formaldehyde; Formic acid; Furfuryl alcohol; Hexone; Hydrazine; Hydrogen cyanide; Hydrogen fluoride; Hydrogen peroxide; Hydroquinone; Iodine; Isoamyl alcohol; Isobutyl acetate; Isobutyl alcohol; Isopropyl alcohol; Isopropyl ether; Lead; Lindane; Limonene; Malathion; Manganese; Mercury; Methyl alcohol; Methyl bromide; Methyl cellosolve acetate; Methyl chloride; Methyl formate; Methyl hydrazine; Methyl iodide; Methyl parathion; Naled; Naphthalene; Nickel; Nickel carbonyl; Nicotine; Nitric acid; p-Nitroaniline; Nitrobenzene; Nitroethane; Nitrophenols; 1-Nitropropane; 2-Nitropropane; N-Nitrosodimethylamine; Oxalic acid; Pentaborane; Pentachlorophenol; Phenol; Phosdrin; Phosgene; Phosphine; Phosphoric acid; Phosphorus; Phosphorus pentasulfide; Picric acid; Pindone; Propane; n-Propyl acetate; n-Propyl alcohol; Propylene dichloride; Propylene imine; Propylene oxide; Pyrethrum; Selenium; Sodium fluoroacetate; Sodium hydroxide; Stibine; Styrene; Sulfur dioxide; Sulfur monochloride; TEDP; TEPP; 1,1,2,2-Tetrachloroethane; Tetraethyl lead; Tetramethyl lead; Thallium; Thiram; Tin; Toluene; Toluene-2,4-diisocyanate; o-Toluidine; 1,1,1-Trichloroethane; Trichloroethylene; Turpentine; Warfarin; Xylenes; Zinc chloride; Zinc oxide.

Vomiting blood Acetic acid; Acetone; Acetonitrile; Cumene; Formaldehyde; Isopropyl alcohol; Phosphorus; n-Propyl alcohol.

Weakness Acetone; Acetonitrile; Acrylonitrile; 2-Aminopyridine; Aniline; Arsenic; Arsine; Azinphos-methyl; Benzene; Benzyl chloride; Beryllium; 2-Butanone; 2-Butoxyethanol; n-Butyl acetate; sec-Butyl acetate; tert-Butyl acetate; Calcium arsenate; Camphor; Carbaryl; Carbon monoxide; Chloropicrin; Chlorpyrifos; Chromium; Cyanides; 2,4-D; Demeton; Diborane; p-Dichlorobenzene; Dimethyl acetamide; Dimethylaniline; Dimethylformamide; Dinitrotoluenes; EPN; 2-Ethoxyethyl acetate; Ethyl acetate; Ethylene dichloride; Hexachloronaphthalene; Hexone; Hydrogen cyanide; Isoamyl acetate; Isobutyl acetate; Isopropyl acetate; Lead; Malathion; Manganese; Manganese; Mercury; Methyl alcohol; Methyl bromide; Methyl cellosolve; Methyl iodide; Methyl methacrylate; Methyl parathion; Methylene chloride; Mica; Monomethyl aniline; Naled; Nickel; Nickel carbonyl; Nicotine; Nitric oxide; p-Nitrochlorobenzene; Nitrophenols; N-Nitrosodimethylamine; Pentachloronaphthalene; Pentachlorophenol; n-Pentane; Phenol; Phosphine; Phosphorus pentasulfide; Picric acid; Stibine; Styrene; TEDP; TEPP; Tetrachloronaphthalene; Tetraethyl lead; Thiram; Tin; Toluene; o-Toluidine; Tributyl phosphate; 1,1,1-Trichloroethane; 2,4,6-Trinitrotoluene; Vinyl chloride; Zinc oxide.

Weakness, suspected of causing Decaborane; Ethyl mercaptan.

Weight loss Aniline; Beryllium; Carbaryl; Carbon disulfide; Chloromethyl methyl ether; Cobalt; Cyanides; Decaborane; Diborane; p-Dichlorobenzene; Dinitro-o-cresol; Ferbam; n-Hexane; Hydrogen cyanide; Lead; Mica; Mercury; Paraldehyde; Pentaborane; Pentachlorophenol; Phenol; Phosphorus; Stibine; 1,1,2, 2-Tetrachloroethane; Tetraethyl lead; Thiram; o-Toluidine.

Weight loss, suspected of causing Cresols; Cyclohexanone; Dibutylphthalate; Molybdenum.

Wheezing Antimony; Azinphosmethyl; Chlorine dioxide; Chloromethyl methyl ether; Chromium; Cobalt; Demeton; Dichlorvos; EPN; Ethylenediamine; Formaldehyde; Malathion; Methyl parathion; Naled; Phosdrin; Phthalic anhydride; Portland cement; Silica; Trimellitic anhydride; Vanadium pentoxide.

Wilson's disease Copper.

Wrist drops/dangles Arsenic; Triorthocresyl phosphate.

Wrists, paralysis of Lead.

Yawning Zinc oxide.

3
Primary Targets for Chemically Induced Damage

Bladder Benzidine.

Blood Aniline; Arsine; Benzene; Benzidine; 2-Butoxyethanol; Carbon monoxide; Chlorpyrifos; Chromic acid; Chromium; Cresols; p-Dichlorobenzene; 1,3-Dichloropropene; Dimethylaniline; 1,1-Dimethylhydrazine; Dinitrobenzenes; Dinitrotoluenes; Endosulfan; Ethylene glycol; Ethylene glycol dinitrate; Ethyl silicate; Lead; Lindane; Manganese; Methyl cellosolve; Methyl hydrazine; Monomethyl aniline; Naphthalene; p-Nitroaniline; Nitrobenzene; p-Nitrochlorobenzene; Nitrophenols; Phenylhydrazine; Phosphorus; Picric acid; Pindone; Polycyclic aromatic hydrocarbons; Selenium; Stibine; Tin; o-Toluidine; 2,4,6-Trinitrotoluene; Triphenyl phosphate; Vinyl chloride; Warfarin; Xylenes; Xylidine.

Blood cells, red Naphthalene.

Blood cholinesterase Azinphosmethyl; Demeton; Dichlorvos; EPN; Malathion; Naled; Phosdrin.

Body hair Thallium.

Bone marrow Benzene.

Brain Methyl cellosolve acetate; Tetrachloroethylene.

Cardiovascular system *also see*

Heart. Acetonitrile; Acrylonitrile; Aniline; Antimony; Azinphos-methyl; Barium; Carbaryl; Carbon dioxide; Carbon disulfide; Carbon monoxide; Cyanides; Demeton; Dichlorodifluoromethane; Dichloromonofluoromethane; Dichlorotetrafluoroethane; Dichlorvos; Dimethylaniline; Dimethylformamide; Dinitro-o-cresol; Dinitrobenzenes; Dinitrotoluenes; EPN; Ethyl bromide; Ethyl chloride; Ethylene glycol dinitrate; Fluorotrichloromethane; Formaldehyde; Hydrogen cyanide; Iodine; Malathion; Methylene chloride; Methyl hydrazine; Naled; Nicotine; p-Nitrochlorobenzene; Nitrogen dioxide; Pentachlorophenol; Phosdrin; Sodium fluoroacetate; TEDP; TEPP; Tetraethyl lead; Tetramethyl lead; o-Toluidine; 2,4,6-Trinitrotoluene; Warfarin; Xylidine.

Endocrine system Dinitro-o-cresol.

Eyes Acetic acid; Acetic anhydride; Acetone; Acetonitrile; Acetylene tetrabromide; Acrolein; Acrylamide; Allyl alcohol; Allyl chloride; Ammonia; Ammonium sulfamate; n-Amyl acetate; sec-Amyl acetate; Antimony; Barium; Benzene; Benzoyl peroxide; Benzyl alcohol; Benzyl chloride; Beryllium; Boron; Boron trifluoride; Bromine; 1,3-Butadiene; 2-Butoxyethanol; n-

Butyl acetate; sec-Butyl acetate; tert-Butyl acetate; n-Butyl alcohol; sec-Butyl alcohol; Butylamine; Calcium arsenate; Calcium oxide; Camphor; Carbon disulfide; Chlorinated diphenyl; Chlorine; Chlorine dioxide; Chloroacetaldehyde; alpha-Chloroacetophenone; Chlorobenzene; o-Chlorobenzylidene malononitrile; Chloroform; Chloromethyl methyl ether; Chloropicrin; beta-Chloroprene; Chromic acid; Cresols; Crotonaldehyde; Cumene; Cyclohexane; Cyclohexanol; Cyclohexanone; Demeton; Diacetone alcohol; p-Dichlorobenzene; 1,3-Dichloro-5,5-dimethylhydantoin; Dichloroethyl ether; 1,2-Dichloroethylene; Dichlorvos; Diethylamine; 2-Diethylaminoethanol; Diglycidyl ether; Diisobutyl ketone; Diisopropylamine; Dimethyl sulfate; Dimethylamine; 1,1-Dimethylhydrazine; Dinitroo-cresol; Dinitrobenzenes; Di-sec octyl phthalate; EPN; Ethanolamine; 2-Ethoxyethyl acetate; Ethyl acetate; Ethyl acrylate; Ethylamine; Ethyl benzene; Ethyl butyl ketone; Ethylene dibromide; Ethylene dichloride; Ethyleneimine; Ethyl ether; Ethyl formate; Ethyl methacrylate; N-Ethylmorpholine; Fluorides; Formaldehyde; Formic acid; Furfural; Glycidol; Hexachloroethane; n-Hexane; Hexone; sec-Hexyl acetate; Hydrazine; Hydrogen chloride; Hydrogen fluoride; Hydrogen peroxide; Hydrogen sulfide; Hydroquinone; Iodine; Isoamyl acetate; Isoamyl alcohol; Isobutyl acetate; Isobutyl alcohol; Isopropyl acetate; Isopropyl alcohol; Isopropylamine; Ketene; Limonene; Lindane; Magnesium oxide; Maleic anhydride; Mercury; Mesityl oxide; Methyl acetate; Methyl acrylate; Methyl alcohol; Methylamine; Methyl n-amyl ketone; Methyl bromide; Methyl cellosolve; Methylene bisphenyl isocyanate; Methyl formate; 5-Methyl-3-heptanone; Methyl hydrazine; Methyl iodide; Methyl isobutyl carbinol; Methyl methacrylate; alpha-Methyl styrene; Morpholine; Naled; Naphtha; Naphthalene; Nitric acid; 1-Nitropropane; Octane; Oxalic acid; Paraquat; Pentachlorophenol; n-Pentane; 2-Pentanone; Petroleum distillates; Phenyl ether; Phenyl ether-biphenyl mixture; Phenyl glycidyl ether; Phosgene; Phosphoric acid; Phosphorus; Phosphorus pentasulfide; Phthalic anhydride; Picric acid; Polychlorinated biphenyls; Portland cement; beta-Propiolactone; n-Propyl acetate; n-Propyl alcohol; Propylene dichloride; Propylene imine; Propylene oxide; Quinone; Selenium; Silver; Sodium hydroxide; Stoddard solvent; Styrene; Sulfur dioxide; Sulfur monochloride; Sulfuric acid; Tetrachloroethylene; Tetraethyl lead; Tetrahydrofuran; Thallium; Tin; o-Toluidine; Tributyl phosphate; 1,1,2-Trichloroethane; 1,2,3-Trichloropropane; Triethylamine; 2,4,6-Trinitrotoluene; Turpentine; Vanadium pentoxide; Vinyl toluene; Xylenes; Zinc chloride.

Gastrointestinal tract Cadmium; Chlorine; Creosotes; Dibutylphthalate; Dichlorobenzene; 1,1-Dimethylhydrazine; Dimethylphthalate; 1,3-Dichloropropene; Di-sec octyl phthalate; 2-Ethoxyethyl acetate; Ferbam; Formaldehyde; Lead; Malathion; Methyl alcohol; Nicotine; Paraquat; n-Propyl alcohol; Pyridine; TEPP; Thallium; Xylenes.

Gingival tissue Lead.

Heart Chloroform; p-Nitroaniline; Paraquat; Trichloroethylene. Trifluorobromomethane.

Immune system 1,3-Dichloropropene; Ethyl methacrylate; Trimellitic anhydride.

Jaw Phosphorus.

Kidneys Acetaldehyde; Acetonitrile; Aniline; Arsenic; Arsine; Benzidine; 2,3-Benzofuran; Boron trifluoride; 2-Butoxyethanol; Cadmium; Carbon disulfide; Carbon tetrachloride; Chloroform; Chromic acid; Copper; Cresols;

Cyanides; p-Dichlorobenzene; 1,1-Dichloroethane; 2,4-Dichlorophenol; Dimethyl sulfate; Dimethylaniline; Dimethylformamide; Epichlorohydrin; Ethyl bromide; Ethyl chloride; Ethylenediamine; Ethylene dibromide; Ethylene dichloride; Ethylene glycol; Ethyleneimine; Ethyl silicate; Formaldehyde; Formic acid; Hydrogen cyanide; Lead; Limonene; Lindane; Manganese; Mercury; Methyl bromide; Methyl cellosolve acetate; Methyl chloride; Monomethyl aniline; Naphthalene; Nitrobenzene; p-Nitrochlorobenzene; N-Nitrosodimethylamine; Oxalic acid; Paraquat; Pentachlorophenol; Phenol; Phenylhydrazine; Phosphorus; Phthalic anhydride; Picric acid; beta-Propiolactone; Propylene dichloride; Propylene imine; Pyridine; Selenium; Sodium fluoroacetate; Stibine; 1,1,2,2-Tetrachloroethane; Tetrachloroethylene; Tetraethyl lead; Tetramethyl lead; Thallium; o-Toluidine; 1,1,2-Trichloroethane; Trichloroethylene; 2,4,6-Trinitrotoluene; Turpentine; Xylenes; Xylidine.

Liver Acetonitrile; Acetylene tetrabromide; Acrylonitrile; Aniline; Arsenic; Arsine; Benzidine; 2,3-Benzofuran; 2-Butoxyethanol; Calcium arsenate; Carbon disulfide; Carbon tetrachloride; Chlorinated diphenyl; Chlorobenzene; Chloroform; Chromic acid; Copper; Cresols; Cyanides; p-Dichlorobenzene; 1,1-Dichloroethane; 2,4-Dichlorophenol; Dimethyl acetamide; Dimethyl sulfate; Dimethylaniline; Dimethylformamide; 1,1-Dimethylhydrazine; Dinitrobenzenes; Dinitrotoluenes; Ethanol; Ethyl bromide; Ethyl chloride; Ethylenediamine; Ethylene dibromide; Ethylene dichloride; Ethyleneimine; Ethyl silicate; Formaldehyde; Formic acid; Hexachloronaphthalene; Hydrogen cyanide; Lindane; Malathion; Methyl chloride; Methyl hydrazine; Monomethyl aniline; Naphthalene; p-Nitroaniline; Nitrobenzene; p-Nitrochlorobenzene; N-Nitrosodimethyla-

mine; Octachloronaphthalene; Paraquat; Pentachloronaphthalene; Pentachlorophenol; Phenol; Phenylhydrazine; Phosphorus; Phthalic anhydride; Picric acid; Polychlorinated biphenyls; Propylene dichloride; Propylene imine; Pyridine; Selenium; Stibine; 1,1,2,2-Tetrachloroethane; Tetrachloroethylene; Tetrachloronaphthalene; Thallium; Tin; o-Toluidine; Toluene; 1,1,2-Trichloroethane; Trichloroethylene; 1,2,3-Trichloropropane; 2,4,-6-Trinitrotoluene; Vinyl chloride; Xylenes; Xylidine.

Lungs Acetonitrile; Arsenic; Asbestos; Beryllium; 2-Butanone; Carbon dioxide; Carbon monoxide; Ethyleneimine; Mica; Nickel carbonyl; Nicotine; p-Nitroaniline; N-Nitrosodimethylamine; beta-Propiolactone; Sodium fluoroacetate; Stibine; Thallium; Titanium dioxide; Xylidine.

Lymphatic system Arsenic; 2-Butoxyethanol; Calcium arsenate; Vinyl chloride.

Mucous membranes Beryllium; Chloromethyl methyl ether.

Nasal cavities Nickel carbonyl; Silver; 1,1,2-Trichloroethane.

Nervous system, central Acetonitrile; Acrylamide; Acrylonitrile; 2-Aminopyridine; Azinphos-methyl; Barium; Benzene; Benzyl alcohol; Bromine; 1,3-Butadiene; 2-Butanone; sec-Butyl alcohol; Calcium arsenate; Camphor; Carbaryl; Carbon disulfide; Carbon monoxide; Carbon tetrachloride; Chlorinated camphene; Chlorobenzene; Chloroform; Chlorpyrifos; Cresols; Cumene; Cyanides; Cyclohexane; Cyclohexanone; 2,4-D; Decaborane; Demeton; Diborane; 1,2-Dichloroethylene; Dichlorvos; Dimethyl sulfate; 1,1-Dimethylhydrazine; Dinitrobenzenes; Endosulfan; EPN; Ethanol; Ethyl benzene; Ethyl bromide; Ethylene dichloride; Ethylene glycol; Ethylene oxide; Ethyl ether; Fluorides; Formaldehyde; Glycidol; Hexone;

sec-Hexyl acetate; Hydrazine; Hydrogen cyanide; Hydroquinone; Iodine; Lead; Linalyl alcohol; Lindane; Malathion; Manganese; Mercury; Methylal; Methyl alcohol; Methyl n-amyl ketone; Methyl bromide; Methyl cellosolve; Methyl cellosolve acetate; Methyl chloride; Methylene chloride; Methyl formate; 5-Methyl-3-heptanone; Methyl hydrazine; Methyl iodide; Methyl mercaptan; Naled; Naphthalene; Nickel; Nicotine; Nitrobenzene; 1-Nitropropane; 2-Nitropropane; Pentaborane; Pentachloronaphthalene; Pentachlorophenol; 2-Pentanone; Petroleum distillates; Phenyl glycidyl ether; Phosdrin; Phosphorus pentasulfide; Propane; n-Propyl acetate; Pyrethrum; Pyridine; Sodium fluoroacetate; Stibine; Stoddard solvent; Styrene; Sulfuryl fluoride; TEDP; Tellurium; TEPP; 1,1,2,2-Tetrachloroethane; Tetrachloroethylene; Tetraethyl lead; Tetrahydrofuran; Tetramethyl lead; Tetramethyl succinonitrile; Thallium; Tin; Toluene; 1,1,1-Trichloroethane; 1,1,2-Trichloroethane; Trichloroethylene; 1,2,3-Trichloropropane; Trifluorobromomethane; 2,4,6-Trinitrotoluene; Triorthocresyl phosphate; Vinyl chloride; Xylenes.

Nervous system, peripheral Acrylamide; Carbon disulfide; Dichlorodifluoromethane; n-Heptane; Methyl n-amyl ketone; Methyl cellosolve acetate; Triorthocresyl phosphate.

Paranasal sinus Nickel.

Prothrombin Pindone.

Respiratory system Acetaldehyde; Acetic acid; Acetic anhydride; Acetone; Acrolein; Allyl alcohol; Allyl chloride; Aluminum; 2-Aminopyridine; Ammonia; Amorphous silica; n-Amyl acetate; sec-Amyl acetate; Antimony; Azinphos-methyl; Barium; Benzene; Benzoyl peroxide; Benzyl chloride; Boron trifluoride; Bromine; 1,3-Butadiene; 2-Butoxyethanol; n-Butyl acetate; sec-Butyl acetate; tert-Butyl acetate; n-Butyl alcohol; Butylamine; Cadmium; Calcium arsenate; Calcium oxide; Camphor; Carbaryl; Chlorinated diphenyl; Chlorine; Chlorine dioxide; Chloroacetaldehyde; alpha-Chloroacetophenone; Chlorobenzene; o-Chlorobenzylidene malononitrile; Chloromethyl methyl ether; Chloropicrin; beta-Chloroprene; Chromic acid; Chromium; Cobalt; Copper; Cresols; Crotonaldehyde; Cyclohexane; Cyclohexanol; Cyclohexanone; Demeton; Diacetone alcohol; Diborane; Dibutylphthalate; o-Dichlorobenzene; p-Dichlorobenzene; 1,3-Dichloro-5,5-dimethylhydantoin; Dichloroethyl ether; 1,2-Dichloroethylene; Dichloromonofluoromethane; Dichlorotetrafluoroethane; Dichlorvos; Diethylamine; 2-Diethylaminoethanol; Diglycidyl ether; Diisobutyl ketone; Diisopropylamine; Dimethyl sulfate; Dimethylamine; 1,1-Dimethylhydrazine; Dimethylphthalate; Epichlorohydrin; EPN; Ethanolamine; 2-Ethoxyethyl acetate; Ethyl acetate; Ethyl acrylate; Ethylamine; Ethyl bromide; Ethyl butyl ketone; Ethyl chloride; Ethylenediamine; Ethylene dibromide; Ethylene oxide; Ethyl ether; Ethyl formate; Ethyl mercaptan; N-Ethylmorpholine; Ethyl silicate; Ferbam; Fluorides; Formaldehyde; Formic acid; Furfural; Furfuryl alcohol; Glycidol; n-Heptane; n-Hexane; Hexone; Hydrazine; Hydrogen chloride; Hydrogen fluoride; Hydrogen peroxide; Hydrogen sulfide; Hydroquinone; Iodine; Isoamyl acetate; Isoamyl alcohol; Isobutyl acetate; Isobutyl alcohol; Isophorone; Isopropyl acetate; Isopropyl alcohol; Isopropyl ether; Isopropylamine; Ketene; Linalyl alcohol; Limonene; Magnesium oxide; Malathion; Maleic anhydride; Manganese; Mercury; Mesityl oxide; Methyl acetate; Methyl acrylate; Methylal; Methylamine; Methyl n-amyl ketone; Methyl bromide; Methylene bisphenyl isocyanate; Methyl formate; 5-Methyl-3-heptanone; Methyl hydrazine; Methyl mercaptan; Methyl methacrylate;

alpha-Methyl styrene; Molybdenum; Monomethyl aniline; Morpholine; Naled; Naphtha; Nickel; Nitric acid; Nitric oxide; Nitrogen dioxide; 2-Nitropropane; Octane; Oxalic acid; Paraquat; Pentachlorophenol; n-Pentane; 2-Pentanone; Petroleum distillates; Phenyl ether; Phenyl ether-biphenyl mixture; p-Phenylene diamine; Phenylhydrazine; Phosdrin; Phosgene; Phosphine; Phosphoric acid; Phosphorus; Phosphorus pentasulfide; Phthalic anhydride; Polychlorinated biphenyls; Portland cement; n-Propyl acetate; n-Propyl alcohol; Propylene dichloride; Propylene imine; Propylene oxide; Pyrethrum; Silica; Sodium hydroxide; Stoddard solvent; Styrene; Sulfur dioxide; Sulfur monochloride; Sulfuric acid; Sulfuryl fluoride; TEDP; TEPP; Tetrahydrofuran; Thiram; Toluene-2, 4-diisocyanate; Tributyl phosphate; Trichloroethylene; 1,2,3-Trichloropropane; Triethylamine; Trimellitic anhydride; Turpentine; Vanadium pentoxide; Vinyl acetate; Vinyl toluene; Zinc chloride; Zinc oxide.

Respiratory system, upper Acetylene tetrabromide; Ammonium sulfamate; Cumene; Di-sec octyl phthalate; Ethyl benzene; Selenium; Tetrachloroethylene.

Skeleton Fluorides.

Skin Acetaldehyde; Acetic acid; Acetic anhydride; Acetone; Acetonitrile; Acrolein; Acrylamide; Acrylonitrile; Allyl alcohol; Allyl chloride; n-Amyl acetate; sec-Amyl acetate; Antimony; Arsenic; Barium; Benzene; Benzidine; Benzoyl peroxide; Benzyl chloride; Beryllium; Boron; Boron trifluoride; 2-Butoxyethanol; n-Butyl acetate; sec-Butyl acetate; tert-Butyl acetate; n-Butyl alcohol; Butylamine; Calcium arsenate; Calcium oxide; Camphor; Carbaryl; Carbon dioxide; Carbon disulfide; Chlorinated camphene; Chlorinated diphenyl; Chlorine; Chloroacetaldehyde; alpha-Chloroacetophenone; Chlorobenzene;

o-Chlorobenzylidene malononitrile; Chloroform; Chloromethyl methyl ether; Chloropicrin; beta-Chloroprene; Chromic acid; Chromium; Cobalt; Copper; Creosotes; Cresols; Crotonaldehyde; Cumene; Cyanides; Cyclohexane; Cyclohexanol; Cyclohexanone; 2,4-D; Demeton; Diacetone alcohol; p-Dichlorobenzene; 1,1-Dichloroethane; Dichloroethyl ether; 2,4-Dichlorophenol; Dichlorvos; Diethylamine; 2-Diethylaminoethanol; Diglycidyl ether; Diisobutyl ketone; Diisopropylamine; Dimethyl acetamide; Dimethyl sulfate; Dimethylamine; Dimethylformamide; 1,1-Dimethylhydrazine; Epichlorohydrin; EPN; Ethanolamine; Ethyl acetate; Ethyl acrylate; Ethylamine; Ethyl bromide; Ethyl butyl ketone; Ethylenediamine; Ethylene dibromide; Ethylene dichloride; Ethylene glycol dinitrate; Ethyleneimine; Ethyl ether; Ethyl methacrylate; N-Ethylmorpholine; Ethyl silicate; Ferbam; Fluorides; Formaldehyde; Formic acid; Furfural; Glycidol; n-Heptane; Hexachloronaphthalene; n-Hexane; Hexone; Hydrazine; Hydrogen chloride; Hydrogen cyanide; Hydrogen fluoride; Hydrogen peroxide; Hydroquinone; Iodine; Isoamyl acetate; Isoamyl alcohol; Isobutyl acetate; Isobutyl alcohol; Isophorone; Isopropyl acetate; Isopropyl alcohol; Isopropyl ether; Isopropylamine; Ketene; Linalyl alcohol; Limonene; Lindane; Maleic anhydride; Mercury; Mesityl oxide; Methyl acetate; Methyl acrylate; Methylal; Methyl alcohol; Methylamine; Methyl n-amyl ketone; Methyl bromide; Methyl cellosolve; Methyl chloride; Methylene chloride; 5-Methyl-3-heptanone; Methyl iodide; Methyl isobutyl carbinol; Methyl methacrylate; alpha-Methyl styrene; Morpholine; Naled; Naphtha; Naphthalene; Nickel carbonyl; Nitric acid; Nitrobenzene; Nitroethane; Nitromethane; Octachloronaphthalene; Octane; Oxalic acid; Pentaborane; Pentachloronaphthalene; Pentachlorophenol;

n-Pentane; 2-Pentanone; Petroleum distillates; Phenol; Phenyl ether; Phenyl ether-biphenyl mixture; p-Phenylene diamine; Phenyl glycidyl ether; Phenylhydrazine; Phosdrin; Phosgene; Phosphoric acid; Phosphorus; Phosphorus pentasulfide; Phthalic anhydride; Picric acid; Polychlorinated biphenyls; Polycyclic aromatic hydrocarbons; Portland cement; beta-Propiolactone; n-Propyl acetate; n-Propyl alcohol; Propylene dichloride; Propylene imine; Propylene oxide; Pyrethrum; Pyridine; Quinone; Selenium; Silver; Stoddard solvent; Styrene; Sulfur dioxide; Sulfur monochloride; Sulfuric acid; Tellurium; Tetrachloronaphthalene; Tetrahydrofuran; Thiram; Tin; o-Toluidine; Toluene; Toluene-2,4-diisocyanate; Tributyl phosphate; Trichloroethylene; 1,2,3-Trichloropropane; Triethylamine; 2,4,6-Trinitrotoluene; Turpentine; Vanadium pentoxide; Vinyl toluene; Xylenes; Zinc chloride; Zinc oxide.

Teeth Acetic acid; Nitric acid; Phosphorus; Sulfuric acid.

Urinary tract Tin.

4

Sources of
Chemical Exposure

Absorbent materials Acrylamide.

Acaricides (kills acaria such as mites, ticks, etc.) n-Amyl acetate; Azinphosmethyl; Carbaryl; Chlorinated camphene; Chlorpyrifos; Creosotes; Demeton; Dichloroethyl ether; 2,4-Dichlorophenol; Di-sec octyl phthalate; Naled; Pentachlorophenol; Propylene oxide; and TEDP.

Acetaminophen Acetic anhydride; Nitrobenzene; and p-Nitrochlorobenzene.

Acne medication Benzoyl peroxide and Hydroquinone.

Acrylic ethers Acrolein.

Acrylic fingernails Ethyl methacrylate.

Acrylic polymers Ethyl methacrylate.

Acrylic resins Cumene and Dimethylphthalate.

Acrylics Acetic acid; Acetone; Acrolein; Acrylonitrile; 1,3-Butadiene; Cyanides; Cumene; Dimethylformamide; Dimethylphthalate; Ethyl acrylate; Ethyl methacrylate; Isophorone; Methyl acrylate; Methyl methacrylate; Nickel carbonyl; Nitrogen dioxide; and Vinyl acetate.

Activated carbon Phosphoric acid and Zinc chloride.

Adhesive cleaners 1,1,1-Trichloroethane.

Adhesives *also see* **listings for Gums, Glues, and Cements.** Acetone; Acrylamide; Allyl chloride; Antimony trioxide; Benzene; 2,3-Benzofuran; 2-Butanone; n-Butyl acetate; n-Butyl alcohol; Butylamine; Carbon disulfide; Chlorinated diphenyl; Chlorobenzene; Chloroform; beta-Chloroprene; Dibutylphthalate; Dichlorodifluoromethane; Dimethyl sulfate; Dimethylformamide; Di-sec octyl phthalate; Ethyl acetate; Ethyl acrylate; Ethylene dichloride; Ethylene glycol; Ethyleneimine; Ethylene oxide; Ethyl mercaptan; Formaldehyde; n-Hexane; Isobutyl alcohol; Manganese; Methyl acrylate; Methylal; Methylene bisphenyl isocyanate; Methylene chloride; Methyl methacrylate; alpha-Methyl styrene; Morpholine; 2-Nitropropane; Phenol; Phenyl glycidyl ether; Polychlorinated biphenyls; Propylene imine; Propylene oxide; Pyridine; Quinone; Styrene; 1,1,2,2-Tetrachloroethane; Tetrachloroethylene; Tetrahydrofuran; Titanium dioxide; Toluene; Toluene-2, 4-diisocyanate; 1,1,1-Trichloroethane; 1,1,2-Trichloroethane; Trichloroethylene; Trimellitic anhydride; Triorthocresyl phosphate; Triphenyl phosphate; Vanadium pentoxide; Vinyl acetate; and Xylenes.

Adhesives for plastics Vanadium pentoxide.

Aerosol cleaning products Tetrachloroethylene.

Aerosol insecticides Isopropyl alcohol.

Aerosol propellents *also see* **Propellents.** Carbon dioxide; Carbon tetrachloride; o-Chlorobenzylidene malononitrile; Dichlorodifluoromethane; Dichloroethyl ether; Dichloromonofluoromethane; Dichlorotetrafluoroethane; Ethyl chloride; Fluorotrichloromethane; Isopropyl alcohol; Methyl bromide; Methyl chloride; Methylene chloride; Methyl iodide; n-Pentane; Propane; Tetrachloroethylene; 1,1,1-Trichloroethane; 1,1,2-Trichloroethane; Trifluorobromomethane; and Turpentine.

Aerosol/Spray degreasers 1,1,1-Trichloroethane.

Aerospace materials Ethyl methacrylate.

After-shave Dibutylphthalate; Isopropyl alcohol; and Linalyl alcohol.

Agricultural chemicals Chromic acid; Hydrazine; Mercury; p-Nitrochlorobenzene; Nitrogen dioxide; Propylene imine; and Trimellitic anhydride.

Agricultural disinfectants Hydrogen sulfide.

Agricultural water retention products Acrylamide.

Air deodorizers/fresheners Camphor; Cresols; p-Dichlorobenzene; Formaldehyde; Isoamyl acetate; Limonene; Linalyl alcohol; Methylene chloride; Naphthalene; Petroleum distillates; Phenol; Turpentine; and Xylenes.

Airplane dopes Acetone; Isoamyl acetate; Methyl cellosolve acetate; and Triphenyl phosphate.

Airplane fumigants Ethylene oxide.

Airplane glue, commercial (not models) Ethylene dichloride and Formaldehyde.

Airplane hydraulic fluids Tributyl phosphate.

Airplane parts Acrylonitrile; Aluminum; Beryllium; Magnesium oxide; Mica; Molybdenum; and Tin.

Alcohols, denatured Acetaldehyde; n-Butyl alcohol; sec-Butyl alcohol; Crotonaldehyde; Ethanol; n-Hexane; Pyridine; 1,1,2,2-Tetrachloroethane; and Zinc chloride.

Algicides Acrolein; Copper; Manganese; and Pentachlorophenol.

Alkaloid Chloroform.

Aluminum alloys Barium and Hexachloroethane.

Aluminum foil Aluminum and 2-Butanone.

Aluminum production Aluminum; Antimony; Arsine; Chlorine; Fluorides; Hydrogen chloride; Hydrogen fluoride; Nickel; and Sodium hydroxide.

Amebicides Iodine.

Amethyst glass Manganese.

Amino acids 1,3-Dichloro-5,5-dimethylhydantoin.

Amino resins Triethylamine.

Ammunition Antimony and Dinitrotoluenes.

Anesthetics Bromine; Dichloroethyl ether; Ethyl chloride; Ethyl ether; Isopropyl alcohol; and Trichloroethylene.

Anesthetics, local Benzyl alcohol and Morpholine.

Anesthetics, topical Camphor.

Animal dips Chlorinated camphene; Chlorpyrifos; and Creosotes.

Animal feed *also see* **listings for Cattle, Poultry, and Petroleum-based feeds.** Acrolein; Calcium oxide; Cobalt; Copper; Formic acid; Iodine; Isoamyl acetate; Magnesium oxide; Methyl mercaptan; Phosphoric acid; n-Propyl alcohol; 2,4,6-Trichlorophenol; and Zinc chloride.

Animal feed fumigants Phosphine.

Animal feed insecticidal adjuvant Zinc oxide.

Animal flea, lice, mite, and tick control Carbaryl.

Animal growth stimulant Arsenic.

Animal insect repellents/sprays Dimethylphthalate; Malathion; Naled; Propylene dichloride; and Pyrethrum.

Animal oil extraction/refining Acetonitrile; Barium; Isopropyl ether; and Methyl alcohol.

Animal repellents Creosotes.

Antacids Aluminum; Calcium oxide; and Magnesium oxide.

Anthelmintic drugs Hexachloroethane and Tin.

Antibiotic extraction n-Butyl alcohol.

Antibiotics n-Amyl acetate; Ethanolamine; Hexone; Methyl hydrazine; and Triethylamine.

Antibiotics, DNA binding n-Amyl acetate.

Anticaking agent Zinc oxide.

Anti-convulsant drugs Ethyl formate.

Antifoaming agent Tributyl phosphate.

Antifreeze Boron; Boron trifluoride; Chlorine; Diacetone alcohol; Ethanol; Ethylenediamine; Ethylene glycol; Ethylene glycol dinitrate; Ethylene oxide; Isopropyl alcohol; Methyl alcohol; and Phosphoric acid.

Antifreeze, commercial Ethylene glycol.

Anti-fungal preparations *also see* **Feet fungicide.** Creosotes and Thiram.

Anti-hemorrhagic drugs n-Butyl alcohol.

Antihistamines 2-Aminopyridine and Pyridine.

Anti-leukemia drugs Methyl formate.

Antiperspirants Aluminum; Formaldehyde; and Propane.

Antipyretics Creosotes.

Antiseptic cleaners Pentachlorophenol.

Antiseptic sprays Thiram.

Antiseptics Acetone; Calcium oxide; Camphor; Chlorine; Chlorine dioxide; Creosotes; Cresols; 2,4-Dichlorophenol; Ethanol; Ethyl ether; Formic acid; Hydrogen peroxide; Iodine; Isopropyl alcohol; Mercury; Morpholine; Naphtha; Naphthalene; Pentachlorophenol; Phenol; Picric acid; n-Propyl alcohol; Sulfur dioxide; 2,4,6-Trichlorophenol; and Zinc oxide.

Antiseptics, topical Naphthalene.

Antispasmodic drugs Bromine and Ethyl acetate.

Antistatic agents/products Dimethylformamide.

Appliances Aluminum; 1,3-Butadiene; 2-Butanone; Cobalt; Styrene; Toluene; and Xylenes.

Aquamephyton (a medication) Benzyl alcohol.

Asparagus Cresols.

Aspartame *also see* **Sweeteners, artificial** Methyl alcohol and Naphtha.

Asphalt Arsenic; Benzene; Beryllium; Cadmium; Chlorinated diphenyl; Chlorine; Chloroform; Chromium; Cyclohexane; o-Dichlorobenzene; Ethyl benzene; Ethylenediamine; Ethylene dibromide; Ethylene dichloride; Ethylene glycol; Formaldehyde; n-Heptane; n-Hexane; Manganese; Mercury; Nickel; Octane; Polychlorinated biphenyls; Polycyclic aromatic hydrocarbons; Toluene; and Zinc chloride.

Asphalt coatings/felts Aluminum; Arsenic; Asbestos; Beryllium; and Cadmium.

Aspirin Acetic anhydride; Aluminum; Carbon dioxide; Ketene; Naphtha; and Phenol.

Astringents Creosotes; Picric acid; Zinc chloride; and Zinc oxide.

Audio tape cassettes Styrene.

Automotive batteries Antimony; Arsenic; Lead; and Sulfuric acid.

Automotive brake anti-icing additives Methyl cellosolve; n-Propyl alcohol; and Propylene oxide.

Automotive brake cleaners Tetrachloroethylene and 1,1,1-Trichloroethane.

Automotive brake fluids n-Butyl alcohol and sec-Butyl alcohol.

Automotive brake quieters Tetrachloroethylene.

Automotive brakes Asbestos.

Automotive bumper covers Acrylonitrile.

Automotive bumpers Styrene.

Automotive carburetor cleaners 1,1,1-Trichloroethane.

Automotive clutches Asbestos.

Automotive exhaust *also see* **Diesel exhaust.** Acrolein; Benzene; 1,3-Butadiene; 2-Butanone; Carbon monoxide; Carbon tetrachloride; Cresols; Cyanides; Ethylene dibromide; Formaldehyde; n-Hexane; Hydrogen cyanide; Methyl bromide; Polycyclic aromatic hydrocarbons; Styrene; Toluene; and Xylenes.

Automotive fluids analysis Dimethyl sulfate.

Automotive grilles Acrylonitrile.

Automotive interiors Dibutylphthalate.

Automotive lacquers 2-Ethoxyethyl acetate.

Automotive paints Methylene bisphenyl isocyanate; Toluene-2,4-diisocyanate; and Turpentine.

Automotive parts/materials Aluminum; Asbestos; 1,3-Butadiene; Copper; Diglycidyl ether; Ethyl methacrylate; Methylene bisphenyl isocyanate; Methylene chloride; Molybdenum; Styrene; Toluene-2,4-diisocyanate; and Vanadium pentoxide.

Automotive polishes Ethanolamine.

Automotive radiator cleaners Oxalic acid.

Automotive transmission components Asbestos.

Automotive upholstery Trimellitic anhydride and Vinyl chloride.

Aviation fuel Cumene and Xylenes.

Aviation fuel additive Methyl cellosolve and n-Pentane.

Bacon Cresols.

Bactericide intermediate/manufacturing Benzyl chloride and Isopropylamine.

Bactericides n-Butyl alcohol; Chlorine dioxide; Cresols; 2,4-Dichlorophenol; Formaldehyde; Iodine; Mercury; Methyl alcohol; Tin; and 2,4,6-Trichlorophenol.

Bacteriostatic saline Benzyl alcohol.

Bacteriostat soaps Thiram.

Bacteriostats Benzyl alcohol; p-Nitrochlorobenzene; Propylene oxide; Pyridine; Silver; Thiram; and Zinc chloride.

Baked goods Acetaldehyde; Benzyl acetate; n-Butyl alcohol; Butylamine;

Camphor; Formic acid; Isoamyl acetate; Isopropyl alcohol; Limonene; Linalyl alcohol; n-Propyl alcohol; and Turpentine.

Baking enamels Methyl cellosolve.

Baking powder Aluminum.

Ball-point pen inks Benzyl alcohol and Ethylene glycol.

Banana flavorings n-Butyl acetate; Isobutyl acetate; and Isobutyl alcohol.

Bandages Methyl methacrylate and Phenol.

Barbiturates Allyl chloride and Quinone.

Bark removal Chloroacetaldehyde.

Bath sponges, swelling Isoamyl acetate.

Bathtubs 2-Butanone; Cobalt; Methylene bisphenyl isocyanate; Toluene; and Xylenes.

Batteries Antimony; Arsenic; Cadmium; Chlorine; Lead; Manganese; Nickel; N-Nitrosodimethylamine; Pentachloronaphthalene; Picric acid; Silver; Sulfuric acid; Tetrachloronaphthalene; 1,1,1-Trichloroethane; and Zinc chloride.

Batteries, high-energy N-Nitrosodimethylamine.

Battery cases Styrene.

Battery terminal protectors 1,1,1-Trichloroethane.

Bearings Antimony.

Beer Cobalt; Ethanol; Isoamyl acetate; and Sulfur dioxide.

Beeswax Chlorine dioxide.

Beet sugar Acetic acid; Calcium oxide; and Sulfur dioxide.

Belt lubricants Tetrachloroethylene and 1,1,1-Trichloroethane.

Belts n-Pentane.

Berry flavorings n-Butyl acetate.

Beverage acidulant Phosphoric acid.

Beverage additives Ammonia; Benzyl acetate; n-Butyl alcohol; Butylamine; Camphor; Carbon dioxide; Ethanol; Ethyl acetate; Formic acid; Isopropyl alcohol; Limonene; Linalyl alcohol; Methyl acetate; n-Propyl alcohol; and Titanium dioxide.

Beverage cans Aluminum.

Beverage flavorings Ethyl formate and Isoamyl acetate.

Beverage mixes, dry Titanium dioxide.

Beverages, alcoholic *also see* **Liquors.** Butylamine and Ethanol.

Beverages, chlorinated Carbon dioxide.

Beverages, grape Ethyl acetate.

Beverages, non-alcoholic n-Butyl alcohol; Camphor; Ethyl acetate; Formic acid; Isopropyl alcohol; Limonene; Linalyl alcohol; Methyl acetate; and n-Propyl alcohol.

Binders Ethyleneimine.

Biological research Polycyclic aromatic hydrocarbons.

Biological stains Benzidine.

Bird repellents Creosotes.

Black walnut fumigants Ethylene oxide.

Blacksmithing Cyanides.

Blasting caps Tellurium.

Bleaches Bromine; Calcium oxide; Chlorine; Chlorine dioxide; Chromium; 1,3-Dichloro-5,5-dimethylhydantoin; Hydrogen peroxide; Linalyl alcohol; Manganese; Morpholine; Nitric oxide; Oxalic acid; Sodium hydroxide; Sulfur dioxide; 1,1,2,2-Tetrachloroethane; and 1,1,1-Trichloroethane.

Blood containers Di-sec octyl phthalate.

Blowing agent for plastics n-Pentane.

Blowtorch/Welding fuel n-Pentane and Propane.

Body dusting powders Titanium dioxide and Zinc oxide.

Body lotions Benzyl alcohol; Ethylene glycol; Formaldehyde; and Methyl n-amyl ketone.

Bonding agents Ethyl silicate and Manganese.

Bone cements Ethyl methacrylate and Methyl methacrylate.

Bookbinding glues Formaldehyde.

Boots *also see* **listings for Shoes.** Acetylene tetrabromide.

Bowls Dibutylphthalate.

Brandy Cresols; Ethanol; and Methyl acetate.

Brass Lead and Tin.

Brazing alloys Silver.

Bricks Barium; Calcium oxide; Chromium; Ethyl silicate; Fluorides; Magnesium oxide; and Phosphoric acid.

Bronchodilator propellents Fluorotrichloromethane.

Bronze Isoamyl acetate; Lead; and Tin.

Brushes Styrene.

Buckles Lead.

Building/Construction materials Aluminum; Calcium oxide; Diglycidyl ether; Di-sec octyl phthalate; Ethyl methacrylate; Formaldehyde; Lead; Manganese; Mica; Naphtha; 2-Nitropropane; Vanadium pentoxide; and Xylenes.

Burn treatment Silver.

Burning batteries Arsine and Polychlorinated biphenyls.

Burning charcoal Methyl chloride.

Burning coal Methyl chloride.

Burning petroleum-based fuels Acrolein; Arsine; Benzene; 1,3-Butadiene; 2-Butanone; Carbon monoxide; Carbon tetrachloride; Cresols; Cyanides; Ethyl benzene; Ethylene dibromide; Formaldehyde; n-Hexane; Hydrogen cyanide; Methyl bromide; Styrene; Toluene; and Xylenes.

Burning wood/plants Acrolein; 1,3-Butadiene; Formaldehyde; Methyl chloride; Polycyclic aromatic hydrocarbons; and Xylenes.

Butter Acetaldehyde and Cresols.

Butter flavorings Isobutyl acetate.

Cabinetry Formaldehyde.

Cable sheathing Antimony.

Caffeine extraction 1,2-Dichloroethylene; Methylene chloride; and Trichloroethylene.

Calibration gas Nitrogen dioxide.

Camp stove fuels Cyclohexane.

Candy Acetaldehyde; Benzyl acetate; n-Butyl alcohol; Butylamine; Formic acid; Isoamyl acetate; Isopropyl alcohol; Limonene; Linalyl alcohol; n-Propyl alcohol; Titanium dioxide; and Turpentine.

Canned food Acetic acid.

Capacitors Chlorinated diphenyl; Mica; and Polychlorinated biphenyls.

Carbohydrate condensation Formaldehyde.

Carbonless (NRC) paper Chlorinated diphenyl; Formaldehyde; and Polychlorinated biphenyls.

Cardboard *also see* **Paperboard.** Mica and Morpholine.

Cardiac imaging Thallium.

Carpet Benzyl alcohol; Formaldehyde; Styrene; 1,1,1-Trichloroethane; and Zinc oxide.

Carpet backing 1,3-Butadiene; Dibutylphthalate; and Styrene.

Carpet cleaners/shampoos Ammonia; Benzyl alcohol; Naphthalene; Tetrachloroethylene; Trichloroethylene; and Triethylamine.

Carpet fumigant Ethylene dichloride.

Carpet glue Benzene; Ethyl benzene; Formaldehyde; and 1,1,1-Trichloroethane.

Casein (Chiefly used as a food additive and to make plastics.) Benzyl alcohol; Ethylenediamine; Formaldehyde; Magnesium oxide; and Morpholine.

Casein, dissolving of Sodium hydroxide.

Cast iron Nickel and Tellurium.

Cast iron alloy Chromium.

Caster oil sec-Butyl alcohol.

Castings Antimony.

Catsup Acetic acid.

Caulking compounds Dibutylphthalate; Ethyl acrylate; and Lead.

Caulking foam Methylene bisphenyl isocyanate and Toluene-2;4-diisocyanate.

Cauterizing agents Nitric acid.

Cellophane Carbon disulfide; Ethyl acetate; Ethylene glycol; and Sodium hydroxide.

Celluloid sec-Amyl acetate; Cyclohexanol; Diacetone alcohol; Dinitrobenzenes; Hexachloroethane; and Triphenyl phosphate.

Celluloid cements Epichlorohydrin.

Cellulose (Chiefly used in making textile fibers; packaging sheets; photographic film; varnishes; explosives; plastics; paper; and rayon.) Acetic anhydride; Acetone; Acrylamide; Ammonium sulfamate; sec-Amyl acetate; Aniline; Benzyl acetate; Benzyl alcohol; n-Butyl acetate; Camphor; Chlorine dioxide; Cyclohexanol; Diacetone alcohol; Dimethylformamide; Dimethylphthalate; Dinitrobenzenes; Epichlorohy-

drin; Ethyl chloride; Ethylene dichloride; Ethyl formate; Formaldehyde; Formic acid; Furfuryl alcohol; Hexachloroethane; Isopropyl acetate; Isopropyl alcohol; Ketene; Mesityl oxide; Methyl cellosolve acetate; Methyl chloride; Nitrobenzene; Nitroethane; Nitrogen dioxide; Nitromethane; 1-Nitropropane; Paraldehyde; n-Propyl acetate; n-Propyl alcohol; Propylene dichloride; 1,1,2,2-Tetrachloroethane; Tributyl phosphate; Triphenyl phosphate; and Zinc chloride.

Cellulose derivatives Propylene imine.

Cement pipes Asbestos.

Cement/Concrete products Asbestos.

Cements *also see* **Adhesives, Glues, and Gums.** Ammonia; sec-Amyl acetate; 2-Butanone; Creosotes; Epichlorohydrin; Ethyl methacrylate; Ethyl silicate; Furfuryl alcohol; n-Hexane; Hydrogen chloride; Magnesium oxide; Methyl methacrylate; Mica; Phosphoric acid; Portland cement; Styrene; Sulfur monochloride; 1,1,2,2-Tetrachloroethane; Triorthocresyl phosphate; Zinc chloride; and Zinc oxide.

Cements, corrosive-resistant Furfuryl alcohol.

Cements, quick-setting Zinc oxide.

Ceramic coatings Diborane.

Ceramic pigments Titanium dioxide.

Ceramics Antimony trioxide; Barium; Beryllium; Fluorides; Lead; Manganese; Mica; Nickel; Oxalic acid; Phosphoric acid; Vanadium pentoxide; and Zinc oxide.

Cesspool cleaners Phenol.

Cheese Aluminum; Cresols; Hexone; and Methyl mercaptan.

Cheese; white Titanium dioxide.

Chelating agents Cyanides; Ethylenediamine, Formaldehyde, Hydrogen cyanide, and Phosphoric acid.

Chelating agents for lead poisoning Phosphoric acid.

Chemexfoliation (skin peeling) Phenol.

Chemical intermediate/manufacturing Acetaldehyde; Acetic anhydride; Acetone; Acetonitrile; Acrylonitrile; Ammonia; Barium; Benzyl chloride; Bromine; Butylamine; Calcium oxide; Chlorine; Chloroacetaldehyde; Creosotes; Cresols; Diborane; 1,1-Dichloroethane; Dichloroethyl ether; 1,2-Dichloroethylene; Dichlorotetrafluoroethane; Diethylamine; Diglycidyl ether; Dimethylamine; Ethanolamine; Ethyl acetate; Ethyl benzene; Ethyl chloride; Ethyleneimine; Ethyl ether; Ethyl mercaptan; Ethyl methacrylate; Fluorides; Furfural; Hydrogen cyanide; Hydrogen sulfide; Isoamyl acetate; Isophorone; Isopropyl alcohol; Maleic anhydride; Mesityl oxide; Methyl acrylate; Methyl alcohol; Methyl formate; Methyl hydrazine; Methyl iodide; Methyl methacrylate; Naphthalene; Nickel; Nickel carbonyl; 1-Nitropropane; n-Pentane; Phenol; Polycyclic aromatic hydrocarbons; beta-Propiolactone; n-Propyl alcohol; and Tetrachloroethylene.

Chemical odor warning agents Acrolein; n-Amyl acetate; Chloropicrin; Crotonaldehyde; Dichlorodifluoromethane; Ethyl mercaptan; Isoamyl acetate; Methyl mercaptan; and Sulfur dioxide.

Chemosurgery for skin cancer Zinc chloride.

Chemotherapeutic agents Crotonaldehyde and Polycyclic aromatic hydrocarbons.

Chewing gum Benzyl acetate; Calcium oxide; Isoamyl acetate; Limonene; Linalyl alcohol; and Turpentine.

Chinaware Tellurium.

Chocolate Butylamine.

Chrome printing Formaldehyde.

Chromium alloy Nickel.

Cigarette filters Acetic anhydride.

Cigarette paper Ammonium sulfamate.

Cigarette smoke *also see* **headings under Tobacco.** Acrolein; Benzene; 2,3-Benzofuran; Beryllium; 1,3-Butadiene; Cadmium; Carbon monoxide; Cresols; Cyanides; Endosulfan; Formaldehyde; Hydrazine; Hydrogen cyanide; Limonene; Methyl chloride; Nickel; Nicotine; n-Nitrosodimethylamine; Phenol; Polycyclic aromatic hydrocarbons; Styrene; Thallium; Toluene; o-Toluidine; Vinyl chloride; and Xylenes.

Circuit board cleaners 1,1,1-Trichloroethane.

Citrus fruits Limonene.

Clay Diglycidyl ether and Silica.

Cleaners, liquid 1,1,1-Trichloroethane.

Cleaning products Ammonia; Ammonium sulfamate; Benzene; Benzyl alcohol; Boron; Boron trifluoride; 2-Butanone; 2-Butoxyethanol; sec-Butyl alcohol; Chlorine; Chloromethyl methyl ether; Cyanides; Cyclohexanol; Diacetone alcohol; o-Dichlorobenzene; p-Dichlorobenzene; Dichlorodifluoromethane; 1,1-Dichloroethane; Dichloroethyl ether; Dichlorotetrafluoroethane; Ethanol; 2-Ethoxyethyl acetate; Ethyl acetate; Ethyl chloride; Ethylene dichloride; Ethylene glycol; Ethyl ether; Fluorotrichloromethane; Formaldehyde; Hexachloroethane; n-Hexane; Hydrogen peroxide; Isoamyl acetate; Isopropyl alcohol; Isopropyl ether; Manganese; Methylal; Methyl alcohol; Methyl cellosolve acetate; Methylene chloride; Morpholine; Naphtha; Naphthalene; Oxalic acid; Pentachlorophenol; Petroleum distillates; Phenol; Phosphoric acid; n-Propyl alcohol;

Silver; Sodium hydroxide; Stoddard solvent; Sulfur dioxide; 1,1,2,2-Tetrachloroethane; Tetrachloroethylene; Tetrahydrofuran; Toluene; 1,1,1-Trichloroethane; Trichloroethylene; 1,2,3-Trichloropropane; Triethylamine; Trifluorobromomethane; Turpentine; Xylenes; and Zinc chloride.

Clear films Dimethylphthalate.

Clothes out-gassing, drying Nitrogen dioxide.

Cloud seeding Carbon dioxide and Silver.

Coal Polycyclic aromatic hydrocarbons.

Coal tar Cresols; Methyl mercaptan; Naphthalene; Phosgene; Polycyclic aromatic hydrocarbons; and Xylenes.

Coatings Acetone; Acrylamide; Asbestos; Benzene; 2-Butoxyethanol; n-Butyl alcohol; Chlorinated diphenyl; Chlorobenzene; Cyclohexanone; 2-Diethylaminoethanol; Dimethylformamide; Dimethylphthalate; Ethanol; Ethyl acrylate; Ethyl methacrylate; Hexone; Isobutyl alcohol; Isopropyl acetate; Methyl acrylate; Methylal; Methyl cellosolve; Methylene bisphenyl isocyanate; Methylene chloride; Methyl isobutyl carbinol; Methyl methacrylate; alpha-Methyl styrene; 2-Nitropropane; 2-Pentanone; Polychlorinated biphenyls; Propylene oxide; Sodium hydroxide; Styrene; Tetrachloroethylene; Tetrachloronaphthalene; Tetrahydrofuran; Titanium dioxide; Toluene; Toluene-2,4-diisocyanate; 1,1,2-Trichloroethane; Trimellitic anhydride; Vinyl acetate; Vinyl chloride; and Vinyl toluene.

Coatings, protective Aluminum; 2-Butoxyethanol; and Ethyl silicate.

Coatings, water-based 2-Butoxyethanol.

Coatings, water-resistant 2,3-Benzofuran.

Cocoa Propylene oxide.

Coffee Cresols.

Coins Nickel and Nickel carbonyl.

Cologne Limonene and Linalyl alcohol.

Colonic irrigation agent Hydrogen peroxide.

Combs Styrene.

Commercial/Industrial fuels Propane.

Computers *also see* listings for **Electronics.**

Concrete Dibutylphthalate; Formaldehyde; Paraldehyde; and Portland cement.

Concrete grout Acrylamide.

Concrete water-proofing Methyl methacrylate.

Condiments Camphor and Linalyl alcohol.

Confectionery panned goods Titanium dioxide.

Contact lense mold releasing agent Ethyl acetate.

Contact lenses Ethyl methacrylate; Methyl methacrylate; and n-Propyl alcohol.

Containers Tin.

Conveyer belts beta-Chloroprene and Styrene.

Cooking oil, heated Formaldehyde and Magnesium oxide.

Cooking utensils Aluminum.

Copper alloy Nickel.

Copper etching Picric acid.

Copper refining Arsenic and Selenium.

Copper soldering Triethylamine.

Corn syrups Sulfur dioxide.

Corrosion inhibitors Ammonia; Creosotes; Decaborane; 1,3-Dichloropropene; Diethylamine; Ethanolamine; Ethylenediamine; Formaldehyde; Hydrazine; Maleic anhydride; Morpholine; Pentaborane; and Zinc chloride.

Cortisone Quinone.

Cosmetic astringents Aluminum.

Cosmetic creams *also see* Lotions. Hydrogen peroxide; Limonene; and Methyl n-amyl ketone.

Cosmetic powders Ethylene glycol.

Cosmetics Acetonitrile; Aluminum; Benzyl acetate; Benzyl alcohol; Boron; Boron trifluoride; Camphor; Dibutylphthalate; Dichlorodifluoromethane; Dichloromonofluoromethane; Dichlorotetrafluoroethane; 2-Diethylaminoethanol; Dimethylphthalate; Di-sec octyl phthalate; Ethanol; Ethanolamine; Ethylene dichloride; Ethyleneimine; Ethylene oxide; Fluorotrichloromethane; Formaldehyde; Glycidol; Hydrogen peroxide; Hydroquinone; Isopropyl alcohol; Magnesium oxide; Mica; Naphtha; 2-Pentanone; n-Propyl alcohol; Quinone; Titanium dioxide; Toluene; Trifluorobromomethane; Zinc chloride; and Zinc oxide.

Cotton, hemostatic Nitrogen dioxide.

Cottonseed oil extraction n-Hexane.

Cough syrup Benzyl alcohol; Ethanol; and Ethyl ether.

Crayons p-Nitroaniline.

Cream n-Butyl alcohol.

Crepe Zinc chloride.

Crude oil Cresols; Methyl mercaptan; and Polycyclic aromatic hydrocarbons.

Crude oil, extraction of aromatic hydrocarbons from Dimethylformamide.

Crystallography 1,1,2,2-Tetrachloroethane.

Cushions, foam Methylene bisphenyl isocyanate and Toluene-2, 4-diisocyanate.

Cutting and grinding fluids Turpentine.

Dairy equipment cleaner Chlorine.

Dairy packaging fumigants Ethylene oxide.

Decongestant aerosols 1,1,2-Trichloroethane.

Defoliants Creosotes; Dinitro-o-cresol; Ethyl mercaptan; Pentachlorophenol; and 2,4,6-Trichlorophenol.

Degreasing products n-Amyl acetate; Benzene; Benzyl alcohol; 2-Butanone; Chlorobenzene; Cresols; Cyclohexanol; o-Dichlorobenzene; Dichlorodifluoromethane; 1,1-Dichloroethane; Dichloromonofluoromethane; Dichlorotetrafluoroethane; Ethylene dichloride; Ethyl formate; Fluorotrichloromethane; Hexachloroethane; n-Hexane; Methyl bromide; Methyl iodide; n-Propyl alcohol; Propylene dichloride; 1,1,2,2-Tetrachloroethane; 1,1,1-Trichloroethane; Trichloroethylene; and 1,2,3-Trichloropropane.

Dehairing agents Calcium oxide; Dimethylamine; Formic acid; and Isopropylamine.

De-icing agents Ethylene glycol; Methyl alcohol; Methyl cellosolve; n-Propyl alcohol; and Propylene oxide.

Dental adhesives/cements 2-Butanone; beta-Chloroprene; Ethyl methacrylate; Methyl methacrylate; Phosphoric acid; Toluene; Zinc chloride; and Zinc oxide.

Dental amalgam Mercury and Silver.

Dental anesthetic Creosotes.

Dental crowns Aluminum.

Dental disclosing waxes Zinc oxide.

Dental disinfectants Chlorine; Formaldehyde; and Hydrogen peroxide.

Dental impression paste Zinc oxide.

Dental industry Chloroacetaldehyde and Methyl acrylate.

Dental lotions n-Propyl alcohol.

Dental materials beta-Chloroprene and Tin.

Dental solution preservatives Benzyl alcohol.

Dentifrices (teeth cleaning products) Calcium oxide; Camphor; Fluorides; Formaldehyde; Hydrogen peroxide; Phosphoric acid; Silica; and Zinc chloride.

Dentures Allyl alcohol; Aluminum; Ethyl methacrylate; and Methyl methacrylate.

Deodorants Aluminum; Camphor; Formaldehyde; Limonene; Linalyl alcohol; and Propane.

Deodorizers see **Air deodorizers/ fresheners.**

Dermatological aerosol sprays Benzyl alcohol.

Desiccants Bromine; Ethanol; and Paraquat.

Detergents Benzene; Boron; n-Butyl alcohol; Chlorine; Chromium; Cumene; Cyclohexanol; Decaborane; Diborane; Dichlorodifluoromethane; Dimethylamine; Epichlorohydrin; Ethanol; Ethanolamine; Ethylamine; Ethylenediamine; Ethyleneimine; Ethylene oxide; Formaldehyde; Glycidol; Limonene; Linalyl alcohol; Methyl alcohol; Methyl n-amyl ketone; Naphtha; Pentaborane; Phenol; Phenyl ether; Phosphoric acid; Propylene oxide; Sodium hydroxide; Tetrachloroethylene; Toluene; and 1,1,1-Trichloroethane.

Detergents, liquid Cumene.

Dextrins Pentachlorophenol.

Dialysis additive Zinc chloride.

Diapers, infant and adult Acrylamide.

Diesel exhaust also see **Automobile exhaust.** Carbon disulfide; Carbon monoxide; Formaldehyde; Nitric oxide; Nitrogen dioxide; and Sulfur dioxide.

Diesel fuel additive Tetramethyl succinonitrile.

Diesel primer Ethyl ether.

Dinnerware, disposable Styrene.

Dish washing detergents Chlorine.

Dish washing disinfectants Chlorine.

Dish washing liquid Acetone; Ethylene oxide; Limonene; and Styrene.

Disinfectant inactive ingredient Phosphoric acid.

Disinfectants Aluminum; Camphor; Carbaryl; Chlorine; Chlorine dioxide; Chloroacetaldehyde; Chloroform; Creosotes; Cresols; Cumene; 1,3-Dichloro-5,5-dimethylhydantoin; 2,4-Dichlorophenol; Ethanol; Ethylene oxide; Fluorides; Formaldehyde; Hydrogen peroxide; Hydrogen sulfide; Iodine; Isopropyl alcohol; Manganese; Methyl alcohol; Methyl bromide; Naphtha; Pentachlorophenol; Phenol; beta-Propiolactone; n-Propyl alcohol; Propylene oxide; Silver; Sodium hydroxide; Sulfur dioxide; Thiram; and 2,4,6-Trichlorophenol.

Disinfectants, topical Camphor.

Diuretics Allyl chloride.

Door spray lubricants 1,1,1-Trichloroethane.

Dough (baking) conditioners Calcium oxide.

Drain cleaners Phenol and 1,1, 1-Trichloroethane.

Drain pipes Acrylonitrile.

Drinking cups Styrene.

Dry-cell batteries Manganese and Zinc chloride.

Dry cleaning n-Amyl acetate; Benzene; 2-Butoxyethanol; Chlorobenzene;

Chloroform; Cyclohexanol; Dichloro-ethyl ether; Ethylene dichloride; Formaldehyde; Hexone; Isoamyl acetate; Propylene dichloride; Stoddard solvent; Tetrachloroethylene; 1,1,1-Trichloroethane; and Trichloroethylene.

Dry ice Carbon dioxide.

Drying agents Zinc chloride.

Dusting agent *also see* **Furniture polish.** Mica.

Dye intermediates Polycyclic aromatic hydrocarbons.

Dye strippers Decaborane.

Dyes Acetaldehyde; Acetic acid; Acrylonitrile; Aniline; Benzene; Benzidine; Benzyl alcohol; Benzyl chloride; Bromine; n-Butyl acetate; n-Butyl alcohol; sec-Butyl alcohol; Butylamine; Chlorobenzene; Chloroform; Chromium; Copper; Cresols; Cyanides; Cyclohexanol; o-Dichlorobenzene; 1,2-Dichloroethylene; Diethylamine; Diisobutyl ketone; Dimethyl sulfate; Dimethylamine; Dimethylaniline; Dimethylphthalate; Dinitrobenzenes; Dinitrotoluenes; Ethanol; Ethyl chloride; Ethylenediamine; Ethylene dibromide; N-Ethylmorpholine; Formaldehyde; Furfuryl alcohol; Glycidol; Hydrogen peroxide; Hydroquinone; Iodine; Isoamyl acetate; Isopropyl ether; Isopropylamine; Maleic anhydride; Methylamine; Morpholine; Naphtha; Naphthalene; Nickel; Nitric acid; p-Nitroaniline; Nitrobenzene; Nitroethane; Nitrophenols; 1-Nitropropane; Oxalic acid; Paraldehyde; Phenol; Phenylhydrazine; Phosgene; Phosphoric acid; Phthalic anhydride; Polycyclic aromatic hydrocarbons; Pyridine; Quinone; Sodium hydroxide; Sulfur monochloride; Tin; Titanium dioxide; Toluene; o-Toluidine; Triethylamine; Trimellitic anhydride; 2,4,6-Trinitrotoluene; Xylidine; and Zinc chloride.

Dyes, black Vanadium pentoxide.

Eatable inks Ethyl acetate.

Elastics beta-Chloroprene; Epichlorohydrin; Ethylene dichloride; Ethylene glycol; n-Hexane; Methylene bisphenyl isocyanate; Toluene-2, 4-diisocyanate; and Zinc oxide.

Electric batteries *see* **Batteries.**

Electric cells Chromium.

Electric shaver cleaner 1,1,1-Trichloroethane.

Electrical cables/wirings Copper and Mica.

Electrical components/devices 2,4-Dichlorophenol; Lead; Mercury; Molybdenum; Nickel; Selenium; and Silver.

Electrical conductors Aluminum.

Electrical insulation Acrolein; Beryllium; Dichlorodifluoromethane; Fluorotrichloromethane; Formaldehyde; Hexachloronaphthalene; Pentachloronaphthalene; Phenyl ether; Tetrachloronaphthalene; Vanadium pentoxide; and Zinc oxide.

Electrical lights Phosphoric acid.

Electrolyte fuel cells Dimethyl acetamide and Phosphoric acid.

Electronic component cleaners 1,1,1-Trichloroethane.

Electronic components/equipment/consumer products Acrylonitrile; Arsenic; Beryllium; Copper; Cyclohexanone; Hydrogen peroxide; Nickel carbonyl; Silver; and Tin.

Electroplating Ammonium sulfamate; Arsenic; Arsine; Cadmium; Carbon disulfide; Chromic acid; Chromium; Copper; Cyanides; Formic acid; Hydrazine; Nickel; Nickel carbonyl; Sodium hydroxide; and Zinc chloride.

Electroplating metal on glass Hydrazine; Mercury; and Nickel carbonyl.

Electro-polishing Phosphoric acid.

Embalming fluids Camphor; Formaldehyde; Methyl alcohol; and Phenol.

Enamel thinners Cumene.

Enamels/Enamel paints Boron trifluoride; 2-Butanone; 2-Butoxyethanol; Cobalt; Cresols; Ethyl acetate; Fluorides; Mesityl oxide; Methyl cellosolve; Stoddard solvent; Tellurium; Titanium dioxide; Toluene; Triethylamine; Trimellitic anhydride; Xylenes; and Zinc oxide.

Enamels for household products/ appliances Boron trifluoride; 2-Butanone; Toluene; and Xylenes.

Engine degreasers *also see* **Metal degreasers.** 1,1,1-Trichloroethane.

Engineering industry Nitric acid.

Engraving Acetic acid; Hydrogen peroxide; Oxalic acid; and Phosphoric acid.

Epoxides Cresols; Diborane; and Isophorone.

Epoxy paints 2-Nitropropane.

Epoxy resin coatings Methyl cellosolve.

Epoxy resins Diglycidyl ether; Phthalic anhydride; Triethylamine; and Trimellitic anhydride.

Erasable inks Di-sec octyl phthalate.

Essential oils Isopropyl alcohol.

Expectorants Creosotes; Ethyl ether; and Turpentine.

Explosives Acetic anhydride; Acetone; Ammonia; Aniline; Camphor; Chromium; Cresols; Dichlorotetrafluoroethane; Dinitrobenzenes; Dinitrotoluenes; Ethanol; Ethylene glycol; Formaldehyde; Hexachloroethane; Hydrazine; Naphtha; Nitric acid; Nitrogen dioxide; Picric acid; Polycyclic aromatic hydrocarbons; Sodium hydroxide; Tetramethyl succinonitrile; Toluene; and 2,4,6-Trinitrotoluene.

Eye drops Zinc chloride.

Eyeglasses Epichlorohydrin and Styrene.

Fabric bleach Bromine; Chlorine; and Morpholine.

Fabric bleach, powdered 1,3-Dichloro-5,5-dimethylhydantoin and Linalyl alcohol.

Fabric coatings n-Butyl alcohol; Di-sec octyl phthalate; Formaldehyde; Hexachloronaphthalene; Methylene bisphenyl isocyanate; Toluene; and Xylenes.

Fabric fumigants Ethylene oxide.

Fabric fungicides Copper.

Fabric preservatives Copper.

Fabric/Textile anti-mildew agents 2,4,6-Trichlorophenol.

Fabric/Textile backcoatings Ethyl acrylate.

Fabric/Textile cleaners n-Hexane.

Fabric/Textile dyes Barium; Dimethylformamide; Formaldehyde; Formic acid; Hydrazine; Methyl cellosolve; and Picric acid.

Fabric/Textile finishes Acetic acid; n-Amyl acetate; Ethyl acrylate; Isoamyl acetate; Oxalic acid; Phosphoric acid; Tetrachloroethylene; 1,1,1-Trichloroethane; and Vinyl acetate.

Fabric/Textile fire-proofing Ethyleneimine and Formaldehyde.

Fabric/Textile printing n-Amyl acetate; Chromium; Isoamyl acetate; Methyl cellosolve acetate; and o-Toluidine.

Fabric/Textile shrink-proofing Bromine; Chlorine; and Ethyleneimine.

Fabric/Textile sizing sec-Amyl acetate; Formaldehyde; Formic acid; Vinyl acetate; and Zinc chloride.

Fabric/Textile softeners 2-Diethylaminoethanol; Dimethyl sulfate; Limonene; Linalyl alcohol; and Morpholine.

Fabric/Textile stiffening Ethyleneimine.

Fabric/Textile water-proofing Di-sec octyl phthalate; Ethyleneimine, Formaldehyde, and Pyridine.

Fabrics/Fibers, acrylic Acetic acid; Acetonitrile; Dimethylformamide; Ethyl acrylate; Methyl acrylate; and Vinyl acetate.

Fabrics/Fibers, synthetic Acetic acid; Acetic anhydride; Acetone; Acetonitrile; Acetylene tetrabromide; Ammonia; Benzidine; 1,3-Butadiene; Carbon disulfide; Chloroform; Cyanides; Cyclohexane; Diacetone alcohol; Decaborane; Dibutylphthalate; Dimethylformamide; Ethyl acetate; Ethyl acrylate; Ethylene dichloride; Ethylene glycol, Ethylene oxide, Formaldehyde; Hydrogen cyanide; Isoamyl acetate; Isoamyl alcohol; Methyl acrylate; Sodium hydroxide; 1,1,2,2-Tetrachloroethane; Titanium dioxide; Vinyl acetate; Xylenes and Zinc oxide.

Fabrics/Textiles Acetic acid; Acetic anhydride; Acrylamide; Ammonium sulfamate; n-Amyl acetate; Antimony trioxide; Asbestos; Benzidine; 2,3-Benzofuran; Benzyl alcohol; Boron; Boron trifluoride; 2-Butoxyethanol; n-Butyl alcohol; Cadmium; Carbon disulfide; Chlorine dioxide; Chlorobenzene; Chromium; Cresols; Crotonaldehyde; Cyclohexanol; 1,1-Dichloroethane; 2-Diethylaminoethanol; Diglycidyl ether; Dimethylamine; Ethanolamine; 2-Ethoxyethyl acetate; Ethyl acrylate; Ethylenediamine; Ethylene oxide; Fluorides; Hydrogen peroxide; Isopropylamine; Mercury; Methyl acrylate; Methylamine; Mica; Naphtha; Pentachloronaphthalene; Phosphoric acid; Picric acid; Propylene imine; Selenium; Sodium hydroxide; Sulfur dioxide; Sulfur monochloride; 1,1,2,2-Tetrachloroethane; Tetrachloroethylene; Tetrachloronaphthalene; Tin; Titanium dioxide; 1,1,1-Trichloroethane; Trichloroethylene; Vanadium pentoxide; Vinyl acetate; Xylidine; Zinc chloride; and Zinc oxide.

Fabrics/Textiles, durable-press Formaldehyde and Maleic anhydride.

Fabrics/Textiles, rubber-coated Sulfur monochloride.

Fabrics/Textiles, wash & wear Ethylamine.

Fabrics/Textiles wet strength additives Ethyleneimine.

Facial creams Hydrogen peroxide and Limonene.

Facial prostheses Acetic acid.

Farm fuel additive n-Pentane.

Fat dissolvers Tetrachloroethylene.

Fat preservatives Maleic anhydride.

Fats Acetone; Acetylene tetrabromide; n-Butyl acetate; n-Butyl alcohol; Carbon disulfide; Cyclohexane; Diacetone alcohol; 1,1-Dichloroethane; Diethylamine; Ethanol; Ethyl chloride; Ethylene dichloride; Ethyl ether; Formaldehyde; Hydrogen peroxide; Hydroquinone; Isoamyl alcohol; Isophorone; Isopropyl acetate; Nitroethane; 1-Nitropropane; Paraldehyde; Propylene dichloride; Sodium hydroxide; 1,1,2,2-Tetrachloroethane; Thiram; and 1,1,2-Trichloroethane.

Fatty acids Ethanol.

Fax machines Zinc oxide.

Feather pillows Zinc chloride.

Feather sterilants Zinc chloride.

Feet fungicides Chlorine.

Felt making Mercury.

Felt-tipped markers n-Hexane.

Feminine hygiene products Aluminum and Zinc chloride.

Fencing Aluminum and Tin.

Fermentation, inhibits 1,2-Dichloroethylene; Hexachloroethane; and Pentachlorophenol.

Fertilizers Ammonia; Arsenic; Carbon dioxide; Copper; 1,1-Dimethylhydrazine; Fluorides; Formaldehyde;

Magnesium oxide; Manganese; Molybdenum; Naphtha; Nitric acid; Nitrophenols; Phosphoric acid; and Phosphorus.

Fiberglass Acetone; Aluminum; Ammonia; Benzoyl peroxide; Boron; Boron trifluoride; Dimethylaniline; Formaldehyde; Methylene bisphenyl isocyanate; Styrene; Sulfuric acid; Titanium dioxide; Toluene; Trimellitic anhydride; and Xylenes.

Fiberglass bathtubs Methylene bisphenyl isocyanate; Toluene; and Xylenes.

Fiberglass insulation Boron and Boron trifluoride.

Fiberglass lamination Styrene.

Fibers, modacrylic Acetone.

Filbert nuts Methyl mercaptan.

Films Naphtha.

Fingernail polish sec-Amyl acetate, Benzyl alcohol, Camphor, Dibutylphthalate, Epichlorohydrin, Ethyl acetate, Ethylenediamine, Formaldehyde, Isoamyl acetate, Tin, and Toluene.

Fingernail polish remover Acetone; Ethyl acetate; Formaldehyde; Limonene; and Linalyl alcohol.

Finish removers Cyclohexanol; 1,1-Dichloroethane; and Ethylene dichloride.

Finishes Acetic acid; n-Amyl acetate; sec-Amyl acetate; Boron; Boron trifluoride; sec-Butyl acetate; Chromium; Dimethyl acetamide; Dimethylformamide; Ethyl acrylate; Ethyl butyl ketone; Hydrogen peroxide; Isoamyl acetate; Isophorone; Methyl acrylate; Methylene bisphenyl isocyanate; Oxalic acid; Phosphoric acid; Pyrethrum; Stoddard solvent; Tellurium; Tetrachloroethylene; Titanium dioxide; 1,1, 1-Trichloroethane; and Vinyl acetate.

Fire bricks Magnesium oxide.

Fire extinguishers Bromine; Carbon dioxide; Chloroform; Dichlorodifluoromethane; 1,1-Dichloroethane; Dichlorotetrafluoroethane; Fluorotrichloromethane; Hexachloroethane; Methyl bromide; Methyl chloride; Methyl iodide; Phosphoric acid; and Trifluorobromomethane.

Fire/Flame retardants Acetylene tetrabromide; Acrylonitrile; Allyl alcohol; Ammonium sulfamate; Antimony trioxide; Boron; Boron trifluoride; Bromine; Chlorine; Cresols; Ethyleneimine; Formaldehyde; Hexachloroethane; Hexachloronaphthalene; Methylene chloride; Octachloronaphthalene; Phosphine; Phosphoric acid; Phosphorus; Trichloroethylene; Triphenyl phosphate; and Zinc oxide.

Fireworks Aluminum; Camphor; Hexachloroethane; Manganese; Mercury; Phosphorus; and Thallium.

Fish oil extraction Acetonitrile.

Flame-speed accelerators Diborane.

Flaxseed oil extraction n-Hexane.

Flexible coatings Vinyl acetate.

Flexible sheeting Vinyl acetate.

Floor coverings Titanium dioxide.

Floor coverings, plastic Vinyl acetate.

Floor polishes Chloroform; Ethanolamine; Ethyl acrylate; and Naled.

Floor sealants, hardwood Ethyl acrylate; Methylene bisphenyl isocyanate; and Toluene-2,4-diisocyanate.

Floor tiles Benzyl chloride; Dibutylphthalate; Di-sec octyl phthalate; Vanadium pentoxide; and Zinc oxide.

Floor tiles, asbestos Asbestos and 2,3-Benzofuran.

Floor tiles, vinyl Styrene and Trimellitic anhydride.

Floor waxes Fluorotrichloromethane.

Flooring Tin.

Flour Aluminum; Benzoyl peroxide; Chlorine dioxide; Hydrogen peroxide; Nitrogen dioxide; Silica; and Sulfur dioxide.

Flowers Linalyl alcohol.

Flowers fresh, used to keep cut 1,3-Dichloro-5,5-dimethylhydantoin.

Fluorescent lamps n-Amyl acetate and Isoamyl acetate.

Fluorocarbon intermediate Tetrachloroethylene.

Fluorocarbon propellents Carbon tetrachloride; Chloroform; and Sodium hydroxide.

Foam blowing agents Dichlorodifluoromethane; Dichloromonofluoromethane; Dichlorotetrafluoroethane; Methylene chloride; and Trifluorobromomethane.

Foam blown insulation *also see* **Insulation.** Methylene bisphenyl isocyanate and Toluene-2,4-diisocyanate.

Foam resins Hydrogen peroxide.

Foams, flexible Methylene bisphenyl isocyanate; Propylene oxide; and Toluene-2,4-diisocyanate.

Foams, rigid Propylene oxide.

Foliage fungicides Copper.

Food acidulants Maleic anhydride and Phosphoric acid.

Food additives Acetaldehyde; Acetic acid; Acetic anhydride; Acetone; Allyl alcohol; Aluminum; Ammonia; n-Amyl acetate; Benzyl acetate; Benzyl alcohol; Benzyl chloride; 2-Butanone; n-Butyl acetate; sec-Butyl alcohol; Butylamine; Calcium oxide; Camphor; Carbon dioxide; alpha-Chloroacetophenone; Cresols; Cyclohexanone; Diglycidyl ether; Diisobutyl ketone; Ethanol; Ethyl acetate; Ethyl acrylate; Ethyl butyl ketone; Ethylene glycol; Ethyl formate; Formaldehyde; Formic acid; Furfural; Furfuryl alcohol; Hexone; Isoamyl acetate; Isobutyl acetate; Isobutyl alcohol; Isopropyl acetate; Isopropyl alcohol; Limonene; Linalyl alcohol; Magnesium oxide; Mesityl oxide; Methyl n-amyl ketone; 5-Methyl-3-heptanone; Methyl mercaptan; Naphtha; Nitrobenzene; 2-Pentanone; Phosphoric acid; n-Propyl acetate; n-Propyl alcohol; Propylene oxide; Pyridine; Styrene; Titanium dioxide; Turpentine; and Zinc chloride.

Food additives, indirect Ethyl methacrylate and Tetrahydrofuran.

Food adjuncts Acetaldehyde; Formic acid; Isopropyl alcohol; and Tetrahydrofuran.

Food bags/wraps, plastic *also see* **Cellophane.** Acrylonitrile and Dibutylphthalate.

Food cans Aluminum.

Food containers Styrene.

Food flavorings Acetaldehyde; Acetic acid; Acetic anhydride; Acetone; Allyl alcohol; n-Amyl acetate; Benzyl acetate; Benzyl alcohol; Benzyl chloride; 2-Butanone; n-Butyl acetate; sec-Butyl alcohol; Butylamine; Camphor; alpha-Chloroacetophenone; Cyclohexanone; Diisobutyl ketone; Ethanol; Ethyl acetate; Ethyl acrylate; Ethyl butyl ketone; Ethylene glycol; Ethyl formate; Formic acid; Furfural; Furfuryl alcohol; Hexone; Isoamyl acetate; Isobutyl acetate; Isobutyl alcohol; Isopropyl acetate; Isopropyl alcohol; Limonene; Linalyl alcohol; Mesityl oxide; Methyl n-amyl ketone; 5-Methyl-3-heptanone; Naphtha; Nitrobenzene; 2-Pentanone; Phosphoric acid; n-Propyl acetate; n-Propyl alcohol; Pyridine; Styrene; and Turpentine.

Food flavorings, synthetic Cresols and Isoamyl alcohol.

Food freezants (freeze dried) Dichloromonofluoromethane and Trifluorobromomethane.

Food fumigant Ethyl formate.

Food odor enhancers Benzyl chloride and Cresols.

Food packaging Di-sec octyl phthalate and Tetrahydrofuran.

Food preservatives Acetic acid; n-Butyl acetate; Carbon dioxide; Formaldehyde; Formic acid; Phosphoric acid; and Sulfur dioxide.

Food processing Chlorine; Fluorotrichloromethane; Isopropyl alcohol; Sodium hydroxide; and Sulfur dioxide.

Food starch Formaldehyde.

Food starch, modified Acetic anhydride; Acrolein; Calcium oxide; and Propylene oxide.

Food sterilants Dichlorodifluoromethane; Ethylene oxide; Hydrogen peroxide; and Propylene oxide.

Foods Boron; Cadmium; Cresols; Cyanides; and Hydrogen cyanide.

Formica Formaldehyde.

Foundry sand Chromium.

Fragrances *also see* **Perfumes.** Acetaldehyde; Benzyl acetate; Camphor; Cresols; Cyclohexanol; Ethyl acetate; Ethyl acrylate; Isobutyl alcohol; Methyl n-amyl ketone; and Phenyl ether.

Friction products Asbestos.

Fruit, peels (Commercially added to peel fruit) Sodium hydroxide.

Fruit coatings 2,3-Benzofuran.

Fruit flavors, artificial n-Amyl acetate; Ethyl acetate; Hexone; Isobutyl acetate; Isobutyl alcohol; and Methyl acetate.

Fruit fumigants Acetaldehyde and Ethyl bromide.

Fruit fungicides Ferbam.

Fruit juices Acetaldehyde.

Fruit preservatives Sulfur dioxide.

Fuel Barium; Benzene; Boron; Boron trifluoride; 1,3-Butadiene; Cumene; Cyclohexane; 2-Diethylaminoethanol; Dimethylamine; 1,1-Dimethylhydrazine; Ethyleneimine; Fluorides; Furfuryl alcohol; Isopropyl alcohol; Methylal; Methyl alcohol; Nitric acid; Nitrogen dioxide; Nitromethane; Pentaborane; n-Pentane; Propane; Tetrahydrofuran; and Xylenes.

Fuel, high energy Boron and Boron trifluoride.

Fuel, liquid Isopropyl alcohol.

Fuel additives Barium; Benzyl chloride; Bromine; tert-Butyl acetate; Chlorine; Decaborane; o-Dichlorobenzene; Dichloroethyl ether; Diborane; 1,1-Dimethylhydrazine; Ethanol; Ethanolamine; Ethyl benzene; Ethyl bromide; Ethylenediamine; Ethylene dibromide; Ethylene dichloride; Isopropyl alcohol; Lead; Manganese; Methylamine; Methyl cellosolve; Methyl mercaptan; p-Nitroaniline; Nitromethane; 1-Nitropropane; Octane; n-Pentane; p-Phenylene diamine; Phosphoric acid; Phosphorus; Propylene dichloride; Tetraethyl lead; Tetramethyl lead; Tetramethyl succinonitrile; Toluene; Xylenes; and Xylidine.

Fuel containers Beryllium.

Fuel oils Creosotes.

Fumigant intermediates Bromine and Methyl chloride.

Fumigants Acetaldehyde; Carbon dioxide; Carbon disulfide; Carbon tetrachloride; Chloroform; Chloropicrin; Cyanides; o-Dichlorobenzene; p-Dichlorobenzene; 1,1-Dichloroethane; Dichloroethyl ether; 1,3-Dichloropropene; Epichlorohydrin; Ethyl bromide; Ethylene dichloride; Ethyl formate; Ethylene oxide; Formaldehyde; Formic acid; Hydrogen cyanide; Methyl chloride; Methylene chloride; Methyl formate; Methyl iodide; Nicotine; Pentachlorophenol; n-Pentane; Phosphine; Propylene dichloride; Stibine; Sulfur dioxide; Sulfuryl fluoride; and TEDP.

Fungicide intermediates/manufacturing Benzyl chloride; 1,3-Butadiene; Calcium oxide; Methylamine; and Quinone.

Fungicides Acetic acid; Allyl alcohol; Aniline; Carbon disulfide; Chloroacetaldehyde; Chloropicrin; Copper; Cresols; Cyclohexane; 2,4-Dichlorophenol; Dinitro-o-cresol; Ethylenediamine; Ferbam; Formaldehyde; Furfural; Hexachloronaphthalene; Iodine; Manganese; Methyl bromide; Morpholine; Nitrophenols; Pentachlorophenol; Picric acid; Polycyclic aromatic hydrocarbons; Propylene oxide; Sodium hydroxide; Thallium; Tin; and 2,4,6-Trichlorophenol.

Fur coats Formaldehyde; Quinone; and 1,1,2,2-Tetrachloroethane.

Fur dyes Hydrogen peroxide and p-Phenylene diamine.

Furniture Cumene; Diglycidyl ether; Ethyl methacrylate; Formaldehyde; Hexone; Naphtha; 2-Nitropropane; Styrene; and Toluene.

Furniture, outdoor Acrylonitrile.

Furniture polishes n-Amyl acetate; Benzene; Ethanolamine; Methyl acrylate; Naphtha; Nitrobenzene; Petroleum distillates; Phenol; and Stoddard solvent.

Furniture/Wood finishes Methylene bisphenyl isocyanate; Stoddard solvent; Toluene-2,4-diisocyanate; and 1,1,1-Trichloroethane.

Gallium Antimony.

Gallstone treatment Limonene.

Games Styrene.

Garbage Polycyclic aromatic hydrocarbons.

Garden hoses beta-Chloroprene.

Gas Polycyclic aromatic hydrocarbons.

Gas drilling Barium.

Gas fires Nitrogen dioxide.

Gasket adhesives 1,1,1-Trichloroethane.

Gasket remover 1,1,1-Trichloroethane.

Gaskets Asbestos and Trimellitic anhydride.

Gasohol Ethanol.

Gasoline Benzene; 1,3-Butadiene; Cumene; 2-Diethylaminoethanol; Dimethylamine; Ethyl benzene; and Toluene.

Gasoline additives Benzyl chloride; Bromine; tert-Butyl acetate; Chlorine; Dichloroethyl ether; 1,1-Dimethylhydrazine; Ethanol; Ethanolamine; Ethyl bromide; Ethylenediamine; Ethylene dibromide; Ethylene dichloride; Isopropyl alcohol; Lead; Manganese; Methyl cellosolve; p-Nitroaniline; Nitromethane; 1-Nitropropane; Octane; n-Pentane; p-Phenylene diamine; Phosphoric acid; Phosphorus; Propylene dichloride; Tetraethyl lead; Tetramethyl lead; Toluene; Xylenes; and Xylidine.

Gasoline-based products n-Hexane.

Gasoline primer Ethyl ether.

Gasoline processing Methyl isobutyl carbinol.

Gauges, fluid in Acetylene tetrabromide.

Gelatin Benzyl acetate; Benzyl alcohol; Butylamine; Formaldehyde; Hydrogen peroxide; Isoamyl acetate; Limonene; Linalyl alcohol; Phosphoric acid; Propylene imine; and Sulfur dioxide.

Gelatin, insoluble Quinone.

Gems, artificial Manganese; Phosphoric acid; and Thallium.

Germicides Creosotes; Cyclohexanol; 2,4-Dichlorophenol; Formaldehyde; Furfural; Iodine; Isopropyl alcohol; Picric acid; and 2,4,6-Trichlorophenol.

Glass, colored Picric acid and Tin.

Glass bonding materials Manganese.

Glass bottles Dichlorodifluoromethane and Dichloromonofluoromethane.

Glass cleaners Ammonia; Isopropyl alcohol; Naphtha; and Naphthalene.

Glass decolorizers Cobalt.

Glass etching Arsine; Formaldehyde; Hydrogen fluoride; Sodium hydroxide; and Zinc chloride.

Glass polishes Hydrogen fluoride.

Glass products/production Arsenic; Barium; Boron; Boron trifluoride; Calcium oxide; Decaborane; Diborane; Diglycidyl ether; Fluorides; Hydrogen chloride; Iodine; Mica; Pentaborane; Selenium; Sulfur dioxide; Tellurium; Tin; Vanadium pentoxide; Vinyl chloride; and Zinc oxide.

Glasses, chilling Dichlorodifluoromethane.

Glazes Boron trifluoride; Manganese; and Silica.

Glazes for household products/ appliances Boron trifluoride.

Glucose Nitrophenols; Oxalic acid; and o-Toluidine.

Glue preservatives 2,4,6-Trichlorophenol.

Glues *also see* listings for Adhesives, Cements, and Gums. Aluminum; Benzene; 2-Butanone; Chromium; Ethyl benzene; Ethylene dichloride; Formaldehyde; n-Hexane; Magnesium oxide; Methyl methacrylate; Pentachlorophenol; Phenol; Stoddard solvent; Styrene; Sulfur dioxide; Tetrachloroethylene; Toluene; 1,1,1-Trichloroethane; 1,1,2-Trichloroethane; 2,4,6-Trichlorophenol; Vinyl acetate; and Zinc oxide.

Glues, white Zinc oxide.

Glycerin Acrolein; Epichlorohydrin; Glycidol; and Hydrogen peroxide.

Glycerol Acetic anhydride; Acrolein; Allyl alcohol; Epichlorohydrin; and Propylene oxide.

Gold alloys Nickel.

Gold extraction/recovery Bromine; Cyanides; Formaldehyde; and Sulfur monochloride.

Golf ball centers Carbon dioxide.

Golf balls Zinc chloride.

Golf clubs Acrylonitrile.

Grain fumigants Carbon disulfide; Carbon tetrachloride; Chloroform; Cyanides; Ethyl bromide; Ethylene dichloride; Formaldehyde; Methylene chloride; and n-Pentane.

Graphite Hydrogen cyanide.

Greases, dissolves Tetrachloroethylene.

Greenhouse fumigants Nicotine and TEDP.

Grenades o-Chlorobenzylidene malononitrile; Hexachloroethane; and 2,4,6-Trinitrotoluene.

Gums *also see* listings for Adhesives, Glues, and Cement. Acetic acid; 2-Butanone; n-Butyl acetate; Chloroform; Cyclohexanol; o-Dichlorobenzene; Dimethyl acetamide; Epichlorohydrin; Ethylene dibromide; Ethylene dichloride; Ethyl ether; Furfuryl alcohol; Isophorone; Isopropyl acetate; Isopropyl alcohol; Mesityl oxide; Methyl cellosolve acetate; Paraldehyde; n-Propyl alcohol; Propylene dichloride; and Toluene.

Gun cleaners o-Dichlorobenzene.

Gun powder Ethyl ether.

Gutters Acrylonitrile.

Gyroscopes Beryllium.

Hair bleach Hydrogen peroxide.

Hair conditioners Epichlorohydrin and Formaldehyde.

Hair dye 2-Aminopyridine; Benzyl alcohol; and p-Phenylene diamine.

Hair gels/setting lotions Dibutylphthalate; Ethylenediamine; and Formaldehyde.

Hair shampoo Dimethylamine; Formaldehyde; Limonene; Linalyl alcohol; Phosphoric acid; and Xylidine.

Hair shampoo, dry Dichlorodifluoromethane.

Hair spray Dibutylphthalate; Dichlorodifluoromethane; Dichloromonofluoromethane; Dichlorotetrafluoroethane; Dimethylphthalate; Formaldehyde; Methylene chloride; Propane; Trifluorobromomethane; and Vinyl acetate.

Hair tonic Isopropyl alcohol.

Hair waving solutions Bromine; Ethanolamine; Ethylenediamine; and Isopropyl alcohol.

Hand lotions Isopropyl alcohol; Limonene; Linalyl alcohol; and Methyl n-amyl ketone.

Hardening agent Formaldehyde.

Hardwood paneling Formaldehyde.

Hardwoods n-Pentane.

Heat-resistant glass Mica.

Heat shields Beryllium.

Heat transfer medium, industrial Phenyl ether-biphenyl mixture.

Hemorrhoid creams Aluminum.

Heprin (a medication) Benzyl alcohol.

Herbal medicine Limonene.

Herbicide intermediates/manufacturing Cresols; 2,4-Dichlorophenol; Ethyl acetate; Ethylamine; Ethylenediamine; Formaldehyde; Isopropylamine; Pyridine; and Triethylamine.

Herbicides Acrolein; Allyl alcohol; Ammonium sulfamate; Aniline; Boron; Boron trifluoride; Calcium arsenate; 2,4-D; o-Dichlorobenzene; 1,3-Dichloropropene; Dinitro-o-cresol; Furfural; Morpholine; Paraquat; Pentachlorophenol; Propylene oxide; 1,1,2, 2-Tetrachloroethane; 2,4,6-Trichlorophenol; and Zinc chloride.

Herbs Linalyl alcohol.

Hiccups, relieves Carbon dioxide.

High-technology ceramics Beryllium.

Highway coatings Methyl methacrylate.

Hobby kits Styrene.

Hops extraction Methylene chloride.

Hormone extraction n-Butyl alcohol.

Hormones Methyl alcohol and Tetrahydrofuran.

Hospital/Health care facilities fumigants Ethylene oxide.

Hospital sterilants Crotonaldehyde and Ethylene oxide.

Household aerosol products Carbon tetrachloride; Dichloromonofluoromethane; Dichlorotetrafluoroethane; and Trifluorobromomethane.

Household cleaners, liquid 2-Butoxyethanol.

Household cleaning products *also see* **Cleaning products.** Ammonia; Boron; Chlorine; Cyclohexanol; Ethanol; Formaldehyde; Isoamyl acetate; Isopropyl alcohol; Methyl alcohol; Morpholine; Naphtha; Phenol; Stoddard solvent; and Trifluorobromomethane.

Household disinfectants *also see* **Disinfectants.** Formaldehyde and Naphtha.

Household equipment Vanadium pentoxide.

Household fungicides Ferbam and Sodium hydroxide.

Household insect sprays Pyrethrum.

Hydraulic fluid Bromine; 2-Butoxyethanol; n-Butyl alcohol; Cresols;

Diacetone alcohol; Dichlorodifluoro-methane; Dichloromonofluoromethane; Ethylene glycol; Isobutyl alcohol; Tributyl phosphate; and Triphenyl phosphate.

Hydraulic fluid additives Isoamyl alcohol.

Hypnotic drugs Allyl chloride.

Ice, artificial n-Pentane.

Ice cream Benzyl acetate; n-Butyl alcohol; Butylamine; Formic acid; Isoamyl acetate; Limonene; Linalyl alcohol; and n-Propyl alcohol.

Icepacks Isopropyl alcohol.

Ices n-Butyl alcohol; Butylamine; Isoamyl acetate; and n-Propyl alcohol.

Icings Titanium dioxide.

Ignition compounds Phosphorus pentasulfide.

Immunotherapy solution Phenol.

Incandescent lamps Mica.

Indigo, synthetic Phthalic anhydride.

Industrial cleaners sec-Butyl alcohol.

Industrial deodorants 1,3-Di-chloro-5,5-dimethylhydantoin.

Industrial humectant Ethylene glycol.

Industrial sterilants Formaldehyde.

Industrial values and fittings Copper.

Inferred detectors Antimony.

Ink thinners Isophorone.

Inks *also see* **Printing inks.** Benzene; Benzyl acetate; Benzyl alcohol; n-Butyl acetate; Chlorinated diphenyl; Diacetone alcohol; Di-sec octyl phthalate; Ethanol; Ethyl acetate; Ethyl benzene; Ethylene glycol; Formaldehyde; n-Hexane; Hexone; Iodine; Isoamyl acetate; Isophorone; Isopropyl alcohol; Mesityl oxide; Methyl alcohol; Methyl cellosolve acetate; Molybdenum;

Naphthalene; Nickel carbonyl; Oxalic acid; Polychlorinated biphenyls; n-Propyl acetate; Propylene imine; Styrene; Sulfur monochloride; Titanium dioxide; Turpentine; Vanadium pentoxide; Vinyl acetate; and Zinc oxide.

Inks, white Zinc oxide.

Insect ointments Benzyl alcohol.

Insect repellents n-Amyl acetate; Benzyl alcohol; Camphor; Copper; Dibutylphthalate; Diethylamine; Dimethylphthalate; Mesityl oxide; and Phthalic anhydride.

Insecticide intermediate/manufacturing Allyl chloride; Benzyl chloride; Butylamine; Calcium oxide; Crotonaldehyde; Cyclohexanol; 1,3-Dichloro-5,5-dimethylhydantoin; Epichlorohydrin; Ethyl chloride; Ethylenediamine; Formic acid; Hexachloroethane; Isopropyl acetate; Methylamine; Phosgene; Phosphorus pentasulfide; n-Propyl acetate; Pyridine; 1,1,2,2-Tetrachloroethane; and Tetrahydrofuran.

Insecticide paste Phosphorus.

Insecticide propellents Fluorotrichloromethane.

Insecticide solids 1,1,1-Trichloroethane.

Insecticide sprays 1,1,1-Trichloroethane.

Insecticides Acetic acid; n-Amyl acetate; Arsenic; Azinphos-methyl; Barium; Boron; Boron trifluoride; Calcium arsenate; Carbaryl; Carbon disulfide; Chlorinated camphene; Chloropicrin; Chlorpyrifos; Copper; Creosotes; Cyanides; Decaborane; Demeton; o-Dichlorobenzene; p-Dichlorobenzene; Dichlorodifluoromethane; 1,1-Dichloroethane; Dichlorvos; Diisobutyl ketone; Dinitro-o-cresol; Endosulfan; EPN; Ethyl benzene; Ethylene oxide; Ethyl mercaptan; Formaldehyde; Furfural; Hexachloronaphthalene; Hydrogen cyanide; Lindane; Malathion; Methyl bromide;

Methylene chloride; Methyl formate; Methyl parathion; Morpholine; Naled; Naphthalene; Nicotine; Nitrophenols; Phosdrin; Phosphine; Phthalic anhydride; Pindone; Polycyclic aromatic hydrocarbons; Propylene dichloride; Propylene oxide; Pyrethrum; Sulfuryl fluoride; TEDP; TEPP; Trichloroethylene; Turpentine; and Xylenes.

Insulations Boron; Boron trifluoride; Formaldehyde; Magnesium oxide; Methyl chloride; Methylene bisphenyl isocyanate; Mica; Styrene; and Toluene-2,4-diisocyanate.

Iron alloys Nickel.

Iron manufacturing 2,4-Dichlorophenol.

Ivory Hydrogen peroxide.

Jellies and preserves Phosphoric acid.

Jet fuel Barium and 1,1-Dimethylhydrazine.

Jet fuel additive Methyl mercaptan.

Jewelry Nickel; Nitric acid; and Silver.

Joint prostheses Chromium.

Kitchen utensils *also see* **Cooking utensils.** Naphtha.

Kraft paper pulp products Calcium oxide.

Lacquer removers 2-Pentanone.

Lacquer thinners sec-Butyl acetate; Cumene; and Isobutyl acetate.

Lacquers Acetone; n-Amyl acetate; sec-Amyl acetate; Aniline; Benzene; Benzyl acetate; Benzyl alcohol; 2-Butanone; 2-Butoxyethanol; n-Butyl acetate; tert-Butyl acetate; Camphor; Chloroform; Cyclohexane; Cyclohexanol; 1,2-Dichloroethylene; Diisobutyl ketone; Dimethylphthalate; Epichlorohydrin; Ethanol; 2-Ethoxyethyl acetate; Ethyl acetate; Ethyl butyl ketone; Ethyleneimine; Ethyl silicate; Formic acid; n-Hexane; Hexone; sec-Hexyl acetate; Isoamyl acetate; Isoamyl alcohol;

Isophorone; Isopropyl acetate; Maleic anhydride; Mesityl oxide; Methyl acetate; Methyl cellosolve; Methyl cellosolve acetate; Molybdenum; Nitric acid; 1-Nitropropane; 2-Nitropropane; Octane; 2-Pentanone; n-Propyl acetate; n-Propyl alcohol; 1,1,2,2-Tetrachloroethane; Tetrahydrofuran; Titanium dioxide; Toluene; Tributyl phosphate; 1,1,2-Trichloroethane; Triorthocresyl phosphate; Triphenyl phosphate; and Xylidine.

Lactic acid Acetaldehyde; Cyanides; and Hydrogen cyanide.

Laminants Formaldehyde and Phenyl glycidyl ether.

Larvicides n-Butyl acetate; Ethyl formate; and Methyl formate.

Laser components Beryllium and Carbon dioxide.

Latex gloves 1,3-Butadiene.

Latex paints Ethyl acrylate; Ethylene glycol; Propylene imine; and Styrene.

Laundry cleaners Cyclohexanol.

Laundry detergents *also see* **Detergents.** Ethylene oxide; Formaldehyde; and Sodium hydroxide.

Laundry disinfectants *also see* **Disinfectants.** Chlorine.

Laundry marking inks Aniline.

Laundry pre-soak cleaners Phosphoric acid.

Law enforcement incapacitating agents o-Chlorobenzylidene malononitrile.

Laxative Magnesium oxide and Polycyclic aromatic hydrocarbons.

Lead crystal Lead.

Lead plating Arsine.

Lead refining Arsenic.

Leather Aluminum; Benzidine; Chlorine dioxide; Diglycidyl ether; Ethanolamine; 2-Ethoxyethyl acetate;

Ethyl acrylate; Formaldehyde; Hydrogen peroxide; Mesityl oxide; Methyl cellosolve; Molybdenum; Oxalic acid; Paraldehyde; Picric acid; Tin; Toluene; and Xylenes.

Leather, artificial/synthetic sec-Amyl acetate; Benzene; Benzyl chloride; 2-Butanone; n-Butyl acetate; Butylamine; Diacetone alcohol; Di-sec octyl phthalate; Ethyl acetate; Isoamyl acetate; Methyl acetate; and 1,1,2, 2-Tetrachloroethane.

Leather bleach Manganese.

Leather cleaners Ethylene dichloride and n-Hexane.

Leather degreasers Cyclohexanol and o-Dichlorobenzene.

Leather dyes Ethylene glycol.

Leather finishes sec-Amyl acetate; Boron; Boron trifluoride; sec-Butyl acetate; Dimethylformamide; Methyl acrylate; and Titanium dioxide.

Leather polishes n-Amyl acetate and Isoamyl acetate.

Leather preservatives Copper and 2,4,6-Trichlorophenol.

Leather tanning Acetic acid; Acrolein; Ammonia; Boron; Boron trifluoride; Chromium; Crotonaldehyde; Cyanides; Dimethylamine; Ethylene dichloride; Formic acid; Furfuryl alcohol; Isopropylamine; Manganese; Methylamine; Nicotine; Nitrophenols; Quinone; and Sulfur dioxide.

Lemonade Ethyl formate.

Library fumigants Ethylene oxide.

Lighter fluid n-Pentane.

Lime manufacturing Arsenic; Cadmium; Chromium; Copper; Formaldehyde; Manganese; and Nickel.

Liniments Isopropyl alcohol and Methyl alcohol.

Linoleum *also see* **Floor coverings.** sec-Amyl acetate and Benzene.

Linseed oil sec-Butyl alcohol.

Liquid propellents Furfuryl alcohol.

Liquors *also see* **Wine; Beer; Beverages, alcoholic; and individual liquors.** Butylamine, Cresols, Ethanol, Hexone, Isoamyl acetate, Methyl acetate, and Sulfur dioxide.

Liquors, artificially aged Hydrogen peroxide.

Lithography Benzene; Carbon disulfide; Chromium; and Phosphoric acid.

Livestock dips *also see* **Animal dips.** Chlorinated camphene and Malathion.

Livestock insect sprays Malathion; Propylene dichloride; and Pyrethrum.

Livestock/Cattle feeds *also see* listing for **Animal feed.** Acrolein and n-Propyl alcohol.

Lotions, personal care *also see* **Cosmetic creams.** Ethylene glycol; Hydrogen peroxide; Isopropyl alcohol; Limonene; Linalyl alcohol; Methyl n-amyl ketone; Naphthalene; and Titanium dioxide.

Lubricant additives Cresols; Isoamyl alcohol; Isobutyl alcohol; Maleic anhydride; Molybdenum; Morpholine; Octachloronaphthalene; Phosphorus pentasulfide; Thiram; and Triorthocresyl phosphate.

Lubricant dewaxing 2-Butanone.

Lubricants Aluminum; Barium; Benzene; Benzyl chloride; 2-Butanone; Calcium oxide; Chlorinated diphenyl; Creosotes; Crotonaldehyde; o-Dichlorobenzene; Dichloroethyl ether; Diisobutyl ketone; Ethylenediamine; Ethyleneimine; Fluorides; Furfural; Hexachloroethane; Hexachloronaphthalene; Hydrogen sulfide; Naphthalene; Nitrobenzene; N-Nitrosodimethylamine; Pentachloronaphthalene; Phenyl ether; Polychlorinated biphenyls; Propylene oxide; Sulfur monochloride; Tetrachloroethylene; Tetrachloronaphthalene; 1,1,1-Trichloroethane; Trichloroethylene; and Zinc oxide.

Lubricants, dry Mica.

Lucite (tn) Ethyl methacrylate and Methyl methacrylate.

Luggage Styrene.

Mace alpha-Chloroacetophenone and Linalyl alcohol.

Machine oils *also see* **Lubricants.** Chromium.

Magnesia cements Zinc chloride.

Magnesium refining Dichloromonofluoromethane.

Magnetic alloys Cobalt.

Magnetic tapes *also see* **Audio and Video cassette.** 2-Butanone; Chromium; Cyclohexanone; Tetrahydrofuran; and Toluene.

Mail boxes Acrylonitrile.

Marble, cultured Methyl methacrylate and Styrene.

Marine coatings 2-Nitropropane.

Mason lime Calcium oxide.

Mastics (Chiefly used in varnish, protective coatings, and cements) Turpentine.

Matches Chromium; Manganese; Phosphorus; Phosphorus pentasulfide; and Zinc oxide.

Mayonnaise Acetic acid.

Medical aerosols Fluorotrichloromethane and Trifluorobromomethane.

Medical fumigants Ethylene oxide.

Medical/Hospital disinfectants *also see* **Disinfectants.** Carbaryl.

Medical spray adhesives Methyl methacrylate.

Medical supplies Vanadium pentoxide.

Medical therapeutic agents Selenium.

Medicine, experimental Diisopropylamine and Hydrazine.

Medicine intermediate Bromine and 1,3-Dichloro-5,5-dimethylhydantoin.

Medicine preservatives Benzyl alcohol and Phenol.

Medicines Acetic acid; Acetic anhydride; 2-Aminopyridine; n-Amyl acetate; Arsenic; Barium; Benzene; Benzoyl peroxide; Bromine; n-Butyl alcohol; Camphor; Chloroform; Cobalt; Dichlorodifluoromethane; Dichloroethyl ether; Diethylamine; 2-Diethylaminoethanol; Dimethyl sulfate; Dinitrobenzenes; Ethanolamine; Ethyl acetate; Ethyl chloride; Ethylene oxide; Ethyl ether; Formaldehyde; Hexachloroethane; Hexone; Hydrazine; Hydroquinone; Iodine; Ketene; Limonene; Lindane; Magnesium oxide; Malathion; Methyl acrylate; Methylene chloride; Methyl hydrazine; Naphtha; Naphthalene; Nitrobenzene; p-Nitrochlorobenzene; Paraldehyde; Phosphoric acid; Pindone; Propylene imine; Pyridine; Quinone; Silver; Thiram; Tin; Toluene; 1,1,1-Trichloroethane; Turpentine; Warfarin; Zinc chloride; and Zinc oxide.

Melmac (tn) dinnerware Formaldehyde.

Mercury alloy Thallium.

Metal, sheet Antimony.

Metal alloys Barium; Cobalt; Chromium; Hexachloroethane; Molybdenum; Nickel; Nickel carbonyl; Selenium; Silver; and Thallium.

Metal cements Zinc chloride.

Metal cleaners 2-Butoxyethanol; Cyanides; Diacetone alcohol; Ethylene dichloride; Ethylene glycol; Hydrogen peroxide; Manganese; Methylene chloride; Naphtha; Oxalic acid; Petroleum distillates; Silver; 1,1,2,2-Tetrachloroethane; and Tetrachloroethylene.

Metal coatings Hexone and Methyl cellosolve.

Metal degreasers 2-Butanone; Cresols; o-Dichlorobenzene; Propylene dichloride; 1,1,2,2-Tetrachloroethane; 1,1,1-Trichloroethane; and Trichloroethylene.

Metal extraction Hexone and Tributyl phosphate.

Metal finishes Chromium; Dimethyl acetamide; and Hydrogen peroxide.

Metal plating/welding Cadmium and Mica.

Metal polishes Chromic acid; o-Dichlorobenzene; Oxalic acid; Petroleum distillates; Phenol; and Silica.

Metal refining/processing Arsenic; Dichloromonofluoromethane; Nickel carbonyl Selenium; Sodium hydroxide; and Trifluorobromomethane.

Metallic paints sec-Amyl acetate and Isoamyl acetate.

Metallurgy Ammonia; Arsenic; Boron trifluoride; Cadmium; Calcium oxide; Carbon disulfide; Carbon monoxide; Cyanides; Epichlorohydrin; Hexone; Hydrazine; Hydrogen peroxide; Hydrogen sulfide; Isopropyl ether; Methyl isobutyl carbinol; Nickel; and Nickel carbonyl.

Microencapsulation Epichlorohydrin and Methyl acrylate.

Microwave ovens Beryllium.

Mildew cleaners Formaldehyde; Pentachlorophenol; and Phenol.

Mildew control p-Dichlorobenzene; Sodium hydroxide; and Zinc oxide.

Military incapacitating agents o-Chlorobenzylidene malononitrile.

Military vehicle armor Beryllium.

Military warfare / poisonous chemicals Acrolein; Allyl alcohol; Benzyl chloride; Bromine; Chloropicrin; Cyanides; Methyl formate; Phosgene; Sulfur monochloride; and Tetramethyl succinonitrile.

Milk, determining the fat in Isoamyl alcohol.

Milk products Acetaldehyde.

Milk sterilants beta-Propiolactone.

Mineral oil extraction Isopropyl ether.

Mineral oils Acetylene tetrabromide; Crotonaldehyde; Dimethyl sulfate; and Hexone.

Mineral processing Sulfur dioxide.

Mineral water Isoamyl acetate.

Mining Bromine; Cyanides; Formaldehyde; Hydrogen peroxide; Sulfur monochloride; and Tin.

Mirrors Acetaldehyde; Acrylonitrile; Beryllium; Formaldehyde; Formic acid; and Silver.

Missile fuels Dimethylamine and Furfuryl alcohol.

Missile parts Beryllium.

Missile propellents Methyl hydrazine.

Miticides *see* **Acaricides.**

Mobile home skirting Acrylonitrile.

Molasses Sulfur dioxide.

Mold cleaners Formaldehyde; Pentachlorophenol; and Phenol.

Mold control p-Dichlorobenzene.

Milk products Acetaldehyde.

Molding powders Dimethylphthalate and Methyl methacrylate.

Molding resins Methyl methacrylate.

Mollusicides (kills molluscoids such as snails) Acrolein; Azinphosmethyl; and Carbaryl.

Molybdenum alloy Nickel.

Mortar Calcium oxide and Ethyl silicate.

Mosquito control Malathion and Naled.

Mosquito repellent Dimethylphthalate.

Moth balls p-Dichlorobenzene and Naphthalene.

Moth proofing Decaborane; 2,4-Dichlorophenol; Formaldehyde; and 1,1,2,2-Tetrachloroethane.

Motor fuels Hydroquinone and Tetrahydrofuran.

Motor oil *also see* **listings for Lubricants.** Hydroquinone.

Motor oil additive o-Dichlorobenzene.

Mouthwash Ethanol; Formaldehyde; and Zinc chloride.

Mushroom disinfectant Thiram.

Mushrooms, toxic Methyl hydrazine.

Nail channels sec-Butyl acetate.

Natural gas additives Ethylene glycol.

Nickel plating Formic acid and Hydrazine.

Nickel refining Nickel carbonyl.

Nitrates Nitric acid.

Nitrocellulose (chiefly used in explosives, plastics, rayon and varnishes) sec-Amyl acetate; 2-Butoxyethanol; n-Butyl acetate; sec-Butyl acetate; Diacetone alcohol; Diisobutyl ketone; Dimethylphthalate; 2-Ethoxyethyl acetate; Ethyl acetate; Ethyl butyl ketone; Ethyl ether; Ethyl formate; Furfural; Hexachloroethane; Hexone; sec-Hexyl acetate; Isoamyl acetate; Isobutyl acetate; Isophorone; Methyl acetate; Methyl cellosolve acetate; Monomethyl aniline; Nitric acid; 2-Nitropropane; n-Propyl acetate; and Triphenyl phosphate.

Nitrocellulose lacquers sec-Butyl acetate; Nitric acid; and 2-Nitropropane.

Nitroparaffin Formaldehyde.

Nuclear fuels Nitric acid.

Nuclear reactor components Beryllium and Tin.

Nuclear weapons Beryllium.

Nut oil extraction Methyl bromide.

Nutrition additives/supplements Cobalt, Manganese, and Zinc oxide.

Nylon Acetic acid; Benzidine; 1,3-Butadiene; Cyanides; Cyclohexane; Ethylene dichloride; Hydrogen cyanide; Phenol; and Titanium dioxide.

Nylon carpet Benzyl alcohol.

Oil additive Barium; Ethylenediamine; Phosphorus; Propylene imine; and Sulfur dioxide.

Oil based paints Stoddard solvent.

Oil cloth Benzene.

Oil colors Isoamyl acetate.

Oil dissolvers Tetrachloroethylene.

Oil extraction Acetonitrile; n-Hexane; Isopropyl ether; Isopropyl ether; Methyl alcohol; and Methyl bromide.

Oil preservative Maleic anhydride.

Oil refining Ethylamine and Zinc chloride.

Oil well drilling Barium and Formaldehyde.

Oils Acetic anhydride; Acetone; Acetylene tetrabromide; Benzene; Benzyl acetate; n-Butyl acetate; n-Butyl alcohol; Carbon disulfide; Chlorine dioxide; Cyclohexanol; Diacetone alcohol; o-Dichlorobenzene; 1,1-Dichloroethane; Diethylamine; 2-Ethoxyethyl acetate; Ethyl chloride; Ethylene dichloride; Ethyl ether; Ethyl formate; N-Ethylmorpholine; Formaldehyde; Glycidol; Hydrogen peroxide; Hydroquinone; Isoamyl alcohol; Isophorone; Isopropyl acetate; Methyl acetate; Methyl cellosolve acetate; 1-Nitropropane; Paraldehyde; Polycyclic aromatic hydrocarbons; Propylene dichloride; Sulfur dioxide; 1,1,2,2-Tetrachloroethane; Tetrahydrofuran; Thiram; 1,1,2-Trichloroethane; and Turpentine.

Oils, air filter Cresols.

Oils, bleaching Benzoyl peroxide.

Oils, quick-drying Vinyl toluene.

Ointments *see* **Topical medicines.**

Onion smut fumigant Methyl alcohol.

Opal glass Phosphoric acid.

Opaque glass Zinc oxide.

Ophthalmic preservatives Benzyl alcohol.

Optical instruments Magnesium oxide.

Organic substances Polycyclic aromatic hydrocarbons.

Orlon Dimethylformamide.

Ornamental crop fungicides Ferbam.

Oven cleaners Ammonia; Chloromethyl methyl ether; 1,1-Dichloroethane; Dichloroethyl ether; 2-Ethoxyethyl acetate; Ethyl acetate; Ethyl chloride; Ethyl ether; Isopropyl ether; Methylal; Methyl cellosolve acetate; Methylene chloride; Petroleum distillates; Sodium hydroxide; Stoddard solvent; and 1,1,1-Trichloroethane.

Oxide coatings Sodium hydroxide.

Oyster beds Carbaryl.

Packaging, loose-fill Styrene and Vinyl chloride.

Pain relievers *also see* **Aspirin and Acetomeniphen.** Acetic anhydride; Aluminum; n-Butyl alcohol; Carbon dioxide; Ketene; Naphtha; Nitrobenzene; p-Nitrochlorobenzene; Phenol; and Trichloroethylene.

Paint brush cleaners Limonene and Toluene.

Paint cleaners Dimethylformamide.

Paint primers 1,1,1-Trichloroethane.

Paint strippers/removers Acetone; Benzene; 2-Butanone; n-Butyl alcohol; sec-Butyl alcohol; Cyclohexane; Cyclohexanone; o-Dichlorobenzene; Dichlorodifluoromethane; 1,1-Dichloroethane; Dimethyl acetamide; Dimethylformamide; Ethylene dichloride; Formic acid; Methyl acetate; Methylamine; Methylene chloride; Oxalic acid; 1,1,2,2-Tetrachloroethane; Toluene; 1,1,1-Trichloroethane; Trichloroethylene; 1,2,3-Trichloropropane; and Turpentine.

Paint thinners Acetone; Benzene; n-Butyl acetate; Cumene; Ethylenediamine; Hexone; Isobutyl acetate; Petroleum distillates; Toluene; and Turpentine.

Paintings, renovating oil Hydrogen peroxide.

Paints Acetonitrile; Acrylonitrile; Aluminum; n-Amyl acetate; Antimony trioxide; Barium; Benzene; 2,3-Benzofuran; Cadmium; Carbon disulfide; Chlorobenzene; Chromium; Cobalt; Cresols; Cyclohexanol; o-Dichlorobenzene; Epichlorohydrin; Ethanol; Ethanolamine; Ethyl acrylate; Ethyl benzene; Ethylene glycol; Ethyl methacrylate; Ethyl silicate; n-Hexane; Hexone; Hydroquinone; Isoamyl acetate; Isobutyl alcohol; Lead; Mesityl oxide; Methylene bisphenyl isocyanate; Mica; Molybdenum; Naphtha; Nickel carbonyl; 2-Nitropropane; Pentachlorophenol; Petroleum distillates; Propylene imine; Pyridine; Silver; Stoddard solvent; Styrene; Sulfur monochloride; 1,1,2,2-Tetrachloroethane; Tin; Titanium dioxide; Toluene; Toluene-2,4-diisocyanate; 1,1,1-Trichloroethane; Trichloroethylene; Triethylamine; Trimellitic anhydride; Turpentine; Vanadium pentoxide; Vinyl acetate; Xylenes; Zinc chloride; and Zinc oxide.

Pancuronium (a medication) Benzyl alcohol.

Paper coatings 1,3-Butadiene; Ethyl acrylate; Styrene; Vinyl acetate; and Xylenes.

Paper finish for food packages Pyrethrum.

Paper/Paper products Acrolein;

Acrylamide; Ammonia; Ammonium sulfamate; sec-Amyl acetate; Aniline; Antimony trioxide; Asbestos; Barium; Benzidine; 2,3-Benzofuran; Chlorine; Chloroform; Cumene; Di-sec octyl phthalate; Epichlorohydrin; Ethyleneimine; Formaldehyde; Hexachloroethane; Hexachloronaphthalene; Hydrogen peroxide; Magnesium oxide; Methyl acrylate; Mica; Morpholine; Oxalic acid; Pentachloronaphthalene; Pentachlorophenol; Propylene dichloride; Propylene imine; Sodium hydroxide; Sulfur dioxide; Tetrachloronaphthalene; Tin; Titanium dioxide; Toluene; Vanadium pentoxide; and Vinyl chloride.

Paper sizing Crotonaldehyde.

Paper towels Formaldehyde.

Paperboard *also see* **Cardboard.** 2,4-Dichlorophenol; Di-sec octyl phthalate; Ethyl acrylate; Morpholine; and Titanium dioxide.

Paraffin (Chiefly used in candle wax, rubber compounds, pharmaceuticals, and cosmetics.) Acetone; 2-Butanone; sec-Butyl alcohol; and Carbon disulfide.

Paraffin heaters Nitrogen dioxide.

Parchment paper Zinc chloride.

Particle board Formaldehyde; Methylene bisphenyl isocyanate; Pentachlorophenol; and Toluene-2; 4-diisocyanate.

Pear flavorings n-Butyl acetate.

Pearl glues Stoddard solvent.

Pearls, artificial sec-Amyl acetate; Isoamyl acetate; and 1,1,2,2-Tetrachloroethane.

Penicillin *also see* **listings for Antibiotics.** Benzyl chloride.

Penicillin extraction n-Amyl acetate; Isoamyl acetate; and Phosphoric acid.

Perfume oils Dibutylphthalate.

Perfumes *also see* **Fragrances.** Ace-

taldehyde; Acetic anhydride; Acetone; Acetonitrile; Acrolein; Allyl alcohol; sec-Amyl acetate; Aniline; Benzyl acetate; Benzyl alcohol; Benzyl chloride; 2-Butanone; n-Butyl acetate; sec-Butyl alcohol; Camphor; alpha-Chloroacetophenone; Cresols; Cyclohexane; Cyclohexanone; 1,2-Dichloroethylene; Diisobutyl ketone; Dimethyl sulfate; Dimethylphthalate; Ethanol; Ethyl acetate; Ethyl butyl ketone; Ethyl chloride; Ethyl ether; Fluorotrichloromethane; Formic acid; Hexone; Isobutyl acetate; Isobutyl alcohol; Isopropyl acetate; Isopropyl alcohol; Limonene; Linalyl alcohol; Mesityl oxide; Methylal; Methyl n-amyl ketone; Methylene chloride; 5-Methyl-3-heptanone; Naphtha; 2-Pentanone; Phenyl ether; n-Propyl acetate; Tetrahydrofuran; Tin; Toluene; and Turpentine.

Pesticide extenders Chlorinated diphenyl and Polychlorinated biphenyls.

Pesticide inert ingredients (includes herbicides, fumigants, insecticides, etc.) Acetic acid; Acetic anhydride; Acetone; Acetonitrile; Acrylamide; Allyl alcohol; Aluminum; Ammonia; Amorphous silica; n-Amyl acetate; Aniline; Antimony trioxide; Arsenic; Asbestos; Barium; Benzene; 2,3-Benzofuran; Benzoyl peroxide; Benzyl acetate; Benzyl alcohol; Boron; Boron trifluoride; 2-Butanone; 2-Butoxyethanol; n-Butyl acetate; n-Butyl alcohol; sec-Butyl alcohol; Calcium oxide; Camphor; Carbon dioxide; Carbon disulfide; Carbon monoxide; Carbon tetrachloride; Chlorinated camphene; Chlorine dioxide; Chloroacetaldehyde; Chlorobenzene; Chloroform; Chromium; Cobalt; Copper; Cresols; Cumene; Cyclohexane; Cyclohexanol; Cyclohexanone; Diacetone alcohol; Dibutylphthalate; o-Dichlorobenzene; p-Dichlorobenzene; Dichlorodifluoromethane; 1,3-Dichloro-5,5-dimethylhydantoin; Dichloromonofluoromethane; Dichlorotetrafluoroethane; Dichlorvos; Diethylamine; 2-Diethylaminoethanol; Diisobutyl ketone; Diisopropylamine; Dimethylamine; Dimethylformamide; Dimethylphthalate; Dinitro-o-cresol; Di-sec octyl phthalate; Epichlorohydrin; Ethanol; Ethanolamine; 2-Ethoxyethyl acetate; Ethyl acetate; Ethyl acrylate; Ethyl benzene; Ethyl chloride; Ethylene dibromide; Ethylene dichloride; Ethylene glycol; Ethylene glycol dinitrate; Ethyl methacrylate; Fluorotrichloromethane; Formaldehyde; Formic acid; n-Hexane; Hexone; Hydrazine; Hydrogen chloride; Hydrogen cyanide; Hydroquinone; Isobutyl acetate; Isobutyl alcohol; Isophorone; Isopropyl acetate; Isopropyl alcohol; Isopropylamine; Lead; Limonene; Magnesium oxide; Malathion; Maleic anhydride; Manganese; Mercury; Mesityl oxide; Methyl alcohol; Methyl n-amyl ketone; Methyl bromide; Methyl cellosolve; Methyl chloride; Methylene chloride; 5-Methyl-3-heptanone; Methyl methacrylate; alpha-Methyl styrene; Mica; Morpholine; Naphtha; Naphthalene; Nickel; Nitroethane; Nitromethane; Nitrophenols; 2-Nitropropane; Oxalic acid; Paraquat; Pentachlorophenol; n-Pentane; Petroleum distillates; Phenol; Phenyl ether; Phenyl ether-biphenyl mixture; Phosphoric acid; Phthalic anhydride; Picric acid; Propane; n-Propyl alcohol; Propylene dichloride; Propylene oxide; Pyrethrum; Stoddard solvent; Styrene; Sulfur dioxide; Sulfur monochloride; Sulfuric acid; 1,1,2,2-Tetrachloroethane; Tetrachloroethylene; Titanium dioxide; Toluene; Tributyl phosphate; 1,1,1-Trichloroethane; 1,1,2-Trichloroethane; Trichloroethylene; Triethylamine; Trimellitic anhydride; Turpentine; Vinyl acetate; Vinyl chloride; Xylenes; and Zinc oxide.

Pesticide intermediate/manufacturing Acetaldehyde; Acetic anhydride; Acetonitrile; Acrylonitrile; Aniline; Arsenic; Benzene; Butylamine;

Chlorinated diphenyl; Chlorine; Chlorobenzene; Chloroform; Cresols; Crotonaldehyde; Diborane; Diisopropylamine; Dimethyl sulfate; Ethanolamine; Ethyleneimine; Ethyl mercaptan; Hydrazine; Hydrogen peroxide; Isobutyl alcohol; Isophorone; Isopropylamine; Maleic anhydride; Methylamine; Methyl chloride; Phosphorus; Phosphorus pentasulfide; Polychlorinated biphenyls; Tetrachloroethylene; o-Toluidine; 1,1,1-Trichloroethane; and Triethylamine.

Pesticide propellent Dimethylamine.

Pesticides Acrolein; Allyl alcohol; n-Amyl acetate; Carbaryl; Carbon dioxide; Chlorinated camphene; Chloropicrin; Cyanides; 1,3-Dichloropropene; Endosulfan; EPN; Ethyl methacrylate; Fluorides; Lindane; Manganese; Methyl acetate; Methyl alcohol; Methyl chloride; Methylene chloride; Methyl iodide; Methyl mercaptan; Naled; Nitrobenzene; Pentachlorophenol; Phosphine; Propylene dichloride; Pyridine; TEDP; Thiram; Tin; Trichloroethylene; 2,4,6-Trichlorophenol; Vanadium pentoxide; Warfarin; and Zinc chloride.

Pesticides, restricted use Creosotes and Methyl parathion.

Pesticides, time-release Methyl acrylate.

Petroleum *also see* **Crude oil.** Xylenes.

Petroleum additives Magnesium oxide.

Petroleum industry Selenium.

Petroleum jelly Carbon disulfide.

Petroleum recovery/refining/processing Acrylamide; Aniline; Benzene; Carbon tetrachloride; Dichlorodifluoromethane; Diethylamine; Ethylamine; Ethyleneimine; Lead; Methyl isobutyl carbinol; Nitrobenzene; Phenol; Propylene imine; Sodium hydroxide; and Sulfur dioxide.

Petroleum-based feed *also see* listing for Animal feed. Isoamyl acetate.

Petroleum-based products Carbon dioxide; Formaldehyde; and n-Hexane.

Petroleum-well cleaning Carbon disulfide.

Pets *see* listings for Animals.

Pewter Antimony and Tin.

Pharmaceutical aids Acetic acid; Acetone; Benzyl alcohol; Cobalt; Dichlorodifluoromethane; Dichlorotetrafluoroethane; Dimethyl acetamide; Ethanolamine; Ethylenediamine; Ethylene glycol; Formaldehyde; and Phenol.

Pharmaceutical dyes Aniline.

Pharmaceutical flavorings Ethyl acetate and Ethyl formate.

Pharmaceutical intermediate/ manufacturing Allyl alcohol; n-Butyl alcohol; Diisopropylamine; Ethyl bromide; Ethyl formate; Ethyl mercaptan; Phthalic anhydride; and Trifluorobromomethane.

Pharmaceutical preservative Diacetone alcohol.

Pharmaceuticals Acetic anhydride; Acetone; Acetonitrile; Acrolein; Acrylonitrile; Allyl chloride; Aluminum; Ammonia; Benzyl chloride; n-Butyl acetate; Butylamine; Carbon tetrachloride; Chlorobenzene; Creosotes; Cresols; Cumene; Cyanides; Dichlorodifluoromethane; Dichloroethyl ether; 2,4-Dichlorophenol; Diethylamine; Diisobutyl ketone; Dimethyl sulfate; Dimethylamine; Dimethylformamide; Epichlorohydrin; Ethanol; Ethyl chloride; Ethylene dibromide; Ethylene dichloride; Ethyleneimine; N-Ethylmorpholine; Glycidol; n-Hexane; Hydrazine; Hydrogen chloride; Hydrogen cyanide; Hydrogen peroxide; Isoamyl alcohol; Isobutyl alcohol; Isopropyl alcohol; Isopropylamine; Maleic anhydride; Methyl acrylate; Methyl alcohol;

Methylamine; Methylene chloride; Morpholine; Nitric acid; p-Nitroaniline; Nitrophenols; 2-Pentanone; Phenylhydrazine; Phosgene; n-Propyl alcohol; Propylene imine; Quinone; Sulfur monochloride; Tetrachloroethylene; Tetrahydrofuran; Tin; Toluene; o-Toluidine; Trichloroethylene; Trimellitic anhydride; Xylenes; and Xylidine.

Phenobarbital injections Benzyl alcohol.

Phonograph records Vinyl acetate.

Photocells Thallium.

Photocells, selenium Selenium.

Photocopier developer Amorphous silica and Methyl methacrylate.

Photocopier ink Amorphous silica and Styrene.

Photocopier toner Amorphous silica, Chromium, and Styrene.

Photocopiers Ethylene dichloride, Selenium, and Zinc oxide.

Photocopy paper Zinc oxide.

Photoengraving Cyanides; Nitric acid; and Phosphoric acid.

Photographic films Acetone; n-Amyl acetate; n-Butyl acetate; Diacetone alcohol; Dimethylformamide; Ethyl acetate; Formaldehyde; Isoamyl acetate; Methyl cellosolve acetate; Methylene chloride; 1,1,2,2-Tetrachloroethane; 1,1,1-Trichloroethane; and Vinyl chloride.

Photography Acetaldehyde; Acetic acid; Acetonitrile; Acrylamide; Acrylonitrile; Aniline; Barium; Benzyl alcohol; Benzyl chloride; Boron; Boron trifluoride; Bromine; Cadmium; Carbon disulfide; Chromium; Cyanides; 2,4-Dichlorophenol; Dimethylamine; 1,1-Dimethylhydrazine; Ethylene dichloride; Ethyleneimine; Formaldehyde; Hydrazine; Hydrogen peroxide; Hydroquinone; Iodine; Mercury; Methylamine; Morpholine; Nitrophenols; Oxalic acid; Phenol; p-Phenylene diamine; Picric acid; Propylene imine; Quinone; Selenium; Silver; Triethylamine; 2,4,6-Trinitrotoluene; Xylenes; and Zinc oxide.

Pickles Acetic acid and Aluminum.

Picnic coolers Styrene.

Pigments Aniline; Antimony trioxide; Arsenic; Barium; Benzidine; Cadmium; Carbon monoxide; Chromium; Cobalt; Cyanides; Diacetone alcohol; Dibutylphthalate; Dimethylformamide; Ethyl acrylate; Lead; Mercury; Methyl cellosolve; Molybdenum; Nickel; p-Nitroaniline; Nitrophenols; Oxalic acid; Phthalic anhydride; Selenium; Tellurium; Titanium dioxide; Tributyl phosphate; Trimellitic anhydride; Vanadium pentoxide; and Zinc oxide.

Pine oil, synthetic Turpentine.

Pineapple flavorings n-Butyl acetate.

Pipe protective linings Polycyclic aromatic hydrocarbons.

Pipes Antimony; Asbestos; 1,3-Butadiene; Copper; Lead; Polycyclic aromatic hydrocarbons; Styrene; Tin; and Vinyl chloride.

Plant growth regulators 1,1-Dimethylhydrazine.

Plant growth stimulant Arsenic and Nitrophenols.

Plant mutations Ethyleneimine.

Plaster Calcium oxide and Formaldehyde.

Plastic bags Di-sec octyl phthalate.

Plastic bottles Ethylene glycol.

Plastic dyes intermediate Polycyclic aromatic hydrocarbons.

Plastic flexible tubing Di-sec octyl phthalate.

Plastic impact-resistant appliances *also see* **Consumer products.** 1,3-Butadiene.

Plastic impact-resistant pipes 1,3-Butadiene.

Plastic paneling/wood/veneer sec-Amyl acetate; Formaldehyde; and Styrene.

Plastic plumbing materials *also see* **PVC.** Di-sec octyl phthalate.

Plastic sheets Methyl acrylate.

Plasticizers Allyl alcohol; Benzyl alcohol; Benzyl chloride; 2-Butoxyethanol; n-Butyl alcohol; Chlorinated diphenyl; Cresols; Cyclohexanol; Dibutylphthalate; Diglycidyl ether; Dimethylamine; Dimethylphthalate; Epichlorohydrin; Ethanol; Ethylamine; Ethylene glycol; Formic acid; Hexachloroethane; Hydrogen peroxide; Isobutyl alcohol; Morpholine; Nitroethane; N-Nitrosodimethylamine; Phenol; Phenyl glycidyl ether; Phosphorus; Phthalic anhydride; Polychlorinated biphenyls; Tributyl phosphate; Trimellitic anhydride; Triorthocresyl phosphate; and Triphenyl phosphate.

Plastics Acetaldehyde; Acetic acid; Acetic anhydride; Acetone; Acetonitrile; Acrolein; Acrylamide; Acrylonitrile; Allyl chloride; Ammonia; Antimony trioxide; Barium; Benzene; Benzidine; 2,3-Benzofuran; Benzoyl peroxide; Benzyl alcohol; Benzyl chloride; Bromine; 1;3-Butadiene; 2-Butanone; n-Butyl acetate; Cadmium; Camphor; Chlorine; Chloroform; alpha-Chloroacetophenone; Cresols; Cyanides; Cyclohexane; Cyclohexanol; Cyclohexanone; Decaborane; Dibutylphthalate; 1,1-Dichloroethane; 1,2-Dichloroethylene; 2,4-Dichlorophenol; Diisobutyl ketone; Dimethyl acetamide; Dimethylphthalate; Di-sec octyl phthalate; Epichlorohydrin; Ethanol; Ethyl acetate; Ethyl acrylate; Ethyl butyl ketone; Ethyl chloride; Ethylene dichloride; Ethylene glycol; Ethyl mercaptan; Ethyl methacrylate; Fluorides; Formaldehyde; n-Hexane; Hexone; Hydrogen peroxide; Hydrogen sulfide; Isophorone; Isopropyl acetate; Lead; Maleic anhydride; Mesityl oxide; Methyl acrylate; Methyl alcohol; Methyl n-amyl ketone; Methyl chloride; Methylene bisphenyl isocyanate; Methylene chloride; 5-Methyl-3-heptanone; Methyl isobutyl carbinol; Methyl mercaptan; Methyl methacrylate; alpha-Methyl styrene; Mica; Naphtha; 2-Nitropropane; N-Nitrosodimethylamine; 2-Pentanone; Phenol; Phosphine; n-Propyl acetate; Propylene dichloride; Sodium hydroxide; Styrene; Tetrahydrofuran; Tin; Titanium dioxide; Toluene; Toluene-2,4-diisocyanate; Tributyl phosphate; Trimellitic anhydride; Vanadium pentoxide; Vinyl acetate; Vinyl chloride; Vinyl toluene; Xylenes; and Zinc oxide.

Plastics, dissolving of n-Amyl acetate and 1,1-Dimethylhydrazine.

Plastics, removing print from Carbon disulfide.

Plastics, soft/flexible Acrylonitrile; Dibutylphthalate; Di-sec octyl phthalate; Ethylene dichloride; Methyl acrylate; and Tin.

Plexiglass (tn) Ethyl methacrylate; Methyl methacrylate; and Naphtha.

Plumbing materials Copper.

Plumbing pipe solders Zinc chloride.

Plywood Formaldehyde; Methylene bisphenyl isocyanate; and Toluene-2, 4-diisocyanate.

Plywood adhesives Carbon disulfide.

Pneumatic tires Mica.

Polishes n-Amyl acetate; Benzene; Benzyl acetate; Benzyl alcohol; sec-Butyl alcohol; Camphor; Chlorobenzene; Chloroform; Chromic acid; Cyclohexanol; Cyclohexanone; Dibutylphthalate; o-Dichlorobenzene; Epichlorohydrin; Ethanolamine; Ethyl acetate; Ethyl acrylate; Ethylenediamine; Ethyl methacrylate; Formaldehyde; Hydrogen fluoride; Isoamyl acetate; Isoamyl acetate; Naled; Naphtha; Nitrobenzene; Oxalic acid; Petroleum distillates; Phenol; Phosphoric acid; n-Propyl alcohol; Silica; Stoddard solvent; Tetrachloroethylene; Tin; Titanium dioxide; Toluene; 1,1,1-Trichloroethane; and Turpentine.

Pollution control Hydrogen peroxide.

Polycarbonated resins Phosgene and Pyridine.

Polyester bottles Ethylene oxide.

Polyester fabrics/fibers Ethylene glycol, Ethylene oxide, and Xylenes.

Polyester films Ethylene oxide.

Polyester resins Cumene and Vinyl toluene.

Polyesters (Chiefly used in making fibers and plastics.) Acrolein; Allyl chloride; Benzoyl peroxide; Cumene; Dimethylaniline; Ethyl acrylate; Ethylene glycol; Ethylene glycol dinitrate; Ethylene oxide; Isophorone; Maleic anhydride; alpha-Methyl styrene; 2-Nitropropane; Phthalic anhydride; Styrene; 1,1,2,2-Tetrachloroethane; 1,1,2-Trichloroethane; Trimellitic anhydride; Vinyl toluene; and Xylenes.

Polyesters, thermoset Benzoyl peroxide.

Polyethylene films (Chiefly used in packaging and insulation.) Benzyl alcohol.

Polymers Acetonitrile; Chloromethyl methyl ether; Hexachloroethane; Nitromethane; Octane; Propylene imine; Quinone; 1,2,3-Trichloropropane; and Trimellitic anhydride.

Polystyrene (Transparent thermoplastic used chiefly in electrical insulation, containers, molded products such a styrene cups, and sheet materials.) Acetylene tetrabromide; 2-Butanone; Dimethylphthalate; Methyl chloride; and Styrene.

Polyurethane (Chiefly used in flexible and rigid foams, elastomers,

and resins for such things as cushions and insulation.) Acetylene tetrabromide; Acrolein; Aniline; 2-Butanone; Cyclohexanone; Ethylene glycol; Ethylene oxide; Methylene bisphenyl isocyanate; Propylene oxide; Tin; Toluene; Toluene-2,4-diisocyanate; and Triethylamine.

Polyurethane coatings Cyclohexanone.

Polyurethane insulation *also see* **Insulation.** Methyl chloride.

Porcelain bathroom/kitchen fixtures 2-Butanone; Cobalt; Toluene; and Xylenes.

Porcelain glazing Titanium dioxide.

Porcelains 2-Butanone; Cobalt; Tellurium; Titanium dioxide; Toluene; Xylenes; and Zinc oxide

Poultry dips Malathion.

Poultry feeds *also see* **listings for Animal feed.** Acrolein; Calcium oxide; and Methyl mercaptan.

Poultry insect sprays Malathion.

Predator elimination Sodium fluoroacetate.

Preservatives Acetic acid; Aluminum; Arsenic; Benzyl alcohol; n-Butyl acetate; Carbon dioxide; Chromium; Copper; Creosotes; Cresols; Diacetone alcohol; o-Dichlorobenzene; 2,4-Dichlorophenol; Formaldehyde; Formic acid; Limonene; Maleic anhydride; Manganese; Methyl alcohol; Naphthalene; Nitrophenols; Pentachlorophenol; Phenol; Phosphoric acid; Sulfur dioxide; Thiram; Tin; 2,4,6-Trichlorophenol; Xylidine; and Zinc chloride.

Printing compounds/materials sec-Amyl acetate; Cadmium; Cyclohexanone; and Xylenes.

Printing inks *also see* **Inks.** Acetone; Aniline; Benzidine; 2-Butanone; alpha-Chloroacetophenone; Cyclohexanone; Diisobutyl ketone; Dimethylformamide; Ethyl acetate; Ethyl butyl ketone; Ethylene glycol; n-Heptane; Isoamyl acetate; Isopropyl acetate; Methyl n-amyl ketone; Methyl cellosolve; 5-Methyl-3-heptanone; 2-Nitropropane; 2-Pentanone; n-Propyl alcohol; Tetrachloroethylene; Tetrahydrofuran; Toluene; Toluene-2,4-diisocyanate; 1,1,1-Trichloroethane; Triethylamine; and Trimellitic anhydride.

Propellents Beryllium; Carbon dioxide; Carbon tetrachloride; o-Chlorobenzylidene malononitrile; Decaborane; Diborane; Dichlorodifluoromethane; Dichloroethyl ether; Dichloromonofluoromethane; Dichlorotetrafluoroethane; Dimethylamine; Dimethylphthalate; Ethyl chloride; Fluorotrichloromethane; Furfuryl alcohol; Hydrazine; Hydrogen peroxide; Isopropyl alcohol; Methylamine; Methyl bromide; Methylene chloride; Methyl hydrazine; Methyl iodide; Nitroethane; Nitromethane; Octane; n-Pentane; Propane; Tetrachloroethylene; Tetramethyl succinonitrile; 1,1,1-Trichloroethane; 1,1,2-Trichloroethane; Triethylamine; Trifluorobromomethane; Turpentine.

Prosthetic devices Acetic acid; Chromium; and Cobalt.

Pudding Butylamine; Isoamyl acetate; Limonene; and Linalyl alcohol.

PVC (polyvinyl chlorinated) pipes Vinyl chloride.

Radios Selenium.

Railroad ties Carbon monoxide; Formaldehyde; Hydrogen chloride; Phenol; and Zinc chloride.

Raincoats Dibutylphthalate and Disec octyl phthalate.

Raspberry flavorings Isobutyl acetate.

Rayon Acetone; Carbon disulfide; Decaborane; Dimethylformamide; Ethylene dichloride; Hydrogen sulfide; Sodium hydroxide; Titanium dioxide; and Zinc oxide.

Rayon bleach *also see* **Bleaches.** Nitric oxide.

Refracting optic glass *also see* **Eyeglasses.** Thallium.

Refrigerants Ammonia; Bromine; Carbon dioxide; Carbon tetrachloride; Chlorine; Chloroform; Dichlorodifluoromethane; 1,2-Dichloroethylene; Dichloromonofluoromethane; Dichlorotetrafluoroethane; Ethyl bromide; Ethyl chloride; Fluorotrichloromethane; Formic acid; Methyl bromide; Methyl chloride; Methyl formate; Methyl iodide; Propane; Sulfur dioxide; Trichloroethylene; and Trifluorobromomethane.

Refrigerator door liners Styrene.

Refrigerators Asbestos.

Reinforced plastics Asbestos.

Research chemical n-Heptane and N-Nitrosodimethylamine.

Residential fuels Propane.

Resins (Chiefly used in varnishes, printing inks, plastics, sizing, and medicine.) Acetaldehyde; Acetic acid; Acetic anhydride; Acetone; Acetonitrile; Acrylonitrile; Allyl alcohol; Allyl chloride; Ammonia; Aniline; Benzene; 2,3-Benzofuran; Benzyl acetate; Benzyl chloride; 2-Butanone; n-Butyl acetate; n-Butyl alcohol; sec-Butyl alcohol; Carbon disulfide; Carbon dioxide; Chlorobenzene; Chlorinated diphenyl; Chlorine; Chloromethyl methyl ether; Cresols; Crotonaldehyde; Cumene; Cyclohexane; Cyclohexanol; Diacetone alcohol; o-Dichlorobenzene; Dichlorodifluoromethane; Dichloromonofluoromethane; 2-Diethylaminoethanol; Diglycidyl ether; Diisobutyl ketone; Dimethyl acetamide; Dimethylphthalate; Dinitro-o-cresol; Epichlorohydrin; Epichlorohydrin; Ethanol; 2-Ethoxyethyl acetate; Ethyl acetate; Ethyl acrylate; Ethylamine; Ethyl chloride; Ethylenediamine; Ethylene dibromide; Ethylene dichloride; Ethylene glycol; Ethyleneimine; Ethyl formate; Ethyl methacrylate; N-Ethylmorpholine; Fluorotrichloromethane; Formaldehyde; Furfuryl alcohol; Hexachloronaphthalene; Hydrogen peroxide; Isoamyl acetate; Isoamyl alcohol; Isophorone; Isopropyl acetate; Isopropyl alcohol; Isopropyl ether; Limonene; Maleic anhydride; Mesityl oxide; Methyl acetate; Methylal; Methyl cellosolve acetate; Methyl methacrylate; alpha-Methyl styrene; Morpholine; Naphthalene; Nitroethane; 1-Nitropropane; 2-Nitropropane; Paraldehyde; Phenol; Phenyl ether; Phenyl glycidyl ether; Phosgene; Phthalic anhydride; Polychlorinated biphenyls; n-Propyl alcohol; Propylene dichloride; Pyridine; Quinone; Sodium hydroxide; Styrene; 1,1,2,2-Tetrachloroethane; Tetrahydrofuran; Toluene; o-Toluidine; Tributyl phosphate; 1,1,2-Trichloroethane; Triethylamine; Trimellitic anhydride; Turpentine; and Vinyl toluene.

Resins, urea Ammonia; Carbon dioxide; and Phosgene.

Respiratory systems, stimulating depressed Carbon dioxide.

Rifle barrels Molybdenum.

Road construction *also see* **Asphalt and Concrete.** Furfural.

Road salts Cyanides.

Rocket fuels 1,1-Dimethylhydrazine; Fluorides; Nitrogen dioxide; Nitromethane; Picric acid; and Propylene imine.

Rocket propellents Beryllium; Decaborane; Diborane; Dimethylamine; Dimethylphthalate; Hydrazine; Hydrogen peroxide; Methylamine; Octane; and Tetramethyl succinonitrile.

Rodent repellents Tin.

Rodenticide Barium; Chloropicrin; Cyanides; Lindane; Methyl bromide; Methyl parathion; Phosphine; Phosphorus; Pindone; Sodium fluoroacetate; Thallium; 1,1,1-Trichloroethane; and Warfarin.

Rodine based products o-Toluidine.

Roofing compounds/products
also see **Asphalt felt.** Aluminum; Asbestos; Creosotes; Lead; Mica; Polycyclic aromatic hydrocarbons; Titanium dioxide; and Triphenyl phosphate.

Room deodorizers *see* **Air deodorizers/fresheners.**

Room dividers Styrene.

Ropes Tin.

Rosins 2-Butanone.

Rotogravure printing Benzene.

Rubber Acetic acid; Acetone; Acetonitrile; Acrylonitrile; Aluminum; Ammonia; sec-Amyl acetate; Aniline; Antimony trioxide; Asbestos; Barium; Benzene; Benzyl chloride; 1,3-Butadiene; n-Butyl alcohol; Butylamine; Calcium oxide; Camphor; Carbon disulfide; Chlorinated diphenyl; Chlorobenzene; Chloroform; beta-Chloroprene; Chromium; Crotonaldehyde; Decaborane; Diborane; o-Dichlorobenzene; 1,2-Dichloroethylene; Diethylamine; Diglycidyl ether; Dimethylamine; Dimethylphthalate; Ethanolamine; Ethylene dichloride; N-Ethylmorpholine; Formaldehyde; Furfural; Hexachloroethane; Hydroquinone; Isopropylamine; Magnesium oxide; Mesityl oxide; Mica; Molybdenum; Morpholine; p-Nitrochlorobenzene; Nitrophenols; n-Nitrosodimethylamine; Oxalic acid; Paraldehyde; p-Phenylene diamine; Phthalic anhydride; Polychlorinated biphenyls; Propylene dichloride; Propylene imine; Pyridine; Quinone; Selenium; Styrene; Sulfur monochloride; Tellurium; 1,1,2,2-Tetrachloroethane; Tetrahydrofuran; Titanium dioxide; Toluene; o-Toluidine; Toluene; 1,1,2-Trichloroethane; Triethylamine; Vanadium pentoxide; Xylenes; Zinc chloride; and Zinc oxide.

Rubber, chlorinated 2-Nitropropane.

Rubber, latex Acetic acid; 1,3-Butadiene; Ethylamine; Ethylenediamine; Formaldehyde; Formic acid; and Phosphoric acid.

Rubber, silicone Benzoyl peroxide.

Rubber, synthetic Acetaldehyde; 2-Butanone; Chlorine; Cyclohexane; 1,1-Dichloroethane; Ethanol; Hydrogen chloride; Methyl chloride; alpha-Methyl styrene; Nitrobenzene; 1-Nitropropane; Phthalic anhydride; Sulfur monochloride; and Thiram.

Rubber cement Acetone; Benzene; 2-Butanone; Carbon disulfide; Ethylene dichloride; n-Hexane; Naphtha; and Toluene.

Rubber coatings Tetrachloroethylene.

Rubber dissolvers Sodium hydroxide.

Rubbing alcohol Ethanol, Hexone, and Isopropyl alcohol.

Rubefacient liniments Ethyl ether.

Rug cleaners/shampoos see listing for Carpet.

Rum Cresols; Ethanol; Hexone; and Methyl acetate.

Rum flavorings Ethyl formate and Isobutyl alcohol.

Rust proofing o-Dichlorobenzene; 2-Diethylaminoethanol; Petroleum distillates; Phosphoric acid; Toluene; and Xylenes.

Rust proofing metals Phosphoric acid.

Rust proofing paints Petroleum distillates and Toluene.

Rust removers Carbon disulfide; 1,1,2,2-Tetrachloroethane; and 1,1,1-Trichloroethane.

Saccharin *also see* **Sweeteners, artificial.** Naphtha.

Safety glass n-Butyl acetate; n-Butyl alcohol; Dimethylphthalate; Ethyl formate; and Vinyl acetate.

Safflower oil extraction n-Hexane.

Sandblasting Silica.

Sanitary lotions Hydrogen peroxide.

Sanitary napkins Acrylamide.

Sanitizers see Disinfectants.

Scotch whiskey Cresols and Ethanol.

Scouring compounds/powders Chlorine; Ethylene dichloride; Propylene dichloride; Silica; and 1,1,1-Trichloroethane.

Seafood Arsenic and Butylamine.

Sealants Asbestos; Ethyl acrylate; Furfuryl alcohol; Isobutyl acetate; Methylene bisphenyl isocyanate; Molybdenum; Tetrachloroethylene; and Toluene-2,4-diisocyanate.

Sealants, corrosion-resistant Furfuryl alcohol.

Sealing metal to glass Molybdenum.

Sedatives Bromine and Paraldehyde.

Seed disinfectants Calcium oxide.

Seed fungicides Copper.

Seed oil extraction Methyl bromide.

Semiconductors *also see* **listings for Electronics.** Ammonia; Antimony; Arsenic; Arsine; Cadmium; Carbon disulfide; Chlorine; Fluorides; Hydrazine; Hydrogen chloride; Phosphine; Polycyclic aromatic hydrocarbons; Selenium; Stibine; Tellurium; Thallium; Titanium dioxide; and Zinc oxide.

Sewage out-gassing Arsine.

Sewage treatment Calcium oxide; Carbaryl; and Formaldehyde.

Sex hormones, synthetic Ethyl formate.

Shaving creams Limonene and Propane.

Sheet lead Lead.

Sheet plastic Benzyl alcohol.

Shellacs Benzyl alcohol; n-Butyl alcohol; Cyclohexanol; Ethanol; Ethyl acetate; Ethylenediamine; Isopropyl acetate; Isopropyl alcohol; and Xylenes.

Shoe adhesive/cements n-Hexane; Trichloroethylene; and Triorthocresyl phosphate.

Shoe black Aniline.

Shoe dyes Furfural and Nitrobenzene.

Shoe polishes Ethyl acrylate; Isoamyl acetate; Titanium dioxide; and 1,1,1-Trichloroethane.

Shoes Acetone; Acetylene tetrabromide; Benzene; Cyclohexane; Di-sec octyl phthalate; Ethyl formate; n-Hexane; and Toluene.

Shower curtain, plastic Dibutylphthalate; Di-sec octyl phthalate; and Ethylene dichloride.

Shower drains Styrene.

Shower stalls Styrene.

Shutters Acrylonitrile and Styrene.

Signs Acrylonitrile and Aluminum.

Silicon carbide fibers Carbon monoxide.

Silicone Chlorobenzene; Cresols; Isophorone; Methyl chloride; Stibine; Tetrachloroethylene; Tin; 1,1,1-Trichloroethane.

Silicone chips Cresols.

Silicone lubricants Tetrachloroethylene and 1,1,1-Trichloroethane.

Silicone resins Chlorobenzene.

Silk Benzidine and Hydrogen peroxide.

Silk, artificial Chloroform; Diacetone alcohol; Ethyl acetate; Formaldehyde; Isoamyl acetate; Isoamyl alcohol; 1,1,2,2-Tetrachloroethane; and Zinc chloride.

Silk dyes Picric acid.

Silkscreening ink *also see* **Fabric/Textile printing.** Methyl cellosolve acetate.

Silver alloy Nickel and Thallium.

Silver extraction/recovery Cyanides and Formaldehyde.

Silver polishes Petroleum distillates.

Silverware Tin.

Silverware finishes, black Tellurium.

Skin freezing for medical purposes Dichlorodifluoromethane and Dichlorotetrafluoroethane.

Skin fresheners Zinc chloride.

Skin lotions *also see* **Body lotions.**

Skin stains Aniline.

Slimicides Acrolein; Methyl alcohol; and Pentachlorophenol.

Smog *also see* **Automotive exhaust and Diesel exhaust.** Nitrogen dioxide.

Smoke bombs Hexachloroethane; Phosphorus; and Zinc chloride.

Smoke screens Hexachloroethane; Phosphorus; and Polycyclic aromatic hydrocarbons.

Smoked foods Cresols.

Smokeless powders Acetone; 2-Butanone; Ethyl acetate; Ethyl ether; Isoamyl acetate; and Isoamyl alcohol.

Soap dishes Styrene.

Soap perfume *also see* **Perfumes and Fragrances.** Nitrobenzene.

Soaps Benzidine; Benzyl acetate; Boron; Boron trifluoride; Carbon dioxide; Cyclohexanol; Diborane; Decaborane; 2-Diethylaminoethanol; Diisobutyl ketone; Dimethylamine; Ethanol; Ethanolamine; Ethylene dichloride; Ethylene oxide; Iodine; Isopropyl alcohol; Limonene; Linalyl alcohol; Methyl n-amyl ketone; Naphtha; Nitrobenzene; Pentaborane; Phenyl ether; Phosphoric acid; Sodium hydroxide; Tetrachloroethylene; and Tin.

Soaps, liquid Isopropyl alcohol.

Soft drink bottles Xylenes.

Soft drinks *also see* **Beverages.**
Acetaldehyde; Isoamyl acetate; and Phosphoric acid.

Soil fumigants Chloropicrin; o-Dichlorobenzene; Dichloroethyl ether; 1,3-Dichloropropene; and Propylene dichloride.

Soil sterilants Formaldehyde; Propylene oxide; and 1,1,2,2-Tetrachloroethane.

Soldering materials Antimony; Arsine; Cadmium; Hydrazine; Lead; Silver; Tin; Triethylamine; and Zinc chloride.

Solid propellents Nitroethane.

Solvents Acetic acid; Acetic anhydride; Acetone; Acetonitrile; Acetylene tetrabromide; n-Amyl acetate; sec-Amyl acetate; Aniline; Benzene; Benzyl acetate; Benzyl alcohol; Bromine; 2-Butoxyethanol; n-Butyl acetate; sec-Butyl acetate; tert-Butyl acetate; n-Butyl alcohol; sec-Butyl alcohol; Carbon disulfide; Carbon tetrachloride; Chlorobenzene; Chloromethyl methyl ether; Crotonaldehyde; Cumene; Cyclohexane; Cyclohexanol; Diacetone alcohol; o-Dichlorobenzene; Dichlorodifluoromethane; 1,1-Dichloroethane; Dichloroethyl ether; 1,2-Dichloroethylene; Dichloromonofluoromethane; Dichlorotetrafluoroethane; Diethylamine; Diisobutyl ketone; Dimethyl acetamide; Dimethyl sulfate; Dimethylamine; Dimethylaniline; Dimethylformamide; Dimethylphthalate; Epichlorohydrin; Ethanol; 2-Ethoxyethyl acetate; Ethyl acetate; Ethylamine; Ethyl butyl ketone; Ethyl chloride; Ethylenediamine; Ethylene dibromide; Ethylene dichloride; Ethylene glycol; Ethyl ether; Ethyl formate; Fluorotrichloromethane; Formic acid; Furfural; Furfuryl alcohol; Hexachloroethane; Hexone; sec-Hexyl acetate; Hydrazine; Isoamyl acetate; Isoamyl alcohol; Isobutyl alcohol; Isophorone; Isopropyl acetate; Isopropyl alcohol; Isopropyl ether; Limonene; Mesityl oxide; Methyl acetate; Methylal; Methyl alcohol; Methylamine; Methyl n-amyl ketone;

Methyl bromide; Methyl cellosolve acetate; Methylene chloride; Methyl formate; Methyl hydrazine; Methyl isobutyl carbinol; Monomethyl aniline; Morpholine; Naphtha; Nitrobenzene; Nitroethane; Nitromethane; 1-Nitropropane; N-Nitrosodimethylamine; Octane; Paraldehyde; n-Pentane; Phenol; Propane; n-Propyl acetate; n-Propyl alcohol; Propylene dichloride; Propylene oxide; Sulfur dioxide; 1,1,2,2-Tetrachloroethane; Tetrahydrofuran; Toluene; 1,1,2-Trichloroethane; Triethylamine; Trifluorobromomethane; Turpentine; and Zinc chloride.

Soot remover Tetrachloroethylene.

Sorbic acid Crotonaldehyde.

Sorbitol Naphtha.

Soybean oil extraction n-Hexane.

Space vehicle windows Beryllium.

Spandex Dinitrobenzenes.

Spark plugs Molybdenum.

Spice extraction Ethylene dichloride and Methylene chloride.

Spice fumigants Ethylene oxide.

Spices Linalyl alcohol.

Spray paints Dichlorodifluoromethane; Dichloromonofluoromethane; Fluorotrichloromethane; and 1,1,1-Trichloroethane.

Stain/Spot cleaners or removers n-Amyl acetate; Benzene; Chloroform; Cyclohexanone; Dichloroethyl ether; Isopropyl ether; Naphtha; Oxalic acid; Propylene dichloride; Sodium hydroxide; Tetrachloroethylene; Toluene; 1,1,1-Trichloroethane; and Trichloroethylene.

Stain/Spot repellents 1,1,1-Trichloroethane.

Stainless steel Chromium; Iodine; Manganese; and Nickel.

Stains Aniline; Benzidine; Diisobutyl ketone; 2-Ethoxyethyl acetate; Ethylene glycol; n-Hexane; Stoddard solvent; and 1,1,1-Trichloroethane.

Stamp-pad inks Ethylene glycol.

Starch Epichlorohydrin.

Starch preservatives Pentachlorophenol.

Steel alloys Molybdenum.

Steel manufacturing 2,4-Dichlorophenol; Fluorides; Manganese; Selenium; and Vanadium pentoxide.

Steels, case hardening Barium.

Stencil inks Benzyl alcohol.

Sterilants Carbon dioxide; Chlorine; Crotonaldehyde; Dichlorodifluoromethane; Ethylene oxide; Formaldehyde; Hydrogen peroxide; beta-Propiolactone; Propylene oxide; 1,1,2,2-Tetrachloroethane; and Zinc chloride.

Sterling ware Silver.

Steroid recrystallization Acetonitrile and Cyclohexane.

Steroids Pyridine.

Storage tanks, lining material to protect Polycyclic aromatic hydrocarbons.

Stoves Asbestos.

Straw hats n-Amyl acetate; Isoamyl acetate; and Oxalic acid.

Straw products Hydrogen peroxide.

Strawberry flavors, artificial Isobutyl acetate.

Stucco Calcium oxide.

Styptic compounds Aluminum and Creosotes.

Sucrose Isobutyl alcohol.

Suede protectors Tetrachloroethylene and 1,1,1-Trichloroethane.

Sugar condensation Formaldehyde.

Sugar refining Acrylamide; Aluminum; Barium; and Calcium oxide.

Sugar syrups Titanium dioxide.

Sugar-bearing juices Phosphoric acid and Sulfur monochloride.

Sulfa drugs Naphtha and Pyridine.

Sunscreens Titanium dioxide.

Surface coatings Chlorinated diphenyl; Chlorobenzene; 2-Diethylaminoethanol; Ethanol; Ethyl acrylate; Ethyl methacrylate; Isobutyl alcohol; alpha-Methyl styrene; 2-Pentanone; Polychlorinated biphenyls; and Vinyl toluene.

Surgical instrument sterilization beta-Propiolactone.

Surgical suture packing Ethanol and Isopropyl alcohol.

Sweeteners, artificial Aniline; Methyl alcohol; Naphtha; and Triethylamine.

Swimming pool cleaners/disinfectants Bromine; Chlorine dioxide; 1,3-Dichloro-5,5-dimethylhydantoin; Iodine; Methyl chloride; and Silver.

Syrups Benzyl alcohol; Ethanol; Ethyl ether; Isoamyl acetate; Sulfur dioxide; and Titanium dioxide.

Tablecloths Di-sec octyl phthalate.

Tablet coatings Titanium dioxide.

Tar removers Chlorobenzene.

Tars o-Dichlorobenzene.

Taxidermy Formaldehyde and Mercury.

Tea, black Cresols.

Tear gas Acrolein; alpha-Chloroacetophenone; o-Chlorobenzylidene malononitrile; Chloropicrin; and Crotonaldehyde.

Teflon tubing 1,1,2-Trichloroethane.

Telecommunications Copper.

Telephones Styrene.

Telephotographic apparatus Selenium.

Television cabinets Styrene.

Television glass Lead.

Televisions Beryllium and Selenium.

Termiticides *see* **Acaricides.**

Terpene resins Limonene.

Theatrical smoke and fumes Carbon dioxide.

Thermocouple tubing Beryllium.

Thermo-electric devices Antimony.

Thermoplastic 1,3-Butadiene and 1,2-Dichloroethylene.

Tile drain cleaners Sulfur dioxide.

Tiles Barium; 2,3-Benzofuran; Benzyl chloride; Di-sec octyl phthalate; Fluorides; Styrene; Vanadium pentoxide; and Zinc oxide.

Tin plating Sodium hydroxide.

Tire cleaners 1,1,1-Trichloroethane.

Tires *also see* listings for **Rubber.** Benzene; 1,3-Butadiene; Mica; Styrene; Titanium dioxide; and Zinc oxide.

Tissue dehydration Acetone.

Tissue hardening Acetone.

Tissue-fixatives Acrolein and Formaldehyde.

Toasters Asbestos.

Tobacco Ethylene glycol.

Tobacco extraction Ethylene dichloride.

Tobacco leaf fumigants Phosphine.

Tobacco smoke *see* **Cigarette smoke.**

Tobacco wrappings Titanium dioxide.

Toilet bowl cleaners o-Dichlorobenzene, p-Dichlorobenzene, Phenol, and Zinc chloride.

Toilet deodorants Nitrobenzene.

Toilet paper Formaldehyde.

Toiletries Ethanol.

Tomatoes Cresols.

Tools Molybdenum.

Toothpaste *see* **Dentifrices.**

Topcoat lacquers Isobutyl acetate.

Topical medicines Benzyl alcohol; Camphor; Ethanol; Ethyl acetate; Hydroquinone; Methylal; Naphthalene; Propane; Titanium dioxide; Turpentine; and Zinc oxide.

Topical protectorates Zinc oxide.

Toys Di-sec octyl phthalate; Naphtha; Phenol; and Styrene.

Tracer bullets Phosphorus.

Transformers Chlorinated diphenyl and Polychlorinated biphenyls.

Transparent paper 2-Butanone.

Trees/wood 2-Butanone; Cresols; Formaldehyde; Limonene; and Linalyl alcohol.

Tungsten steel Carbon monoxide and Molybdenum.

Typesetting Cyclohexanone.

Typewriter correction fluids Ethylene dichloride; 1,1,1-Trichloroethane; and Trichloroethylene.

Typewriter ribbons Benzidine.

Underclothes Acetylene tetrabromide.

Upholstery *also see* **Fabrics/Textiles.** Di-sec octyl phthalate; Formaldehyde; Titanium dioxide; Trimellitic anhydride; Triphenyl phosphate; and Vinyl chloride.

Upholstery backcoatings Styrene.

Upholstery fumigants Ethylene dichloride and Ethylene oxide.

Upholstery shampoo Ammonia; Naphthalene; and Tetrachloroethylene.

Urethane Aniline; Ethylenediamine; N-Ethylmorpholine; Hydrazine; and Methylene chloride.

Vaccine preservatives Phenol.

Vaccine sterilants beta-Propiolactone.

Vaccines Ethyl acetate and Formaldehyde.

Varnish strippers/removers Acetone; Benzyl acetate; 2-Butoxyethanol; n-Butyl alcohol; Cyclohexane; Dichlorodifluoromethane; 1,1-Dichloroethane; 2-Ethoxyethyl acetate; Ethylene dichloride; Isobutyl alcohol; Mesityl oxide; Oxalic acid; and 1,2,3-Trichloropropane.

Varnish thinners Isobutyl acetate.

Varnish water-proofing Isoamyl acetate.

Varnishes Acetone; Allyl chloride; Aniline; Benzene; 2,3-Benzofuran; 2-Butanone; 2-Butoxyethanol; n-Butyl alcohol; Camphor; Carbon disulfide; Cyclohexanol; Dimethylphthalate; Epichlorohydrin; Ethyl acetate; Ethyl benzene; Ethyleneimine; Formaldehyde; Furfural; n-Hexane; Hexone; Hydroquinone; Isoamyl acetate; Manganese; Mesityl oxide; Methyl cellosolve; Naphtha; Stoddard solvent; Sulfur monochloride; 1,1,2,2-Tetrachloroethane; Titanium dioxide; 1,1,1-Trichloroethane; Trichloroethylene; Triorthocresyl phosphate; Triphenyl phosphate; Turpentine; Vanadium pentoxide; and Xylenes.

Vegetable fungicides Ferbam.

Vegetable oil, saturated 2-Nitropropane.

Vegetable oil extraction Acetonitrile; n-Hexane; Isopropyl ether; and Methyl alcohol.

Vegetable oil refining Barium, n-Butyl alcohol, n-Propyl alcohol, Sodium hydroxide, and Sulfur monochloride.

Vegetable preservatives Sulfur dioxide.

Vegetables, peeling Sodium hydroxide.

Vermicides Creosotes.

Veterinary deodorants Creosotes.

Veterinary medicines Acetic acid; Benzoyl peroxide; Benzyl alcohol; n-

Butyl alcohol; Carbon disulfide; Carbaryl; Creosotes; Dichlorotetrafluoroethane; Ethyl chloride; Ethylenediamine; Ethyl ether; Hexachloroethane; Hydrogen peroxide; Iodine; Lindane; Malathion; Naled; Nicotine; Nitric acid; p-Nitroaniline; Phenol; Phosphoric acid; Sodium hydroxide; Sulfur dioxide; and Zinc chloride.

Video tape cassettes Styrene.

Vinegar Acetic acid.

Vinyl 2-Butanone; n-Butyl acetate; Dibutylphthalate; Isophorone; Nitroethane; 1-Nitropropane; 2-Nitropropane; Tributyl phosphate; and Trimellitic anhydride.

Vinyl coatings 2-Nitropropane.

Vinyl fabrics Dibutylphthalate.

Vinyl films 2-Butanone.

Vinyl resins Ethyl acetate; 1-Nitropropane; and Tributyl phosphate.

Vitamin A Formaldehyde.

Vitamin B1 Methyl acrylate.

Vitamin B12 Cobalt.

Vitamin E Formaldehyde.

Vitamin extraction n-Butyl alcohol.

Vitamin intermediate Acetone.

Vitamins Formaldehyde; Methyl acrylate; Methyl alcohol; Pyridine; Tetrahydrofuran; and Xylenes.

Waferboard Formaldehyde; Methylene bisphenyl isocyanate; and Phenol.

Wall coverings *also see* **Wallpaper.** Vinyl chloride.

Wall paneling *see* **Plastic paneling.**

Wallboard Formaldehyde and Magnesium oxide.

Wallboard joint cement Mica.

Wallpaper sec-Amyl acetate and Chromium.

Wallpaper glue Mica and 1,1,1-Trichloroethane.

Wart removers Acetic acid; Carbon dioxide; and Nitric acid.

Wastewater disinfectants/treatments Chlorine dioxide; Chloroacetaldehyde; Hydrazine; and Hydrogen peroxide.

Water-based paints Naled and Titanium dioxide.

Water chlorination Chlorine and Methyl chloride.

Water clarification, drinking Acrylamide.

Water disinfectants Silver.

Water disinfectants, drinking Chloroform and Iodine.

Water purification Aluminum; Ammonia; Calcium oxide; Chlorine; Chlorine dioxide; Dichlorodifluoromethane; and Silver.

Water softening Calcium oxide and Ethylene dichloride.

Water sterilants beta-Propiolactone.

Water treatment Acrylamide; Aluminum; Ammonia; Bromine; Calcium oxide; Carbon dioxide; Chlorine; Chlorine dioxide; Chloroform; Dichlorodifluoromethane; 1,3-Dichloro-5,5-dimethylhydantoin; Dimethylamine; Epichlorohydrin; Iodine; Methyl chloride; Phosphoric acid; beta-Propiolactone; Silver; Sodium hydroxide; Sulfur dioxide; and Zinc chloride.

Waterless dyes Trichloroethylene.

Waterproofing/repellents Chlorinated diphenyl; Chloromethyl methyl ether; Creosotes; Di-sec octyl phthalate; Ethyleneimine; Formaldehyde; Hexachloronaphthalene; Isoamyl acetate; Methylene bisphenyl isocyanate; Methyl methacrylate; Octachloronaphthalene; Petroleum distillates; Polychlorinated biphenyls; Pyridine; Tetrachloroethylene; Toluene-2,4-diisocyanate; 1,1,1-Trichloroethane; and Triethylamine.

Waxes Acetone; Acetylene tetrabromide; Benzene; n-Butyl acetate; n-Butyl alcohol; Carbon disulfide; Chlorinated diphenyl; Chlorobenzene; Chloroform; Cyclohexane; Diacetone alcohol; o-Dichlorobenzene; Diethylamine; Ethyl chloride; Ethylenediamine; Ethylene dibromide; Ethylene dichloride; Ethyl ether; Isopropyl ether; Methyl cellosolve acetate; alpha-Methyl styrene; Morpholine; Nitroethane; Nitromethane; 1-Nitropropane; Paraldehyde; Pentachloronaphthalene; Phosphoric acid; Polychlorinated biphenyls; n-Propyl acetate; Propylene dichloride; 1,1,2,2-Tetrachloroethane; and 1,1,2-Trichloroethane.

Waxes, dissolving of Tetrachloroethylene.

Waxes, synthetic Hexachloronaphthalene and Tetrachloronaphthalene.

Weatherstripping Styrene.

Well water Arsenic.

Whiskey Ethanol; Isoamyl acetate; and Methyl acetate.

Wicker ware *also see* **listings for Straw.** Sulfur dioxide.

Wigs 1,1,1-Trichloroethane.

Windsurfing boards Acrylonitrile.

Wine Acetic acid; Cresols; Ethanol; Hydrogen peroxide; and Sulfur dioxide.

Wire coatings Tin and Vinyl chloride.

Wire enamels Cresols and Trimellitic anhydride.

Wire insulations *also see* **Electrical insulation.** beta-Chloroprene and Trimellitic anhydride.

Wire stripping compounds Formic acid.

Wood, hardening of Sulfur monochloride.

Wood cleaners Oxalic acid; Tetrachloroethylene; and 1,1,1-Trichloroethane.

Wood coatings Tetrachloronaphthalene.

Wood finish removers 1,1-Dichloroethane and Methylene bisphenyl isocyanate.

Wood fire retardants Ammonium sulfamate and Zinc chloride.

Wood fungicides Copper.

Wood industry Pentachloronaphthalene.

Wood preservatives Aluminum; Arsenic; Chromium; Copper; Creosotes; Cresols; o-Dichlorobenzene; 2,4-Dichlorophenol; Formaldehyde; Methyl alcohol; Naphthalene; Nitrophenols; Pentachlorophenol; Thiram; Tin; 2,4,6-Trichlorophenol; Xylidine; and Zinc chloride.

Wood putty/dough Benzidine and Turpentine.

Wood stains Aniline; Benzidine; 2-Ethoxyethyl acetate; Ethylene glycol; Stoddard solvent; and 1,1,1-Trichloroethane.

Wool Benzidine and Dichloroethyl ether.

Wool, carbonizing Zinc chloride.

Wool degreasers o-Dichlorobenzene and Methyl bromide.

Wool dyes Picric acid.

Wool fat extraction Acetic anhydride and Methyl bromide.

Wool moth-proofing Formaldehyde.

Wool shrink-proofing Bromine and Chlorine.

Wound covering gels Epichlorohydrin.

Wound sterilants Chlorine.

X-ray transmissions Beryllium.

Yeast Phosphoric acid.

Yeast growth medium Ethanol.

Zinc alloy Nickel.

5
Chemical Directory

Abbreviations

ACGIH	American Conference of Governmental Industrial Hygienists
ATSDR	Agency for Toxic Substances and Disease Registry
CDC	Center for Disease Control
EPA	Environmental Protection Agency
IDLH	Immediately dangerous to life and health. Unless otherwise noted NIOSH IDLH data are used.
LOAEL	Lowest observable adverse effects level
MG/M³	Milligrams per cubic meter
MRL	Minimal risk level (non-cancer)
NAS	National Academy of Science
NE	No evidence could be found for the existence of an IDLH
NIOSH	National Institute for Occupational Safety and Health
NOAEL	No observable adverse effects level
NRC	National Research Council
OSHA	Occupational Safety and Health Administration
OTS	Office of Toxic Substances
PEL	Permissible exposure level
PP/S	Personal protective equipment and/or sanitary measures required for PEL exposure
PPB	Part(s) per billion
PPM	Part(s) per million
REL	Recommended exposure level
TLV	Threshold Value Limits
TN	Trade names
µG/KG	Microgram per kilogram
µG/DL	Microgram per deciliter
Unknown	Lack of data

AA *see* **Allyl alcohol.**

Absolute ethanol *see* **Ethanol.**

Acetaldehyde *TN/synonyms:* Acetic aldehyde; Ethanal; Ethyl aldehyde; Methyl formaldehyde. *NIOSH:* Carcinogen at any exposure level. Reduce exposure to lowest feasible concentration. *OSHA PEL:* 100 ppm or 180 mg/m³ (8hr/day-40hr/wk-PP/S); 150 ppm or 270 mg/m³ (15 min not to be exceeded). *IDLH:* 10,000 ppm. *Symptoms:* Eye, nasal, and throat irritation; Cough; Conjunctivitis; Central nervous system depression; Eye and skin burns; Dermatitis; Delayed pulmonary edema; Tearing; Eyes become sensitive to light; Nasal mucosa inflammation; Bronchitis; Drowsiness; Nausea; Vomiting; Diarrhea; Albumin in urine; Respiratory paralysis and failure; Loss of sensation; Death; Auditory sensitivity changes; Chromosomal aberrations; DNA damage. Suspected of causing Cancer. *End-point Targets:* Respiratory system; Skin; Kidneys. *Usage:* Food flavoring and adjunct; Resins; Dyes; Perfumes; Plastics; Synthetic rubber; Silvering mirrors; Butter; Fruit juices; Milk products; Candy; Denatured alcohol; Pesticide intermediate; Lactic acid; Baked goods; Soft drinks; Fragrances; Chemical manufacturing; Photography; Fruit fumigant. *Synergistic effects:* Alcohol may increase the potential adverse health effects. *Note:* Symptoms of chronic exposure may resemble those of chronic alcoholism. There is no tolerance level on the amount of residue which may remain on the food after fumigation. *References:* 94, 279, 299, 304, 392.

p-Acetaldehyde *see* **Paraldehyde.**

Acetic acid *TN/synonyms:* Ethanoic acid; Glacial acetic acid; Methanecarboxlic acid. *NIOSH REL:* 10 ppm or 25 mg/m³ (10hr/day-40hr/wk); 15 ppm or 37 mg/m³ (15 min not to be exceeded). *OSHA PEL:* 10 ppm or 25 mg/m³ (8hr/day-40hr/wk). *IDLH:* 1,000

ppm. *Symptoms:* Nasal and throat irritation; Pharyngeal, eyelid, glottis, and pulmonary edema; Conjunctivitis; Tearing; Chronic bronchitis; Eye and nasal burns; Sensitive dermatitis; Dental erosion; Black skin; Cornea overgrowth; Heartburn; Constipation; Vomiting blood; Low blood pressure; Cardiac arrhythmias; Esophagus perforation; Bronchial pneumonia; Vomiting; Diarrhea; Destruction of red blood cells; Hemoglobin in urine; Absence of urine formation; Inability or difficulty swallowing; Circulatory shock; Respiratory inflammation; Lymph node hypertrophy; Gastric hemorrhage; Thirst; Membrane and tissue ulceration; Clammy skin; Weak and rapid pulse; Death; Esophageal, gastric, and pyloric strictures. *End-point Targets:* Respiratory system; Skin; Eyes; Teeth. *Usage:* Pesticide inert ingredient; Latex; Engraving; Plastics; Rubber; Leather tanning; Food preservative; Gums; Resins; Pharmaceutical aids; Insecticides; Photography; Canned foods; Food additive and flavoring; Dyes; Textiles; Fabric finishes; Nylon; Acrylic fabrics; Catsup; Mayonnaise; Pickles; Fungicide; Beet sugar; Wine; Vinegar; Facial prostheses; Wart removers; Solvent; Veterinary medicine; Medicine. *Contaminant:* Acetaldehyde. *References:* 46, 304, 305, 423.

Acetic acid anhydride *see* **Acetic anhydride.**

Acetic acid, ethenyl ester *see* **Vinyl acetate.**

Acetic acid, vinyl ester *see* **Vinyl acetate.**

Acetic aldehyde *see* **Acetaldehyde.**

Acetic anhydride *TN/synonyms:* Acetic acid anhydride; Acetic oxide; Acetyl oxide; Ethanoic anhydride. *OSHA PEL:* 5 ppm or 20 mg/m³ (ceiling limit, PP/S). *IDLH:* 1,000 ppm. *Symptoms:* Eye, nasal, pharyngeal, and skin irritation; Conjunctivitis; Tearing; Corneal swelling, opacity, and burns;

Eyes become sensitive to light; Cough; Labored or difficulty breathing; Bronchitis; Skin burns and vesiculation; Sensitive dermatitis; Mucous membrane corrosion; Inability or difficulty swallowing; Inhibits blood clotting; Epigastric pain; Nausea; Vomiting; Gastric hemorrhaging; Thirst; Ulceration of all tissue and membranes; Circulatory collapse; Shock; Glottis and conjunctiva swelling; Esophageal, gastric, and pyloric strictures; Renal failure; Liver and heart ischemic lesions; Clammy skin; Weak, rapid pulse; Shallow respiration; Asphyxia; Burning sensation in nasal and throat. *End-point Targets:* Respiratory system; Eyes; Skin. *Usage:* Pesticide inert ingredient; Cellulose; Solvent; Extracting wool fat; Glycerol; Oils; Resins; Synthetic fabrics; Plastics; Explosives; Perfumes; Food flavorings; Textiles; Acetanilide; Medicine; Aspirin; Acetaminophen; Modified food starch; Pharmaceuticals; Pesticide intermediate; Cigarette filters; Chemical intermediate and manufacturing. *Contaminant:* Acetaldehyde. Toxic by inhalation, ingestion, and dermal contact. *References:* 111, 304, 305, 423.

Acetic ester *see* **Ethyl acetate.**

Acetic ether *see* **Ethyl acetate.**

Acetic oxide *see* **Acetic anhydride.**

Acetone *TN/synonyms:* Dimethyl ketone; Ketone propane; Propanone; 2-Propanone; beta-Ketopropane; Methyl ketone. *NIOSH REL:* 250 ppm or 590 mg/m^3 (10hr/day-40hr/wk). *OSHA PEL:* 750 ppm or 1,800 mg/m^3 (8hr/day-40hr/wk-PP/S); 1,000 ppm or 2,400 mg/m^3 (not to exceed 15 min). *IDLH:* 1,000 ppm. *Symptoms:* Eye, nasal, and throat irritation; Belligerence; Blood poisoning; Alcoholic psychosis; Boastfulness; Bronchitis; Circulatory failure; Cold, pale skin; Coma; Collapse; Conjunctivitis; Convulsions; Death; Defatting dermatitis; Dilated pupils; Dizziness; Double vision; Drowsiness; Emotional effects; Exhilaration; Flushed face; Gastritis;

Gastroduodenitis; Headaches; Hearing loss; Heart rate over 100 beats per minute; Hypothermia; Impaired or absent tendon reflexes; Incontinence; Incoordination; Increased susceptibility to infection; Inflammation of airway, stomach, and duodenum; Liver injury; Loss of sensation; Low blood pressure; Nausea; Peripheral vascular collapse; Pharyngitis; Pneumonia; Profuse sweating; Rapid pulse; Remorse; Renal lesions; Respiratory failure; Restlessness; Sensory disturbances; Shock; Slowed reaction time; Slurred speech; Stupor; Talkativeness; Vertigo; Vomiting blood; Vomiting; Weakness. Suspected of causing adverse spermatogenic effects; Low birth weight; Neonate lethality. *End-point Targets:* Respiratory system; Eyes; Skin. *Usage:* Acetic acid; Acetic anhydride; Adhesives; Airplane dopes; Antiseptic; Bromoform; Cellulose; Chemical intermediate; Chloroform; Coatings; Diacetone alcohol; Dishwashing liquid; Explosives; Fats; Fiberglass; Fingernail polish remover; Food flavoring; Hardening and dehydrating tissues; Isoprene; Lacquers; Mesityl oxide; Modacrylic fibers; Oils, Paint and varnish removers; Paint thinner; Paraffin; Perfumes; Pesticide inert ingredient; Pharmaceutical aids; Pharmaceuticals; Photographic films; Plastics; Printing ink; Rayon; Resins; Rubber cement; Rubber; Shoes; Smokeless powder; Solvent; Varnishes; Vitamin intermediate; Waxes. *Classification:* Organic solvent (Ketone compound); Polar volatile organic compounds. *Note:* Found in the blood and urine in diabetes and other metabolic disorders. Neurotoxin. *References:* 61, 299, 304, 305, 384, 388, 423, 427, 429, 452, 463.

Acetonitrile *TN/synonyms:* Cyanomethane; Ethyl nitrile; Methyl cyanide. *NIOSH REL:* 20 ppm or 34 mg/m^3 (10hr/day-40hr/wk). *OSHA PEL:* 40 ppm or 70 mg/m^3 (8hr/day-40hr/wk-PP/S); 60 ppm or 105 mg/m^3 (not to exceed 15 min). *IDLH:* 4,000 ppm.

Symptoms: Eye irritation; Albumin in cerebrospinal fluid; Albumin in urine; Anxiety; Asphyxia; Bitter almond breath; Bitter taste; Cardiac and respiratory arrest; Chest pains; Coma; Confusion; Conjunctivitis; Constriction or numbness in throat; Death; Dermatitis; Dilated pupils; Dizziness; Excessive salivation; Foamy and bloodstained mouth; Foamy sputum; Gastric distress; Giddiness; Headaches; Incontinence; Increased blood pressure; Increased rate or depth of respiration; Labored or difficulty breathing; Lockjaw; Loss of appetite; Low blood pressure; Lower jaw stiffness; Nausea; Olfactory fatigue; Paralysis; Profuse sweating; Rapid, weak, and irregular pulse; Respiratory depression; Slow pulse and heart rate under 60 beats per minute; Stupor; Tonic, epileptiform, and opisthotono convulsions; Unconsciousness; Urine retention; Vertigo; Vomiting blood; Vomiting; Weakness. *End-point Targets:* Kidneys; Liver; Cardiovascular system; Central nervous system; Lungs; Skin; Eyes. *Usage:* Acrylic fibers; Chemical intermediate; Cosmetics; Fish, animal, and vegetable oil extraction; Paint; Perfumes; Pesticide inert ingredient; Pesticide intermediate; Pharmaceuticals; Photography; Plastics; Polymers; Resins; Rubber; Solvent; Steroid recrystallization. Found in the urine of cigarette smokers. Toxic by inhalation; ingestion; and skin contamination. *Classification:* Organic solvents (Nitrile compound). *Note:* Neurotoxin. *References:* 95, 299, 304, 383, 388, 423, 429, 463.

3-(alpha-Acetonyl)-benzyl-4-hydroxycoumarin *see* **Warfarin.**

1-Acetoxyethylene *see* **Vinyl acetate.**

alpha-Acetoxytoluene *see* **Benzyl acetate.**

Acetylene dichloride *see* **1,2-Dichloroethylene.**

Acetylene tetrabromide *TN/synonyms:* Symmetrical tetrabromoethane; TBE; Tetrabromoacetylene; Tetrabromoethane; 1,1,2,2-Tetrabromoethane. NIOSH found OSHA's documentation inadequate for PELs. *OSHA PEL:* 1 ppm or 14 mg/m³ (8hr/day-40hr/wk-PP/S). *IDLH:* 10 ppm. *Symptoms:* Eye and nasal irritation; Loss of appetite; Nausea; Severe headaches; Abdominal pain; Jaundice; Excessive monocytes in the blood; Delayed liver injury; Vomiting; Excess urobilin in urine; Bilirubin in urine; Kidney and lung damage; Central nervous system depression; Skin blistering. *End-point Targets:* Eyes; Upper respiratory system; Liver. *Usage:* Solvent; Fats; Oils; Waxes; Fluid in liquid gauges; Synthetic fibers; Fire retardant; Boots; Shoes; Underclothes; Polystyrene; Polyurethane; Polylefins; Terephthalic acid; Mineral oils. *References:* 91, 304, 388.

Acetylene tetrachloride *see* **1,1,2,2-Tetrachloroethane.**

Acetylene trichloride *see* **Trichloroethylene.**

Acetyl oxide *see* **Acetic anhydride.**

Acintene DP *see* **Limonene.**

Acquinite (tn) *see* **Chloropicrin.**

Acraldehyde *see* **Acrolein.**

Acritet *see* **Acrylonitrile.**

Acrolein *TN/synonyms:* Acraldehyde; Acrylaldehyde; Acrylic aldehyde; Allyl aldehyde; Propenal; 2-Propenal; Prop-2-en-1-al; 2-Propen-1-one; Aqualin; NSC 8819. *OSHA PEL:* 0.10 ppm or 0.25 mg/m³ (8hr/day-40hr/wk-PP/S); 0.30 ppm or 0.80 mg/m³ (15 min exposure limit). *ATSDR MRL:* 0.00005 ppm-less than 14 days 0.000009 ppm-more than 14 days *IDLH:* 5 ppm. *Symptoms:* Eye, skin, throat, mucous membranes, and upper respiratory irritation; Abnormal pulmonary function; Delayed pulmonary edema; Chronic respiratory disease; Tearing; Upper respiratory and pulmonary congestion; Airway occlusion; Death; Asphyxia; Emphysema; Epidermal tissue death; Tissue damage. Suspected of causing Cancer, Birth defects, Spontaneous abortions. *End-point Targets:* Eyes; Skin; Respiratory System. *Usage:* Livestock feeds; Pesticides; Slimicide; Paper; Herbicides; Algicide; Tear gas; Perfumes; Warning agent in refrigerant; Leather tanning; Electrical insulation; Poultry feed; Modified food starch; Military poison gas; Plastics; Glycerin; Acrylic acids and ethers; Glycerol; Polyurethane; Polyesters; Pharmaceuticals; Mollusicides; Tissue-fixative; Glutaraldehyde; Methinonine. Found naturally in burning trees and other plants, when fuels such as gasoline and oil are burned, and in cigarette smoke. *Metabolites:* Acrylic acid; Methyl acrylate; S-Carboxyethyl mercapturic acid methyl ester. *Additive:* Usually inhibited with hydroquinone. *Note:* The drug cycolphosphanide metabolizes into acrolein in the body. *References:* 96, 279, 299, 304, 319, 388, 392.

Acrylaldehyde *see* **Acrolein.**

Acrylamide *TN/synonyms:* Acrylamide monomer; Acrylic amide; Propenamide; 2-Propenamide. *NIOSH:* Carcinogen at any exposure level. *NIOSH REL:* 0.03 mg/m^3 (10hr/day-40hr/wk). *OSHA PEL:* 0.03 mg/m^3 (8hr/day-40hr/wk-PP/S). *ACGIH:* Suspected human carcinogen. *IDLH:* unknown. *Symptoms:* Eye and skin irritation; Incoordination; Numb limbs; Numbness, tingling, or prickling sensation; Muscle weakness; Absent deep tendon reflex; Hand sweats; Fatigue; Lethargy; Polyneuropathy; Brain dysfunction; Hallucinations; Tremors; Irritability; Nervousness; Anxiety; Depression; Headaches; Insomnia; Sexual disorders; Staggering gait. Suspected of causing Cancer. *End-point Targets:* Central nervous system; Peripheral nervous system; Skin; and Eyes. *Usage:*

Plastics; Paper; Sugar processing; Textiles; Concrete grout; Adhesives; Coatings; Diapers (infant and adult); Sanitary napkins; Agricultural water retention products; Petroleum processing; Absorbant materials; Drinking water clarification; Cellulose; Pesticide inert ingredient; Photography. Derivative of Acrylonitrile. *Note:* Historically established as a neurotoxin. *References:* 299, 304, 305, 388, 413, 423.

Acrylamide monomer *see* **Acrylamide.**

Acrylic aldehyde *see* **Acrolein.**

Acrylic amide *see* **Acrylamide.**

Acrylonitrile *TN/synonyms:* Acrylonitrile monomer; AN; Cyanoethylene; Propenenitrile; 2-Propenenitrile; VCN; Vinyl cyanide; Acritet; Caswell No. 101; ENT 54; Fumigran; Ventox. *NIOSH:* Carcinogen at any exposure level. *NIOSH REL:* 1 ppm (8hr/day-40hr/wk); 10 ppm (Ceiling limit, 15 min exposure). *OSHA PEL:* 2 ppm (8hr/day-40hr/wk-PP/S); 10 ppm (ceiling limit, 15 min exposure). *ACGIH:* Suspected human carcinogen. *ATSDR MRL:* 0.1 ppm (Inhalation, less than 15 days); 3.0 ppm (Ingestion, less than 15 days); 1.4 ppm (Ingestion, more that 14 days). *IDLH:* 500 ppm. *Symptoms:* Eye and nasal irritation; Headaches; Sneezing; Irritability; Apprehension; Impaired judgment; Asphyxia; Death; Upper respiratory oppression and congestion; Low grade anemia; Liver damage; Brain tumors; Mild jaundice; Skin itching, erythema, and desquamation; Slow healing; Collapse; Convulsions; Weakness in limbs; Labored, irregular breathing; Cyanosis; Vomiting; Weakness; Nausea; Lightheadedness; Skin vesiculation; Scaling dermatitis. Suspected of causing Birth defects, Reproductive effects, Cancer (lungs, prostate, intestines). *End-point Targets:* Cardiovascular system; Liver; Central nervous system; Skin. *Usage:* Plastics; Plastic food bags; Dyes; Pharmaceuti-

nervous system; Skin. *Usage:* Plastics; Plastic food bags; Dyes; Pharmaceuticals; Rubber; Paints; Fire retardant; Photography; Office and consumer electronics; Gutters; Drain pipes; Shutters; Mail boxes; Signs; Mobile home skirting; Outdoor furniture; Windsurfer boards; Side view mirrors; Vehicle grilles; Bumper covers; Aircraft parts; Golf clubs; Pesticide intermediate; Resins; Acrylics; Chemical manufacturing. No longer used as a Pesticide or Grain fumigants. *Metabolites:* Epoxide hydrase; Thiocyanate; 2-Cyanoethylene oxide; Rhodanase; Glutathionases; Hydroxyethyl mercapturic acid; Cyanorthylated mercapturic acid; Thiodiglycolic acid; Cuanohydroxethl mercapturic acid. *Additive:* Usually inhibited with methylhydroquinone. *Note:* Plastic food bags will leach Acrylontrile into food at 1 ppb. *References:* 304, 306, 329, 388, 412, 433.

Acrylonitrile monomer *see* **Acrylonitrile.**

Actinolite *see* **Asbestos.**

Actomar (tn) *see* **Iodine.**

Adronal *see* **Cyclohexanol.**

Adronol *see* **Cyclohexanol.**

Aerothene TT (tn) *see* **1,1,1-Trichloroethane.**

Aethylbenzyl *see* **Ethyl benzene.**

Ageflex FM-1 (tn) *see* **Ethyl methacrylate.**

Agricide Maggot Killer (tn) *see* **Chlorinated camphene.**

A-Gro (tn) *see* **Methyl parathion.**

AI3-08544 (tn) *see* **Iodine.**

Alcohol *see* **Ethanol.**

Alcohol anhydride *see* **Ethanol.**

Alcohol benzylique (tn) *see* **Benzyl alcohol.**

Algrain (tn) *see* **Ethanol.**

Algylen (tn) *see* **Trichloroethylene.**

Aliphatic petroleum naphtha *see* **Petroleum distillates.**

Allo-ocimenol *see* **Linalyl alcohol.**

Alltox (tn) *see* **Chlorinated camphene.**

Allyl alcohol *TN/synonyms:* AA; Allylic alcohol; 1-Propene-3-ol; Propenol; 2-Propenol; Vinyl cabinol. *OSHA PEL:* 2 ppm or 5 mg/m³ (8hr/day-40hr/wk-PP/S); 4 ppm or 10 mg/m³ (not exceed 15 min). *IDLH:* 150 ppm. *Symptoms:* Eye, upper respiratory, and skin irritation; Pulmonary edema; Dermatitis; Death; Skin burns; Tissue or bone death; Tissue damage; Corneal tissue death; Temporary blindness; Liver congestion; Blood in urine; Kidney inflammation; Tearing; Photosensitivity; Blurred vision; Pain behind the eyes. *End-point Targets:* Eyes; Skin; Respiratory system. *Usage:* Herbicides; Pesticides; Pesticide inert ingredient; Food flavorings; Perfumes; Dentures; Resins; Fungicide; Plasticizers; Fire retardants; Pharmaceutical intermediate; Glycerol; Acrolein; Military poison. *References:* 51, 304, 388, 423.

Allyl aldehyde *see* **Acrolein.**

Allyl chloride *TN/synonyms:* 3-Chloropropene; 1-Chloro-2-propene; 3-Chloropropylene. *OSHA PEL:* 1 ppm or 3 mg/m³ (8hr/day-40/wk-PP/S); 2 ppm or 6 mg/m³ (not to exceed 15 minutes). *IDLH:* 300 ppm. *Symptoms:* Eye, nasal, respiratory, and skin irritation; Pulmonary edema; Eye pains; Liver and kidney injury; Conjunctivitis; Reddening of eyelids; Corneal burns; Excess sodium in blood; Potassium in blood; Excessive protein in blood; Polyneuropathy; Peripheral nerve degeneration of axons and myelin sheaths; Death; Unconsciousness; Corneal burns. *End-point Targets:* Respiratory system; Skin; Eyes. *Usage:* Resins; Plastics; Varnishes; Adhesives; Insecticide manufacturing; Polyesters; Pharmaceuticals; Diuretics; Barbiturates; Aprobatbital; Butalbital methohexital sodium; Secobarbital; Talbutal; Thiamyl sodium; Hypnotic drugs; Epichlorohydrin; Allyl ethers; Allyl isocyanate; Dibromochloropropane. *Classification:* Organic solvent. *References:* 47, 304, 383, 388.

Allylic alcohol *see* **Allyl alcohol.**

Allyl trichloride *see* **1,2,3-Trichloropropane.**

Alnico *see* **Nickel.**

Aluminum *Compounds:* Aluminum chloride; Aluminum chorohydrate; Aluminum hydroxide; Aluminum lactate; Aluminum nitrate; Aluminum oxide; Aluminum phosphate; Aluminum isopro-pylate; Aluminum fluoride; Stearic acid (aluminum salt); Sulfuric acid (aluminum sodium salt); Aluminum ammonium sulfate; Aluminum palmitate; Triethyl aluminum; Aluminum phosphide. *OSHA PEL:* 10 mg/m^3 (metal dust) or 5 mg/m^3 (powders and welding fumes) or 2 mg/m^3 (salts and alkyls) (8hr/day-40hr/wk); 20 mg/m^3 (metals and oxides) (exposure not to exceed 15 minutes). *Symptoms:* Cough; Pulmonary fibrosis; Bone diseases; Increase in softness in bones; Skin sensitization; Brain dysfunction; Interferes with DNA; Alters sister chromatic exchange; Decreases cell division; Interacts with DNA in the formation of neurofibrillary tangles in the brain; Developmental effects. Suspected of causing Alzheimer's Disease. *Endpoint Targets:* Respiratory system. *Usage:* Cooking utensils; Appliances; Building materials; Aluminum foil; Deodorants; Antiperspirants; Antacids; Aspirin; Cosmetics; Pharmaceuticals; Hemorrhoid creams; Feminine hygiene products; Automotive parts; Aircraft parts; Electrical conductors; Highway signs; Fencing; Food and beverage cans; Food additive; Pickles; Cheese; Flour; Baking powder; Dental crowns; Dentures; Paint; Protective coatings; Fireworks; Water purification; Sugar refining; Rubber; Lubricants;

Wood preservatives; Cosmetic astringents; Leather; Glues; Disinfectants; Asphalt felts and coatings; Pesticide inert ingredient; Roofing compounds; Fiberglass; Styptic compounds. *Note:* Aluminum exposure may occur during dialysis. Historically established as a neurotoxin. *Natural aluminum minerals:* bentonite and zeolite. *References:* 340, 388, 413, 423, 429.

4-Amino aniline *see* **p-Phenylene diamine.**

Aminobenzene *see* **Aniline.**

1-Aminobutane *see* **Butylamine.**

Aminodimethylbenzene *see* **Xylidine.**

Aminoethane *see* **Ethylamine or Methylamine.**

2-Aminoethanol *see* **Ethanolamine.**

beta-Aminoethyl alcohol *see* **Ethanolamine.**

Aminoethylene *see* **Ethyleneimine.**

para-Aminonitrobenzene *see* **p-Nitroaniline.**

2-Aminopropane *see* **Isopropylamine.**

alpha-Aminopyridine *see* **2-Aminopyridine.**

2-Aminopyridine *TN/synonyms:* alpha-Aminopyridine; alpha-Pyridylamine. *OSHA PEL:* 0.5 ppm or 2.0 mg/m^3 (8hr/day-40hr/wk-PP/S). *IDLH:* 5 ppm. *Symptoms:* Headaches; Dizziness; Excitement; Nausea; High blood pressure; Respiratory distress; Weakness; Stupor; Convulsions; Intense sweating; Thirst; Psychotic-like behavior; Tremors; Labored or difficulty breathing; Respiratory arrest; Hyperexcitability; Periorbital numbness, tingling, or prickling sensations; Elevated blood pressure; Disagreeable taste; Burning throat; Abdominal discomfort; Acidosis; Coma; Paralysis; Death. *Endpoint Targets:* Central nervous system;

Respiratory system. *Usage:* Medicine; Antihistamines; Hair coloring; Pyridine; Sodamide. Derivatives are used in hair coloring products. *References:* 44, 304, 388.

o-Aminotoluene *see* **o-Toluidine.**

2-Aminotoluene *see* **o-Toluidine.**

Aminoxylene *see* **Xylidine.**

Ammate herbicide *see* **Ammonium sulfamate.**

Ammonia *TN/synonyms:* Anhydrous ammonia; Aqua ammonia; Aqueous ammonia; Ammonium hydroxide; Spirits of hartshorn. *NIOSH REL:* 25 ppm or 18 mg/m³ (10hr/day-40hr/wk); 35 ppm or 27 mg/m³ (exposure not to exceed 15 min). *OSHA PEL:* 35 ppm or 27 mg/m³ (exposure not to exceed 15 min-PP/S). *ATSDR MRL:* 0.5 ppm (Inhalation, less than 14 days); 0.3 ppm (Inhalation, more than 365 days); 10.0 ppm (Ingestion, more than 15 days). *IDLH:* 500 ppm. *Symptoms:* Eye, nasal, throat, and respiratory irritation; Eye, skin, and respiratory burns; Labored or difficulty breathing; Bronchial spasms; Chest pain; Pulmonary edema; Pink frothy sputum; Skin burns and vesiculation; Upper gastrointestinal damage and hemorrhaging; Renal failure; Liver damage; Death; Airway occlusion; Respiratory failure; Bronchial pneumonia; Laryngeal swelling; Mucous membrane secretions; Blurred vision; Nonspecific brain dysfunction; Loss of consciousness; Decreased deep tendon reflexes. *End-point Targets:* Respiratory system; Eyes. *Usage:* Fertilizer; Synthetic fibers; Plastics; Explosives; All-purpose cleaning products; Oven cleaners; Urea resins; Refrigerant; Corrosion inhibitor; Water purification; Paper products; Metallurgy; Rubber; Food; Beverages; Leather tanning; Pharmaceuticals; Fiberglass; Semiconductors and related devices; Chemical manufacturing; Cement; Pesticide inert ingredient; Rug, carpet, and upholstery shampoo; Glass cleaners. *Note:* Neurotoxin. *References:* 8, 304, 323, 384, 388, 423, 429, 463.

Ammonium aminosulfonate *see* **Ammonium sulfamate.**

Ammonium hydroxide *see* **Ammonia.**

Ammonium sulfamate *TN/synonyms:* Ammate herbicide; Ammonium aminosulfonate; Monoammonium salt of sulfamic acid; Sulfamate. *OSHA PEL:* 10 mg/m³ (Total); 5 mg/m³ (Respiratory). *IDLH:* 5,000 mg/m³. *Symptoms:* Eye, nasal, and throat irritation; Cough; Breathing difficulty; Gastrointestinal disturbances. *End-point Targets:* Upper respiratory system; Eyes. *Usage:* Herbicide; Cigarette paper; Fire retardant; Cellulose; Textiles; Paper; Flame-proofing wood; Cleaners; Electroplating. *Note:* Added to cigarette paper to reduce the risk of tumor formation. *References:* 92, 304, 388.

Amorphous silica *TN/synonyms:* Diatomaceous earth; Diatomaceous silica; Diatomite; Silica gel; Silicon dioxide (amorphous). *NIOSH:* No REL, notified OSHA that documentation doesn't support the worker's safety at established PELs. *OSHA PEL:* 6 mg/m³ (8hr/day-40hr/wk). *IDLH:* NE. *Symptoms:* Pneumoconiosis. *End-point Targets:* Respiratory system. *Usage:* Pesticide inert ingredient; Photocopy ink, toner, and developer. *References:* 304, 388, 423, 459, 460.

Amosite *see* **Asbestos.**

AMS *see* **alpha-Methyl styrene.**

n-Amyl acetate *TN/synonyms:* Amyl acetic ester; Amyl acetic ether; 1-Pentanol acetate; Pentyl ester of acetic acid; Primary amyl acetate. *OSHA PEL:* 100 ppm or 525 mg/m³ (8hr/day-40hr/wk-PP/S). *IDLH:* 4,000 ppm. *Symptoms:* Eye, nasal, throat, and skin irritation; Unconsciousness due to narcotic effects; Dermatitis; Headaches; Muscle weakness; Giddiness; Incoordination; Confusion; Delirium; Coma;

Nausea; Vomiting; Diarrhea; Cough; Labored or difficulty breathing; Respiratory failure; Death; Gastrointestinal hemorrhage; Renal damage; Glucose in urine; Liver damage; Hemoglobin oxidizes into ferric form; Vision disturbances. *End-point Targets:* Eyes; Skin; Respiratory system. *Usage:* Pesticide inert ingredient; Solvent; Lacquers; Paints; Penicillin extraction; Photographic film; Leather polish; Warning agent; Food flavorings; Fabric printing and finishes; Textiles; Fluorescent lamps; Spot remover; Dry cleaning; Artificial fruit flavoring; Straw hats; Dissolves plastics; Degreaser; Medication; Insect repellents; Pesticide; Miticide; Furniture polish; DNA binding antibiotics. *Note:* Neurotoxin. *References:* 8, 175, 304, 388, 423, 463.

sec-Amyl acetate *TN/synonyms:* 1-Methylbutyl acetate; 2-Pentanol acetate; 2-Pentyl ester of acetic acid; 2-Pentyl acetate. *OSHA PEL:* 125 ppm or 650 mg/m³ (8hr/day-40hr/wk-PP/S). *IDLH:* 9,000. *Symptoms:* Eye, nasal, and upper respiratory irritation; Unconsciousness due to narcotic effects; Dermatitis; Central nervous system depression; Neurotic effects. *End-point Targets:* Respiratory system; Eyes; Skin. *Usage:* Solvent; Nitrocellulose; Cellulose; Artificial leather; Celluloid; Cements; Paper; Lacquers; Leather finishes; Linoleum; Fingernail polish; Plastic wood; Textile sizing; Printing compounds; Washable wallpaper; Rubber; Metallic paint; Perfumes; Pearlescent coating on artificial pearls. *References:* 224, 304, 388.

Amyl acetic ester *see* **n-Amyl acetate.**

Amyl acetic ether *see* **n-Amyl acetate.**

Amyl ethyl ketone *see* **5-Methyl-3-heptanone.**

Amyl methyl ketone *see* **Methyl n-amyl ketone.**

n-Amyl methyl ketone *see* **Methyl n-amyl ketone.**

AN *see* **Acrylonitrile.**

Anamenth (tn) *see* **Trichloroethylene.**

Anhydrol (tn) *see* **Ethanol.**

Anhydrotrimellitic acid *see* **Trimellitic anhydride.**

Anhydrous ammonia *see* **Ammonia.**

Anhydrous hydrogen chloride *see* **Hydrogen chloride.**

Anhydrous hydrogen fluoride *see* **Hydrogen fluoride.**

Anhydrous methylamine *see* **Methylamine.**

Aniline *TN/synonyms:* Aminobenzene; Aniline oil; Benzenamine; Phenylamine. *NIOSH:* Carcinogen at any exposure level. *OSHA PEL:* 2 ppm or 8 mg/m³ (8hr/day-40hr/wk-PP/S). *IDLH:* 100 ppm. *Symptoms:* Eye irritation; Anemia; Bladder wall ulceration and tissue death; Blood or hemoglobin in urine; Cardiovascular collapse; Chocolate colored blood; Coma; Confusion; Convulsions; Cyanosis; Death; Dermatitis; Destruction of red blood cells; Diminished amount of urine; Disorientation; Dizziness; Drowsiness; Dry throat; Granules in red blood cells; Headaches; Heart rate over 100 beats per minute; Incoordination; Irritability; Kidney, liver, spleen, and corneal damage; Labored or difficulty breathing; Lethargy; Loss of appetite; Nausea; Navy blue or blue lips, tongue, and mucous membrane; Painful urination; Photosensitivity; Respiratory paralysis; Ringing or tingling in the ear; Slate gray skin; Vertigo; Vision weakness; Vomiting; Weakness; Weight loss. Suspected of causing Cancer (bladder). *End-point Targets:* Blood; Cardiovascular system; Liver; Kidneys. *Usage:* Pesticide inert ingredient; Resins; Varnishes; Perfumes; Shoe black; Solvent; Printing inks; Cloth (laundry) marking ink; Photography; Explosives; Herbicide; Fungicide; Dyes; Paper; Lacquers; Wood stains; Skin stains; Cellulose; Polyurethanes; Urethane foams; Petroleum refining; Pigment; Rubber; Artificial sweeteners; Pharmaceutical dyes; Pesticide intermediate. Derivative of Benzene. *Classification:* Aromatic amine. *Note:* Infant deaths have occurred from exposure to laundry marking ink on diapers. Aniline has antipyretic action but is too toxic to use as medicine. Historically established as a neurotoxin. *References:* 109, 304, 385, 388, 413, 423, 463.

Aniline oil *see* **Aniline.**

Ankilostin (tn) *see* **Tetrachloroethylene.**

Annulene *see* **Benzene.**

Anol *see* **Cyclohexanol.**

Anprolene (tn) *see* **Ethylene oxide.**

Anthophyllite *see* **Asbestos.**

Antimony *TN/synonyms:* Antimony powder; Stibium; Antimony black. *Compound:* Antimony trioxide-Antimonious oxide; Antimony oxide; Diantimony trioxide; Flowers of Antimony; Antimony sesquioxide; Senmarmontite; Valentinite; HP (tn); LP (tn); White Star (tn); White Star M (tn); KR-LTS (tn); Thermoguard S (tn); Thermoguard L (tn); H grade (tn); L Grade (tn); Fire Shield H (tn); Fire Shield L (tn); Montana Brand (tn). *OSHA PEL:* 0.5 mg/m³ (8hr/day-40hr/wk). *IDLH:* 80 mg/m³. *Symptoms:* Eye, nasal, throat, mouth, skin, and respiratory irritation; Cough; Dizziness; Headaches; Nausea; Vomiting; Diarrhea; Stomach cramps; Insomnia; Loss of appetite; Inability to smell properly; Pneumoconiosis; Altered Electrocardiogram reading; Increased blood pressure; Abnormal stress and ulcers; Dermatosis; Airway occlusion; Bronchial spasms; Wheezing; Spontaneous abortions; Menstruation disturbances;

Metallic taste; Cardiac depression; Sweating; Metal fume fever; Suspected of causing DNA damage; Chromosomal breakage and aberrations; and Viral transformation. *End-point Targets:* Respiratory system; Cardiovascular system; Skin; Eyes. *Usage:* Automobile batteries; Solder; Sheet metal; Pipes; Bearing metal; Bearings; Castings; Ammunition; Cable sheathing; Pewter; Semiconductors; Aluminum; Gallium; Inferred detectors; Thermoelectric devices. *Antimony trioxide:* Fire retardant; Plastics; Textiles; Rubber; Adhesives; Paper; Pigments; Paint; Ceramics; Pesticide inert ingredient. *References:* 283, 299, 304, 305, 370, 385, 423, 429.

Antimony black *see* **Antimony.**

Antimony hydride *see* **Stibine.**

Antimony powder *see* **Antimony.**

Antimony trihydride *see* **Stibine.**

Antisal 1 (tn) *see* **Tetrachloroethylene.**

Aqua ammonia *see* **Ammonia.**

Aqua fortis *see* **Nitric acid.**

Aqualin *see* **Acrolein.**

Aqueous ammonia *see* **Ammonia.**

Aqueous hydrogen chloride *see* **Hydrogen chloride.**

Aqueous hydrogen fluoride *see* **Hydrogen fluoride.**

Aqueous methylamine *see* **Methylamine.**

Argentum *see* **Silver.**

Argentum crede *see* **Silver.**

Aroclor (tn) *see* **Polychlorinated biphenyls.**

Arsenic *TN/synonyms:* Arsenic black; Colloidal arsenic; Gray arsenic. *Compounds:* Arsenic acid; Arsenic pentoxide; Arsenic trioxide; Calcium arsenate; Gallium arsenide; Sodium arsenate; Sodium arsenite; Arsenilic acid; Arsenobetaine; Dimethylarsinic acid; Disodium methanearsonate; Methanearsonic acid; 3-Nitro-4-hydroxy-phenylarsonic acid; Sodium arsenilate; Sodium dimethylarsinate; Sodium methanearsonate. *NIOSH:* Carcinogen at any exposure level. *NIOSH REL:* 0.002 mg/m³ (ceiling exposure of 15 min). *OSHA PEL:* 0.010 mg/m³ (8hr/day-40hr/wk-PP/S). *NOAEL:* Between 0.0005 and 0.01 ug/kg/day (Ingestion). *IDLH:* 100 mg/m³. *Symptoms:* Nasal, throat, lung, skin, respiratory, and gastrointestinal mucosa irritation; Abnormal decrease in white blood cells; Altered electrocardiograms; Anemia; Anxiety; Birth defects; Blackfoot disease (loss of circulation in fingers and toes); Brain dysfunction; Bronchitis; Cancer (skin, lung); Cardiac arrhythmias; Cardiopulmonary collapse; Chromosomal aberrations; Coma; Confusion; Contact dermatitis; Convulsions; Cyanosis; Death; Dehydration; Depression; Depression of red or white blood cells; Dermatitis; Destruction of red blood cells; Diarrhea; Distal axon degeneration; Elevated serum enzyme levels; Emotional lability; Fatigue; Garlic breath; Gastrointestinal disturbances; Hallucinations; Headaches; Heart rate over 100 beats per minute; Hoarseness; Hyperpigmentation of skin with interspersed spots of hypopigmentation; Impaired memory; Impaired respiratory function; Insomnia; Irritability; Kidney inflammation; Lassitude; Loss of reflexes; Low birth weight; Metal fume fever; Metallic taste; Nasal mucosa inflammation; Nausea; Nervousness; Numbness in hands and feet; Numbness, tingling, or prickling sensation; Overgrowths of the skin; Painful pins and needles sensation; Paralysis; Peripheral and central neuropathy; Premature ventricular contractions; Pulmonary edema and hemorrhagic lesions; Raynaud's Disease; Removes the myelin sheath from nerves; Respiratory distress; Sexual disorders; Shock; Skin diseases and lesions; Spontaneous abortions; Swollen and tender liver; Tissue damage; Ulceration of nasal septum; Vascular lesions; Vomiting; Weakness; Wrist or ankle drop. *End-point Targets:* Liver; Kidneys; Skin; Lungs; Lymphatic system. *Usage:* Medicine; Lime manufacturing; Automobile batteries; Asphalt; Asphalt felts and coatings; Lead and copper refining; Wood preservative; Pesticides; Insecticides; Pesticide, herbicide, and algicide inert ingredients; Growth stimulants for plants and animals; Lead oxide; Glass; Electronics; Semiconductors; Metallurgy; Pigments; Electroplating. Found in well water and seafood. *Synergistic effects:* Reacts with hydrogen gas to form the highly toxic gas arsine. *Note:* Humans appear to be more susceptible to arsenic than animals. Animal studies suggest that low levels of arsenic may be beneficial. Historically established as a neurotoxin. *References:* 284, 299, 304, 306, 357, 388, 410, 413, 423, 429, 449.

Arsenic black *see* **Arsenic.**

Arsenic hydride *see* **Arsine.**

Arsenic trihydride *see* **Arsine.**

Arseniuretted hydrogen *see* **Arsine.**

Arsenous hydride *see* **Arsine.**

Arsine *TN/synonyms:* Arsenic hydride; Arsenic trihydride; Arseniuretted hydrogen; Arsenous hydride; Hydrogen arsenide. *NIOSH:* Carcinogen at any exposure level. *NIOSH REL:* 0.002 mg/m³ (ceiling exposure of 15 min). *OSHA PEL:* 0.05 ppm or 0.2 mg/m³ (8hr/day-40hr/wk). *IDLH:* 6 ppm. *Symptoms:* Headaches; Malaise; Weakness; Dizziness; Labored or difficulty breathing; Abdominal and back pain; Nausea; Vomiting; Bronze skin; Blood in urine; Destruction of red blood cells; Jaundice; Peripheral neuropathy; Inability to urinate; Liver damage; Cardiac damage; Diarrhea; Dermatitis; Thickening of skin on hands and feet; Electrocardiogram abnormalities;

Decrease in red and white blood cells; Cancer (skin). *End-point Targets:* Blood; Kidneys; Liver. *Usage:* Semiconductors and related devices; Soldering; Glass etching; Lead plating; Aluminum manufacturing. Found in Sewage out-gassing; Burning coal or batteries. *Note:* Symptoms are generally delayed from 2 to 48 hours after exposure. Historically established as a neurotoxin. *References:* 304, 306, 308, 388, 413, 429.

Artic (tn) *see* **Methyl chloride.**

Artificial ant oil *see* **Furfural.**

Asbestos *TN/synonyms:* Actinolite; Amosite; Cummingtonitegrunerite; Anthophyllite; Chrysotile; Crocidolite; Tremolite. *NIOSH:* Carcinogen at any exposure rate. *NIOSH REL:* 0.1 fiber/cm³ (10hr/day-40hr/wk). *OSHA PEL:* 0.2 fiber/cm³ (8hr/day-40hr/wk). *ACGIH:* Confirmed human carcinogen. *ACGIH TLV:* Amosite-0.5 fiber/cm³ or Chrysotile-2.0 fiber/cm³ or Crocidolite-0.2 fiber/cm³ or Other forms-2.0 fiber/cm³ (8hr/day-40/wk). *IDLH:* Carcinogen. *Symptoms:* Labored or difficulty breathing; Interstitial fibrosis; Restricted pulmonary function; Finger clubbing; Cancer; Immune system depression; Asbestosis; Mesothelioma; Pleural disease. *Endpoint Targets:* Lungs. *Usage:* Friction products such as automobile clutch, brake, and transmission components; Paper products; Cement products (pipe); Textiles; Packing and gaskets; Coatings and sealants; Asbestos-reinforced plastics; Roofing products; Asphalt felt and coatings; Consumer products such as toasters, stoves, refrigerators, etc.; Pesticide inert ingredient; Rubber. *References:* 304, 306, 322, 388, 407, 423.

Asymmetrical dichloroethane *see* **1,1-Dichloroethane.**

Aurum paradoxum *see* **Tellurium.**

Azabenzene *see* **Pyridine.**

Azine *see* **Pyridine.**

Azinphos-methyl *TN/synonyms:* Guthion; O,O-Dimethyl-S-4-oxo-1,2, 3-benzotriazan-3(4H)-ylmethyl phosphorodithioate; Methyl azinphos. *OSHA PEL:* 0.2 mg/m³ (8hr/day-40hr/wk-PP/S). *IDLH:* 20 mg/m³. *Symptoms:* Abdominal cramps; Apathy; Asphyxia; Blurred vision; Bronchial constriction; Cardiac arrhythmias; Cardiac irregularities; Coma; Confusion; Constricted pupils; Convulsions; Cyanosis; Death; Diarrhea; Difficulty in breathing; Dilated pupils; Dimness of vision; Disorientation; Drowsiness; Emotional instability; Excessive dreaming; Excessive salivation; Eye pain; Giddiness; Headaches; Heart rate over 100 beats per minute; Heart rate under 60 beats per minute; High blood pressure; Hypothermia; Incontinence; Incoordination; Inhibits cholinesterase; Insomnia; Laryngeal spasms; Loss of appetite; Low blood pressure; Muscle twitching and involuntary contractions; Nasal discharge; Nausea; Neurosis; Nightmares; Paralysis; Profuse sweating; Pulmonary rales; Respiratory failure; Restlessness; Slurred speech; Tearing; Tight chest; Vertigo; Vomiting; Weakness; Wheezing. *End-point Targets:* Respiratory system; Central nervous system; Cardiovascular system; Blood cholinesterase. *Usage:* Insecticide; Acaricide; Mollusicide. *Classification:* Organophosphate. *Note:* Historically established as a neurotoxin. *References:* 48, 304, 388, 413, 463.

Azirane *see* **Ethyleneimine.**

Aziridine *see* **Ethyleneimine.**

Azofos (tn) *see* **Methyl parathion.**

Azophos (tn) *see* **Methyl parathion.**

Banana oil *see* **Isoamyl acetate.**

Barion ion *see* **Barium.**

Barium *TN/synonyms:* Elemental barium; Barion ion. *Compounds:* Barium acetate; Barium carbonate;

Barium nitrate; Barium dinitrate; Barium dichloride; Barium chloride; Barium cyanide; Barium hydroxide; Barium oxide; Barium sulfate; Barium sulfide. *OSHA PEL:* 0.5 mg/m³ (8hr/day-40hr/wk-PP/S). *OSHA IDLH:* 1,100 mg/m³. *NIOSH IDLH:* 250 mg/m³). *Symptoms:* Eye, skin, and upper respiratory irritation; Absence of deep tendon reflexes; Brain congestion and swelling; Cardiac arrhythmias and failure; Changes in heart physiology; Changes in metabolism; Convulsions; Death; Decreased and increased blood potassium levels; Diarrhea; Gastrointestinal hemorrhages and inflammation; Increased blood pressure; Liver degeneration; Muscle spasms, weakness, and paralysis; Myocardial damage; Numbness and tingling of the mouth and neck; Pneumonoconiosis; Premature constriction of the heart; Renal failure, insufficiency, and degeneration; Respiratory failure; Skin burns; Slow pulse; Vomiting. *End-point Targets:* Cardiovascular system; Central nervous system; Skin; Respiratory system; Eyes. *Usage:* Medicine; Oil and gas drilling; Paint; Plastics; Case hardening steels; Bricks; Tiles; Lubricating oils; Jet fuel; Pesticide inert ingredient; Insecticides; Glass; Rubber; Ceramics; Photography; Chemical manufacturing; Rodenticide; Paper; Pigments; Textile dyes; Sugar refining; Animal and vegetable oil refining; Oils and fuels additive; Aluminum alloys. *Note:* Historically established as a neurotoxin. Chemically pure barium sulfate which is used for making x-rays is reported to be non-toxic. *References:* 304, 358, 388, 413, 429.

Battery acid *see* **Sulfuric acid.**

Bay E-601 (tn) *see* **Methyl parathion.**

Bay 11405 (tn) *see* **Methyl parathion.**

BEHP *see* **Di-sec octyl phthalate.**

Benzal alcohol *see* **Benzyl alcohol.**

Benzeen *see* **Benzene.**

Benzenamine *see* **Aniline.**

1,4-Benzendiol *see* **Hydroquinone.**

Benzene *TN/synonyms:* Benzol; Benzole; Annulene; Benzeen; Phenyl hydride; Coal naphtha; Cyclohexatriene; Fenzen; Phene; Pyrobenzol; Pyrobenzole; Polystream (tn); Benzol 90 (tn). *NIOSH:* Carcinogen at any exposure level. *NIOSH REL:* 0.1 ppm (10hr/day-40hr/wk); 1 ppm (exposure not to exceed 15 min). *OSHA PEL:* 1 ppm (8hr/day-40hr/wk-PP/S); 5 ppm (exposure not to exceed 15 min). *ACGIH:* Suspected human carcinogen. *ATSDR MRL:* .001 ppm (inhalation, less than 15 days). *IDLH:* 3,000 ppm. *Symptoms:* Eye, nasal, and respiratory system irritation; Eye, skin, DNA, immune system, and chromosomal damage; Abnormal decrease in white blood cells; Affects brain catecholamines; Anemia; Antibody formation; Aplastic anemia; Asphyxia; Blood diseases; Blurred vision; Bone marrow depression; Bronchitis; Cancer (leukemia); Cardiac collapse; Central nervous system depression; Cerebral swelling; Congestive gastritis; Convulsions; Death; Decreased antibodies, leukocytes, erythrocytes, and platelets; Decreased coordination; Delirium; Dermatitis; Dizziness; Drowsiness; Euphoria; Fatigue; Gastritis; Giddiness; Granular tracheitis; Headaches; Impaired judgment; Kidney congestion; Laryngitis; Lassitude; Leukocyte chromosomal aberrations; Lightheadedness; Loss of appetite; Loss of balance; Menstrual pain and disorders; Nausea; Nervousness; Non-lymphocytic leukemia; Ovarian atrophy; Pallor; Paralysis; Premature births; Pulmonary hemorrhage; Pyloric strictures; Respiratory arrest; Ringing or tingling in the ear; Skin swelling; Spleen infarction; Spontaneous abortions; Staggering gait; Tight chest; Tremors; Unconsciousness;

Underdevelopment of organs or body; Vertigo; Vomiting; Weakness. Suspected of causing Birth defects. *Endpoint Targets:* Blood; Central nervous system; Bone marrow; Skin; Eyes; Respiratory system. *Usage:* 1 to 2% of Gasoline; Adhesives; Aniline; Artificial leather; Asphalt; Carpet glue; Chlorobenzene; Coatings; Cumene; Cyclohexane; Degreasing cleaners; Detergents; Dry cleaning; Dyes; Ethylbenzene; Furniture polish (wax); Glues; Inks; Lacquers; Linoleum; Lithographic printing; Lubricants; Maleic anhydride; Medicines; Nitrobenzene; Oil cloth; Oils; Paint remover and thinners; Paints; Pesticide inert ingredients; Pesticide intermediate; Petroleum refining; Phenol; Plastics; Resins; Rotogravure printing; Rubber cement; Rubber; Shoes; Solvent; Styrene; Tires; Varnishes; Waxes; Spot remover. Cancelled as an active pesticide ingredient. Found in tobacco smoke and automobile exhaust. *Metabolites:* Benzene oxide oxepin; Muconic acid; Phenyl mercapturic acid; Pre-phenyl mercapturic acid; Benzene oxide; Benzene glycol; Muconaldehyde; Benzoquinone; Hydroquinone; Phenol; Catechol; Trihydroxy benzene; Glucuronide; Sulfate. *Classification:* Organic solvent. *Note:* Historically established as a neurotoxin. *References:* 8, 75, 304, 305, 356, 383, 388, 389, 413, 423, 429, 432, 463.

Benzene chloride *see* **Chlorobenzene.**

1,4-Benzenediamine *see* **p-Phenylene diamine.**

1,2-Benzene-dicarboxylic acid *see* **Dibutylphthalate.**

1,2-Benzenedicarboxylic anhydride *see* **Phthalic anhydride.**

Benzene hexahydride *see* **Cyclohexane.**

Benzenemethanol *see* **Benzyl alcohol.**

1,2,4-Benzenetricarboxylic acid *see* **Trimellitic anhydride.**

1,2,4-Benzenetricarboxlic acid anhydride *see* **Trimellitic anhydride.**

cyclic 1,2-anhydride, Benzenetricarboxlic anhydride: *see* **Trimellitic anhydride.**

Benzidine *TN/synonyms:* 4,4'-Bianiline; 4,4'-Biphenyldiamine; 1,1'-Biphenyl-4,4'-diamine; 4,4-Diaminobiphenyl; p-Diaminodiphenyl. *NIOSH:* Carcinogen at any exposure level. Reduce exposure to the lowest feasible concentration. *OSHA:* No PEL, 1 of 13 chemicals recognized as an occupational carcinogen. Exposure of workers is to be controlled through required engineering controls, work practices, and personal protective equipment. *ACGIH:* Confirmed human carcinogen. No threshold value limit will insure prevention of hypersensitive responses. *IDLH:* Carcinogen. *Symptoms:* Blood in urine; Anemia; Destruction of red blood cells; Acute bladder inflammation; Acute liver disorders; Dermatitis; Painful and irregular urination; Chemical hypersensitivities; and Cancer (bladder). *End-point Targets:* Bladder; Kidneys; Liver; Skin; and Blood. *Usage:* Printing inks; Pigments; Biological stains; Wood stains; Wood putty or dough; Dyes; Textiles such as nylon, silk, cotton, and wool; Typewriter ribbons; Leather; Plastics; Paper; Soap. *References:* 304, 306, 388, 397, 418.

Benzinol (tn) *see* **Trichloroethylene.**

Benzo(b)furan *see* **2,3-Benzofuran.**

Benzofuran *see* **2,3-Benzofuran.**

2,3-Benzofuran *TN/synonyms:* Benzofuran; Cumaron; Coumarone; Benzo(b)furan; Benzofurfuran; 1-Oxindene. *OSHA PEL:* None. *Symptoms:* None confirmed. Suspected of causing adrenal and thyroid damage and lesions; Lung, kidney, and liver damage; Excessive proliferation of normal cells; Stomach inflammation; Bone degeneration; Cancer; Lymphatic tissue and nervous system lesions; Male and female reproductive organs effects. *End-point Targets:* Liver; Kidneys. *Usage:* Resins; Fruit coatings; Pesticide inert ingredient; Plastics; Paints; Varnishes; Water-resistant coatings; Paper; Fabrics; Adhesives; Asphalt floor tiles. Found in cigarette smoke. *References:* 355, 423.

Benzofurfuran *see* **2,3-Benzofuran.**

Benzol *see* **Benzene.**

Benzol 90 (tn) *see* **Benzene.**

Benzole *see* **Benzene.**

Benzoperoxide *see* **Benzoyl peroxide.**

p-Benzoquinone *see* **Quinone.**

1,4-Benzoquinone *see* **Quinone.**

Benzoyl peroxide *TN/synonyms:* Benzoperoxide; Dibenzoyl peroxide. *OSHA PEL:* 5 mg/m^3 (8hr/day-40hr/wk-PP/S). *IDLH:* 7,000 mg/m^3. *Symptoms:* Skin, eye, and mucous membrane irritation; Contact dermatitis; Dry, peeling skin. *End-point Targets:* Skin; Respiratory system; Eyes. *Usage:* Bleaching oils; Flour; Plastics; Fiberglass; Silicone rubber; Veterinary medicine; Medicine; Acne medications; Thermoset polyesters; Vinyl chloride; Pesticide inert ingredient. *References:* 49, 304, 388, 423.

Benzyl acetate *TN/synonyms:* alpha-Acetoxytoluene; Benzyl ethanoate; Ivoir (tn). *OSHA PEL:* None. *Symptoms:* Skin, eye, respiratory, and gastrointestinal irritation; Vomiting; Diarrhea; Death; Tissue damage. Suspected of causing Cerebral dysfunction, Blurred vision, Impaired speech, Involuntary eye movement, Tremors, Staggering gait, Abnormal electroencephalogram. *End-point Targets:* No data. *Usage:* Solvent; Cellulose; Varnish remover; Fragrances; Soaps; Perfumes; Cosmetics; Food flavoring;

Chewing gum; Candy; Gelatin; Ice cream; Beverages; Baked goods; Resins; Oils; Lacquers; Polishes; Inks; Pesticide inert ingredient. *Note:* Capable of causing death or permanent injury due to exposures from normal use. *Classification:* Polar volatile organic compounds. *References:* 89, 144, 423, 452.

Benzyl alcohol *TN/synonyms:* (Hydroxymethyl)benzene; alpha-Hydroxytoluene; alpha-Toluenol; Benzal alcohol; Benzenemethanol; Hydroxytoluene; Phenolcarinol; Phenylmethanol; Phenylmethyl alcohol; Euxyl K 100 (tn); Benzylicum (tn); Alcohol benzylique (tn). *OSHA PEL:* None. *Symptoms:* Vomiting; Diarrhea; Central nervous system depression; Convulsions; Respiratory paralysis; Loss of sensation; Calcium deposits in the superficial layer of the cornea; Corneal swelling; Tissue or bone death; Delirium; Visual disturbances; Blurred vision. Suspected of causing Cerebral dysfunction; Impaired speech; Involuntary eye movement; Tremors; Staggering gait; Abnormal electroencephalogram. *End-point Targets:* Eyes; Central nervous system. *Usage:* Solvent; Cellulose acetate; Perfumes; Food flavorings; Sheet plastic; Polyethylene films; Gelatin; Casein; Shellac; Veterinary medicine; Lacquers; Plasticizers; Photography; Dyes; Ball point pen ink; Stencil ink; Ophthalmic preservative; Medicine preservative; Bacteriostatic saline; Heprin; Phenobarbital injections; Pancuronium; Aquamephyton; Rug cleaners; Degreasing agent; Dental solution preservative; Cough syrup; Ointments; Nylon carpeting; Cosmetics; Fingernail polish; Hair dyes; Textiles; Insect ointments and repellents; Dermatological aerosol sprays; Local anesthetic for minor surgery; Pesticide inert ingredient; Body lotions. *References:* 29, 90, 144, 423.

Benzyl chloride *TN/synonyms:* Chloromethylbenzene; alpha-Chlorotoluene. *NIOSH:* Carcinogen at any exposure level. *NIOSH REL:* 1 ppm or 5 mg/m³ (Ceiling limit, 15 min exposure). *OSHA PEL:* 1 ppm or 5 mg/m³ (-8hr/day-40hr/wk). *IDLH:* 10 ppm. *Symptoms:* Eye, nasal, skin, upper respiratory irritation; Weakness; Irritability; Headaches; Skin eruptions; Pulmonary edema; Cough; Conjunctivitis; Dizziness; Tremors in eyelids and fingers; Increase bilirubin; Decrease leukocytes; Pulmonary and eye damage (permanent); Central nervous system depression; Feeling of being hot; Insomnia; Loss of appetite; Nausea; Vomiting; Abdominal cramps; Diarrhea; Allergic nasal mucosa inflammation; Cold-like illness; Gastrointestinal damage; Skin burns. Suspected of causing Cancer; Genetic mutations; Cerebral dysfunction; Blurred vision; Impaired speech; Involuntary eye movement; Staggering gait; Abnormal electroencephalogram. *End-point Targets:* Eyes; Respiratory system; Skin. *Usage:* Perfumes; Pharmaceuticals; Dyes; Military warfare chemical; Photography; Rubber; Gasoline additive; Chemical intermediate; Bactericide, insecticide, and fungicide manufacturing; Food flavoring and odor enhancer; Lubricants; Plastics; Plasticizers; Floor tiles; Artificial leather; Penicillin; Resins; Benzyl phthalates and alcohols. Toxic by inhalation, ingestion, and skin absorption. Synergistic effects; Hydrolyzes in water to form benzyl alcohol. *Classification:* Organic solvent. *References:* 50, 144, 304, 306, 383, 388.

Benzyl ethanoate *see* **Benzyl acetate.**

Benzylicum (tn) *see* **Benzyl alcohol.**

Beosit (tn) *see* **Endosulfan.**

Beryllium *TN/synonyms:* Beryllium-9; Glucinium; Glucinum; Beryllium metallic. *Compounds:* Beryllium chloride; Beryllium fluoride; Beryllium oxide; Beryllium hydroxide; Beryllium phosphate; Beryllium nitrate; Beryllium sulfate; Beryllium carbonate. *NIOSH:* Carcinogen at any exposure level. *NIOSH REL:* 0.0005 mg/m³ (not to exceed at any time). *OSHA PEL:* 0.002 mg/m³ (8hr/day-40hr/wk); 0.005 mg/m³ (Ceiling limit); 0.025 mg/m³ (30 min max peak). *ACGIH:* Suspected human carcinogen. *ATSDR LOAEL:* 0.0012 mg/m³ (Inhalation, more than 365 days). *IDLH:* 10 mg/m³. *Symptoms:* Respiratory disease; Chemical pneumonia; Cough; Substernal burning; Shortness of breath; Loss of appetite; Pulmonary granulomas and fibrosis; Emphysema; Arterial hypoxemia; Weakness; Fatigue; Weight loss; Right atrial and ventricular hypertrophy; Enlarged heart; Liver tissue death; Kidney congestion; Skin lesions and granulomas; Conjunctivitis; Contact dermatitis; Adrenal gland congestion and cellular vacuolization; Cell-mediated immune response; Delayed skin hypersensitivity. Suspected of causing Cancer (lung), Macrocytic anemia, Rickets, Osteoporosis. *End-point Targets:* Lungs; Skin; Eyes; Mucous membranes. *Usage:* Asphalt; Asphalt felts and coatings; Televisions; Computers; Aircraft disc brakes; X-ray transmission and space vehicle windows; Missile parts; Nuclear reactors and weapons; Fuel containers; Rocket propellents; Heat shields; Mirrors; High-technology ceramics; Electrical insulators; Microwave ovens; Gyroscopes; Military vehicle armor; Thermocouple tubing; Laser components. Naturally found in tobacco. *References:* 304, 305, 354, 388, 429.

Beryllium-9 *see* **Beryllium.**

Beryllium metallic *see* **Beryllium.**

BHC *see* **Lindane.**

4,4'-Bianiline *see* **Benzidine.**

Biethylene *see* **1,3-Butadiene.**

4,4'-Biphenyldiamine *see* **Benzidine.**

1,1'-Biphenyl-4,4'-diamine *see* **Benzidine.**

bis(2-Chloroethyl)ether *see* **Dichloroethyl ether**

bis(Dimethylthiocarbarnoyl) disulfide *see* **Thiram**

bis (2,3-Epoxypropyl) ether *see* **Diglycidyl ether**

S-[1,2-bis(Ethoxycarbonyl)ethyl]0, 0-demethyl-phosphorodithioate *see* **Malathion**

bis-(2-Ethylhexyl) phthalate *see* **Disec octyl phthalate**

Bisoflex 81 (tn) *see* **Di-sec octyl phthalate.**

Bivinyl *see* **1,3-Butadiene.**

Black leaf 40 (tn) *see* **Nicotine.**

Blacosolv (tn) *see* **Trichloroethylene.**

Bladan-M (tn) *see* **Methyl parathion.**

Blancosolv (tn) *see* **Trichloroethylene.**

Boric acid *see* **Boron.**

Boroethane *see* **Diborane.**

Boron *TN/synonyms:* Boric acid; Sodium borates (borax). *Compounds:* Borate; Boric oxide; Boron trioxide; Borax decahydrate; Anhydrous borax; Elemental boron; Boron tribromide; Boron trofluoride. *OSHA PEL:* 10 mg/m³ (8hr/day-40hr/wk-PP/S). *ATSDR MRL:* 3.20 ppm (Ingestion; more than 14 days); 4.10 mg/m³ (Inhalation, more than 14 days). *IDLH:* NE. *Symptoms:* Eye, nasal, throat, and upper respiratory irritation; Conjunctivitis; Skin erythema and lesions; Eye and skin damage; Abdominal pain; Liver, kidney, and brain damage; Death; Respiratory failure; Gastrointestinal disorders; Vomiting; Diarrhea; Liver congestion and degeneration; Exfoliative dermatitis; Degenerative changes in brain neurons; Vascular congestion; Perivascular hemorrhage; Intravascular thrombosis. Suspected of causing Testicular damage, Altered metabolism. *End-point Targets:* Skin; Eyes. *Usage:* Glass; Fiberglass insulation; Fire retardant; Leather tanning and finishes; Cosmetics; Photography; High-energy fuel; Soaps; Household cleaners; Antifreeze; Herbicides; Insecticides; Pesticide inert ingredient; Textiles; Detergents. *Synergistic effects:* Reacts with water to form boric acid. Found naturally in food. *Note:* Infants appear to be more susceptible. Ingestion appears to be the most dangerous route of exposure. Historically established as a neurotoxin. *References:* 304, 353, 388, 413, 423.

Boron fluoride *see* **Boron trifluoride.**

Boron hydride *see* **Decaborane or Diborane.**

Boron trifluoride *TN/synonyms:* Boron fluoride; Trifluoroborane. *OSHA PEL:* 1 ppm or 3 mg/m³ (ceiling limit). *IDLH:* 100 ppm. *Symptoms:* Nasal irritation; Nosebleeds; Burns eyes and skin. Suspected of causing Pneumonia; Kidney damage. *End-point Targets:* Respiratory system; Kidneys; Eyes; Skin. *Usage:* Glass; Fiberglass insulation; Fire retardant; Leather tanning and finishes; Cosmetics; Photography; High-energy fuel; Metallurgy; Enamels and glazes for household and industrial products; Soaps; Cleaners; Antifreeze; Herbicides; Insecticides; Pesticide inert ingredient; Textiles. *Synergistic effects:* Hydrolyzes in moist air or hot water to form boric acid, hydrogen fluoride, and fluoboric acid. *References:* 304, 353, 388, 423.

Bottled gas *see* **Propane.**

BPL *see* **beta-Propiolactone.**

Brick Oil *see* **Creosotes.**

Brodan (tn) *see* **Chlorpyrifos.**

Bromine *TN/synonyms:* Molecular bromine. *OSHA PEL:* 0.1 ppm or 0.7

mg/m³ (8hr/day-40hr/wk-PP/S); 0.3 ppm or 2.0 mg/m³ (exposure not to exceed 15 min). *IDLH:* 10 ppm. *Symptoms:* Abdominal pain; Asthma; Choking; Circulatory collapse; Collapse; Corrosive gastrointestinal inflammation; Cough; Cyanosis; Death; Delirium; Diarrhea; Dizziness; Excessive proliferation of normal cells in the thyroid; Eye, skin, and pulmonary burns; Eyelid spasms; Fecal bleeding; Feeling of oppression; Glottis and pulmonary edema; Headaches; Heart rate over 100 beats per minute; Hemorrhagic kidney inflammation; Indigestion; Intravascular destruction of red blood cells; Irritability; Joint pain; Loss of appetite; Loss of corneal reflexes; Low blood pressure; Measle-like skin eruptions; Myocardial degeneration; Nosebleeds; Pharyngitis; Photosensitivity; Pneumonia; Reduced and absence of urine formation; Shock; Stupor; Tearing; Thyroid dysfunction; Vegetative disorders; Vomiting. *End-point Targets:* Respiratory system; Eyes; Central nervous system. *Usage:* Gold extraction; Military gas; Fabric bleach; Medicine and medicine intermediate; Gasoline additive; Flame retardant; Plastics; Photography; Shrink-proofing wool; Solvent; Fire extinguishers; Dyes; Fumigant intermediate; Chemical intermediate; Sedatives; Anesthetics; Antispasmodic drugs; Hydraulic fluid; Refrigeration; Dehumidifying agent; Hair-waving solutions (permanents); Swimming pool and water treatments. No longer used as a topical antiseptic or in deodorants. *Classification:* Halogen. *References:* 98, 304, 388, 432.

Bromoethane *see* **Ethyl bromide.**

Bromofume *see* **Ethylene dibromide.**

Bromomethane *see* **Methyl bromide.**

Bromotrifluoromethane *see* **Trifluorobromomethane.**

Burned lime *see* **Calcium oxide.**

Burnt lime *see* **Calcium oxide.**

Butadiene *see* **1,3-Butadiene.**

Buta-1,3-diene *see* **1,3-Butadiene.**

a,a-Butadiene *see* **1,3-Butadiene.**

trans-Butadiene *see* **1,3-Butadiene.**

1,3-Butadiene *TN/synonyms:* Biethylene; Bivinyl; Butadiene; Divinyl; Erythrene; Vinylethylene; a,a-Butadiene; trans-Butadiene; Pyrrolylene; Buta-1,3-diene. *NIOSH:* Carcinogen at any exposure level. Reduce exposure to lowest feasible concentration. *OSHA PEL:* 1,000 ppm or 2,200 mg/m³ (8hr/day-40hr/wk-PP/S). *ACGIH:* Suspected human carcinogen. *ACGIH TLV:* 10 ppm or 22 mg/m³ (8hr/day-40hr/wk). *IDLH:* 20,000 ppm. *Symptoms:* Eye, nasal, throat, and skin irritation; Drowsiness; Cough; Fatigue; Dermatitis; Lightheadedness; Frostbite; Heart disease; Unconsciousness due to narcotic effects; Affects production and development of blood cells; Respiratory disease; Respiratory paralysis; Death; Emphysema; Arteriosclerosis; Chronic rheumatic heart disease; Nausea; Dry mouth and nasal passage; Headaches; Low blood pressure and pulse rate; Decreased levels of red blood cells, hemoglobin, platelets, hematocrit, white blood cells, erythrocytes, and neutrophils; Diabetes. Suspected of causing Cancer, Birth defects, Reproductive effects, Genetic mutations. *End-point Targets:* Eyes; Respiratory system; Central nervous system. *Usage:* Tires; Carpet backing; Paper coating; Latex gloves; Thermoplastics; Plastic impact resistant pipes; automobile parts, and appliances; Acrylics; Gasoline; Nylon; Fungicide intermediate; Latex rubber. Found in cigarette smoke, gasoline vapors, and wood smoke. *Additive:* May contain inhibitors such as tri-butylcatechol. *Metabolites:* 1,2-Epoxybutene; Epoxide hydratase; 3-butene-1,2 diol; DLdiepoxybutane; 3,4-Epoxy-1,2-butane diol. *References:* 304, 314, 352, 388, 429.

n-Butanol *see* **n-Butyl alcohol.**

1-Butanol *see* **n-Butyl alcohol.**

2-Butanol *see* **sec-Butyl alcohol.**

2-Butanone *TN/synonyms:* Ethyl methyl ketone; MEK; Methyl acetone; Methyl ethyl ketone. *OSHA PEL:* 200 ppm or 590 mg/m³ (8hr/day-40hr/wk-PP/S); 300 ppm or 885 mg/m³ (exposure not to exceed 15 min). *ATSDR MRL:* 0.1 ppm (Inhalation, less than 15 days). *IDLH:* 3,000 ppm. *Symptoms:* Eye, nasal, throat, and upper respiratory irritation; Headaches; Weakness; Lightheadedness; Dizziness; Vomiting; Numbness of extremities; Muscle weakness; Nausea; Loss of coordination; Respiratory system effects; Temporary blindness; Fatigue; Nerve inflammation behind the eyes. Suspected of causing Developmental effects. *End-point Targets:* Central nervous system; Lungs. *Usage:* Synthetic rubber; Adhesives; Magnetic tapes; Lube oil dewaxing; Printing ink; Rubber cement; Paint remover; Vinyl films; Paraffin wax; Plastic; Lubricating oils; Cement; Glue; Lacquer; Varnish; Gums; Resins; Rosins; Polystyrene; Polyurethane; Cleaning products; Synthetic leather; Transparent paper; Aluminum foil; Degreasing metals; Smokeless powders; Food flavoring; Perfumes; Porcelain enameling of steel (bathtubs and appliances); Pesticide inert ingredient; Dental adhesive. Found in vehicle exhaust and off-gasses naturally from trees. *Potentiation:* In combination with other solvents it becomes a very hazardous neurotoxin. *Synergistic effect:* Off-gasses formaldehyde when burned. *Note:* Research suggests that humans are more sensitive than other species tested. *Classification:* Organic solvent (Ketone compound). *References:* 15, 304, 372, 383, 388, 423, 429, 432.

trans-2-Butenal *see* **Crotonaldehyde.**

2-Butenal *see* **Crotonaldehyde.**

cis-Butenedioic anhydride *see* **Maleic anhydride.**

2-Butoxyethanol *TN/synonyms:* Butyl cellosolve; Butyl oxitol; Dowanol EB (tn); Ektasolve EB (tn); Ethylene glycol monobutyl ether; Jeffersol EB (tn). *OSHA PEL:* 25 ppm or 120 mg/m³ (8hr/day-40hr/wk-PP/S). *IDLH:* 700 ppm. *Symptoms:* Eye, nasal, and throat irritation; Destruction of red blood cells; Hemoglobin in urine; Acidosis; Central nervous system depression; Kidney injury; Albumin in urine; Blood in urine; Low blood pressure; Nausea; Vomiting; Diarrhea; Headaches; Abdominal and lumbar pain; Absence of urine formation; Deficiency in number of red blood cells; Increase in reticulocytes in the blood; Abnormal increase in granulocytes in the blood; Increase in leukocytes in the blood; Bone marrow damage; Drowsiness; Weakness; Staggering gait; Slurred speech; Tremors; Blurred vision; Changes in personality. Suspected of causing Conjunctivitis, Liver tissue death, Fetal toxicity. *End-point Targets:* Liver; Kidneys; Lymphoid system; Skin; Blood; Eyes; Respiratory system. *Usage:* Pesticide inert ingredient; Hydraulic fluids; Protective coatings; Metal cleaners; Liquid household cleaners; Water-based coatings; Di-(2-butoxyethyl) phthalate; 2-Butoxyethyl acetate; Plasticizers; Nitrocellulose; Lacquers; Varnishes; Enamels; Dry cleaning; Varnish remover; Textiles; Solvent. *Note:* Poisoning is often misdiagnosed as schizophrenia or narcolepsy. *References:* 43, 304, 388, 423.

Butyl acetate *see* **n-Butyl acetate.**

n-Butyl acetate *TN/synonyms:* Butyl acetate; n-Butyl ester of acetic acid; Butyl ethanoate. *OSHA PEL:* 150 ppm or 710 mg/m³ (8hr/day-40hr/wk-PP/S); 200 ppm or 950 mg/m³ (exposure not to exceed 15 min). *IDLH:*

10,000 ppm. *Symptoms:* Eye, throat, upper respiratory, and skin irritation; Headaches; Drowsiness; Dry eyes; Muscle weakness; Giddiness; Incoordination; Confusion; Delirium; Coma; Nausea; Vomiting; Diarrhea; Cough; Labored or difficulty breathing; Death; Respiratory failure; Cardiac arrhythmias; Kidney and liver damage; Glucose in urine; Pulmonary edema; Corneal inflammation; Inebriation; Hallucinations; Anemia; Dizziness; Behavioral effects; Impaired performance; Central nervous system depression; Weakness; Unconsciousness. *End-point Targets:* Eyes; Skin; Respiratory system. *Usage:* Pesticide inert ingredient; Lacquers; Artificial leather; Photographic films; Plastics; Safety Glass; Vinyl; Perfumes; Food preservative; Solvent; Adhesives; Nitrocellulose; Oils; Fats; Waxes; Camphor; Gums; Resins; Dyes; Cellulose; Larvicide; Food flavoring for banana, pear, pineapple and berry flavors; Inks; Pharmaceuticals; Paint thinner. *Note:* Behavioral effects and impaired performance occur below TLVs/PELs. Neurotoxin. *References:* 17, 176, 304, 388, 423.

sec-Butyl acetate *TN/synonyms:* sec-Butyl ester of acetic acid; 1-Methylpropyl acetate. *OSHA PEL:* 200 ppm or 950 mg/m³ (8hr/day-40hr/wk-PP/S). *IDLH:* 10,000 ppm. *Symptoms:* Eye, nasal, throat, and skin irritation; Headaches; Drowsiness; Upper respiratory and skin dryness; Weakness; Unconsciousness; Central nervous system depression; Vertigo; Cardiac palpitations; Gastrointestinal disorders; Anemia; Skin lesions; Dermatitis; Liver effects. *End-point Targets:* Eyes; Skin; Respiratory system. *Usage:* Nitrocellulose lacquers; Lacquer thinners; Nail channels; Leather finishes; Solvent. *References:* 225, 304, 388.

tert-Butyl acetate *TN/synonyms:* tert-butyl ester of acetic acid. *OSHA PEL:* 200 ppm or 950 mg/m³ (8hr/day-40hr/wk-PP/S). *IDLH:* 10,000 ppm.

Symptoms: Eye, nasal, throat, and upper respiratory irritation; Itchy, inflamed eyes; Headaches; Unconsciousness due to narcotic effects; Dermatitis; Weakness; Drowsiness; Nervous system disorders; Cardiovascular disorders; Central nervous system depression; Vertigo; Cardiac palpitations; Anemia; Gastrointestinal disorder; Skin lesions; Liver effects. *End-point Targets:* Respiratory system; Eyes; Skin. *Usage:* Gasoline additive; Solvents; Lacquers. *References:* 237, 305, 388.

Butyl alcohol *see* n-Butyl alcohol.

n-Butyl alcohol *TN/synonyms:* 1-Butanol; n-Butanol; Butyl alcohol; 1-Hydroxybutane; n-Propyl carbinol. *OSHA PEL:* 50 ppm or 150 mg/m³ (ceiling limit-PP/S). *IDLH:* 8,000 ppm. *Symptoms:* Eye, nasal, and throat irritation; Headaches; Vertigo; Drowsiness; Corneal inflammation; Blurred vision; Tearing; Photosensitivity; Dry, cracked skin; Muscle weakness; Giddiness; Incoordination; Confusion; Delirium; Coma; Nausea; Vomiting; Diarrhea; Cough; Labored or difficulty breathing; Respiratory failure; Death; Cardiac arrhythmias; Gastrointestinal hemorrhage; Kidney damage; Glucose in urine; Liver damage; Cardiac failure; Pulmonary edema; Corneal inflammation; Contact dermatitis; Dizziness; Chemical sensitivity. Suspected of causing Impaired motor control; Decreased levels of testosterone. *End-point Targets:* Skin; Eyes; Respiratory system. *Usage:* Adhesives; Anti-hemorrhagic drugs for cancer patients; Bactericide; Baked goods; Brake fluids; Candy; Coatings; Cream; Denatured alcohol; Detergents; Dyes; Extraction of antibiotics, vitamins, and hormones; Fabric coatings; Fats; Hydraulic fluids; Ice cream; Ices; Medicine; Non-alcoholic beverages; Oils; Pain relievers; Paint and varnish strippers; Pesticide inert ingredient; Pharmaceutical intermediate; Plasticizer; Resins; Rubber; Safety glass; Shellacs; Solvent; Textiles; Varnishes; Vegetable oil; Veterinary medicine; Waxes. *Note:* Occupationally acquired sensitivity to isopropyl alcohol also caused reactions to n-propyl alcohol, n-butyl alcohol; 2-Propanol. Neurotoxin. *References:* 17, 177, 304, 388, 423, 426.

sec-Butyl alcohol *TN/synonyms:* 2-Butanol; Butylene hydrate; 2-Hydroxybutane; Methyl ethyl carbinol. *NIOSH REL:* 100 ppm or 305 mg/m³ (10hr/day-40hr/wk); 150 ppm or 455 mg/m³ (exposure not to exceed 15 min). *OSHA PEL:* 100 ppm or 305 mg/m³ (8hr/day-40hr/wk-PP/S). *IDLH:* 10,000 ppm. *Symptoms:* Eye, throat, and skin irritation; Cardiac arrhythmias; Cardiac failure; Chemical hypersensitivity; Coma; Confusion; Cough; Death; Delirium; Dermatitis; Diarrhea; Dizziness; Drowsiness; Dry, cracking skin; Gastrointestinal hemorrhage; Giddiness; Glucose in urine; Headache; Incoordination; Kidney damage; Labored or difficulty breathing; Liver damage; Muscle weakness; Nausea; Pulmonary edema; Respiratory failure; Unconsciousness due to narcotic effects; Vomiting. *End-point Targets:* Eyes; Central nervous system. *Usage:* Food flavoring; Perfumes; Dyes; Industrial cleaners; Paint removers; Solvent; Resins; Linseed oil; Caster oil; Brake fluids; Polishes; Dewaxing paraffin; Methyl ethyl ketone; Denatured alcohol; Adhesives; Pesticide inert ingredient. *Note:* Occupationally acquired sensitivity to isopropyl alcohol also caused reactions to 1-Propanol; 1-Butanol; 2-Propanol; 2-Butanol. *References:* 226, 304, 388, 423.

Butylamine *TN/synonyms:* 1-Aminobutane; n-Butylamine. *OSHA PEL:* 5 ppm or 15 mg/m³ (Ceiling limit-PP/S). *IDLH:* 2,000 ppm. *Symptoms:* Eye, nasal, throat, and mucous membrane irritation; Headaches; Flushed skin; Skin burns and erythema; Faintness; Cough; Chest pains; Dizziness; Depression; Convulsions; Unconsciousness due to narcotic effects; Blindness; Nausea; Vomiting; Shock; Death. *End-point Targets:* Respiratory system; Skin; Eyes. *Usage:* Food flavoring; Seafood; Chocolate; Alcoholic beverages; Ice cream; Ices; Candy; Baked goods; Gelatins; Pudding; Chemical intermediate; Pesticide and insecticide intermediate; Pharmaceuticals; Dyes; Synthetic leather; Rubber. *Note:* Used in food at 0.1 ppm. *References:* 99, 304, 388.

n-Butylamine *see* **Butylamine.**

Butyl cellosolve *see* **2-Butoxyethanol.**

Butylene hydrate *see* **sec-Butyl alcohol.**

n-Butyl ester of acetic acid *see* **n-Butyl acetate.**

sec-Butyl ester of acetic acid *see* **sec-Butyl acetate.**

tert-butyl ester of acetic acid *see* **tert-Butyl acetate.**

Butyl ethanoate *see* **n-Butyl acetate.**

Butyl ethyl ketone *see* **Ethyl butyl ketone.**

Butyl oxitol *see* **2-Butoxyethanol.**

Butyl phosphate *see* **Tributyl phosphate.**

tri-n-Butyl phosphate *see* **Tributyl phosphate.**

Butylphthalate *see* **Dibutylphthalate.**

tert-Butyl valone *see* **Pindone.**

BVF *see* **Formaldehyde.**

Cadmium *TN/synonyms:* Colloidal cadmium. *Compounds:* Cadmium carbonate; Cadmium chloride; Cadmium oxide; Cadmium sulfate; Cadmium sulfide. *NIOSH:* Carcinogen at any exposure level. Reduce exposure to the lowest feasible concentration. *OSHA PEL:* 5.0 ug/m³ (8hr/day-40hr/wk-PP/S); 2.5 ug/m³ (exposure monitoring and medical surveillance required). *ATSDR MRL:* 0.0002 ug/kg/day (Ingestion; more than 365 days). *IDLH:* 50 mg/m³ (dust); 9 mg/m³ (fumes). *Symptoms:* Lung and gastrointestinal irritation; Abdominal pain; Anemia; Behavioral problems; Cancer (lung, prostate); Cardiac lesions; Chills; Contact dermatitis; Cough; Death; Destruction of cell membranes; Diarrhea; Emphysema; Headaches; Impaired and decreased respiratory function; Increase blood pressure; Increased softness of the bone; Kidney damage; Labored or difficulty breathing; Liver destruction; Loss of smell; Metal fume fever; Muscle aches; Nausea; Osteoporosis; Pneumonia; Protein in urine; Pulmonary edema and fibrosis; Renal dysfunction; tissue death, and tubular lesions; Substernal pain; Tight chest; Tracheobronchitis; Vomiting; Autoimmue disease; Immune-complex glomerulonephritis. Suspected of causing Liver damage; Immune system suppression or activation; Nerve cell and brain damage; Birth defects; Low birth weight; Impaired neurological development of fetuses; Testicular damage; Chromosomal aberrations; Genetic mutations; Altered libido; Infertility. *End-point Targets:* Gastrointestinal tract; Respiratory system; Kidneys. *Usage:* Asphalt; Asphalt felts and coatings; Lime manufacturing; Batteries; Metal plating; Pigments; Plastics; Paints; Metal soldering and welding; Electroplating; Semiconductors; Metallurgy; Photography; Printing; Textiles. Found in food and cigarettes. *Note:* Historically established as a neurotoxin. *References:* 17, 280, 299, 304, 315, 351, 388, 389, 416A, 429, 432, 449.

Cajeputen *see* **Limonene.**

Cajeputene *see* **Limonene.**

Calcium arsenate *TN/synonyms:* Calcium salt (2:3) of arsenic acid; Cucumber dust; Tricalcium arsenate; Tricalcium ortho-arsenate. *NIOSH:* Carcinogen at any exposure level. *NIOSH REL:* 0.002 mg/m³ (ceiling limit 15 min exposure). *OSHA PEL:* 0.010 mg/m³ (8hr/day-40hr/wk-PP/S). *IDLH:* 100 mg/m³. *Symptoms:* Abnormal decrease in white blood cells; Absence of urine formation; Blood, albumin, protein, or glucose in urine; Cholera; Cirrhosis; Cold extremities; Coma; Conjunctivitis; Constipation; Convulsions; Corneal inflammation; Cyanosis; Death; Delirium; Dermatitis; Diarrhea; Difficulty swallowing; Excessive salivation; Fecal blood; Frontal headaches; Garlic breath; Gastrointestinal cramps and distress; Heart rate over 100 beats per minute; Itching and burning eyes; Jaundice; Liver damage and tissue death; Mania; Mucous membrane inflammation; Muscle cramps; Myocardial hemorrhage; Numb, burning, or tingling extremities; Palmar planter hyperkeratoses; Peripheral neuropathy; Photosensitivity; Profuse sweating; Shock; Skin hyperpigmentation; Sore throat; Stomach inflammation; Stupor; Sweet, metallic taste; Tearing; Thirst; Throat constriction; Unconsciousness due to inadequate blood flow; Vascularity of bone marrow; Vertigo; Vomiting; Weak pulse; Weakness. Suspected of causing Cancer (lung); Birth defects. *End-point Targets:* Eyes; Respiratory system; Liver; Skin; Lymphatic system; Central nervous system. *Usage:* Insecticide; Herbicide. *Synergistic effects:* When heated produces arsenic fumes. *References:* 52, 304, 388.

Calcium oxide *TN/synonyms:* Burned lime; Burnt lime; Lime; Pebble lime; Quick lime; Unslaked lime. *NIOSH REL:* 2 mg/m³ (10hr/day-40hr/wk). *OSHA PEL:* 5 mg/m³ (8hr/day-40hr/wk-PP/S). *IDLH:* Unknown. *Symptoms:* Eye, skin, gastric, and upper respiratory irritation; Cold, clammy skin; Collapse; Death; Dermatitis; Esophageal and gastric perforation; Esophageal strictures; Excessive salivation; Fever; Mediastinum tissue inflammation; Nasal septum perforation and ulcers; Pharyngeal, esophageal, and glottis swelling; Pneumonia; Rapid pulse; Respiratory inflammation; Shock; Substernal pain; Vomiting. *Endpoint Targets:* Respiratory system; Skin; Eyes. *Usage:* Antacids; Antiseptic; Bleaching agent; Bricks; Building materials; Cane and beet sugar refining; Chemical manufacturing; Chewing gums; Dehairing hides (leather); Dentifrices; Dough (baking) conditioner; Food additive; Fungicides and insecticides intermediate; Glass; Kraft paper pulp products; Lubricants; Mason lime; Metallurgy; Modified starches; Mortar; Pesticide inert ingredient; Plaster; Poultry feed; Rubber; Seed disinfectant; Sewage treatment; Stucco; Water purification and softening. *Synergistic effects:* Reacts with water to form calcium hydroxide. *References:* 53, 304, 388, 423.

Calcium salt (2:3) of arsenic acid *see* **Calcium arsenate.**

Camphofene Huilex (tn) *see* **Chlorinated camphene.**

Camphor *TN/synonyms:* 2-Camphonone; Gum camphor; Laurel camphor; Synthetic camphor. *OSHA PEL:* 2 mg/m³ (8hr/day-40hr/wk-PP/S). *IDLH:* 200 mg/m³. *Symptoms:* Eye, skin, and mucous membrane irritation; Absence of urine formation; Albumin in urine; Central nervous system depression; Central neuronal tissue death; Clammy skin; Coma; Confusion; Convulsions and epileptiform convulsions; Death; Delirium; Depression; Diarrhea; Dizziness; Excitement; Feeling warm; Gastric distress; Hallucinations; Headaches; Increased muscular excitement; Irrationality; Jerky muscle movements; Kidney lesions; Loss of sensation; Nausea; Noise in ears; Respiratory failure; Restlessness; Tremors; Unexpanded fetal lungs at birth; Urinary retention; Vertigo; Visual disturbances; Vomiting; Weak; rapid pulse; Weakness; Widespread hemorrhaging. *End-point Tar-*

gets: Central nervous system; Eyes; Skin; Respiratory system. *Usage:* Pesticide inert ingredient; Nail polish; Solid air fresheners; Rubber; Antiseptic; Perfumes; Fragrances; Plastics; Lacquers; Varnishes; Explosives; Fireworks; Embalming fluids; Medicines; Topical disinfectant and anesthetic; Food flavoring; Insect repellent; Cosmetics; Deodorant; Non-alcoholic beverages; Baked goods; Condiments; Cellulose; Linalool; Camphorated parachlorophenol; Dentifrices. *Classification:* Polar volatile organic compounds. *References:* 54, 304, 388, 423, 452.

Carbaryl *TN/synonyms:* Sevin; alpha-Naphthyl-N-methylcarbamate; 1-Naphthyl N-Methylcarbamate. *OSHA PEL:* 5 mg/m³ (8hr/day-40hr/wk-PP/S). *IDLH:* 600 mg/m³. *Symptoms:* Skin irritation; Abdominal cramps; Asphyxia; Blurred vision; Bronchial constriction; Chest tightness; Cholinesterase poisoning; Coma; Constricted pupils; Convulsions; Cyanosis; Death; Diarrhea; Difficulty breathing; Dilated pupils; Dimness of vision; Excessive salivation; Eye pain; Headaches; High blood pressure; Incontinence; Jerky movements; Lassitude; Loss of appetite; Memory loss; Muscle cramps, twitching, spasms, and involuntary contractions; Nasal discharge; Nausea; Mouth and nasal frothing; Profuse sweating; Progressive peripheral neuropathy; Proximal muscle weakness; Pulmonary rales; Respiratory arrest and paralysis; Slurred speech; Sympathoadrenal discharge; Tearing; Temporary cessation of breathing during sleep; Tremors; Vomiting; Weakness; and Weight loss. *End-point Targets:* Central nervous system; Skin; Respiratory system; Cardiovascular system. *Usage:* Pesticide; Insecticide; Acaricide; Mollusicide; Animal flea, lice, mite, and tick control; Medical/hospital disinfectant; Veterinary medicine; Sewage treatment; Oyster beds. *References:* 55, 304, 388.

Carbinol *see* **Methyl alcohol.**

Carbolic acid *see* **Phenol.**

Carbomethene *see* **Ketene.**

2-Carbomethoxy-1-methylvinyl dimethyl phosphate *see* **Phosdrin.**

Carbon bichloride *see* **Tetrachloroethylene.**

Carbon bisulfide *see* **Carbon disulfide.**

Carbon chloride *see* **Carbon tetrachloride.**

Carbon dichloride *see* **Tetrachloroethylene.**

Carbon dioxide *TN/synonyms:* Carbonic acid gas; Dry ice. *NIOSH REL:* 5,000 ppm or 9,000 mg/m³ (10hr/day-40hr/wk); 30,000 ppm or 54,000 mg/m³ (exposure not to exceed 15 min). *OSHA PEL:* 10,000 ppm or 18,000 mg/m³ (8hr/day-40hr/wk); 30,000 ppm or 54,000 mg/m³ (exposure not to exceed 15 min). *IDLH:* 50,000 ppm. *Symptoms:* Asphyxia; Central nervous system damage; Coma; Confusion; Convulsions; Death; Dimness of vision; Disorientation; Dizziness; Frostbite; Headaches; High blood pressure; Increased heart rate and pulse pressure; Labored or difficulty breathing; Malaise; Numbness, tingling, or prickling sensation; Profuse sweating; Restlessness; Skin blisters; Temporary blindness; Tremors; Unconsciousness; Vomiting; Metabolic stress. *End-point Targets:* Lungs; Skin; Cardiovascular system. *Usage:* Pesticides; Pesticide inert ingredient; Aerosol propellant; Refrigerant; Food preservatives; Carbonated beverages; Theatrical smoke and fumes; Fire extinguisher; Petroleum-based products; Fertilizer; Dry ice; Golf ball centers; Cloud seeding; Lasers; Aspirin; Food additive; Used to stimulate depressed respiratory systems; Relieves hiccups; Wart destruction; Soap; Fumigant; Sterilizing agent; Urea resins; Methanol; Carbonic acid; Lead carbonate; Potassium carbonate;

Water treatment. Found in diesel exhaust. *References:* 56, 304, 384, 388, 394, 423.

Carbon disulfide *TN/synonyms:* Weeviltox (tn); Carbon bisulfide; Carbon disulphide; Carbon sulfide; Carbon sulphide; Dithiocarbonic anhydride; Sulphocarbonic anhydride; Sulphuret of carbon. *NIOSH REL:* 1 ppm or 3 mg/m³ (10hr/day-40hr/wk); 10 ppm or 30 mg/m³ (exposure not to exceed 15 min). *OSHA PEL:* 4 ppm or 12 mg/m³ (8hr/day-40hr/wk-PP/S); 12 ppm or 36 mg/m³ (exposure not to exceed 15 min). *ATSDR MRL:* 0.003 ppm- Inhalation, more than 14 days *IDLH:* 500 ppm. *Symptoms:* Dizziness; Headaches; Poor sleep; Fatigue; Nervousness; Tissue or bone death; Loss of appetite; Weight loss; Psychosis; Polyneuropathy; Parkinson-like syndrome; Ocular changes; Coronary heart disease; Gastritis; Kidney and liver damage; Eye and skin burns; Dermatitis; Elevated blood pressure; Skin blisters; Behavioral changes; Altered menstrual cycles; Altered libido; Sperm abnormalities; Peripheral neuropathy; Pyschomotor deficits; Impaired IQ; Brain dysfunction; Vision disturbances; Central nervous system effects; Cranial neuropathy; Tremors; Memory impairment; Emotional instability. Suspected of causing birth defects. *End-point Targets:* Central nervous system; Peripheral nervous system; Cardiovascular system; Eyes; Kidneys; Liver; and Skin. *Usage:* Rayon; Cellophane; Carbon tetrachloride; Rubber; Rubber accessories; Petroleum jelly; Paraffins; Fibers; Pesticide inert ingredient; Resins; Plywood adhesives; Solvent; Vinyl chloride; Petroleum-well cleaning; Electroplating; Metallurgy; Photography; Lithography; Removing print on plastics; Insecticide; Fungicide; Grain fumigant; Rust removal from metals; Semiconductors; Animal medicine; Fats; Oils; Waxes; Paints; Textiles; Varnishes; Rubber cement;

Preservative. Contaminates breast milk. *Classification:* Organic solvent. *Note:* Historically established as a neurotoxin. *References:* 17, 304, 359, 383, 388, 413, 423, 449.

Carbon disulphide *see* **Carbon disulfide.**

Carbon hexachloride *see* **Hexachloroethane.**

Carbonic acid gas *see* **Carbon dioxide.**

Carbon monoxide *TN/synonyms:* Carbon oxide; Flue gas; Monoxide. *OSHA PEL:* 35 ppm or 40 mg/m³ (8hr/day-40hr/wk-PP/S); 200 ppm or 229 mg/m³ (ceiling limit). *IDLH:* 1,500 ppm. *Symptoms:* Albumin in urine; Angina; Brain and heart lesions; Brain damage; Brain function depression; Coma; Confusion; Congestive heart failure; Bronchial pneumonia; Convulsions; Cyanosis; Death; Defective memory; Depressed or absent reflexes; Depressed S-T segment of electrocardiogram; Dimness of vision; Dizziness; Emotional instability; Enlarged liver; Fatigue; Fetal brain damage and death; Fever above 106 degrees; Hallucinations; Headaches; Heart rate over 100 beats per minute; Impaired judgment; Incontinence; Incoordination; Irritability; Multiple sclerosis–like symptoms; Myocardial infarction; Nausea; Parkinson-like symptoms; Profuse sweating; Pulmonary edema; Rapid breathing; Rapid respiration; Reduced urine formation; Respiratory arrest; Shortness of breath; Skin lesions; Unconsciousness due to inadequate blood flow to the brain; Vision disturbances; Vomiting; Weak pulse; Weakness. *Endpoint Targets:* Cardiovascular system; Lungs; Blood; Central nervous system. *Usage:* Acetic acid; Acrylic acid; Dimethylformamide; Ethylene glycol; Metallurgy; Methanol; Methyl formate; Nickel; Phosgene; Pigments; Railroad ties; Silicon carbide fibers; Tungsten steel; Pesticide inert ingredient. Found in petroleum products; exhaust; cigarette smoke. *Note:* Signs of nerve or brain injury may appear at any time within 3 weeks following exposure. Historically established as a neurotoxin. *References:* 17, 57, 304, 307, 388, 389, 394, 413, 423, 429, 449.

Carbon oxide *see* **Carbon monoxide.**

Carbon oxychloride *see* **Phosgene.**

Carbon sulfide *see* **Carbon disulfide.**

Carbon sulphide *see* **Carbon disulfide.**

Carbon tet *see* **Carbon tetrachloride.**

Carbon tetrachloride *TN/synonyms:* Carbon chloride; Carbon tet; Freon 10; Halon 104; Tetrachloromethane. *NIOSH:* Carcinogen at any exposure level. *NIOSH REL:* 2 ppm or 12.5 mg/m³ (exposure not to exceed 60 min). *OSHA PEL:* 2 ppm or 12.6 mg/m³ (8hr/day-40hr/wk-PP/S). *ACGIH:* Suspected human carcinogen. *IDLH:* 300 ppm. *Symptoms:* Skin, eye, nasal, and throat irritation; Central nervous system depression; Nausea; Headaches; Dizziness; Loss of coordination; Unconsciousness; Vomiting; Liver and kidney damage; Abdominal pain; Diarrhea; Coma; Cardiac failure; Death. Suspected of causing Cancer (skin). *End-point Targets:* Central nervous system; Liver; Kidneys. *Usage:* Pharmaceuticals; Petroleum refining; Pesticide inert ingredient; Fluorocarbon propellants; Solvent; Refrigerants; Grain fumigant; Household aerosol products. Found in engine exhaust. *Classification:* Organic solvent; Halogenated organic compound. *Note:* Historically established as a neurotoxin. *References:* 17, 286, 304, 383, 388, 413, 423, 432.

Carbonyl chloride *see* **Phosgene.**

4-Carboxyphthalic anhydride *see* **Trimellitic anhydride.**

Caswell No. 101 (tn) *see* Acrylonitrile.

Caswell No. 183A (tn) *see* Chlorobenzene.

Caswell No. 292 (tn) *see* Dibutylphthalate.

Caswell No. 501 (tn) *see* Iodine.

Caswell No. 600 (tn) *see* Nitrobenzene.

Caswell No. 880C (tn) *see* 2,4, 6-Trichlorophenol.

Caustic soda *see* Sodium hydroxide.

Cecolene (tn) *see* Trichloroethylene.

Cekumethion (tn) *see* Methyl parathion.

Cellosolve acetate *see* 2-Ethoxyethyl acetate.

Celluflex DBP (tn) *see* Dibutylphthalate.

Cement *see* Portland cement.

2-Champhonone *see* Camphor.

Chlorilen (tn) *see* Trichloroethylene.

Chlorinated camphene *TN/synonyms:* Chlorocamphene; Octachlorocamphene; Polychlorocamphene; Toxaphene; Agricide Maggot Killer (tn); Alltox (tn); Camphofene Huilex (tn); Geniphene (tn); Hercules 3956 (tn); Hercules Toxaphene (tn); Motox (tn); Penphene (tn); Phenicide (tn); Phenatox (tn); Strobane-T (tn); Synthetic 3956 (tn); Toxakil (tn). *NIOSH:* Carcinogen at any exposure level. Reduce exposure to lowest feasible level. *OSHA PEL:* 0.5 mg/m³ (8hr/day-40hr/wk-PP/S); 1.0 mg/m³ (exposure not to exceed 15 min). *ATSDR MRL:* 0.18 ppm (Ingestion, less than 15 days); 0.002 ppm (Ingestion, more than 14 days). *IDLH:* 200 mg/m³. *Symptoms:* Skin irritation; Agitation; Aplastic anemia; Behavioral changes; Brain hemorrhages; Bronchial pneumonia; Bronchitis; Cancer; Chromosomal aberrations; Confusion; Convulsions; Death; Dry, red eyes; Excessive salivation; Muscle spasms; Nausea; Pulmonary congestion and edema; Reflex hyperexcitability; Respiratory failure; Tremors; Unconsciousness; Vomiting. Suspected of causing Thyroid injury; Renal swelling; Congestion; Tubular degeneration; Focal tissue death, lesions, and enlargement; Immune system damage. *End-point Targets:* Central nervous system; Skin. *Usage:* Pesticide inert ingredient; Pesticide; Insecticide; Miticide; Livestock dip. *Note:* Man-made from 670 chemicals. *References:* 58, 304, 327, 388, 423.

Chlorinated diphenyl *TN/synonyms:* Hexachlorodiphenyl oxide; Hexachlorophenyl ether. *OSHA PEL:* 0.5 mg/m³ (8hr/day-40hr/wk-PP/S). *IDLH:* Unknown. *Symptoms:* Eye and skin irritation; Acne-form dermatitis; Cancer (liver, skin, and gastrointestinal); Chest tightness; Chloracne; Death; Decreased fertility; Depression; Dizziness; Epigastric distress and pain; Fatigue; Fatty food intolerance; Fetal neurobehavioral deficits; Gastritis; Headaches; High blood pressure; Impaired lung function; Joint pain; Liver damage; Loss of appetite; Low birth weight; Nausea; Premature births. Suspected of causing Pericardial swelling; Gastric ulcers, cysts, and hemorrhages; Increased erythrocytes and hemoglobin counts; Anemia; Kidney damage; Antibody production; Immunosuppression. *End-point Targets:* Respiratory system; Skin; Eyes; Liver. *Usage:* Plasticizer; Surface coatings; Inks; Adhesives; Pesticide extenders; Carbonless paper; Capacitors; Transformers; Asphalt; Waterproofing; Coatings; Lubricants; Rubber; Resins; Waxes; Pesticide manufacturing. Also see polychlorinated biphenyls. *Note:* Fire resistant. *References:* 59, 304, 388.

Chlorinated hydrochloric ether *see* 1,1-Dichloroethane.

Chlorine *TN/synonyms:* Molecular chlorine. *OSHA PEL:* 0.5 ppm or 1.5 mg/m³ (8hr/day-40hr/wk-PP/S); 1.0 ppm or 3.0 mg/m³ (exposure not to exceed 15 min). *IDLH:* 30 ppm. *Symptoms:* Anxiety; Bleeding gums; Bloody expectoration; Bronchial constriction; Bronchial pneumonia; Bronchitis; Burning of eyes, nasal passages, and mouth; Cardiac arrest; Choking; Conjunctivitis; Corneal inflammation; Cough; Death; Dental corrosion; Dermatitis; Dizziness; Emphysema; Fatigue; Headaches; Heart rate over 100 beats per minute; Huskiness or loss of voice; Insufficient oxygenation of blood; Labored or difficult breathing; Myasthenia gravis; Nasal discharge and ulceration; Nausea; Nosebleeds; Pharyngitis; Pneumonia; Predisposition to tuberculosis; Pulmonary blood vessel damage; Pulmonary edema; Skin inflammation and blisters; Sneezing; Substernal pain; Tearing; Tender and painful skin; Tissue or bone death; Unconsciousness due to inadequate blood flow to the brain; Unexpanded fetal lungs at birth; Vomiting. *End-point Targets:* Respiratory system; Skin; Eyes; Gastrointestinal tract. *Usage:* Aluminum production; Antifreeze; Antiseptic; Asphalt; Chemical manufacturing; Cleaning dairy equipment; Dental disinfectant; Dish washing detergent; Dish washing and laundry disinfectant; Disinfectant; Fabric bleach; Feet fungicide; Flame retardant; Food processing; Gasoline additive; Household cleaning products; Lithium or zinc batteries; Paper; Pesticide manufacturing; Plastics; Refrigerants; Resins; Scouring powder; Semiconductors and related devices; Shrink-proofing wool; Synthetic rubber; Used in cooling systems; Water purification; Water treatment for odor control; Wound sterilization. *Classification:* Halogen. *References:* 100, 304, 388, 429, 432.

Chlorine dioxide *TN/synonyms:* Chlorine oxide; Chlorine peroxide.

OSHA PEL: 0.1 ppm or 0.3 mg/m³ (8hr/day-40hr/wk-PP/S); 0.3 ppm or 0.9 mg/m³ (exposure not to exceed 15 min). *IDLH:* 10 ppm. *Symptoms:* Eye, nasal, throat, gastrointestinal, and respiratory irritation; Cough; Wheezing; Bronchial spasms; Pulmonary edema; Bronchitis; Death; Emphysema; Labored or difficulty breathing; Asthmatic bronchitis; Headaches; Light-headedness; Abdominal discomfort; Nausea. Suspected of causing Premature births. *End-point Targets:* Respiratory system; Eyes. *Usage:* Pesticide inert ingredient; Cellulose; Flour; Leather; Oils; Textiles; Beeswax; Water treatment; Swimming pools disinfectant; Bactericide; Antiseptic; Bleach; Chlorine salts; Wood pulp; Tallow; Wastewater disinfectant. *References:* 60, 304, 388, 423.

Chlorine oxide *see* **Chlorine dioxide.**

Chlorine peroxide *see* **Chlorine dioxide.**

Chloroacetaldehyde *TN/synonyms:* 2-Chloroacetaldehyde; 2-Chloroethanol. *OSHA PEL:* 1 ppm or 3 mg/m³ (ceiling limit-PP/S). *IDLH:* 100 ppm. *Symptoms:* Skin, eye, nasal, throat, and mucus membrane irritation; Skin burns; Eye damage; Pulmonary edema; Respiratory system sensitivity; Sensitive dermatitis; Unconsciousness due to narcotic effects; Coma. *End-point Targets:* Eyes; Skin; Respiratory system. *Usage:* Bark removal; Fungicide; Water disinfectant; Dentistry; Chemical intermediate; Pesticide inert ingredient. *Classification:* Organic solvent. *References:* 101, 279, 304, 383, 388, 423.

2-Chloroacetaldehyde *see* **Chloroacetaldehyde.**

alpha-Chloroacetophenone *TN/synonyms:* 2-Chloroacetophenone; Chloromethyl phenyl ketone; Mace; Phenacyl chloride; Phenyl chloromethyl ketone; Tear gas. *OSHA PEL:*

0.30 ppm or 0.05 mg/m³ (8hr/day-40hr/wk-PP/S). *IDLH:* 100 mg/m³. *Symptoms:* Eye, skin, and respiratory irritation; Pulmonary edema. *End-point Targets:* Eyes; Skin; Respiratory system. *Usage:* Mace; Tear gas; Food flavoring; Perfumes; Plastics; Printing ink. *References:* 272, 304, 388.

2-Chloroacetophenone *see* **alpha-Chloroacetophenone.**

2-Chlorobenzalmalononitrile *see* **o-Chlorobenzylidene malononitrile.**

Chlorobenzene *TN/synonyms:* Benzene chloride; Chlorobenzol; MCB; Monochlorobenzene; Phenyl chloride; Caswell No. 183A (tn). *NIOSH:* No REL, notified OSHA that documentation doesn't support the worker's safety at established PEL. *OSHA PEL:* 75 ppm or 350 mg/m³ (8hr/day-40hr/wk-PP/S). *ATSDR MRL:* 15 ppm (Ingestion, more than 14 days). *IDLH:* 2,400 ppm. *Symptoms:* Skin, eye, and nasal irritation; Central nervous system depression; Chest pains; Dizziness; Drowsiness; Electrocardiogram irregularities; Eye and skin burns and inflammation; Headaches; Incoordination; Lung, liver, and kidney damage; Muscle spasms; Nausea; Numbness; Sleepiness; Slow heart rate; Unconsciousness; Vomiting. Suspected of causing immune system, liver, lung, and kidney damage. *End-point Targets:* Respiratory system; Eyes; Skin; Central nervous system; Liver. *Usage:* Pesticide manufacturing; Pesticides inert ingredient; Tar and grease removers; Silicone resin; Solvent; Paint; Dry cleaning; Dyes; Adhesives; Polishes; Waxes; Textiles; Pharmaceuticals; Rubber; Phenol; DDT; Aniline; Surface coatings; Diisocyantes. *Note:* Neurotoxin. *References:* 17, 68, 286, 304, 330, 388, 423.

Chlorobenzol *see* **Chlorobenzene.**

o-Chlorobenzylidene malononitrile *TN/synonyms:* 2-Chlorobenzalmalononitrile; CS; OCBM. *OSHA PEL:* 0.05 ppm or 0.4 mg/m³ (ceiling limit-PP/S). *IDLH:* 2 mg/m³. *Symptoms:* Eye, nasal, and throat irritation; Painful, burning eyes; Tearing; Conjunctivitis; Eyelid redness and spasms; Cough; Chest constriction; Headaches; Skin redness and vesiculation; Pulmonary edema; Pneumonia; Cardiac failure; Liver cell damage; Increase in leukocytes in the blood; Dermatitis. *End-point Targets:* Respiratory system; Skin; Eyes. *Usage:* Military & law enforcement incapacitating agent; Grenades; Tear gas; Aerosol sprays; Methylene chloride; Acetone. *References:* 195, 304, 388.

Chlorobutadiene *see* **beta-Chloroprene.**

2-Chloro-1,3-butadiene *see* **beta-Chloroprene.**

Chlorocamphene *see* **Chlorinated camphene.**

1-Chloro-2,2-dichloroethylene *see* **Trichloroethylene.**

Chlorodiphenyl *see* **Polychlorinated biphenyls.**

1-Chloro-2,3-epoxypropane *see* **Epichlorohydrin.**

Chloroethane *see* **Ethyl chloride.**

2-Chloroethanol *see* **Chloroacetaldehyde.**

Chloroethene *see* **Vinyl chloride.**

Chloroethylene *see* **Vinyl chloride.**

1-Chloroethylene *see* **Vinyl chloride.**

Chloroform *TN/synonyms:* Methane trichloride; Trichloromethane; Methenyl chloride; Methyl trichloride; Formyl trichloride. *NIOSH:* Carcinogen at any exposure level. *NIOSH REL:* 2.00 ppm (exposure not to exceed 15 min); 9.78 mg/m³ (exposure not to exceed 60 min). *OSHA PEL:* 2.00 ppm or 9.78 mg/m³ (8hr/day-40hr/wk-PP/S). *ATSDR MRL:* 0.001 (Inhalation, less than 15 days); 0.0009 (Inhalation, more than 14 days). *ACGIH:* Suspected human carcinogen. *IDLH:* 1,000 mg/m³. *Symptoms:* Eye, skin, and gastrointestinal irritation; Albumin in urine; Cancer (gastrointestinal, colon, bladder); Cardiac arrhythmias and failure; Central nervous system depression; Coma; Convulsions; Death; Decreased erythrocytes and hemoglobin in the blood; Depression; Disorientation; Dizziness; Enlarged liver; Excessive gamma globin in blood; Exhaustion; Fatigue; Fatty degeneration of liver and kidneys; Gastric distress and pain; Genetic mutations; Hallucinations; Headaches; Hepatitis; Impaired liver function; Inability to concentrate; Inability to utilize oxygen; Jaundice; Irritability; Kidney damage; Liver injury; Loss of sensation; Low blood pressure; Mental dullness; Nausea; Psychotic episodes; Pulmonary hemorrhage and congestion; Respiratory paralysis and failure; Testicular atrophy; Vomiting. Suspected of causing Immune system damage; Low birth weight; Birth defects; Unconsciousness due to narcotic effects; Brain hemorrhage; Abnormal sperm. *End-point Targets:* Central nervous system; Liver; Kidneys; Heart; Eyes; Skin. *Usage:* Adhesives; Alkaloids; Artificial silk; Asphalt; Drinking water disinfectant; Dry cleaning; Dyes; Fire extinguishers; Floor polishes; Fluorocarbon-22; Fluoropolymers; Gums; Intermediate for pesticides and fumigants; Lacquers; Medicines; Paper; Pesticide inert ingredient; Plastics; Refrigerants; Rubber; Spot remover; Waxes. *Synergistic effect:* When heated it forms phosgene gas. Natural by-product of chlorination. *Classification:* Organic solvent; Organochlorine; Halogenated organic compound. *Note:* Historically established as a neurotoxin. *References:* 286, 304, 350, 383, 388, 409, 413, 423, 429, 432.

Chloroformyl chloride *see* **Phosgene.**

Chloromethane *see* **Methyl chloride.**

Chloromethylbenzene *see* **Benzyl chloride.**

Chloromethyl ether *see* **Chloromethyl methyl ether.**

Chloromethyl methyl ether *TN/ synonyms:* Chloromethyl ether; CMME; Dimethylchloroether; Methoxychloromethyl ether; Monochlorodimethyl ether; Monochloromethyl methyl ether. *NIOSH:* Carcinogen at any exposure level. Reduce exposure to lowest feasible concentration. *OSHA:* No PEL, 1 of 13 chemicals recognized as an occupational carcinogen. Exposure of workers is to be controlled through required engineering controls, work practices, and personal protective equipment. *ACGIH:* Suspected human carcinogen. *IDLH:* Carcinogen. *Symptoms:* Eye, skin, and mucus membrane irritation; Pulmonary edema and congestion; Pneumonia; Skin burns; Tissue or bone death; Cough; Wheezing; Blood stained sputum; Weight loss; Bronchial secretions; Sore throat; Chills; Fever; Difficulty breathing; Unconsciousness; Dermatitis; Bronchitis; DNA damage; Cancer (lung). *End-point Targets:* Respiratory system; Skin; Eyes; Mucus membrane. *Usage:* Solvent; Water repellent; Resins; Polymers; Chloromethylated compounds; Oven cleaners. *Synergistic effects:* Reacts with water to form hydrochloric acid and formaldehyde. *Contaminant:* bis(chloromethyl) ether. *References:* 71, 304, 306, 388.

Chloromethyl phenyl ketone *see* **alpha-Chloroacetophenone.**

p-Chloronitrobenzene *see* **p-Nitrochlorobenzene.**

1-Chloro-4-nitrobenzene *see* **p-Nitrochlorobenzene.**

4-Chloronitrobenzene *see* **p-Nitrochlorobenzene.**

p-Chlorophenyl chloride *see* **p-Dichlorobenzene.**

Chlor-O-Pic (tn) *see* **Chloropicrin.**

Chloropicrin *TN/synonyms:* Nitrochloroform; Nitrotrichloromethane; Trichloronitromethane; Acquinite (tn); Chlor-O-Pic (tn); Dojyopicrin (tn); Dolochlor (tn); G 25 (tn); Larvacide (tn); Larvacide 100 (tn); Microlysin (tn); NCI-C00533 (tn); Pic-Chlor (tn); Picfume (tn); Picride (tn); Profume A (tn); PS (tn); S 1 (tn); Tri-Chlor (tn). *OSHA PEL:* 0.1 ppm or 0.7 mg/m^3 (8hr/day-40hr/wk-PP/S). *IDLH:* 4 ppm. *Symptoms:* Eye, mucous membrane, upper respiratory, and skin irritation; Alveoli swelling and congestion; Anemia; Asthma; Bronchial pneumonia; Bronchioles inflammation; Chemical sensitivity (lowered sensitivity to concentrations of fumes); Colic; Conjunctivitis; Cough; Diarrhea; Eyelid swelling; Fatigue; Gastrointestinal inflammation; Headaches; Low blood pressure; Nausea; Pneumonia; Pulmonary edema; Respiratory inflammation; Tearing; Tissue or bone death; Vertigo; Vomiting; Weak, irregular heart beat; Weakness. Suspected of causing fatal lung diseases. *End-point Targets:* Respiratory system; Skin; Eyes. *Usage:* Pesticide; Insecticide; Rodenticide; Tear gas; Soil fumigant; Fungicide; Chemical warfare agent; Methyl violet; Warning agent. *References:* 72, 304, 388.

Chloroprene *see* **beta-Chloroprene.**

beta-Chloroprene *TN/synonyms:* 2-Chloro-1,3-butadiene; Chlorobutadiene; Chloroprene. *NIOSH:* Carcinogen at any exposure level. *NIOSH REL:* 1.0 ppm (ceiling limit); 3.6 mg/m^3 (exposure not to exceed 15 min). *OSHA PEL:* 10.0 ppm or 35.0 mg/m^3 (8hr/day-40hr/wk-PP/S). *IDLH:* 400 ppm. *Symptoms:* Eye, skin, mucous

membrane, and respiratory irritation; Altered enzyme activities; Cardiac palpitations; Central and peripheral nervous system dysfunction; Central nervous system depression; Chest pain; Chromosomal aberrations; Conjunctivitis; Corneal tissue death; Dental erosion; Dermatitis; Dizziness; Enlarged liver; Fatigue; Gastrointestinal disorders; Gingivitis; Hair loss; Headaches; Impotency; Insomnia; Irritability; Loss of libido; Lung, liver, and kidney injury; Mental and physical birth defects; Myocardium dystrophy; Periodintitis; Periodontum; Reduced liver function; Respiratory difficulty; Spermatogenous disturbances; Spontaneous abortions; Tissue or bone death; Toxic hepatitis. Suspected of causing Cancer. *End-point Targets:* Respiratory system; Skin; Eyes. *Usage:* Rubber; Garden hoses; Wire insulation; Conveyer belts; Adhesive; Elastic; Dental material; Dental adhesive. *Additives/Contaminants:* Inhibited with antioxidants. *Classification:* Organic solvent. *Note:* Wives of exposed workers also have an increased rate of spontaneous abortions. Historically established as a neurotoxin. *References:* 17, 97, 304, 383, 388, 403, 413, 449.

1-Chloro-2-propene *see* **Allyl chloride.**

3-Chloropropene *see* **Allyl chloride.**

3-Chloropropylene *see* **Allyl chloride.**

gamma-Chloropropylene oxide *see* **Epichlorohydrin.**

2-Chloropropylene oxide *see* **Epichlorohydrin.**

Chloropyrifos *see* **Chlorpyrifos.**

Chlorothene (tn) *see* **1,1,1-Trichloroethane.**

alpha-Chlorotoluene *see* **Benzyl chloride.**

Chlorpyrifos *TN/synonyms:* Chloropyrifos; Chlorpyrifos-ethyl; ENT 27; 311 (tn); O,O-Diaethyl 0-3,5,6-trichlor-2-pyridyl phosphorothioate; DOWCO 179 (tn); Brodan (tn); Detmel UA (tn); Dursban (tn); Dursban 4E (tn); Dursban F (tn); Eradex (tn); Killmaster (tn); Pyrinex (tn); Suscon (tn); Lorsban (tn). *OSHA PEL:* None. *ACGIH TLV:* 0.2 mg/m³ (8hr/day-40hr/wk). *Symptoms:* Abdominal cramps; Anxiety; Apathy; Asphyxia; Breath difficulty; Bronchial constriction; Cardiac arrhythmias; Coma; Confusion; Convulsions; Cyanosis; Death; Diarrhea; Dilated pupils; Dimness of vision; Disorientation; Drowsiness; Emotional instability; Excessive dreaming; Giddiness; Headaches; Heart rate over 100 beats per minute; Heart rate under 60 beats per minute; High blood pressure; Hypothermia; Immune system activation; Incontinence; Incoordination; Inhibits cholinesterase enzymes; Insomnia; Leg weakness; Muscle twitching and involuntary contraction; Nausea; Neurosis; Nightmares; Numbness, tingling, or prickling sensation; Peripheral and lymphocytic neuropathy; Profuse sweating; Pulmonary rales; Restlessness; Slurred speech; Tremors; Vertigo; Vomiting; Weakness. *End-point Targets:* Blood; Central nervous system. *Usage:* Insecticide; Animal dip; Acaricide. *Toxic* by inhalation, ingestion, and contact. *Classification:* Organophosphate. *Note:* Historically established as a neurotoxin. *References:* 9, 17, 65, 159, 282, 413.

Chlorpyrifos-ethyl *see* **Chlorpyrifos.**

Chlorthiepan (tn) *see* **Endosulfan.**

Chlorthiepin (tn) *see* **Endosulfan.**

Chlorylea (tn) *see* **Trichloroethylene.**

Chlorylen (tn) *see* **Trichloroethylene.**

Chorylen (tn) *see* **Trichloroethylene.**

Chrom *see* **Chromium.**

Chrome (tn) *see* **Chromium.**

Chromic acid *TN/synonyms:* Potassium chromate; Chromium(VI); Dipotassium salt. *NIOSH:* Carcinogen at any exposure level. *NIOSH REL:* 0.001 mg/m³ (8hr/day-40hr/wk). *OSHA PEL:* 0.100 mg/m³ (8hr/day-40hr/wk); 0.500 mg/m³ (8hr/day-40hr/wk Chromium II, III). *ACGIH TLV:* 0.500 mg/m³-8hr/day-40hr/wk *IDLH:* 30 mg/m³. *Symptoms:* Respiratory irritation; Perforated nasal septum; Liver and kidney damage; Increased leukocytes in blood; Abnormal decrease in white blood cells; Excessive monocytes and eosinophils in blood; Eye injury; Conjunctivitis; Skin ulcers; Sensitive dermatitis. Suspected of causing Cancer. *End-point Targets:* Blood; Respiratory system; Liver; Kidneys; Eyes; Skin. *Usage:* Electroplating; Agricultural chemicals; Metal polishes. *References:* 8, 304, 388, 429, 432.

Chromium *TN/synonyms:* Chromium(O); Chrome (tn); Chrom. *Compounds:* Chromium(III) acetate monohydrate; Chromium(III) nitrate nonahydrate; Chromium(III) chloride; Chromium(III)chloride hexahydrate; Ferrochromite; Chromium(III) oxide; Chromium(III) phosphate; Chromium (III) sulfate; Sodium chromite; Chromium(VI) oxide; Ammonium dichromate; Calcium chromate; Chromium (VI) trioxide; Lead chromate; Chromic acid. *NIOSH REL:* Chromium(VI) 25 ug/m³ (10hr/day-40hr/wk). *OSHA PEL:* Chromium(O) 1.0 mg/m³ or Chromium(II) 0.5 mg/3 or Chromium (III) 0.5 mg/3 (8hr/day-40hr/wk-PP/S); Chromium(VI) 0.1 mg/m³ (ceiling limit). *ACGIH TLV:* Chromium(O) 0.5 mg/m³ or Chromium(II) 0.5 mg/m³- or Chromium(III) 0.5 mg/m³- or Chromium(VI) 0.05 mg/m³-(8hr/day-40hr/wk). *ATSDR MRL:* Chromium(VI) 0.002 mg/m³ (Inhalation, more than 14 days). *IDLH:* N.E. *Symptoms:* Skin and mucous membrane irritation, burns, and ulcers; Nasal irritation and atrophy; Abdominal and stomach pain; Abnormal decrease in blood platelets; Abnormal decrease in white blood cells; Anemia; Asthma; Bronchial spasms; Bronchitis; Cancer (lung); Cerebral and pulmonary edema; Changes in the myocardium of the heart; Chromosomal aberrations; Conjunctiva congestion; Contact dermatitis; Convulsions; Corneal blistering; Cough; Death; Decreased hemoglobin in the blood; Decreased pulmonary function; Dermatitis; Diarrhea; Dizziness; Eczema; Enlarged brain; Facial angioedema; Gastric and duodenal ulcers; Gastric mucosa congestion; Gastrointestinal hemorrhage; Headaches; Heart's left ventricle muscle hemorrhage; Hemolytic anemia; Immune system sensitization; Impaired balance; Increase in leukocytes in the blood; Increased sedimentation rate of red blood cells; Inhibits blood clotting; Intravascular destruction of red blood cells; Kidney inflammation, damage, impairment, and failure; Liver damage; Nasal and pharyngeal itching; Nasal discharge; Nasal itching and soreness; Nasal septum perforation and ulceration; Nausea; Nosebleeds; Pneumonia; Pneumonoconiosis; Respiratory and cardiopulmonary arrest; Skin tissue death; Stomach inflammation; Unconsciousness; Vomiting; Weak pulse; Weakness; Wheezing. Suspected of causing Birth defects; Low birth weight. *End-point Targets:* Respiratory tract; Blood; Skin. *Usage:* Alloy cast iron; Asphalt; Bleach; Bricks; Copy machine toner; Detergents; Dyes; Electric cells; Electroplating; Explosives; Foundry sand; Glues; Joint prostheses; Leather tanning; Lime manufacturing; Lithography; Machine oils; Magnetic tapes; Match heads; Metal finishes; Paint; Pesticide inert ingredient; Photography; Pigments; Rubber based products; Stainless steel; Textile printing; Textiles; Wallpaper; Wood preservatives. *Note:* Recommended daily intake is 50 to 200 ug/day. Chromium oxides are neurotoxins. *References:* 17, 304, 349, 388, 406, 423, 429, 432.

Chromium(O) *see* **Chromium.**

Chromium(VI) *see* **Chromic acid.**

Chrysotile *see* **Asbestos.**

CI44320 (tn) *see* **Cobalt.**

CI77575 (tn) *see* **Lead.**

CI77775 (tn) *see* **Nickel.**

CI77820 (tn) *see* **Silver.**

Cinen *see* **Limonene.**

Cinene *see* **Limonene.**

Cinerin I or II *see* **Pyrethrum.**

Cinnamene *see* **Styrene.**

Circosolv (tn) *see* **Trichloroethylene.**

CMME *see* **Chloromethyl methyl ether.**

Coal naphtha *see* **Benzene.**

Coal tar creosote *see* **Creosotes.**

Coal tar oil *see* **Creosotes.**

Cobalt: (nonradioactive) *TN/Synonyms:* CI44320 (tn); Cobalt-59. *Compounds:* Cobalt chloride; Cobalt oxide; Cobalt sulfate; Cobalt oxide; Cobalt nitrate; Cobalt carbonate. *OSHA PEL:* 0.05 mg/m^3 (8hr/day-40hr/wk-PP/S). *ATSDR:* 0.038 mg/m^3 (6 hrs: breathing problems); 0.003 mg/m^3 (more than 14 days: lung disease); 0.007 mg/m^3 (more than 14 days; allergies that result in asthma). *IDLH:* 20 mg/m^3. *Symptoms:* Acidosis; Antibodies formation; Asthma; Blood supply deficiency to the liver; Cardiac failure; Cardiogenic shock; Cough; Deafness; Death; Decreased iodine uptake by the thyroid; Decreased pulmonary function; Dermatitis; Diarrhea; Diffused nodular fibrosis; Excess of red blood cells; Excessive proliferation on normal thyroid cells; Immune system sensitization; Impaired choroidal perfusion; Labored or difficult breathing; Liver injury; Liver, kidney, and conjunctiva congestion; Loss of appetite; Metal fume fever; Myocardium diseases of the heart; Nausea; Optic atrophy; Pneumonia; Pulmonary rales and edema; Respiratory hypersensitivity and irritation; Vision disturbances; Vomiting; Weight loss; Wheezing. Suspected of causing Testicular degeneration and atrophy, Chromosomal aberrations. *End-point Targets:* Respiratory system; Skin. *Usage:* Beer; Medicine; Paint; Magnetic alloy; Porcelain enameling of steel (bathtubs and appliances); Pigments; Animal feed additive; Nutrition additive; Glass decolorizer; Prosthetic devices; Pesticide inert ingredient; Pharmaceutical aids. Naturally part of the vitamin B12. *Note:* Historically established as a neurotoxin. *References:* 299, 304, 373, 388, 413, 423.

Cobalt-59 *see* **Cobalt.**

Colloidal arsenic *see* **Arsenic.**

Colloidal cadmium *see* **Cadmium**

Colloidal manganese *see* **Manganese.**

Colloidal mercury *see* **Mercury.**

Cologne spirits (tn) *see* **Ethanol.**

Columbian spirits *see* **Methyl alcohol.**

Copper *Compounds:* Black copper oxide; Copper monoxide; Copper hydroxide; Copper carbonate; Copper ammonium carbonate; Copper oxychloride; Copper oxychloride sulfate; Copper oxide; Copper(II) oxide; Cupric oxide. *OSHA PEL:* 1 mg/m³ (8hr/day-40hr/wk-PP/S). *IDLH:* NE. *Symptoms:* Eye, nasal, mucous membrane, and throat irritations; Central nervous system degeneration; Death; Dermatitis; Diarrhea; Disturbed gait; Dizziness; Immune system damage; Liver and kidney damage; Metallic taste; Muscle rigidity; Nasal perforation; Nausea; Poor coordination; Psychological impairment; Stomach cramps; Tremors; Vomiting; Wilson's disease. Suspected

of causing Anemia; Spontaneous abortions; Birth defects; Decreased fertility; Genetic mutations; Chromosomal aberrations; Sperm abnormalities. *End-point Targets:* Respiratory system; Skin; Liver; Kidneys. *Usage:* Air conditioning; Algicide; Animal feed; Automotive parts; Dyes; Electrical wiring; Electronics; Electroplating; Fertilizers; Fungicide for foliage, seeds, wood, and fabric; Industrial values and fittings; Insect Repellents; Insecticides; Lime manufacturing; Pesticide inert ingredient; Plumbing; Power utilities; Preservative for wood, leather, and fabric; Telecommunications. *Note:* Copper deficiency may cause anemia; Weakness; Impaired respiration and growth; and Poor utilization of iron. *References:* 304, 324, 388, 423, 429.

Coumarone *see* **2,3-Benzofuran.**

Crawhaspol (tn) *see* **Trichloroethylene.**

Creosote Oil *see* **Creosotes.**

Creosote PL *see* **Creosotes.**

Creosotes *TN/synonyms:* Preserv-O-Sote (tn); Creosote Oil; Brick Oil; Coal Tar Oil; Creosote PL; Heavy Oil; Liquid Pitch Oil; Wash Oil; Dead Oil; Wood Creosote; Coal Tar Creosote. *NIOSH REL:* 0.1 mg/m³ (10hr/day-40hr/wk). *OSHA PEL:* 0.2 mg/m³ (8hr/day-40hr/wk). *IDLH:* 400 mg/m³. *Symptoms:* Eye and skin irritation; Allergic dermatitis; Cancer (skin); Conjunctivitis; Convulsions; Cyanosis; Death; Excessive salivation; Gastrointestinal lesions; Headaches; Hypothermia; Kidney damage; Liver failure; Loss of pupillary reflexes; Mouth, pharyngeal, and skin hemorrhages; Muscle twitching; Respiratory distress; Skin becomes sensitive to light; Skin redness, burns, and lesions; Thready pulse; Tissue or bone death; Vertigo; Vomiting. Suspected of causing Excessive proliferation of normal cells; Stomach distention; Kidney degeneration.

End-point Targets: Gastrointestinal system; Skin. *Usage:* Wood creosote-Antipyretic; Styptic; Astringent; Lubricant; Waterproofing; Chemical manufacturing; Veterinary medicine and deodorant; Antiseptic; Wood preservative; Expectorant; Dental local anesthetic. Coal tar creosote-Antiseptic; Disinfectant; Antipyretic; Germicide; Fuel oil ingredient; Defoliant; Antifungal preparations; Vermicide; Wood preservative; Pharmaceuticals; Animal dip; Roofing pitch; Animal and bird repellent; Miticide; Insecticide; Restricted use pesticide; Cement; Corrosion inhibitor; Carbon black. Ingredients: Coal tar creosote-phenol, cresols, xylenols, pyridine and lutidine derivatives; polycyclic aromatic hydrocarbons. Wood-phenol, cresol, guaiacol, xylenol, and creosol. *Note:* Neurotoxin. *References:* 17, 73, 74, 332, 388, 429.

Cresols *TN/synonyms:* Methylphenol; Hydroxytoluene; Cresylic acid. *Isomers:* o-cresol: ortho-Cresol; 2-Methylphenol; 2-Hydroxytoluene; o-Cresylic acid. m-cresol: meta-Cresol; 4-Methyl phenol; 4-Hydroxytoluene; m-Cresylic acid. p-Cresol: para-Cresol; 3-Methyl phenol; 3-Hydroxytoluene; p-Cresylic acid. *NIOSH REL:* 2.3 ppm or 10.0 mg/m³ (10hr/day-40hr/wk). *OSHA PEL:* 5.0 ppm or 22.0 mg/m³ (8hr/day-40hr/wk-PP/S). *ATSDR MRL:* 2 ppm (Ingestion, all exposure durations). *IDLH:* 250 ppm. *Symptoms:* Skin, eye, nasal, mouth, throat, and gastrointestinal irritation; Absence of urine formation; Blindness; Central nervous system disorders; Coma; Confusion; Death; Depression; Dermatitis; Facial paralysis; Hemolytic anemia; Impaired kidney function; Irregular, rapid respiration; Kidney failure; Labored or difficulty breathing; Lung, liver, and kidney damage; Lung, pancreas, liver, and kidney lesions; Pneumonia; Respiratory failure; Skin and pancreas inflammation; Vomiting; Weak pulse. Suspected of causing Weight loss; Liver inflammation; Reduced hemoglobin, red blood count, and hematocrit; Lethargy; Convulsions; Incoordination; Muscle tremors; Cerebral dysfunction; Blurred vision; Involuntary eye movement; Abnormal electroencephalogram; Staggering gait. *End-point Targets:* Central Nervous system, Respiratory system, Liver, Kidneys, Skin, Eyes, Blood. *Usage:* Air filter oils; Antiseptics; Bactericides; Chemical intermediate; Deodorizer/Air fresheners; Disinfectants; Dyes; Epoxy; Explosives; Flame retardant; Food odor enhancer; Fragrances; Fungicides; Herbicide and pesticide manufacturing; Hydraulic fluids; Lubricant additive; Metal degreasers; Paint; Perfumes; Pesticide inert ingredient; Pharmaceuticals; Phenol-formaldehyde resins; Plasticizer; Plastics; Preservatives; Resins; Silicone chips; Synthetic food flavors; Textiles; Wire enamels; Wood preservative. Found in wood; tobacco smoke; crude oil; coal tar; vehicle exhaust; and foods such as tomatoes, asparagus, cheeses, butter, bacon, smoked foods, coffee, black tea, wine, Scotch whiskey, brandy, and rum. *Classification:* Organic solvent. *Note:* As a disinfectant it should not come into direct contact with food. Neurotoxin. *References:* 17, 144, 286, 304, 305, 382, 383, 388, 423.

Cresylic acid *see* **Cresols.**

Cristobalite *see* **Silica.**

Crocidolite *see* **Asbestos.**

Crotonal *see* **Crotonaldehyde.**

Crotonaldehyde *TN/synonyms:* Crotonal; Crotonic aldehyde; Crotylaldehyde; trans-2-Butenal; 2-Butenal; beta-Methylacrolein; Propylene aldehyde. *OSHA PEL:* 2 ppm or 6 mg/m³ (8hr/day-40hr/wk-PP/S). *IDLH:* 400 ppm. *Symptoms:* Eye, nasal, skin, and respiratory irritation; Tearing; Conjunctivitis; Corneal damage; Decrease in surface sulfydryls and polymorphphonuclear leukocytes; Inhibits super-oxide production; Chemical sensitivities. Suspected of causing labored or difficult breathing; Pulmonary edema. *End-point Targets:* Respiratory system; Eyes; Skin. *Usage:* Insecticide and pesticide manufacturing; Resins; Rubber; Tear gas; Leather tanning; Alcohol denaturant; Solvent; Warning agent; Mineral oil; Hospital sterilant; Textile and paper sizing; Lubricating oils; Chemotherapeutic agent; Vinyl chloride; n-Butanol; n-Butylaldehyde; Sorbic acid. *Note:* Workers exposed to Dimethoxane became cross sensitized to crotonaldehyde. *References:* 69, 279, 304, 388, 392.

Crotonic aldehyde *see* **Crotonaldehyde.**

Crotylaldehyde *see* **Crotonaldehyde.**

Crude solvent coal tar naphtha *see* **Naphtha.**

Crystalline silica *see* **Silica.**

CS *see* **o-Chlorobenzylidene malononitrile.**

Cucumber dust *see* **Calcium arsenate.**

Cumaron *see* **2,3-Benzofuran.**

Cumene *TN/synonyms:* Cumol (tn); Isopropyl benzene; 2-Phenyl propane; Isopropylbenzene; Isopropylbenzol. *OSHA PEL:* 50 ppm or 245 mg/m³ (8hr/day-40hr/wk-PP/S). *IDLH:* 8,000 ppm. *Symptoms:* Eye and mucous membrane irritation; Abnormal tension of arteries or muscles; Central nervous system depression; Coma; Confusion; Cough; Death; Dermatitis; Dizziness; Drowsiness; Euphoria; Excessive salivation; Giddiness; Headaches; Hemorrhagic pneumonia; Hoarseness; Hyperactive reflexes; Incoordination; Involuntary muscle movement; Motor restlessness; Mucous membrane lesions and hemorrhaging; Nausea; Respiratory failure; Ringing or tingling in ear; Skin redness and blis-

ters; Stupor; Substernal pain; Tremors; Unconsciousness due to narcotic effects; Ventricular fibrillation; Vertigo; Vomiting blood; Vomiting. Suspected of causing Cataracts; Birth defects. *End-point Targets:* Eyes; Upper respiratory system; Skin; Central nervous system. *Usage:* Liquid detergent; Disinfectants; Aviation fuel; Gasoline; Paint, enamel, and lacquer thinner; Furniture; Paper; Pharmaceuticals; Pesticide inert ingredient; Petroleum-based solvent; Styrene; Phenol; Acetone; alpha-Methylstyrene; Acetophenone; Acrylic and polyester resins. A natural component of naphtha. *Toxic* by inhalation, ingestion, and skin absorption. *References:* 70, 304, 388, 423, 441.

Cummingtonitegrunerite *see* **Asbestos.**

Cumol (tn) *see* **Cumene.**

Cyanides *Compounds: Sodium cyanide:* Cyanide of sodium; Sodium salt of Hydrocyanic acid; Cyanogran (tn). *Potassium cyanide:* Cyanide of potassium; Potassium salt of hydro-cyanic acid. *Calcium cyanide:* Calcid; Calcyan; Cyanide of calcium; Caswell No. 143 (tn). *Copper(I) cyanide:* Cuprous cyanide; Cupricin; A13-23745 (tn). *Cyanogen:* Carbon nitride; Dicyanogen. *Cyanogen chloride:* Chlorine cyanide; Chlorocyan; Caswell No. 267 (tn). Also see Hydrogen cyanide. *NIOSH REL:* 5.0 mg/m³ (ceiling limit); 4.7 ppm (exposure not to exceed 10 min). *OSHA PEL:* Cyanogen-20.0 mg/m³ (8hr/day-40hr/wk PP/S); Cyanides-5.0 mg/m³ (8hr/day-40hr/ wk). *IDLH:* 50 mg/m³. *Symptoms:* Eye, skin, and upper respiratory irritation; Abdominal spasms; Altered sense of smell; Asphyxia; Blindness in half the field of vision involving one or both eyes; Bloody expectoration; Cardiac arrhythmia, irregularities, and palpitations; Coma; Confusion; Convulsions; Cough; Death; Depression; Dimness of vision; Dizziness; Endemic goiters; Enlarged thyroid; Fatigue; Gastric tissue death; Gastrointestinal spasms; Headaches; Hearing disturbances; Heart rate under 60 beats per minute; Hyper-reflexia; Impaired speech; Incoordination; Increased hemoglobin and lymphocyte in the blood; Increased respiratory rate; Inhibition of cytochrome oxidase and other metallioenzymes; Inhibits cellular respiration; Insufficient oxygen to cells causing a poisonous condition; Labored or difficulty breathing; Leber's hereditary optic atrophy; Low blood pressure; Muscular rigidity; Nasal congestion; Nausea; Neural system degenerative lesions; Nosebleeds; Numbness, tingling, or prickling sensations of extremities; Paralysis on one side of the body; Parkinson-like symptoms; Partial paralysis of lower limbs; Rapid respiration; Respiratory failure; Ringing or tingling in the ear; Shortness of breath; Skin rashes; Slow, gasping respiration; Spastic muscle movement; Stupor; T-wave abnormalities of the heart; Temporary cessation of breathing; Thyroid effects; Topical neuropathy; Tremors; Unconsciousness due to inadequate blood flow to the brain; Vomiting; Vision disturbances; Weakness; Weight loss. Suspected of causing Behavioral changes; Birth defects. *End-point Targets:* Cardiovascular system; Central nervous system; Liver; Kidneys; Skin. *Usage:* Acrylics; Acrylonitrile; Adiponitrile; Blacksmithing; Chelating agent; Chemical warfare gas; Dyes; Electroplating; Ferrocyanide; Gold and silver extraction; Grain fumigant; Insecticide; Lactic acid; Leather tanning; Metal cleaning; Metallurgy; Nylon; Pesticides; Pharmaceuticals; Photoengraving; Pigments; Photography; Plastics; Road salts; Rodenticide. Found in food, tobacco smoke, vehicle exhaust. *Note:* Historically established as a neurotoxin. *References:* 304, 348, 388, 413, 432.

Cyanoethylene *see* **Acrylonitrile.**

Cyanomethane *see* **Acetonitrile.**

Cyclodan (tn) *see* **Endosulfan.**

1,4-Cyclohexadiene dioxide *see* **Quinone.**

Cyclohexane *TN/synonyms:* Benzene hexahydride; Hexahydrobenzene; Hexamethylene; Hexanaphthene. *OSHA PEL:* 300 ppm or 1,050 mg/m^3 (8hr/day-40hr/wk-PP/S). *IDLH:* 10,000 ppm. *Symptoms:* Eye, skin, mucous membrane, and respiratory irritation; Drowsiness; Dermatitis; Unconsciousness due to narcotic effects; Coma; Central nervous system depression; Loss of sensation. *End-point Targets:* Eyes; Respiratory system; Skin; Central nervous system. *Usage:* Nylon; Asphalt; Pesticide inert ingredient; Solvent; Lacquers; Resins; Paint and varnish remover; Camp stove fuel; Fungicides; Synthetic rubber; Perfumes; Fats; Waxes; Plastics; Shoes; Benzene; Cyclohexanol; Cyclohexyl chloride; Nitrocyclohexane; Recrystallization of steroids; Adipic acid; Caprolactam. *References:* 67, 304, 388, 423, 429.

Cyclohexanol *TN/synonyms:* Anol; 1-Cyclohexanol; Adronal; Adronol; Cyclohexyl alcohol; Hexahydrophenol; Hexalin; Hydralin; Hydroxcyclohexane; Naxol. *OSHA PEL:* 50 ppm or 200 mg/m^3 (8hr/day-40hr/wk-PP/S). *IDLH:* 3,500 ppm. *Symptoms:* Eye, nasal, throat, conjunctiva, and skin irritation; Unconsciousness due to narcotic effects; Nausea; Tremors; Headaches. Suspected of causing Chromosomal aberrations. *End-point Targets:* Eyes; Respiratory system; Skin. *Usage:* Pesticide inert ingredient; Resins; Ethyl cellulose; Celluloid; Insecticide manufacturing; Soaps; Detergents; Textiles; Dyes; Solvent; Lacquers; Paints; Varnishes; Finish removers; Leather degreasing; Polishes; Plasticizers; Plastics; Germicides; Oils; Shellac; Laundry and household cleaners; Gums; Fragrances; Dry cleaning. *Note:* Neurotoxin. *References:* 17, 66, 304, 388, 423.

1-Cyclohexanol *see* **Cyclohexanol.**

Cyclohexanone *TN/synonyms:* Cyclohexyl ketone; Pimelic ketone. *OSHA PEL:* 25 ppm or 100 mg/m³ (8-hr/day-40hr/wk-PP/S). *IDLH:* 5,000 ppm. *Symptoms:* Eye and mucus membrane irritation; Headaches; Unconsciousness due to narcotic effects; Coma; Dermatitis. Suspected of causing Birth defects; Reproductive effects; Developmental effects; Neonatal lethality; Tearing; Weight loss; Lethargy; Unexpanded fetal lungs at birth; Pulmonary damage; edema, and hemorrhaging; Intestinal congestion; Incoordination; Tremors; Hypothermia. *Endpoint Targets:* Respiratory system; Eyes; Skin; Central nervous system. *Usage:* Electronic components; Magnetic tapes; Pesticide inert ingredient; Printing; Polyurethane coatings; Paint strippers; Polishes; Spot/stain removers; Typesetting; Food flavoring; Perfumes; Plastics; Printing inks. *Classification:* Organic solvent (Ketone compound). *Note:* Neurotoxin. *References:* 17, 304, 305, 383, 388, 420, 423, 424, 429, 431, 438, 439.

Cyclohexatriene *see* **Benzene.**

Cyclohexyl alcohol *see* **Cyclohexanol.**

Cyclohexyl ketone *see* **Cyclohexanone.**

Cyclone B (tn) *see* **Hydrogen cyanide.**

2,4-D *TN/synonyms:* 2,4-Dichlorophenoxyacetic acid; Dichlorophenoxyacetic acid. *OSHA PEL:* 10 mg/m³ (8hr/day-40hr/wk-PP/S). *IDLH:* 500 mg/m³. *Symptoms:* Skin, eye, nasal, throat, and respiratory irritation; Abdominal pain; Aching, tender muscles; Acidosis; Albumin in urine; Bronchitis; Cardiac arrhythmias; Chloracne; Coma; Contact dermatitis; Convulsions; Cough; Cyanosis; Death; Dermatitis; Diarrhea; Difficulty breathing; Diminished reflexes; Dizziness; DNA damage; Dulled sensitivity to touch;

Emphysema; Eye pain and swelling; Eyes become sensitive to light; Fatigue; Flaccid paralysis; Headaches; Heart rate over 100 beats per minute; High fever; Hyperventilation; Hyperglycemia; Increased nitrogenous bodies (esp. urea) in blood; Lethargy; Liver injury, pain, and tissue death; Loss of appetite; Loss of sensation; Loss of sexual potency; Low blood pressure; Lowered sensitivity to taste and smell; Malaise; Mental and physical birth defects; Mouth, esophagus and stomach burns; Muscle damage, twitching, spasms, and weakness; Myoglobin in urine; Numbness, tingling, or prickling sensations; Pneumonia; Polyneuropathy; Profuse sweating; Protein in urine; Pulmonary edema; Reduced urine formation; Reduction in body temperature; Respiratory depression; Rhabdomyolysis (a disease characterized by destruction of skeletal muscles); Stupor; Tearing; Temporary muscle rigidity; Unconsciousness; Vasodilatation; Vertigo; Vomiting; Weakness. Suspected of causing Cancer. *End-point Targets:* Skin; Central nervous system. *Usage:* Herbicide. *Classification:* Organochlorine. *Note:* Historically established as a neurotoxin. *References:* 41, 304, 388, 413.

Dactin *see* **1,3-Dichloro-5,5-dimethylhydantoin.**

Dalf (tn) *see* **Methyl parathion.**

DBP *see* **Dibutylphthalate.**

o-DCB *see* **o-Dichlorobenzene.**

p-DCB *see* **p-Dichlorobenzene.**

DD (r) (Nemafene) *see* **1,3-Dichloropropene.**

DD-92 (r) *see* **1,3-Dichloropropene.**

DDH *see* **1,3-Dichloro-5,5-dimethylhydantoin.**

DDVP *see* **Dichlorvos.**

Dead oil *see* **Creosotes.**

Decaborane *TN/synonyms:* Boron

hydride; Decarboron tetradecahydride. *OSHA PEL:* 0.3 mg/m³ or 0.05 ppm (8hr/day-40hr/wk-PP/S); 0.9 mg/m³ or 0.15 ppm (exposure not to exceed 15 min). *IDLH:* 100 mg/m³. *Symptoms:* Dizziness; Headaches; Nausea; Lightheadedness; Drowsiness; Incoordination; Local muscle spasms; Tremors; Convulsions; Fatigue; Central nervous system damage; Delayed fever; Decreased performance at mental and motor tasks; Loss of appetite; Weight loss; Vomiting; Diarrhea; Skin rashes; Hair loss; Anemia; Nervousness. Suspected of causing Labored or difficulty breathing; Weakness; Liver and kidney damage. *End-point Targets:* Central nervous system. *Usage:* Insecticide; Rocket propellents; Rubber; Corrosion inhibitor; Plastics; Mothproofing; Dye stripping; Rayon; Fuel additive; Soap; Detergents; Boron; Glass. *References:* 102, 304, 388.

Decarboron tetradecahydride *see* **Decaborane.**

Dee-Solv (tn) *see* **Tetrachloroethylene.**

DEHP *see* **Di-sec octyl phthalate.**

Demeton *TN/synonyms:* O-O-Diethyl-(O and S)-2-(ethylthio)ethyl phosphorothioate mixture; Systox. *OSHA PEL:* 0.1 mg/m³ (8hr/day-40hr/wk-PP/S). *IDLH:* 20 mg/m³. *Symptoms:* Eye and skin irritation; Abdominal cramps; Apathy; Cardiac irregularities; Coma; Confusion; Constricted pupils; Convulsions; Cyanosis; Depression; Diarrhea; Dizziness; Excessive salivation; Eye aches; Facial and muscle twitching; Giddiness; Headaches; Heart rate under 60 beats per minute; Incoordination; Inhibits cholinesterase enzymes; Involuntary contraction of muscles; Lightheadedness; Localized sweating; Loss of appetite; Low blood pressure; Monotone speech; Nasal discharge; Nausea; Paralysis; Shallow respiration; Somnolence; Sore abdominal area; Tearing; Tight chest; Unscheduled DNA synthesis; Visual disorders; Vomiting; Weakness; Wheezing. *End-point Targets:* Cardiovascular system; Respiratory system; Central nervous system; Skin; Eyes; Blood cholinesterase. *Usage:* Insecticide; Acaricide. *Note:* Easily absorbed through the skin. *References:* 138, 304, 388.

Densinfluat (tn) *see* **Trichloroethylene.**

Detmel UA (tn) *see* **Chlorpyrifos.**

Devithion (tn) *see* **Methyl parathion.**

DGE *see* **Diglycidyl ether.**

Diacetone *see* **Diacetone alcohol.**

Diacetone alcohol *TN/synonyms:* Diacetone; 4-Hydroxy-4-methyl-2-pentanone; 2-Methyl-2-pentanol-4-one. *OSHA PEL:* 50 ppm or 240 mg/m³ (8hr/day-40hr/wk-PP/S). *IDLH:* 2,100 ppm. *Symptoms:* Eye, nasal, and throat irritation; Corneal tissue damage; Unconsciousness due to narcotic effects; Central nervous system depression; Kidney inflammation and lesions; Defatting dermatitis; Dermatitis; Respiratory failure; Death; Kidney and liver injury; Decreased blood pressure; Excitement; Sleepiness. Suspected of causing liver and kidney damage and changes in blood. *End-point Targets:* Eyes; Skin; Respiratory system. *Usage:* Pesticide inert ingredient; Solvent; Cellulose; Nitrocellulose; Celluloid; Fats; Oils; Waxes; Resins; Antifreeze; Hydraulic fluids; Pharmaceutical preservative; Pigments; Inks; Photographic films; Metal cleaning compounds; Artificial silk and leather. *Note:* Neurotoxin. *References:* 17, 103, 304, 305, 388, 423.

O,O-Diethyl O-3,5,6-trichlor-2-pyridyl phosphorothioate *see* **Chlorpyrifos.**

Diallyl ether dioxide *see* **Diglycidyl ether.**

Diamide *see* **Hydrazine.**

Diamine *see* Hydrazine.

p-Diaminobenzene *see* p-Phenylene diamine.

1,4-Diaminobenzene *see* p-Phenylene diamine.

4,4-Diaminobiphenyl *see* Benzidine.

p-Diaminodiphenyl *see* Benzidine.

1,2-Diaminoethane *see* Ethylenediamine.

Diatomaceous earth *see* Amorphous silica.

Diatomaceous silica *see* Amorphous silica.

Diatomite *see* Amorphous silica.

Dibenzoyl peroxide *see* Benzoyl peroxide.

DIBK *see* Diisobutyl ketone.

Diborane: *TN/synonyms:* Boroethane; Boron hydride; Diboron hexahydride. *OSHA PEL:* 0.1 ppm or 0.1 mg/m³ (8hr/day-40hr/wk). *IDLH:* 40 ppm. *Symptoms:* Pulmonary irritation and edema; Anemia; Chemical hypersensitivity; Chest tightness, heaviness, and burning; Chills; Convulsions; Cough; Diarrhea; Difficulty focusing; Dizziness; Double vision; Drowsiness; Fatigue; Fever; Hair loss; Headaches; Hemorrhaging; Kidney damage; Lassitude; Lightheadedness; Loss of appetite; Metal fume fever; Muscular involuntary contractions, fatigue, and weakness; Nausea; Pericardial pain; Pneumonia; Respiratory distress; Shivering; Shortness of breath; Skin rashes; Tremors; Vertigo; Vomiting; Weakness; Weight loss. Suspected of causing Liver damage. *End-point Targets:* Respiratory system; Central nervous system. *Usage:* Ceramic coatings; Rocket propellants; Rubber; Chemical intermediate; Glass production; Soaps; Detergents; Pesticide intermediate; Styrene; Butadiene; Epoxides; Flame-speed accelerator; Fuel additive. *Synergistic effects:* Reacts with water to form hydrogen and boric acid. *References:* 267, 299, 304, 388.

Diboron hexahydride *see* Diborane.

Dibrom *see* Naled.

1,2-Dibromo-2,2-dichloroethyl dimethyl phosphate *see* Naled.

1,2-Dibromoethane *see* Ethylene dibromide.

Dibutyl 1,2-benzene-dicarboxylate *see* Dibutylphthalate.

Dibutyl ester *see* Dibutylphthalate.

Dibutylphthalate *TN/synonyms:* DBP; Dibutyl 1,2-benzene-dicarboxylate; Di-n-butyl phthalate; Butylphthalate; 1,2-Benzene-dicarboxylic acid; Dibutyl ester; Caswell No. 292 (tn); Celluflex DBP (tn); Polycizer DBP (tn); Uniflex DBP (tn). *OSHA PEL:* 5 mg/m³ (8hr/day-40hr/wk). *ATSDR MRL:* 22 ppm (Ingestion, after 20 days). *IDLH:* 9,300 mg/m³. *Symptoms:* Eye, throat, upper respiratory, and stomach irritation; Eyes become sensitive to light; Nausea; Conjunctivitis; Decrease in sperm density; Dizziness; Headaches; Numbness. Suspected of causing Neonate lethality; Spontaneous abortions; Weight loss; Decreased sperm count; Testicular degeneration. *End-point Targets:* Respiratory system; Gastrointestinal tract. *Usage:* Soft and flexible plastics; Shower curtains; Raincoats; Food wraps; Bowls; Car interiors; Vinyl fabrics; Floor tiles; Nail polish; Hair spray and gels; After-shave lotion; Carpet backing; Insect repellent; Adhesives; Caulking; Plasticizer; Concrete additive; Pigments; Perfume oils; Pesticide inert ingredient; Cosmetics. *References:* 286, 304, 321, 388, 423.

Di-n-butyl phthalate *see* Dibutylphthalate.

o-Dichlorobenzene *TN/synonyms:* o-DCB; 1,2-Dichlorobenzene; ortho-Dichlorobenzene; o-Dichlorobenzol. *OSHA PEL:* 50 ppm or 300 mg/m³ (ceiling limit-PP/S). *IDLH:* 1,000 ppm. *Symptoms:* Eye, nasal, and skin irritation; Skin blisters and lesions; Liver and kidney damage; Cataracts; Headaches; Nausea; Vomiting; Drowsiness; Respiratory depression; Anemia; Chromosomal breaks; Loss of sensation; Stomach pain; Diarrhea; Hemoglobin oxides to ferric iron; Jaundice. Suspected of causing Cancer (leukemia). *End-point Targets:* Respiratory system; Gastrointestinal tract. *Usage:* Herbicide; Pesticide inert ingredient; Solvent; Waxes; Gums; Resins; Tars; Rubbers; Oils; Asphalts; Insecticide; Dyes; Degreaser leather and wool; Toilet bowl cleaners; Metal polishes and degreaser; Soil fumigant; Rust proofing; Wood preservatives; Toluene diisocyantes; Motor-oil additive; Paints; Paint removers; Gun cleaners; Lubricants. *Note:* Neurotoxin. *References:* 8, 17, 197, 286, 304, 388, 423.

ortho-Dichlorobenzene *see* **o-Dichlorobenzene.**

p-Dichlorobenzene *TN/synonyms:* p-DCB; 1,4-Dichlorobenzene; para-Dichlorobenzene; Paradichlorobenzene; Dichlorocide; p-Chlorophenyl chloride; Paracide (tn). *NIOSH:* Carcinogen at any exposure level. Reduce exposure to lowest feasible concentration. *OSHA PEL:* 75 ppm or 450 mg/m³ (8hr/day-40hr/wk-PP/S). 110 ppm or 675 mg/m³ (exposure not to exceed 15 min). *IDLH:* 1,000 ppm. *Symptoms:* Eye, skin, and respiratory irritation; Anemia; Blood disorders; Blotchy skin discoloration; Burning sensation on skin; Cirrhosis; Death; Difficulty breathing; Dizziness; Genetic mutations; Granules in red blood cells; Headaches; Hemolytic anemia; Hemorrhagic spots on skin; Hemorrhaging; Hyperactivity; Incoordination; Jaundice; Kidney damage; Liver disorders and atrophy; Loss of appetite; Marked delays of certain brain waves; Methemoglobin in urine; Multicolored skin; Nausea; Numbness; Profuse nasal mucosa inflammation; Pulmonary congestion and damage; Pulmonary granulomatosis and fibrosis; Speech difficulties; Swelling of hands, feet, and around eyes; Vomiting; Weakness; Weight loss. Suspected of causing Cancer (liver); Immune system damage; Abnormal sperm heads; Reduced male fertility. *End-point Targets:* Liver; Respiratory system; Eyes; Kidneys; Skin; Blood. *Usage:* Insecticide; Mothballs; Household deodorizers; Solid air fresheners; Mold and Mildew control; Fumigant; Pesticide inert ingredient; Toilet bowl cleaner. *Classification:* Polar volatile organic compounds. *References:* 8, 286, 304, 347, 388, 423, 452.

para-Dichlorobenzene *see* **p-Dichlorobenzene.**

1,2-Dichlorobenzene *see* **o-Dichlorobenzene.**

1,4-Dichlorobenzene *see* **p-Dichlorobenzene.**

o-Dichlorobenzol *see* **o-Dichlorobenzene.**

1,1-Dichloro-2-chloroethylene *see* **Trichloroethylene.**

Dichlorocide *see* **p-Dichlorobenzene.**

2,2'-Dichlorodiethyl ether *see* **Dichloroethyl ether.**

Dichlorodifluoromethane *TN/synonyms:* Difluorodichloromethane; Fluorocarbon 12; Freon 12; Halon 122; Propellent 12; Refrigerant 12. *OSHA PEL:* 1,000 ppm or 4,950 mg/m³ (8hr/day-40hr/wk-PP/S). *IDLH:* 50,000 ppm. *Symptoms:* Pulmonary irritation; Dizziness; Tremors; Unconsciousness; Cardiac arrhythmias and arrest; Bronchial pneumonia; Coma; Defatting dermatitis; Apprehension; Humming in ears; Tingling sensation; Speech changes; Amnesia; Cardiac palpitations; Lightheadedness; Peripheral neuropathy; Death; Confusion; Psychomotor impairment; Electrocardiographic changes; Psychological impairment; Decreased level of consciousness; Distal axonopathy. *End-point Targets:* Cardiovascular system; Peripheral nervous system. *Usage:* Refrigerant; Spray paint; Pesticide inert ingredient; Aerosol propellents; Fuel warning agent; Chilling cocktail glasses; Cosmetics; Pharmaceuticals; Insecticide; Adhesives; Cleaners; Solvent; Paints and varnish removers; Food sterilization; Hair spray; Dry hair shampoo; Fire extinguishers; Detergents; Water purification; Petroleum recovery; Glass bottles; Electrical insulation; Pharmaceutical aids (skin freezing); Medicine; Resins; Degreaser; Foam blowing agent; Freons; Hydraulic fluids. *Note:* As of 1986 over 100 deaths have been recorded related to the use of dry hair shampoo and chilling cocktail glasses. Physicians using medication containing dichlorodifluoromethane propellents are advised to counsel patients on potential dangers; especially if a preexisting respiratory or cardiac condition exists. Neurotoxin. *References:* 17, 104, 304, 388, 423.

1,3-Dichloro-5,5-dimethylhydantoin *TN/synonyms:* Dactin; DDH; Halane. *OSHA PEL:* 0.2 mg/m³ (8hr/day-40hr/wk-PP/S); 0.4 mg/m³ (exposure not to exceed 15 min). *IDLH:* Unknown. *Symptoms:* Eye, mucous membrane, and respiratory irritation; Tissue or bone death. Suspected of causing Gastrointestinal hemorrhaging; Sex linked recessive lethal mutations. *End-point Targets:* Respiratory system; Eyes. *Usage:* Bleach; Swimming pool disinfectant; Used to keep flowers fresh in vases; Powder laundry bleach; Disinfectant; Industrial deodorant; Water treatment; Amino acids, medicines, and insecticide intermediate; Vinyl chloride; Pesticide inert ingredient. *References:* 42, 304, 388, 423.

1,1-Dichloroethane *TN/synonyms:* Asymmetrical dichloroethane; Ethylidene; 1,1-Ethylidene dichloride; alpha, alpha-Dichloroethane; Chlorinated

hydrochloric ether; S-dichloroethane; Dutch oil; Ethylidene chloride; Ethylidene dichloride. *OSHA PEL:* 100 ppm or 400 mg/m³ (8hr/day-40hr/wk-PP/S). *ACGIH TLV:* 200 ppm (8hr/day-40hr/wk). *IDLH:* 4,000 ppm. *Symptoms:* Central nervous system depression; Dizziness; Headaches; Nausea; Fatigue; Skin irritation; Liver and kidney damage; Cardiac arrhythmias; Loss of sensation; Excessive spontaneous contraction of the heart. Suspected of causing Gene mutations and Cancer. *End-point Targets:* Skin; Liver; Kidneys. *Usage:* Solvent; Chemical manufacturing; Synthetic rubber; Plastics; Oils; Fats; Cleaning and degreasing products; Fabrics; Paint remover; Varnish remover; Wood finish removers; Fire extinguisher; Fumigant; Insecticide; Oven cleaners. *Metabolites:* Acetic acid; 2,2-Dichloroethane; Chloroacetic acid; Dichloroacetic acid; Chloroacetaldehyde. *Classification:* Chlorinated organic compound. *References:* 304, 334, 388, 399, 429.

alpha; alpha-Dichloroethane *see* **1,1-Dichloroethane.**

S-dichloroethane *see* **1,1-Dichloroethane.**

1,2-Dichloroethene *see* **1,2-Dichloroethylene and Ethylene dichloride.**

1,2-Dichloroethylene *TN/synonyms:* Acetylene dichloride; 1,2-Dichloroethene; syn-1,2-Dichloroethylene; Dioform (TN). Isomers *cis-1,2-Dichloroethene:* (Z)-1,2-Dichloroethene; (Z)-1,2-Dichloroethylene; cis-Acetylene dichloroethylene; cis-1,2-Dichloroethylene; cis-Dichloroethylene. *trans-1,2-Dichloroethene:* (E)-1,2-Dichloroethene; (E)-1,2-Dichloroethylene; trans-Acetylene dichloride; trans-1,2-Dichloroethylene; trans-Dichloroethylene. *OSHA PEL:* 200 ppm or 790 mg/m³ (8hr/day-40hr/wk-PP/S). *ATSDR MRL:* 35 ppm (Ingestion, less than 15 days); 11 ppm (Ingestion, more than 14 days). *IDLH:* 4,000 ppm. *Symptoms:* Eye and respiratory system irritation; Central nervous system depression; Dizziness; Nausea; Headaches; Fatigue; Drowsiness; Intracranial pressure; Vertigo. Suspected of causing Lesions to the heart, lungs, and liver; Organ congestion; Alveolar septal distension; Fibrous swelling of the myocardium; Fatty degeneration of the liver. *End-point Targets:* Respiratory system; Eyes; Central nervous system. *Usage:* Dyes; Perfumes; Lacquers; Thermoplastics; Chemical intermediate; Solvent; Retards fermentation; Rubber; Refrigerant; Decaffeinated coffee; Phenol; Camphor. *Note:* Neurotoxin. *References:* 17, 106, 304, 333, 388.

syn-1,2-Dichloroethylene *see* **1,2-Dichloroethylene.**

Dichloroethyl ether *TN/synonyms:* bis(2-Chloroethyl)ether; 2,2'-Dichlorodiethyl ether. *NIOSH:* Carcinogen at any exposure level. *OSHA PEL:* 5 ppm or 30 mg/m³ (8hr/day-40hr/wk-PP/S); 10 ppm or 60 mg/m³ (exposure not to exceed 15 min). *IDLH:* 250 ppm. *Symptoms:* Eye, nasal, throat, mucous membrane, and respiratory irritation; Tearing; Cough; Nausea; Vomiting; Death; Delayed pulmonary edema; Hysteria. Suspected of causing Cancer; Liver damage. *End-point Targets:* Respiratory system; Skin; Eyes. *Usage:* Solvent; Spot cleaner; Dry cleaning; Gasoline additive; Anesthetic; Acaricide; Medicine; Pharmaceuticals; Soil fumigant; Lubricating oils; Chemical intermediate; Aerosol propellents; Wool; Oven cleaners. Formerly used as a pesticide. *References:* 105, 304, 388.

Dichlorofluoromethane *see* **Dichloromonofluoromethane.**

1,3-Dichloro-4-hydroxybenzene *see* **2,4-Dichlorophenol.**

Dichloromethane *see* **Methylene chloride.**

Dichloromonofluoromethane *TN/synonyms:* Dichlorofluoromethane; Fluorodichloromethane; Freon 21; Halon 112; Refrigerant 21. *OSHA PEL:* 10 ppm or 40 mg/m³ (8hr/day-40hr/wk-PP/S). *IDLH:* 50,000 ppm. *Symptoms:* Pulmonary irritation; Asphyxia; Cardiac arrhythmias; Cardiac arrest; Confusion; Tremors; Coma; Laryngeal swelling and spasms; Oxygen deprivation; Collapse; Death; Defatting dermatitis; Central nervous system depression; Peripheral neuropathy; Cardiac palpitations; Lightheadedness. *End-point Targets:* Respiratory system; Cardiovascular system. *Usage:* Refrigerant; Aerosol propellant; Spray paint; Pesticide inert ingredient; Solvent; Glass bottles; Hair spray; Cosmetics; Household aerosol products; Foam blowing agent; Hydraulic fluids; Magnesium refining; Resins; Degreasers; Freeze dried foods. *Note:* Physician are advised to counsel patients on the potential dangers of using dichloromonofluoromethane aerosol medication; especially if the patient has a preexisting respiratory or cardiac condition. *References:* 107, 304, 388, 423.

2,4-Dichlorophenol *TN/synonyms:* 1,3-Dichloro-4-hydroxybenzene; 2,4-DPC; 4,6-Dichlorophenol. *OSHA PEL:* None. *ATSDR MRL:* 3 ppm (Ingestion, more than 14 days). *Symptoms:* Liver and kidney damage; Chloracne; Porphyria cutanea tarda; Elevated serum transaminase levels; Skin hyperpigmentation; Excessive hair growth or hair growth in unusual places. Suspected of causing Liver tissue death; Respiratory failure; Central nervous system depression; Impaired immune function; Bone marrow atrophy; Kidney and spleen damage; Lung hemorrhage; Diarrhea; Immune system damage; Lethargy; Tremors; Muscle weakness; Incoordination; Clonic convulsions; Labored or difficulty breathing; Coma; Respiratory arrest; Spontaneous abortion; Neonate lethality. *End-point Targets:* Liver; Kidneys; Skin. *Usage:* Wood preservative; Disinfectant; Fungicides; Miticides; Bactericides; Antiseptics; Mothproofing; Germicide; Iron and steel manufacturing; Photography; Electrical components; Pharmaceuticals; Plastics; Paperboard; Herbicide intermediate. *Reference:* 374.

4,6-Dichlorophenol *see* **2,4-Dichlorophenol.**

Dichlorophenoxyacetic acid *see* **2,4-D.**

2,4-Dichlorophenoxyacetic acid *see* **2,4-D.**

Dichloro-1,2-propane *see* **Propylene dichloride.**

1,2-Dichloropropane *see* **Propylene dichloride.**

1,3-Dichloropropene *TN/synonyms:* 1,3-Dichloro-1-propene; 1,3-Dichloropropylene; Telone (r); Telone II (r) (M-3993); Telone C-17 (r); DD (r) (Nemafene); DD-92 (r); Terr-O-Cide 15-D (tn); Terr-O-Cide 30-D (tn); Terr-O-Gas 57/43T (tn); Vorlex (tn); Trapex (tn); Ditrapex (tn); MENCS (tn); MIC (tn); MITC (tn). Isomers *cis-1,3-Dichloropropene:* cis-1,3-Dichloro-1-propene; cis-1,3-Dichloropropylene. *trans- 1,3-Dichloropropene:* trans-1,3-Dichloro-1-propene; trans-1,3-Dichloropropylene. *OSHA PEL:* 1 ppm (8-hr/day-40hr/wk). *ATSDR MRL:* 0.002 ppm (Inhalation, more than 14 days); 2.000 ppm (Ingestion, less than 15 days); 0.500 ppm (Ingestion, more than 14 days). *Symptoms:* Mucous membrane irritation; Headaches; Nausea; Vomiting; Abdominal discomfort; Malaise; Blood malignancies; Chest pains; Cough; Skin redness and swelling; Subcutaneous and skeletal muscle hemorrhaging; Chemical sensitivity (delayed-type hypersensitivity); Delayed contact dermatitis. Suspected of causing Gene mutations; Liver effects; Urinary tract effects; and Cancer (Myelonmocytic and histiocytic leukemia). *End-point Targets:* Immune system; Gastrointestinal track; Blood. *Usage:* Soil fumigant; Pesticide; Herbicides; Corrosion inhibitor. *Synergistic:* It can form when chloride is added to water. **Contami-**

nates breast milk. *References:* 38, 361, 388.

1,3-Dichloro-1-propene *see* **1,3-Dichloropropene.**

1,3-Dichloropropylene *see* **1,3-Dichloropropene.**

Dichlorotetrafluoroethane *TN/synonyms:* 1,2-Dichlorotetrafluoroethane; Freon 114; Halcon 242; Refrigerant 114. *OSHA PEL:* 1,000 ppm or 7,000 mg/m³ (8hr/day-40hr/wk-PP/S). *IDLH:* 50,000 ppm. *Symptoms:* Respiratory irritation; Asphyxia; Cardiac arrhythmias, palpitations, and arrest; Confusion; Tremors; Coma; Laryngeal spasms and swelling; Defatting dermatitis; Lightheadedness; Central nervous system depression; Collapse; Death. *End-point Targets:* Respiratory system; Cardiovascular system. *Usage:* Refrigerant; Aerosol propellent; Pesticide inert ingredient; Pharmaceutical aid (skin freezes); Solvent; Cleaning; Degreasing; Household aerosol products; Explosives; Fire extinguishers; Hair spray; Cosmetics; Veterinary medicine; Foam blowing agent; Chemical intermediate and manufacturing. *Note:* Neurotoxin. *References:* 17, 108, 304, 388, 423.

1,2-Dichlorotetrafluoroethane *see* **Dichlorotetrafluoroethane.**

2,2-Dichlorovinyl dimethyl phosphate *see* **Dichlorvos.**

Dichlorvos *TN/synonyms:* DDVP; 2,2-Dichlorovinyl dimethyl phosphate. *OSHA PEL:* 1 mg/m³ (8hr/day-40hr/wk-PP/S). *IDLH:* 200 mg/m³. *Symptoms:* Skin and eye irritation; Constricted pupils; Aching eyes; Nasal discharge; Headaches; Tight chest; Wheezing; Laryngeal spasms; Excessive salivation; Cyanosis; Loss of appetite; Nausea; Vomiting; Diarrhea; Profuse sweating; Muscle involuntary contractions; Paralysis; Giddiness; Incoordination; Convulsions; Low blood pressure; Inhibits cholinesterase enzymes; Cardiac irregularities. *End-point Targets:* Respiratory system; Cardiovascular system; Central nervous system; Eyes; Skin; Blood cholinesterase. *Usage:* Insecticide; Pesticide inert ingredient. *References:* 304, 388, 423.

Didakene (tn) *see* **Tetrachloroethylene.**

Diethamine *see* **Diethylamine.**

Diethylamine *TN/synonyms:* Diethamine; N,N-Diethylamine; N-Ethylethanamine. *OSHA PEL:* 10 ppm or 30 mg/m³ (8hr/day-40hr/wk-PP/S); 25 ppm or 75 mg/m³ (exposure not to exceed 15 min). *IDLH:* 2,000 ppm. *Symptoms:* Eye, skin, and respiratory irritation; Skin redness and vesiculation; Abdominal pain; Vomiting; Diarrhea; Collapse; Death; Delayed gastric and esophageal perforation; Corneal swelling; Vision disturbances; Blurred vision; Eyes become sensitive to light. *End-point Targets:* Respiratory system; Skin; Eyes. *Usage:* Solvent; Dyes; Pharmaceuticals; Corrosion inhibitor; Oils; Fats; Waxes; Petroleum industry; Rubber; Medicine; Insect repellent; Chemical manufacturing; Pesticide inert ingredient. *References:* 76, 304, 388, 423.

N,N-Diethylamine *see* **Diethylamine.**

Diethylaminoethanol *see* **2-Diethylaminoethanol.**

2-Diethylaminoethanol *TN/synonyms:* Diethylaminoethanol; 2-Diethylaminoethyl alcohol; N,N-Diethylethanolamine; Diethyl-(2-hydroxy-ethyl)-amine; 2-Hydroxytriethylamine. *OSHA PEL:* 10 ppm or 50 mg/m³ (8hr/day-40hr/wk-PP/S). *IDLH:* 500 ppm. *Symptoms:* Eye, skin, and respiratory irritation; Nausea; Vomiting; Eye injury. Suspected of causing Mild tremors; Corneal opacity; Bronchitis. *End-point Targets:* Respiratory system; Skin; Eyes. *Usage:* Soaps; Gasoline; Cosmetics; Surface coatings; Textiles; Fab-

rics; Medicines; Procaine; Chloroquine; Fabric softeners; Anti-rust agents; Resins; Pesticide inert ingredient. *References:* 45, 304, 388, 423.

2-Diethylaminoethyl alcohol *see* **2-Diethylaminoethanol.**

Diethyl (dimethoxyphosphinothioylthio) succinate *see* **Malathion.**

Diethylene imidoxide *see* **Morpholine.**

Diethylene oxide *see* **Tetrahydrofuran.**

Diethylene oximide *see* **Morpholine.**

N,N-Diethylethanolamine *see* **2-Diethylaminoethanol.**

Diethyl ether *see* **Ethyl ether.**

O-O-Diethyl-(O and S)-2-(ethylthio)ethyl phosphorothioate mixture *see* **Demeton.**

di(2-Ethylhexyl) phthalate *see* **Di-sec octyl phthalate.**

Diethyl-(2-hydroxy-ethyl)-amine *see* **2-Diethylaminoethanol.**

Diethyl oxide *see* **Ethyl ether.**

Difluorodichloromethane *see* **Dichlorodifluoromethane.**

Diglycidyl ether *TN/synonyms:* Diallyl ether dioxide; DGE; 2-Epoxypropyl ether; bis(2,3-Epoxypropyl) ether; dis(2,3-Epoxypropyl) ether. *NIOSH:* Carcinogen at any exposure level. *OSHA PEL:* 0.1 ppm or 0.5 mg/m³ (8hr/day-40hr/wk-PP/S). *IDLH:* 25 ppm. *Symptoms:* Eye and respiratory irritation; Skin burns. Suspected of causing Cancer; Effects production and development of blood cells; Lung, liver, and kidney damage; Testicular tissue death; Bone marrow cytotoxicity; Decreased white blood count. *End-point Targets:* Skin; Eyes; Respiratory system. *Usage:* Textiles; Epoxy resins; Chlorinated organic compounds; Leather; Plastics; Building materials;

Rubber; Food processing; Glass; Clay; Automotive parts; Chemical manufacturing. *References:* 77, 304, 305, 388, 401.

1,3-Dihydro-1,3-dioxo-5-isobenzofurancarboxylic acid; 1,3-Dioxo-5-Phthalacarboxylic acid *see* **Trimellitic anhydride.**

1,2-Dihydronxyethane *see* **Ethylene glycol.**

Dihydro-oxirene *see* **Ethylene oxide.**

Dihydroxybenzene *see* **Hydroquinone.**

1,4-Dihydroxybenzene *see* **Hydroquinone.**

Diiodine (tn) *see* **Iodine.**

Diisobutyl ketone *TN/synonyms:* DIBK; sym-Diisopropyl acetone; 2, 6-Dimethyl-4-heptanone; Isovalerone; Valerone. *OSHA PEL:* 25 ppm or 150 mg/m³ (8hr/day-40hr/wk-PP/S). *IDLH:* 2,000 ppm. *Symptoms:* Eye, nasal, and throat irritation; Headaches; Dizziness; Dermatitis; Tearing. Suspected of causing Central nervous system depression. *End-point Targets:* Respiratory system; Skin; Eyes. *Usage:* Food flavoring; Perfumes; Nitrocellulose; Pesticide inert ingredient; Plastics; Printing inks; Resins; Pharmaceuticals; Dyes; Insecticide; Stains; Solvent; Lacquers; Soap; Lubricating oils; Diisobutyl carbinol. *Classification:* Organic solvent. *References:* 78, 304, 305, 383, 388, 423.

sym-Diisopropyl acetone *see* **Diisobutyl ketone.**

Diisopropylamine *TN/synonyms:* N-(1-Methylethyl)-2-propanamine. *OSHA PEL:* 5 ppm or 20 mg/m³ (8hr/day-40hr/wk-PP/S). *IDLH:* 1,000 ppm. *Symptoms:* Eye and pulmonary irritation; Nausea; Vomiting; Headaches; Vision disturbances; Dermatitis. *End-point Targets:* Respiratory system; Skin; Eyes. *Usage:* Pesticide inert ingredient; Experimental medicine; Phar-

maceutical and pesticide intermediate; Mesityl oxide. *References:* 79, 304, 388, 423.

Diisopropyl ether *see* **Isopropyl ether.**

Diisopropyl oxide *see* **Isopropyl ether.**

Dimazin *see* **1,1-Dimethylhydrazine.**

Dimethoxymethane *see* **Methylal.**

Dimethyl acetamide *TN/synonyms:* N,N-Dimethyl acetamide; DMAC. *OSHA PEL:* 10 ppm or 35 mg/m³ (8hr/day-40hr/wk-PP/S). *IDLH:* 400 ppm. *Symptoms:* Skin irritation; Jaundice; Renal and liver damage; Depression; Lethargy; Visual and auditory hallucinations; Delusions; Confusion; Disorientation; Perceptual distortions; Emotional detachment; Dizziness; Sleepiness; Weakness; Excessive proliferation of normal epidermal cells; Effects cell division; Contact dermatitis. *End-point Targets:* Liver; skin. *Usage:* Solvent; Plastics; Resins; Gums; Paint remover; Metal finishes; Pharmaceutical aid; Polyacrylonitrile; Electrolytes. **Toxic** by inhalation, ingestion, and skin absorption. *Note:* The health effects have a tendency to be cumulative. *References:* 80, 304, 388.

N,N-Dimethyl acetamide *see* **Dimethyl acetamide.**

Dimethylamine *OSHA PEL:* 10 ppm or 18 mg/m³ (8hr/day-40hr/wk-PP/S). *IDLH:* 2,000 ppm. *Symptoms:* Eye, nasal, throat, mucous membrane, and skin irritation; Sneezing; Cough; Labored or difficulty breathing; Corneal and pulmonary edema; Conjunctivitis; Dermatitis; Skin and mucous membrane burns; Blurred vision; Vision becomes misty and halos appear (visual disturbances); Photosensitivity. *End-point Targets:* Respiratory system, Skin, Eyes. *Usage:* Pesticide inert ingredient; Rubber; Leather tanning; Detergents; Solvent; Chemical intermediate; Dyes; Gasoline additive;

Rocket propellent; Textiles; Dehairing agent; Photography; Plasticizer; Pesticide propellent; Pharmaceuticals; Missile fuels; Soaps; Chemical manufacturing; Magnesium; Water treatment; Shampoo. **Metabolizes** as formaldehyde and nitrosamines. *References:* 82, 304, 388, 423.

Dimethylaminobenzene *see* **Xylidine.**

Dimethylaniline: *TN/synonyms:* N,N-Dimethylaniline; N,N-Dimethylbenzeneamine; N,N-Dimethylphenylamine. *OSHA PEL:* 5 ppm or 25 mg/m³ (8hr/day-40hr/wk-PP/S); 10 ppm or 50 mg/m³ (exposure not to exceed 15 min). *IDLH:* 100 ppm. *Symptoms:* Central nervous system depression; Collapse; Coma; Confusion; Convulsions; Cyanosis; Delayed hemoglobin oxidizing into to ferric form; Disorientation; Dizziness; Inability to utilize oxygen; Incoordination; Lethargy; Ringing or tingling in the ear; Unconsciousness; Vertigo; Visual disturbances; Weakness. *End-point Targets:* Blood; Kidneys; Liver; Cardiovascular system. *Usage:* Fiberglass; Dyes; Polyesters; Solvent; Vanillin; Methanol; Methyl furfural; Hydrogen peroxide; Nitrate; Alcohol; Formaldehyde; Michler's ketone. *References:* 83, 304, 388.

N,N-Dimethylaniline *see* **Dimethylaniline.**

Dimethylbenzene *see* **Xylenes.**

N,N-Dimethylbenzeneamine *see* **Dimethylaniline.**

N,N'-Dimethyl-4,4'-bipyridinium dichloride *see* **Paraquat.**

1,1'-Dimethyl-4-4'-bipyridium dichloride *see* **Paraquat.**

1,3-Dimethylbutyl acetate *see* **sec-Hexyl acetate.**

Dimethyl carbinol *see* **Isopropyl alcohol.**

Dimethylchloroether *see* **Chloromethyl methyl ether.**

Dimethyl-1,2-dibromo-2,2-dichloroethyl phosphate *see* **Naled.**

tris(Dimethyldithiocarbamate)-iron *see* **Ferbam.**

Dimethyleneimine *see* **Ethyleneimine.**

Dimethylene oxide *see* **Ethylene oxide.**

Dimethylenimine *see* **Ethyleneimine.**

Dimethyl ester of 1,2-benzenedicarboxylic acid *see* **Dimethylphthalate.**

Dimethylformamide: *TN/synonyms:* N,N-Dimethylformamide; DMF. *OSHA PEL:* 10 ppm or 30mg/m³ (8hr/day-40hr/wk-PP/S). *IDLH:* 3,500 ppm. *Symptoms:* Alcohol intolerance; Colic; Constipation; Dermatitis; Difficulty sleeping; Dizziness; Enlarged liver; Epigastric cramps; Facial congestion; Flushed face; Headaches; High blood pressure; Liver and kidney damage; Nausea; Nervousness; Stomach pain; Vomiting; Weakness. Suspected of causing Cancer (testicular); Birth defects. *End-point Targets:* Liver; Kidneys; Cardiovascular system; Skin. *Usage:* Solvent; Orlon; Rayon; Synthetic fabrics; Polyacrylic fiber; Cellulose; Antistatic agent; Photographic film; Textile dyes; Paint remover and cleaner; Leather finishing; Ethylene dichloride; Extraction of aromatic hydrocarbons from crude oil; Acrylic fibers; Pharmaceuticals; Pigments; Coatings; Adhesives; Printing ink; Pesticide inert ingredient. *Classification:* Organic solvent. *References:* 85, 304, 383, 386, 388, 423.

N,N-Dimethylformamide *see* **Dimethylformamide.**

2,6-Dimethyl-4-heptanone *see* **Diisobutyl ketone.**

as-Dimethylhydrazine *see* **1,1-Dimethylhydrazine.**

Asym Dimethylhydrazine *see* **1,1-Dimethylhydrazine.**

N,N-Dimethylhydrazine *see* 1,1-Dimethylhydrazine.

U-Dimethylhydrazine *see* 1,1-Dimethylhydrazine.

1,1-Dimethylhydrazine: *TN/synonyms:* Dimazine; DMH; UDMH; Unsymmetrical dimethylhydrazine; as-Dimethylhydrazine; Asym Dimethylhydrazine; N,N-Dimethylhydrazine; U-Dimethylhydrazine; Dimazin. *NIOSH:* Carcinogen at any exposure level. *NIOSH REL:* 0.06 ppm or 0.15 mg/m³ (ceiling limit, 2 hr exposure). *OSHA PEL:* 0.5 ppm or 1.0 mg/3 (8hr/day-40hr/wk-PP/S). *ACGIH:* Suspected human carcinogen. *IDLH:* 50 ppm. *Symptoms:* Eye, skin, and mucous membrane irritation and burns; Bronchial mucous destruction; Cardiac depression; Chest pains; Choking; Conjunctivitis; Convulsions; Death; Destruction of red blood cells; Excessive salivation; Facial swelling; Inability to utilize oxygen; Labored or difficult breathing; Lethargy; Liver and kidney damage; Loss of appetite; Low blood pressure; Nausea; Pulmonary edema; Respiratory distress; Vomiting. Suspected of causing Cancer; Depression; Diarrhea; Incoordination; Hemolytic anemia; Decrease in hematocrit, hemoglobin, and red blood cells; Lethargy; Anemia; Pulmonary hemorrhage; Birth defects; Immunosuppression; DNA damage. *End-point Targets:* Central nervous system; Liver; Blood; Skin; Gastrointestinal tract; Respiratory system; Eyes. *Usage:* Rocket fuel; Jet fuel; Gasoline additive; Photography; Plant growth regulator (fertilizer); Dissolving plastic. *References:* 268, 304, 306, 388.

Dimethyl ketone *see* Acetone.

Dimethyl methane *see* Propane.

Dimethyl monosulfate *see* Dimethyl sulfate.

Dimethylnitromethane *see* 2-Nitropropane.

Dimethyl p-nitrophenyl phos-phorothioate *see* Methyl parathion.

Dimethyl 4-nitrophenyl phosphorothioate *see* Methyl parathion.

Dimethyl p-nitrophenyl thiophosphate *see* Methyl parathion.

Dimethylnitrosamine *see* N-Nitrosodimethylamine.

N,N,-Dimethylnitrosamine *see* N-Nitrosodimethylamine.

2,6-Dimethyl-2,7-octadiene-6-ol *see* Linalyl alcohol.

3,7-Dimethyl-1,6-octadien-3-ol *see* Linalyl alcohol.

3,7-Dimethylocta-1,6-dien-3-ol *see* Linalyl alcohol.

2,6-Dimethylocta-2,7-doen-6-ol *see* Linalyl alcohol.

O,O-Dimethyl-S-4-oxo-1,2,3-benzotriazan-3(4H)-ylmethyl phosphorodithioate *see* Azinphos-methyl.

Dimethyl parathion; o,o-dimethyl o-(p-nitrophenyl) phosphorothioate *see* Methyl parathion.

N,N-Dimethylphenylamine *see* Dimethylaniline.

Dimethylphthalate: *TN/synonyms:* Dimethyl ester of 1,2-benzenedicarboxylic acid; DMP. *OSHA PEL:* 5 mg/m³ (8hr/day-40hr/wk). *IDLH:* 9,300 mg/m³. *Symptoms:* Mucous membrane, upper respiratory, and gastrointestinal irritation; Esophageal and gastric inflammation and hemorrhage; Stomach pains; Low blood pressure; Dizziness; Unconsciousness; Coma. *End-point Targets:* Respiratory system; Gastrointestinal tract. *Usage:* Pesticide inert ingredient; Solvent; Plasticizer; Varnishes; Clear films; Rocket propellent; Lacquers; Coatings; Safety glass; Perfumes; Mosquito, leech, flea, chigger, mite, and fly repellents; Rubber; Dyes; Hair spray; Cosmetics; Resins; Cellulose; Molding powders; Polyvinyl acetate; Polystyrene; Acrylic resins;

Plastics; Nitrocellulose; Animal insect repellent. *References:* 86, 286, 304, 388, 423.

Dimethyl sulfate: *TN/synonyms:* Dimethyl monosulfate; DMS; DMS (methyl sulfate); Methyl sulfate; Dimethyl sulphate. *NIOSH:* Carcinogen at any exposure level. *OSHA PEL:* 0.1 ppm or 0.5 mg/ m³ (8hr/ day-40hr/wk). *ACGIH:* Suspected human carcinogen. *IDLH:* 10 ppm. *Symptoms:* Eye and nasal irritation; Absence of normal sense of pain; Absolute exhaustion; Albumin in urine; Blood in urine; Cardiac damage; Chest pains and oppression; Circulatory failure; Coma; Conjunctiva, tongue, lips, larynx, glottis, and pulmonary edema; Conjunctivitis; Convulsions; Cough; Cyanosis; Dark urine; Death; Delirium; Diarrhea; Swelling around the eyes; Enlarged, tender liver; Eyelid spasms; Eyes become sensitive to light; Fever; Giddiness; Headaches; Hoarseness; Inability or difficulty speaking; Inability or difficulty swallowing; Jaundice; Labored or difficulty breathing; Lethargy; Liver and kidney injury; Liver failure; Loss of appetite; Malaise; Nausea; Painful or difficult urination; Paralysis; Severe itching; Skin and eye burns; Skin tissue death; Tearing; Vomiting. Suspected of causing Hypoglycemia; Cancer (lung). *End-point Targets:* Eyes; Respiratory system; Liver; Kidneys; Central nervous system; Skin. *Usage:* Dyes; Perfumes; Solvent; Mineral oils; Auto fluids analysis; Amines; Phenols; Adhesives; Pesticide manufacturing; Fabric softeners; Pharmaceuticals; Medicine. Formerly used as a chemical warfare gas. *Contaminant:* Paraquat. *Synergistic effects:* Decomposes in water to form sulfuric acid. *Note:* Symptoms may be delayed. *References:* 93, 304, 388.

Dimethyl sulphate *see* **Dimethyl sulfate.**

Dinitrobenzenes: *Isomers:* ortho-Dinitrobenzene; 1,2-Dinitrobenzene. meta-Dinitrobenzene; 1,3-Dinitrobenzene. para-Dinitrobenzene; 1,4-Dinitrobenzene. *OSHA PEL:* 1 mg/m³ (8hr/ day-40hr/wk-PP/S). *IDLH:* 200 mg/ m³ *Symptoms:* Anemia; Apathy; Aplastic anemia; Bad taste; Birth defects; Burning mouth; Cardiac palpitations; Central blind spots in vision; Constricted field of vision; Cyanosis; Dry throat; Fatigue; Headaches; Hemoglobin oxides to ferric form; Hemolytic anemia; Inability to utilize oxygen; Incoordination; Jaundice; Liver damage and tissue death; Numbness, tingling, or prickling sensation in feet, ankles, hands, and forearms; Peripheral nerve disturbances; Shortness of breath; Thirst; Tremors; Vision disturbances; Yellowing of hair, eyes, and skin. *Endpoint Targets:* Blood; Liver; Cardiovascular system; Eyes; Central nervous system. Usage: 1,2-Dinitrobenzene: Dyes; Explosives; Celluloid; Cellulose nitrate; Aniline; Medicine. 1,3-Dinitrobenzene: Spandex; Dyes; Explosives; Medicine; Cellulose; Aramid fibers; Aniline; m-Phenylenediamine; Aminocresols; Aromatic amines. 1,4-Dinitrobenzene: Dyes; Cellulose nitrate; Aniline; Medicine. *Note:* Neurotoxin. *References:* 17, 36, 87, 260, 269, 304, 388.

Dinitro-o-cresol: *TN/synonyms:* 4,6-Dinitro-o-cresol; 3,5-Dinitro-2-hydroxytoluene; 4,6-Dinitro-2-methyl phenol; DN; DNOC. *OSHA PEL:* 0.2 mg/m³ (8hr/day-40hr/wk-PP/S). *IDLH:* 5 mg/m³. *Symptoms:* Acidosis; Albumin, pus, or blood in urine; Anxiety; Cataracts; Chromosomal aberrations; Coma; Cough; Cyanosis; Death; Depression; Fatigue; Fever above 106 degrees; Fever; Flushed skin; Gastric upset; Glaucoma; Headaches; Heart rate over 100 beats per minute; Inability to utilize oxygen; Increased rate or depth of respiration; Intestinal mucosa hemorrhages; Kidney injury; Lassitude; Lung and brain swelling; Malaise; Nausea; Profuse sweating; Pulmonary edema; Rapid respiration; Renal insufficiency; Respiratory and circulatory collapse; Restlessness; Sensation of heat; Sense of well being; Shortness of breath; Skin tissue death; Thirst; Toxic hepatitis; Vomiting; Weak heartbeat; Weight loss; Yellow staining of skin and hair. Suspected of causing Genetic mutations; Cerebral dysfunction; Blurred vision; Involuntary eye movement; Tremors; Abnormal electroencephalogram; Staggering gait. *End-point Targets:* Cardiovascular system; Endocrine system; Eyes. *Usage:* Insecticide; Fungicide; Herbicide; Defoliant; Pesticide inert ingredient. No longer used in medicines or dyes. *References:* 88, 144, 304, 305, 388, 423.

4,6-Dinitro-o-cresol *see* **Dinitro-o-cresol.**

Dinitrogen tetroxide *see* **Nitrogen dioxide.**

3,5-Dinitro-2-hydroxytoluene *see* **Dinitro-o-cresol.**

4,6-Dinitro-2-methyl phenol *see* **Dinitro-o-cresol.**

Dinitrotoluenes: *TN/synonyms:* Dinitrotoluol; DNT; Methyldinitrobenzene. *Isomers:* 2,4-Dinitrotoluene-2, 4-Dinitrotoluol; 1-Methyl-2,4-dinitrobenzene. 2,6-Dinitrotoluene-2,6-Dinitrotoluol; 1-Methyl-2,6-dinitrobenzene. *NIOSH:* Carcinogen at any exposure level. *OSHA PEL:* 1.5 mg/m^3 (8hr/day-40hr/wk-PP/S). *IDLH:* 200 mg/m^3. *Symptoms:* Anemia; Central nervous system depression; Cyanosis; Death; Dizziness; Drowsiness; Headaches; Hemoglobin oxidizes to ferric form; Inability to utilize oxygen; Irritability; Jaundice; Labored or difficulty breathing; Muscle incoordination; Nausea; Respiratory depression; Spontaneous abortions; Unconsciousness; Vertigo; Vomiting; Weakness. Suspected of causing Cancer (liver); Testicular degeneration and atrophy; Nonfunctional ovaries; Decreased sperm count; Cerebral dysfunction; Blurred vision;

Birth defects; Involuntary eye movement; Tremors; Abnormal electroencephalogram; Staggering gait. *End-point Targets:* Blood; Liver; Cardiovascular system. *Usage:* Dyes; Ammunition; Explosives; Toluene diamine. *References:* 125, 144, 304, 317, 388.

Dinitrotoluol *see* **Dinitrotoluenes.**

Dioform (TN) *see* **1,2-Dichloroethylene.**

1,3-Dioxo-2-pivaloylindane *see* **Pindone.**

Dipenten *see* **Limonene.**

Dipentene *see* **Limonene.**

Dipentene 200 *see* **Limonene.**

4,4'-Diphenylmethane diisocyanate *see* **Methylene bisphenyl isocyanate.**

Diphenylmethane-4,4'-diisocyanate-trimellic anhydride-ethomid ht polymer *see* **Trimellitic anhydride.**

Diphenyl ether *see* **Phenylether.**

Diphenyl oxide *see* **Phenyl ether.**

Diphenyl oxide-diphenyl mixture *see* **Phenyl ether-biphenyl mixture.**

Dipotassium salt *see* **Chromic acid.**

Di-sec octyl phthalate: *TN/synonyms:* DEHP; DOP; bis-(2-Ethylhexyl) phthalate; di(2-Ethylhexyl) phthalate; Octyl phthalate; BEHP; Bisoflex 81 (tn); Eviplast 80 (tn); Octoil (tn); Platinol AH (tn); Sicol 150 (tn). *NIOSH:* Carcinogen at any exposure level. *OSHA PEL:* 5 mg/m^3 (8hr/day-40hr/wk); 10 mg/m^3 (exposure not to exceed 15 min). *IDLH:* Unknown. *Symptoms:* Eye and mucous membrane irritation. Suspected of causing Liver, kidney, testicular, thyroid, and pancreas damage; Birth defects; Decreased male and female fertility; Cancer (liver). *End-point Targets:* Eyes; Upper respiratory system; Gastrointestinal tract. *Usage:* Plastic; Rain gear; Footwear; Upholstery materials; Imitation leather; Waterproof clothing; Tablecloths; Shower curtains; Food packaging; Floor tiles; Children's toys; Flexible tubing with medical applications; Plastic bags; Containers for blood; Polyvinyl chloride; Plastic plumbing materials; Adhesives; Paper; Paperboard; Erasable ink; Acaricide; Pesticide inert ingredient; Cosmetics; Fabric coatings. *Classification:* Organic solvent. *References:* 304, 306, 362, 383, 388, 423, 429.

Dithiocarbonic anhydride *see* **Carbon disulfide.**

Dithion *see* **TEDP.**

Ditrapex (tn) *see* **1,3-Dichloropropene.**

Divanadium pentoxide *see* **Vanadium pentoxide.**

Divinyl *see* **1,3-Butadiene.**

DMAC *see* **Dimethyl acetamide.**

DMF *see* **Dimethylformamide.**

DMH *see* **1,1-Dimethylhydrazine.**

DMNA *see* **N-Nitrosodimethylamine.**

DMP *see* **Dimethylphthalate.**

DMS *see* **Dimethyl sulfate.**

DMS(methyl sulfate) *see* **Dimethyl sulfate.**

DN *see* **Dinitro-o-cresol.**

DNOC *see* **Dinitro-o-cresol.**

DNT *see* **Dinitrotoluenes.**

Dojyopicrin (tn) *see* **Chloropicrin.**

Dolochlor (tn) *see* **Chloropicrin.**

DOP *see* **Di-sec octyl phthalate.**

Dowanol EB (tn) *see* **2-Butoxyethanol.**

Dowclene EC (tn) *see* **Tetrachloroethylene.**

DOWCO 179 (tn) *see* **Chlorpyrifos.**

Dowfume EDB (tn) *see* **Ethylene dibromide.**

Dowfume MC-2 (tn) *see* **Ethylene dibromide.**

Dowfume W85 (tn) *see* **Ethylene dibromide.**

Dowfume 40, W-10, W-15, W-40 (tn) *see* **Ethylene dibromide.**

Dowicide 2S(tn) *see* **2,4,6-Trichlorophenol.**

Dowper (tn) *see* **Tetrachloroethylene.**

Dowtherm A (tn) *see* **Phenyl ether-biphenyl mixture.**

Dow-Tri (tn) *see* **Trichloroethylene.**

2,4-DPC *see* **2,4-Dichlorophenol.**

Drexel Methyl Parathion 4E (tn) *see* **Methyl parathion.**

Dry cleaning safety solvent *see* **Stoddard solvent.**

Dry ice *see* **Carbon dioxide.**

Dukeron (tn) *see* **Trichloroethylene.**

Dursban (tn) *see* **Chlorpyrifos.**

Dursban F (tn) *see* **Chlorpyrifos.**

Dursban 4E (tn) *see* **Chlorpyrifos.**

Dutch oil *see* **1,1-Dichloroethane.**

E 601 (tn) *see* **Methyl parathion.**

EB *see* **Ethyl benzene.**

EDB-85 (tn) *see* **Ethylene dibromide.**

EGDN *see* **Ethylene glycol dinitrate.**

EGEEA *see* **2-Ethoxyethyl acetate.**

EGME *see* **Methyl cellosolve.**

EGMEA *see* **Methyl cellosolve acetate.**

Ektasolve EB (tn) *see* **2-Butoxyethanol.**

Elaldehyde *see* **Paraldehyde.**

Elemental barium *see* **Barium.**

Elemental manganese *see* **Manganese.**

Elemental selenium *see* **Selenium.**

Elemental white phosphorus *see* **Phosphorus.**

Embafume (r) *see* **Methyl bromide.**

Endosulfan: *TN/synonyms:* 6,7,8, 9,10,10-Hexachloro-1,5,5a,6,9,9a-hexahydro-6,9-methano-2,4,3-benzodiaoxathiepin; 3-oxide; Chlorthiepin (tn); Endosulfan technical; 5-Norbornene-2, 3-di-methanol-1,4,5,6,7,7-hexachlorocyclic sulfite; Thiodan (tn); Thionex (tn); Thionax (tn); Malix (tn); HOE 02671 (tn); FMA 5462 (tn); Cyclodan (tn); Thifor (tn); Beosit (tn); Chlorthiepan (tn). *OSHA PEL:* 0.1 mg/m³ (8 hr/day-40hr/wk). *ATSDR MRL:* 0.014 ppm (Ingestion, less than 15 days); 0.004 ppm (Ingestion, more than 14 days). *Symptoms:* Brain swelling, Convulsions, Cyanosis, Damage to red blood cells, Death, Decreased respiration, Excessive salivation, Heart rate over 100 beats per minute, Hemorrhaging, High blood pressure, Hyperactivity, Labored or difficulty breathing, Respiratory arrest, Tonic-Clonic convulsions, Tremors. Suspected of causing Reduced kidney function and injury, Immune system damage, Birth defects, and Fetal toxicity. *End-point Targets:* Central nervous system and Blood. *Usage:* Insecticide, Pesticide. Found in cigarette smoke if tobacco has been contaminated. *References:* 375, 388.

Endosulfan technical *see* **Endosulfan.**

Engravers acid *see* **Nitric acid.**

ENT 15, 349 (tn) *see* **Ethylene dibromide.**

ENT 17, 292 (tn) *see* **Methyl parathion.**

ENT 27, 311 (tn) *see* **Chlorpyrifos.**

ENT 54 (tn) *see* **Acrylonitrile.**

ENT 1860 (tn) *see* **Tetrachloroethylene.**

Epichlorohydrin: *TN/synonyms:* 1-Chloro-2,3-epoxypropane; 2-Chloropropylene oxide; gamma-Chloropropylene oxide. *NIOSH:* Carcinogen at any exposure level. Reduce exposure to lowest feasible concentration. *OSHA PEL:* 2 ppm or 8 mg/m³ (8hr/day-40hr/wk-PP/S). *IDLH:* 250 ppm. *Symptoms:* Skin irritation with deep pain; Eye irritation; Abdominal pain; Asthmatic bronchitis; Chemical sensitization; Chromosomal aberrations; Chronic bronchitis; Conjunctivitis; Corneal clouding, tissue death, and opacity; Cough; Cyanosis; Death; Dermatitis; Fatigue; Genetic mutation; Liver and kidney damage; Nasal inflammation with profuse discharge; Nausea; Pulmonary inflammation; Respiratory distress and paralysis; Skin burns; Tearing; Vomiting. Suspected of causing Cancer; Birth defects; Sterility. *End-point Targets:* Respiratory system; Skin; Kidneys. *Usage:* Pesticide inert ingredient; Insecticide manufacturing; Solvent; Resins; Gums; Cellulose; Paints; Varnishes; Fingernail polish; Lacquers; Starch; Microencapsulation; Plastics; Resins; Hair conditioner; Elastic; Paper; Pharmaceuticals; Insect fumigant; Cement for celluloid; Glycerol; Allyl glycidyl ether; Glycerin; Eyeglass lenses; Detergents; Trichloroethylene; Wound covering gel; Cyclodextrins; Aryloxypropanolamine; Metallurgy; Plasticizers; Water treatment. *Classification:* Organic solvent. *References:* 127, 286, 304, 383, 388, 402, 423.

EPN: *TN/synonyms:* O-Ethyl O-P-nitrophenyl benzenephosphonothioate; O-Ethyl O-P-nitrophenyl benzenethiophosphonate. *OSHA PEL:* 0.5 mg/m³ (8hr/day-40hr/wk-PP/S). *IDLH:* 50 mg/m³. *Symptoms:* Skin and eye irritation; Abdominal cramps; Asphyxia; Blurring or dimness of vision; Cardiac irregularities; Coma; Confusion; Constricted pupils; Convulsions; Cyanosis; Death; Diarrhea; Difficulty breathing; Dilated pupils; Disorientation; Drowsiness; Excessive salivation; Eye pain; Giddiness; Headaches; High blood pressure; Incontinence; Incoordination; Inhibits cholinesterase enzymes; Laryngeal spasms; Loss of appetite; Low blood pressure; Muscle spasms, twitching, and involuntary contractions; Nasal discharge; Nausea; Paralysis; Respiratory arrest; Slurred speech; Tearing; Tight chest; Vertigo; Vomiting; Weakness; Wheezing. *End-point Targets:* Respiratory system; Cardiovascular system; Central nervous system; Eyes; Skin; Blood cholinesterase. *Usage:* Pesticide; Insecticide. *References:* 112, 304, 388.

1,4-Epoxybutane *see* **Tetrahydrofuran.**

Epoxyethane *see* **Ethylene oxide.**

1,2-Epoxy ethane *see* **Ethylene oxide.**

1,2-Epoxy-3-phenoxy propane *see* **Phenyl glycidyl ether.**

1,2-Epoxy propane *see* **Propylene oxide.**

2,3-Epoxy-1-propanol *see* **Glycidol.**

Epoxypropyl alcohol *see* **Glycidol.**

2-Epoxypropyl ether *see* **Diglycidyl ether.**

dis(2,3-Epoxypropyl) ether *see* **Diglycidyl ether.**

Eradex (tn) *see* **Chlorpyrifos.**

Eranol *see* **Iodine.**

Erythrene *see* **1,3-Butadiene.**

Essence of mirbane *see* **Nitrobenzene.**

Ethanal *see* **Acetaldehyde.**

1,2-Ethanediamine *see* **Ethylenediamine.**

Ethanedioic acid *see* **Oxalic acid.**

1,2-Ethanediol *see* **Ethylene glycol.**

1,2-Ethanediol dinitrate *see* **Ethylene glycol dinitrate.**

Ethanethiol *see* **Ethyl mercaptan.**

Ethanoic acid *see* **Acetic acid or Vinyl acetate.**

Ethanoic anhydride *see* **Acetic anhydride.**

Ethanol: *TN/synonyms:* Absolute ethanol; Alcohol; Alcohol anhydride; Ethyl alcohol; Ethanol 200 Proof; Ethyl hydrate; Ethyl hydroxide; Fermentation alcohol; Grain alcohol; Methylcarbinol; Molasses alcohol; Potato alcohol; Spirits of wine; Jaysol S (tn); Tecsol (tn); Tecsol C (tn); Algrain (tn); Anhydrol (tn); Cologne spirits (tn). *OSHA PEL:* 1,000 ppm (8hr/day-40hr/wk). *IDLH:* NE. *Symptoms:* Eye and skin irritation; Amnesia; Birth defects; Central nervous system dysfunction; Cerebellar atrophy; Changes in mood, personality, and behavior; Circulatory collapse; Cirrhosis; Clumsiness; Cold, clammy skin; Coma; Congenital abnormally small head; Death; Decreased sense of smell and taste; Dizziness; Double vision; Euphoria; Fetal Alcohol Syndrome; Heavy breathing; Hypothermia; Impaired mental activity; Impaired sensory function; Incoordination; Liver and heart damage; Loss of ability to speak; Loss of sensation; Lowered IQ; Muscular incoordination; Nausea; Pancreatic disorders; Pneumonia; Reduced visual acuity; Spontaneous and induced involuntary eye movement; Staggering gait; Stupor; Vomiting. Suspected of causing Impotence; Sperm abnormalities. *End-point Targets:* Central nervous system; Liver. *Usage:* Acetaldehyde; Acetic acid; Alcoholic beverages; Anti-freeze; Antiseptic; Cosmetics; Dehydrating agent; Denatured alcohols; Detergents; Disinfectant; Dyes; Ethylacetate; Ethylchloride; Ethylether; Explosives; Fats; Fatty acid; Food additive and flavorings; Gasohol; Gasoline additive; Household cleaners; Inks; Lacquer; Oils; Paint; Perfume; Pharmaceuticals; Plasticizers; Plastics; Resins; Soap; Solvent; Surface coatings; Surgical suture packing; Synthetic rubber; Toiletries; Vinegar; Yeast growth medium; Pesticide inert ingredient; Mouthwash; Cough syrup; Alcoholic beverages; Topical mediciation; Mouthwash; Shellac; Rubbing alcohol. *Classification:* Polar volatile organic compounds. *Note:* Neurotoxin. *References:* 16, 17, 62, 388, 423, 429, 449, 452, 457.

Ethanol 200 Proof *see* **Ethanol.**

Ethanolamine: *TN/synonyms:* 2-Aminoethanol; beta-Aminoethyl alcohol; Ethylolamine; 2-Hydroyethylamine; Monoethanolamine. *OSHA PEL:* 3 ppm or 8 mg/m³ (8hr/day-40hr/wk-PP/S); 6 ppm or 15 mg/m³ (exposure not to exceed 15 min). *IDLH:* 1,000 ppm. *Symptoms:* Eye, skin, respiratory irritation; Lethargy. *End-point Targets:* Skin; Eyes; Respiratory system. *Usage:* Pesticide inert ingredient; Pharmaceutical aids; Leather; Pesticide manufacturing; Medicine; Antibiotics; Polishes; Hair wave solution (permanents); Soaps; Detergents; Corrosion inhibitor; Rubber; Textiles; Gasoline additive; Chemical intermediate; Cosmetics; Furniture polish; Floor polishes; Automobile polishes; Paints. *References:* 114, 304, 388, 423.

Ethene oxide *see* **Ethylene oxide.**

Ethenone *see* **Ketene.**

Ethenyl acetate *see* **Vinyl acetate.**

Ethenyl benzene *see* **Styrene.**

Ethenyl ester *see* **Vinyl acetate.**

Ethenyl ethanoate *see* **Vinyl acetate.**

Ethenylmethylbenzene *see* **Vinyl toluene.**

Ether *see* **Ethyl ether.**

Ethinyl trichloride *see* **Trichloroethylene.**

2-Ethoxyethyl acetate: *TN/synonyms:* Cellosolve acetate; EGEEA; Ethylene glycol monoethyl ether acetate; Glycol monoethyl ether acetate. *NIOSH:* Reduce exposure to lowest feasible concentration. *OSHA PEL:* 100 ppm or 540 mg/m³ (8hr/day-40hr/wk-PP/S). *IDLH:* 2,500 ppm. *Symptoms:* Eye and nasal irritation; Abdominal pain; Absence of urine formation; Albumin and blood in urine; Blurred vision; Brain, liver, meninges, and heart lesions; Central nervous system depression; Costervertebral angle tenderness; Diarrhea; Drowsiness; Headache; Kidney damage and failure; Lumbar pain; Nausea; Paralysis; Personality changes; Recrudescent stuttering; Reduced urine formation; Slurred speech; Staggering gait; Transient excessive discharge of urine; Tremors; Vomiting; Weakness. Suspected of causing Pulmonary edema; Intravascular destruction of red blood cells; Bone marrow depression. *End-point Targets:* Respiratory system; Eyes; Gastrointestinal tract. *Usage:* Pesticide inert ingredient; Automobile lacquer; Solvent; Nitrocellulose; Oils; Resins; Varnish removers; Wood stains; Textiles; Leather; Lacquers; Oven cleaners. *Note:* Patients may be misdiagnosed with Schizophrenia or Narcolepsy. *References:* 120, 304, 388, 423.

Ethyl acetate: *TN/synonyms:* Acetic ester; Acetic ether; Ethyl ester of acetic acid; Ethyl ethanoate. *OSHA PEL:* 400 ppm or 1,400 mg/m³ (8hr/day-40hr/wk-PP/s). *IDLH:* 10,000 ppm. *Symptoms:* Eye, nasal, throat, and respiratory irritation; Belligerence;

Boastfulness; Cold, painful skin; Coma; Convulsions; Corneal abnormalities; Death; Dermatitis; Dilated pupils; Double vision; Drowsiness; Emotional instability; Exhilaration; Flushed face; Gastritis; Headaches; Heart rate over 100 beats per minute; Hypoglycemia; Hypothermia; Impaired motor skills; Impaired or absent tendon reflexes; Incontinence; Incoordination; Low blood pressure; Lung, liver, kidney, and heart damage; Nausea; Partial or complete loss of sensation; Peripheral vascular collapse; Pneumonia; Profuse sweating; Rapid pulse; Remorse; Shock; Slowed reaction time; Slowed respiration; Slurred speech; Stupor; Talkativeness; Unconsciousness due to narcotic effects; Vertigo; Vomiting; Weakness. Suspected of causing Central nervous system depression; Death. *End-point Targets:* Eyes; Skin; Respiratory system. *Usage:* Adhesives; Antispasmodic drugs; Artificial fruit flavoring, leather, and silk; Cellophane; Chemical intermediate; Contact lenses mold release; Enamel paints; Fingernail polish remover; Fingernail polish; Food flavoring; Fragrances; Fruit and vegetable inks; Grape beverages; Herbicide intermediate; Inks; Lacquer thinner; Lacquers; Medicines; Nitrocellulose; Perfumes; Pesticide inert ingredient; Pharmaceutical flavoring; Photographic films; Plastics; Printing; Shellac; Smokeless powders; Solvent; Topical medicine; Vaccines; Varnishes; Vinyl resins; Oven cleaners. *Classification:* Polar volatile organic compounds. *Note:* Neurotoxin. *References:* 17, 113, 304, 388, 423, 452.

Ethyl acetone *see* **2-Pentanone.**

Ethyl acrylate: *TN/synonyms:* Ethyl acrylate (inhibited); Ethyl ester of acrylic acid; Ethyl propenoate. *NIOSH:* Carcinogen at any exposure level. Reduce exposure to lowest feasible concentration. *OSHA PEL:* 5 ppm or 20 mg/m³ (8hr/day-40hr/wk-PP/S); 25 ppm or 100 mg/m³ (exposure not to exceed 15 min). *IDLH:* 2,000 ppm. *Symptoms:* Eye, skin, mucous membrane, gastrointestinal, and respiratory irritation; Tearing; Lethargy; Death; Convulsions; Pulmonary edema; Blindness; Headaches; Nausea; Neurotic symptoms; Chemical sensitization; Rapid respiration; Blue lips; Drowsiness; Autonomic symptoms; Cough; Itching skin. Suspected of causing Cancer (colon, rectal). *End-point Targets:* Respiratory system; Eyes; Skin. *Usage:* Pesticide inert ingredient; Food flavoring; Fragrances; Textiles; Fabric backcoatings; Fabric finishes; Shoe polishes; Floor polishes; Surface coatings; Pigments; Paper coatings; Floor sealants; Leather; Caulking compounds; Adhesives; Resins; Plastics; Acrylic fabrics; Latex paint; Paperboard; Polyesters. *Additives:* Inhibitors such as hydroquinone. *References:* 116, 304, 388, 423.

Ethyl acrylate (inhibited) *see* **Ethyl acrylate.**

Ethyl alcohol *see* **Ethanol.**

Ethyl aldehyde *see* **Acetaldehyde.**

Ethylamine: *TN/synonyms:* Aminoethane; Monoethylamine. *OSHA PEL:* 10 ppm or 18 mg/m³ (8hr/day-40hr/wk-PP/S). *IDLH:* 4,000 ppm. *Symptoms:* Eye, mucous membrane, and respiratory irritation; Skin burns; Dermatitis; Corneal swelling; Hazy blue vision. *End-point Targets:* Respiratory system; Eyes; Skin. *Usage:* Resins; Latex rubber; Petroleum and oil refining; Herbicide intermediate; Wash & wear fabrics; Detergents; Solvent; Plasticizer. *References:* 137, 304, 388.

Ethyl amyl ketone *see* **5-Methyl-3-heptanone.**

Ethyl benzene: *TN/synonyms:* Ethylbenzol; Phenylethane; Aethylbenzyl; EB; Etilbenzene; Etylobenzene. *OSHA PEL:* 100 ppm or 435 mg/m³ (8hr/day-40hr/wk-PP/S); 125 ppm or 545 mg/m³ (exposure not to exceed 15 min). *ATSDR MRL:* 0.29 ppm

(Inhalation, more than 15 days). *IDLH:* 2,000 ppm. *Symptoms:* Mucous member, eye, nasal, throat, and upper respiratory irritation; Skin irritation, inflammation, blisters, and burns; Headaches; Dermatitis; Sleepiness; Unconsciousness due to narcotic effects; Coma; Difficulty breathing; Central nervous system depression; Nausea; Dizziness; Vomiting; Vertigo; Chest constriction. Suspected of causing Lung inflammation; Liver and kidney damage. *End-point Targets:* Eyes; Upper respiratory system; Central nervous system. *Usage:* Insecticides; Paint; Varnish; Glue; Carpet glue; Ink; Gasoline (2% by weight); Pesticide inert ingredient; Asphalt; Petroleum based fuels; Chemical manufacturing. *References:* 286, 304, 335, 388, 423, 429.

Ethylbenzol *see* **Ethyl benzene.**

Ethyl bromide: *TN/synonyms:* Bromoethane. *NIOSH:* No REL, notified OSHA that documentation doesn't support the worker's safety at established PEL. *OSHA PEL:* 200 ppm or 890 mg/m³ (8hr/day-40hr/wk-PP/S); 250 ppm or 1,100 mg/m³ (exposure not to exceed 15 min). *IDLH:* 3,500 ppm. *Symptoms:* Eye, respiratory, and skin irritation; Blindness; Cardiac arrhythmias and arrest; Central nervous system depression; Collapse; Conjunctiva and intestinal congestion and hemorrhages; Cyanosis; Death; Dilated pupils; Facial redness; Liver and kidney disease; Liver, kidney, and heart degeneration; Partial or complete loss of sensation; Pulmonary edema; Rapid pulse; Respiratory disorders and paralysis. *End-point Targets:* Skin; Liver; Kidneys; Respiratory system; Cardiovascular system; Central nervous system. *Usage:* Refrigerant; Pharmaceutical intermediate; Gasoline additive; Grain and fruit fumigant. *References:* 115, 304, 388.

Ethyl butyl ketone: *TN/synonyms:* Butyl ethyl ketone; 3-Heptanone. *OSHA PEL:* 50 ppm or 230 mg/m³

(8hr/day-40hr/wk-PP/S). *IDLH:* 3,000 ppm. *Symptoms:* Eye and mucus membrane irritation; Headaches; Unconsciousness due to narcotic effects; Coma; Dermatitis. *End-point Targets:* Eyes; Skin; Respiratory system. *Usage:* Food flavoring; Perfumes; Plastics; Printing ink; Lacquers; Solvent; Finishes; Polyvinyl and nitrocellulose resins. *References:* 117, 304, 388.

Ethyl carbinol *see* **n-Propyl alcohol.**

Ethyl chloride: *TN/synonyms:* Chloroethane; Hydrochloric ether; Monochloroethane; Muriatic ether. *NIOSH:* No REL, notified OSHA that documentation doesn't support the worker's safety at established PELs *OSHA PEL:* 1,000 ppm or 2,600 mg/m³ (8hr/day-40hr/wk-PP/S). *IDLH:* 20,000 ppm. *Symptoms:* Eye and mucous membrane irritation; Nausea; Incoordination; Inebriate; Abdominal cramps; Vomiting; Nervous system dysfunction; Blood cell disorders; Cardiac arrhythmias and arrest; Liver and kidney damage; Frostbite; Stupor; Central nervous system depression; Dizziness; Weak or absent of normal sense of pain; Unconsciousness due to narcotic effects; Death. Suspected of causing Cancer. *End-point Targets:* Liver; Kidneys; Respiratory system; Cardiovascular system. *Usage:* Pesticide inert ingredient; Chemical intermediate; Solvent; Tetraethyl lead; Medicine; Topical anesthetic; Fats; Oils; Resins; Waxes; Insecticide manufacturing; Dyes; Perfumes; Refrigerant; Solvent; Veterinary medicine; Aerosol propellents; Cellulose; Plastics; Pharmaceuticals; Oven cleaners. *Synergistic effects:* Reacts with water to form hydrochloric acid. *Classification:* Chlorinated aliphatic hydrocarbon; Chlorinated organic compound. *References:* 119, 286, 304, 388, 399, 423, 429.

Ethylene *see* **Ethylene glycol.**

Ethylene alcohol *see* **Ethylene glycol.**

Ethylene bromide *see* **Ethylene dibromide.**

Ethylenediamine: *TN/synonyms:* Ethylenediamine anhydrous; 1,2-Diaminoethane; 1,2-Ethanediamine. *OSHA PEL:* 10 ppm or 25 mg/m³ (8hr/day-40hr/wk-PP/S). *ACGIH:* No threshold value limit will insure prevention of hypersensitive responses. *IDLH:* 2,000 ppm. *Symptoms:* Nasal and respiratory irritation; Asthma; Liver and kidney damage; Facial tingling; Wheezing; Heaviness in chest; Allergic nasal inflammation with profuse discharge; Contact dermatitis; Chemical hypersensitivity. Suspected of causing Cancer (mycosis fungoides). *End-point Targets:* Respiratory system; Liver; Kidneys; Skin. *Usage:* Fungicide; Solvent; Casein; Shellac; Latex rubber; Antifreeze; Lubricants; Pharmaceutical aids; Dyes; Waxes; Resins; Asphalt; Insecticide and herbicide manufacturing; Detergents; Corrosion inhibitors; Gasoline and oil additive; Paint thinner; Hair setting lotion; Cold hair lotions (permanents); Fingernail polish; Textiles; Urethane; Veterinary medicine; Chelating agent. *References:* 133, 304, 388.

Ethylenediamine anhydrous *see* **Ethylenediamine.**

Ethylene dibromide: *TN/Synonyms:* 1,2-Dibromoethane; Ethylene bromide; Glycol dibromide; Bromofume; Dowfume W85 (tn); Dowfume EDB (tn); Dowfume 40, W-10, W-15, W-40 (tn); Dowfume MC-2 (tn); Iscobrome D (tn); ENT 15, 349 (tn); Netis (tn); Pestmaster EDB-85 (tn); Santryuum (tn); Unifume (tn); EDB-85 (tn); Fumogas (tn); Icopfume soilbrom-85 (tn); Soilfume (tn). *NIOSH:* Carcinogen at any exposure level. *NIOSH REL:* 0.045 ppm (10hr/day-40hr/wk); 0.13 ppm (ceiling limit not to exceed 15 min). *OSHA PEL:* 20 ppm (8hr/day-40hr/wk-PP/S); 30 ppm (ceiling exposure); 50 ppm (exposure not exceed 5 min). *ACGIH:* Suspected human carcinogen. *ATSDR MRL:*

0.0006 ppm (Inhalation, less than 15 days); 0.1 ppm (Ingestion, more than 14 days). *IDLH:* 400 ppm. *Symptoms:* Eye and respiratory irritation; Acute myocardial lesions; Binds to DNA; Cardiopulmonary arrest; Collapse; Death; Depression; Dermatitis with vesiculation; Diarrhea; Disorientation; Headaches; Kidney damage and failure; Liver cell death, damage, and disease; Nausea; Pharyngeal ulcers; Pulmonary edema; Skin blisters, redness, and inflammation; Tissue or bone death; Vomiting. Suspected of causing Respiratory tract lesions; Affects production and development of blood cells; Corneal damage; Decreased sperm count; Sperm abnormalities; Genetic mutation; Inheritable genetic mutations; Chromosomal aberrations; Cancer. *End-point Targets:* Respiratory system; Liver; Kidneys; Skin; Eyes. *Usage:* Pesticide inert ingredient; Gasoline additive; Dyes; Pharmaceuticals; Resins; Waxes; Gums; Asphalt; Vinyl bromide; Solvent. Banned as an insecticide and fumigant in 1984. Found in Engine exhaust. *Note:* Humans are more susceptible than animals to the acute toxic effects. *Classification:* Organic solvent. *References:* 136, 304, 312, 360, 383, 388, 396, 405, 423, 429, 434, 449.

Ethylene dichloride: *TN/synonyms:* 1,2-Dichloroethane; Ethylene chloride; Glycol dichloride. *NIOSH:* Carcinogen at any exposure level. *OSHA PEL:* 1 ppm or 4 mg/m³ (8hr/day-40hr/wk-PP/S); 2 ppm or 8 mg/m³ (exposure not to exceed 15 min). *IDLH:* 1,000 ppm. *Symptoms:* Eye and skin irritation; Adrenal tissue death; Anemia; Central nervous system depression; Circulatory and respiratory failure; Coma; Confusion; Conjunctiva congestion; Corneal abrasions and opacity; Death; Defatting dermatitis; Deficiency of thrombin enzymes in blood; Dermatitis; Diarrhea; Excessive calcium in the blood; Eyes become sensitive to light; Gastrointestinal hemorrhage; Headaches; Heart rate over 100 beats per minute; Hypoglycemia; Insomnia; Involuntary eye movement; Jaundice; Labored or difficulty breathing; Lightheadedness; Kidney damage and hemorrhaging; Liver damage, hemorrhaging, pain, tissue death, and failure; Low blood pressure; Memory disorders; Metallic taste; Nausea; Nervousness; Poor equilibrium; Reduced blood clotting factor; Reduced urine formation; Stupor; Tremors; Vertigo; Vomiting; Weakness; Widespread internal hemorrhaging. Suspected of causing Cancer; Genetic mutations. *End-point Targets:* Kidneys; Liver; Eyes; Skin; Central nervous system. *Usage:* Adhesives; Aircraft manufacturing glues; Asphalt; Cellulose; Cosmetics; Degreasers; Dry cleaning; Elastics; Extraction of spices; Fats; Fumigant for grain, upholstery, and carpet; Gasoline additive; Gums; Leather tanning and cleaning; Metal cleaners; Nylon; Oils; Paints, varnish, and finish remover; Pesticide inert ingredient; Pharmaceuticals; Photocopying; Photography; Plastics; Rayon; Resins; Rubber cement; Rubber products; Rubber; Scouring compounds; Shower curtains; Soaps; Solvent; Tobacco extraction; Trichlorethane; Trichloroethylene; Typewriter correction fluid; Vinyl chloride; Vinylidene chloride; Water softener; Waxes. *Synergistic effects:* Exposed smokers may be more prone to emphysema. *Classification:* Organic solvent; Polar volatile organic compounds; Chlorinated organic compound. *Note:* Historically established as a neurotoxin. *References:* 17, 135, 286, 304, 306, 383, 388, 398, 399, 413, 423, 452.

Ethylene dinitrate *see* **Ethylene glycol dinitrate.**

Ethylene ester *see* **Vinyl acetate.**

Ethylene glycol: *TN/synonyms:* 1,2-Dihydronxyethane; 1,2-Ethanediol; Glycol; Glycol alcohol; Ethylene alcohol; Ethylene; Lutrol-9 (tn); Macrogol 400 BPC (tn); Monoethylene glycol. *OSHA PEL:* None. *ACGIH TLV:* 50 ppm. *Symptoms:* Throat irritation; Absence of reflexes; Absence of urine formation; Albumin and blood in urine; Brain and meninges inflammation; Central nervous system depression; Cerebral swelling; Coma; Convulsions; Cyanosis; Death; Drowsiness; Excess of lymphocytes in the blood; Headaches; Inability to utilize oxygen; Involuntary eye movement; Kidney damage, failure, and hemorrhagic tissue death; Lower backaches; Nausea; Perivascular swelling; Respiratory failure; Tremors; Unconsciousness; Uremia; Vomiting. *End-point Targets:* Blood; Central nervous system; Kidneys. *Usage:* Commercial antifreeze; Hydraulic; Industrial humectant; Solvent; Paints; Plastics; Printing ink; Stamp pad ink; Ball-point pens; Cellophane; Explosives; Resins; Plasticizers; Elastics; Pharmaceutical aids; Food flavoring; Skin lotion; Cosmetic powders; Asphalt; Polyester fibers; Wood stains; Adhesives; Leather dyes; Tobacco; Deicing; Polyurethanes; Latex paints; Pesticide inert ingredient; Natural gas additive; Metal cleaning; Plastic bottles. *Classification:* Organic solvent. *Note:* Neurotoxin. *References:* 17, 259, 383, 423.

Ethylene glycol dinitrate: *TN/synonyms:* EGDN; 1,2-Ethanediol dinitrate; Ethylene dinitrate; Ethylene nitrate; Glycol dinitrate; Nitroglycol. *OSHA PEL:* 0.1 mg/m^3-exposure not to exceed 15 min. *IDLH:* 500 mg/m^3. *Symptoms:* Throbbing headaches; Dizziness; Nausea; Vomiting; Abdominal pain; Low blood pressure; Flushed skin; Cardiac palpitations; Hemoglobin oxides to ferric form; Delirium; Central nervous system depression; Angina; Skin irritation. Suspected of causing Anemia; Mild liver and kidney damage. *End-point Targets:* Cardiovascular system; Blood; Skin. *Usage:* Antifreeze; Polyesters; Pesticide inert ingredient. *Classification:* Organic solvent. *References:* 134, 304, 306, 383, 388, 423.

Ethylene glycol monobutyl ether *see* **2-Butoxyethanol.**

Ethylene glycol monoethyl ether acetate *see* **2-Ethoxyethyl acetate or Methyl cellosolve acetate.**

Ethylene glycol monomethyl ether *see* **Methyl cellosolve.**

Ethyleneimine: *TN/synonyms:* Aminoethylene; Azirane; Aziridine; Dimethyleneimine; Dimethylenimine; Ethylenimine; Ethylimine. *NIOSH:* Carcinogen at any exposure level. Reduce exposure to lowest feasible concentration. *OSHA:* No PEL, 1 of 13 chemicals recognized as an occupational carcinogen. Exposure of workers is to be controlled through required engineering controls, work practices, and personal protective equipment. *IDLH:* 100 ppm. *Symptoms:* Nasal and throat irritation; Albumin and blood in urine; Bronchial pneumonia; Bronchitis; Cancer; Conjunctivitis; Corneal inflammation; Coughing; Dizziness; DNA damage; Excess of red blood cells; Excessive eosinophils in blood; Eye and skin burns; Facial swelling; Headaches; Increased in leukocytes; Liver and kidney damage; Nausea; Pulmonary and laryngeal edema; Septum ulceration; Shortness of breath; Skin sensitivity; Vomiting. Suspected of causing Genetic mutations. *End-point Targets:* Eyes; Lungs; Skin; Liver; Kidneys. *Usage:* Paper; Adhesives; Binders; Petroleum refining; Fuels; Lubricants; Resins; Varnishes; Lacquers; Pesticide manufacturing; Cosmetics; Photography; Detergents; Chemical manufacturing; Textile flame-proofing; improving wet strength; shrink-proofing; stiffening, and water-proofing; Plant mutations; Pharmaceuticals. *References:* 132, 304, 305, 388.

Ethylene monochloride *see* **Vinyl chloride.**

Ethylene nitrate *see* **Ethylene glycol dinitrate.**

Ethylene oxide: *TN/synonyms:* Dimethylene oxide; 1,2-Epoxy ethane; Oxirane; Dihydro-oxirene; Epoxyethane; Ethene oxide; ETO; Anprolene (tn); Oxyfume (tn); T-Gas (tn). *NIOSH:* Carcinogen at any exposure level. *NIOSH REL:* (means less than) 0.1 ppm or 0.18 mg/m³ (10hr/day-40hr/wk); 5 ppm (ceiling limit); 9 mg/m³ (15 min/day). *OSHA PEL:* 1 ppm (8hr/day-40hr/wk); 5 ppm (15-min Excursion). *ACGIH:* Suspected human carcinogen. *ATSDR MRL:* 0.09 ppm (Inhalation, more than 14 days). *IDLH:* 800 ppm. *Symptoms:* Eye, nasal, and throat irritation; Bronchitis; Burns skin and eyes; Cancer (leukemia, stomach, pancreatic); Cataracts; Chromosomal aberrations; Corneal burns; Cyanosis; Decreased sperm count; Diarrhea; Electrocardiogram abnormalities; Emphysema; Frostbite; Headaches; Hodgkin's disease; Impaired hand/eye coordination; Labored or difficulty breathing; Memory loss; Nausea; Neuropathy; Numbness, tingling, or prickling sensation; Peculiar taste; Peripheral neuropathy; Pulmonary edema; Spontaneous abortion; Vomiting. Suspected of causing Nasal mucosa inflammation; Epithelial tissue death; Respiratory lesions; Low birth weight; Neonate lethality; Birth defects; Testicular degeneration; Convulsions; Liver and kidney damage. *End-point Targets:* Respiratory system; Central nervous system. *Usage:* Adhesives; Antifreeze; Choline; Cosmetics; Dishwashing liquids; Disinfectant; Ethanolamines; Ethylene glycol; Food sterilant; Fumigant for health care facilities; medical products manufacturing; libraries; museums; beekeeping; spices; seasonings; black walnuts; diary packaging; aircraft; buses; railroad cars; clothing, furs, and furniture; Glycol ethers; Hospital sterilant; Hydroxyethyl starch; Insecticides; Laundry detergents; Medicine; Polyester fibers; film and bottles; Polyurethane foam; Soaps; Textiles. *References:* 304, 306, 310, 325, 388, 390, 413, 429, 449.

Ethylenimine *see* **Ethyleneimine.**

Ethyl ester *see* **Ethyl methacrylate.**

Ethyl ester of acetic acid *see* **Ethyl acetate.**

Ethyl ester of acrylic acid *see* **Ethyl acrylate.**

Ethyl ester of formic acid *see* **Ethyl formate.**

N-Ethylethanamine *see* **Diethylamine.**

Ethyl ethanoate *see* **Ethyl acetate.**

Ethyl ether: *TN/synonyms:* Diethyl ether; Ethyl oxide; Ether; Diethyl oxide; Solvent ether. *NIOSH:* No REL, notified OSHA that documentation doesn't support the worker's safety at established PEL. *OSHA PEL:* 400 ppm or 1,200 mg/m^3 (8hr/day-40hr/wk-PP/S); 500 ppm or 1,500 mg/m^3 (exposure not to exceed 15 min). *IDLH:* 19,000 mg/m^3. *Symptoms:* Eye, nasal, skin, and upper respiratory irritation; Albumin in urine; Bladder inflammation; Bronchial dilation and secretions; Cardiac arrhythmias; Central nervous system depression; Constipation; Convulsions; Cough; Death; Depression; Dizziness; Drowsiness; Dry, cracked skin; Excess of red blood cells; Excessive salivation; Excitement; Exhaustion; Fatigue; Headaches; Hyperglycemia; Increased heart rate; Irregular respiration; Kidney damage and inflammation; Laryngeal spasms; Loss of appetite; Loss of sensation; Mania; Mental disorders; Metabolic acidosis; Myocardial depression; Nausea; Painful or difficult urination; Pallor; Profuse sweating; Psychotic disturbances; Respiratory paralysis; Sleepiness; Unconsciousness due to narcotic effects; Vomiting. *End-point Targets:* Central nervous system; Skin; Eyes; Respiratory system. *Usage:* Medicine; Anesthetic; Chemical intermediate; Diesel and gasoline primer; Antiseptic; Cough and expectorant syrups; Smokeless powder; Solvent; Fats; Oils; Waxes; Perfumes; Gums; Nitrocellulose; Gun powder; Veterinary medicine; Rubefacient liniments; Oven cleaners. *Note:* Historically established as a neurotoxin. *References:* 118, 304, 388, 413.

Ethyl formate: *TN/synonyms:* Ethyl ester of formic acid; Ethyl methanoate. *OSHA PEL:* 100 ppm or 300 mg/m^3 (8hr/day-40hr/wk-PP/S). *IDLH:* 8,000 ppm. *Symptoms:* Eye, nasal, skin, mucous membrane, and upper respiratory irritation; Unconsciousness due to narcotic effects; Central nervous system depression. *End-point Targets:* Eyes; Respiratory system. *Usage:* Food and beverage flavoring; Food fumigant; Solvent; Nitrocellulose; Pharmaceutical flavoring; Safety glass; Shoes; Oils; Degreasers; Lemonade; Artificial rum; Larvicide; Resins; Synthetic sex hormones; Pharmaceutical intermediate; Cellulose; Anticonvulsant drugs (Estazolam). *Synergistic effects:* Decomposed slowly in water to form ethyl alcohol and formic acid. *Classification:* Chlorinated aliphatic hydrocarbons. *References:* 122, 304, 388.

Ethyl hydrate *see* **Ethanol.**

Ethyl hydroxide *see* **Ethanol**

Ethylidene *see* **1,1-Dichloroethane.**

Ethylidene chloride *see* **1,1-Dichloroethane.**

Ethylidene dichloride *see* **1,1-Dichloroethane.**

1,1-Ethylidene dichloride *see* **1,1-Dichloroethane.**

Ethylimine *see* **Ethyleneimine.**

Ethyl mercaptan: *TN/synonyms:*

Ethanethiol; Ethyl sulfhydrate; Mercaptoethane. *NIOSH REL:* 0.5 ppm or 1.3 mg/m^3 (ceiling limit, 15 min exposure). *OSHA PEL:* 0.5 ppm or 1.0 mg/m^3 (8hr/day-40hr/wk-PP/S). *IDLH:* 2,500 ppm. *Symptoms:* Headaches; Nausea; Mucus membrane irritation; Central nervous system depression; Bitter or sweet taste. Suspected of causing Incoordination; Weakness; Pulmonary irritation; Liver and kidney damage; Cyanosis. *End-point Targets:* Respiratory system. *Usage:* Plastics; Insecticides; Warning agent for natural gas; Chemical and pesticide intermediate; Adhesives; Defoliants; Pharmaceutical intermediate. *Classification:* Organic solvent (Thiol compounds). *References:* 121, 304, 305, 383, 388.

Ethyl methacrylate: *TN/synonyms:* Ethyl ester; 2-Propenic acid; Ethyl 2-methacrylate; Ethyl 2-methyl-2-propenoate; Ethyl alpha-methyl acrylate; Rhoplex AC-33 (tn); Ageflex FM-1 (tn). *OSHA PEL:* None. *Symptoms:* Eye irritation, pain, and swelling; Mucous membrane irritation; Tearing; Dizziness; Suffocation; Death; Low blood pressure; Headaches; Irritability; Allergic contact dermatitis; Dystrophic fingernail changes; Vomiting; Coma; Convulsions; Eyes become sensitive to light; Central nervous system effects. Suspected of causing Respiratory depression. *End-point Targets:* Eyes; Skin; Immune system. *Usage:* Acrylic polymers; Acrylic fingernails; Hard contact lenses; Paints; Surface coatings; Dentures; Dental cement; Bone cement; Cements; Plastics; Lucite (tn); Plexiglass (tn); Perspex (tn); Pesticides; Pesticide inert ingredient; Indirect food additive; Resins; Building materials; Automotive materials; Aerospace materials; Furniture; Polishes; Chemical intermediate. *Additive:* Usually inhibited with hydroquinone. *Metabolite:* Alcohol; Methacrylic acid; Acetyl CoA derivatives. *Note:* In animals, ethyl methacrylate has caused cross sensitization to other methacry-lates. Exempt from pesticide tolerance regulations if applied to growing crops using good agricultural practices. *References:* 34, 423.

Ethyl 2-methacrylate *see* **Ethyl methacrylate.**

Ethyl methanoate *see* **Ethyl formate.**

Ethyl alpha-methyl acrylate *see* **Ethyl methacrylate.**

Ethyl methyl ketone *see* **2-Butanone.**

Ethyl 2-methyl-2-propenoate *see* **Ethyl methacrylate.**

N-Ethylmorpholine: *TN/synonyms:* 4-Ethylmorpholine. *OSHA PEL:* 5 ppm or 23 mg/m^3 (8hr/day-40hr/wk-PP/S). *IDLH:* 2,000 ppm. *Symptoms:* Eye, nasal, and throat irritation; Vision disturbances; Olfactory fatigue; Drowsiness. *End-point Targets:* Respiratory system; Eyes; Skin. *Usage:* Urethane foam; Dyes; Pharmaceuticals; Rubber; Resins; Oils. *References:* 179, 304, 388.

4-Ethylmorpholine *see* **N-Ethylmorpholine.**

Ethyl nitrile *see* **Acetonitrile.**

O-Ethyl O-P-nitrophenyl benzenephosphonothioate *see* **EPN.**

O-Ethyl O-P-ntirophenyl benzenethiophosphonate *see* **EPN.**

Ethylolamine *see* **Ethanolamine.**

Ethyl orthosilicate *see* **Ethyl silicate.**

Ethyl oxide *see* **Ethyl ether.**

Ethyl propenoate *see* **Ethyl acrylate.**

Ethyl pyrophosphate *see* **TEPP.**

Ethyl silicate: *TN/synonyms:* Ethyl orthosilicate; Tetraethoxysilane; Tetraethyl silicate. *OSHA PEL:* 10 ppm or 85 mg/m^3 (8hr/day-40hr/wk-PP/S). *IDLH:* 1,000 ppm. *Symptoms:* Eye, nasal, and mucous membrane irritation;

Central nervous system depression; Tearing. Suspected of causing labored or difficult breathing; Tremors; Unconsciousness due to narcotic effects; Liver and kidney damage; Anemia. *End-point Targets:* Respiratory system; Liver; Kidneys; Blood; Skin. *Usage:* Mortars; Cements; Paint; Bricks; Lacquers; Bonding agents; Protective coatings for stone and industrial buildings; Silicon oxide. *References:* 110, 304, 388.

Ethyl sulfhydrate *see* **Ethyl mercaptan.**

Etilbenzene *see* **Ethyl benzene.**

ETO *see* **Ethylene oxide.**

Etylobenzene *see* **Ethyl benzene.**

Eulimen *see* **Limonene.**

Euxyl K 100 (tn) *see* **Benzyl alcohol.**

Eviplast 80 (tn) *see* **Di-sec octyl phthalate.**

Fannoform *see* **Formaldehyde.**

Fedal-Un (tn) *see* **Tetrachloroethylene.**

Fenclor (tn) *see* **Polychlorinated biphenyls.**

Fenzen *see* **Benzene.**

Ferbam: *TN/synonyms:* tris(Dimethyldithiocarbamate)iron; Ferric dimethyl dithiocarbamate. *OSHA PEL:* 10 mg/m³ (8hr/day-40hr/wk-PP/S). *IDLH:* NE. *Symptoms:* Eye, nasal, throat, skin, mucous membrane, and respiratory irritation; Dermatitis; Gastrointestinal distress; Nausea; Vomiting; Diarrhea; Loss of appetite; Weight loss; Headaches; Lethargy; Dizziness; Confusion; Incoordination; Drowsiness; Emotional liability; Coma; Reduced blood pressure; Tendon reflex suppression; Loss of muscle tone; Flaccid paralysis; Respiratory paralysis; Death; Hepatitis. Suspected of causing Kidney damage; Hypersensitive reactions. *End-point Targets:* Respiratory

system; Skin; Gastrointestinal tract. *Usage:* Fungicide on fruits; vegetables; ornamental crops and household applications. *References:* 131, 304, 388.

Fermentation alcohol *see* **Ethanol.**

Fermentation amyl alcohol *see* **Isoamyl alcohol.**

Ferric dimethyl dithiocarbamate *see* **Ferbam.**

Fifanon (tn) *see* **Malathion.**

Fleck-Flip (tn) *see* **Trichloroethylene.**

Flock Flip (tn) *see* **Trichloroethylene.**

Fluate (tn) *see* **Trichloroethylene.**

Flue gas *see* **Carbon monoxide.**

Fluorides: *Compounds:* Sodium fluoride; Calcium fluoride; Fluorine; Hydrogen fluoride; Hydrofluoric acid. *OSHA PEL:* 2.5 mg/m³ (8hr/day-40hr/wk-PP/S). *IDLH:* 500 mg/m³. *Symptoms:* Eye and respiratory irritation; Abdominal pain; Abnormally low blood calcium; Calcification of ligaments of ribs and pelvis; Cardiac arrhythmias; Death; Decreased respiratory function; Dermatitis; Diarrhea; Excessive salivation; Gastric discomfort and hemorrhaging; Headaches; Nausea; Numbness, tingling, or prickling sensation; Profuse sweating; Pulmonary edema; Stiff spine; Thirst; Vertigo; Vomiting. Suspected of causing Anemia; Male reproductive system damage; Chromosomal aberrations. *End-point Targets:* Eyes; Respiratory system; Central nervous system; Skeleton; Skin. *Usage:* Pesticide; Rocket fuel; Glass; Enamel; Bricks; Dental Care; Aluminum; Plastics; Tiles; Disinfectant; Steel; Textiles; Ceramics; Fertilizers; Lubricants; Semiconductors; Manufacture of other chemicals. Found in volcanic eruptions; coal; clay. *Classification:* Florine, halogen. *References:* 304, 363, 388, 429, 432.

Fluorocarbon 12 *see* **Dichlorodifluoromethane.**

Fluorocarbon 1301 *see* **Trifluorobromomethane.**

Fluorodichloromethane *see* **Dichloromonofluoromethane.**

Fluorotrichloromethane: *TN/synonyms:* Freon 11; Monofluorotrichloromethane; Trichlorofluoromethane; Trichloromonofluoromethane; Refrigerant 11. *OSHA PEL:* 1,000 ppm or 5,600 mg/m^3 (ceiling limit-PP/S). *IDLH:* 10,000 ppm. *Symptoms:* Upper respiratory and pulmonary irritation; Incoordination; Tremors; Dermatitis; Frostbite; Confusion; Coma; Defatting dermatitis; Excitement; Collapse; Cardiac arrhythmias and arrest; Bronchial constriction; Death; Heart rate under 60 beats per minute; T-wave inversion in the heart. Suspected of causing Central nervous system depression. *Endpoint Targets:* Cardiovascular system. *Usages:* Refrigerant; Pesticide inert ingredient; Cleaning products; Fire extinguishers; Food processing; Solvent; Degreasing agent; Electrical insulation; Aerosol propellent; Insecticide propellent; Floor waxes; Spray paint; Cosmetics; Perfumes; Medicine propellent in bronchodilators and corticosteroids; Resins. *Note:* Neurotoxin. *References:* 17, 130, 304, 388, 423.

FMA 5462 (tn) *see* **Endosulfan.**

Folodol-80/M (tn) *see* **Methyl parathion.**

Formal *see* **Methylal.**

Formaldehyde: *TN/synonyms:* Quaternium-15; Methanal; Methyl aldehyde; Methylene oxide; Formalin; Formic aldehyde; Formalith; Formol; Fyde; BVF; Morbicid; Oxymethylene; Oxomethane; Lysoform; Superlysoform; Fannoform; Ivalon. *NIOSH:* Carcinogen at any exposure level. *NIOSH REL:* 0.016 ppm (10 hr/day-40hr/wk); 0.100 ppm (ceiling limit not to exceed 15 min). *OSHA PEL:* 0.750 ppm (8hr/day-40hr/wk-PP/S); 2.000 ppm (exposure not to exceed 15 min); 0.500 ppm (requires medical surveillance). *NAS:* There is no population threshold for irritation effects. *NRC:* Fewer than 20% but perhaps more than 10% of the general population may be susceptible to formaldehyde and may react acutely at any exposure level. *ACGIH:* Suspected human carcinogen. *IDLH:* 30 ppm. *Symptoms:* Eye, nasal, throat, and pulmonary irritation; Acidosis; Acute sense of smell; Altered tissue proteins; Anemia; Antibodies formation; Apathy; Blindness; Blood in urine; Blurred vision; Body aches; Bronchial spasms; Bronchitis; Burns, nasal and throat; Cardiac impairment, palpitations, and arrhythmias; Central nervous system depression; Changes in higher cognitive functions; Chemical sensitivity; Chest pains and tightness; Chronic vaginitis; Colds; Coma; Conjunctivitis; Constipation; Convulsions; Corneal erosion; Cough; Death; Depression; Dermatitis; Diarrhea; Difficulty concentrating; Disorientation; Dizziness; DNA damage; Drowsiness; Ear aches; Eczema; Emotional upsets; Ethmoid polyps; Fatigue; Fecal bleeding; Fetal asphyxiation; Flu-like or cold-like illness; Frequent urination with pain; Gastritis; Gastrointestinal inflammation; Headaches; Hemolytic anemia; Hoarseness; Hyperactive airway disease; Hyperactivity; Hypomenstrual syndrome; Immune system sensitizer; Impaired (short) attention span; Impaired capacity to focus attention; Inability or difficulty swallowing; Inability to recall words and names; Inconsistent IQ profiles; Inflammatory diseases of the reproductive organs; Intestinal pain; Intrinsic asthma; Irritability; Jaundice; Joint pains, aches, and swelling; Kidney pain; Laryngeal spasm; Loss of memory; Loss of sense smell; Loss of taste; Malaise; Menstrual and testicular pain; Menstrual irregularities; Metallic taste; Muscle spasms and cramps; Nasal congestion, crusting, and mucosa inflammation; Nausea; Nosebleeds; Numbness and tingling of the forearms and finger tips; Pale, clammy skin; Partial laryngeal paralysis; Pneumonia; Post nasal drip; Pulmonary edema; Reduced body temperature; Retarded speech pattern; Ringing or tingling in the ear; Schizophrenic-type symptoms; Sensitivity to sound; Shock; Short term memory loss; Shortness of breath; Skin lesions; Sneezing; Sore throat; Spacey feeling; Speaking difficulty; Sterility; Swollen glands; Tearing; Thirst; Tracheitis; Tracheobronchitis; Vertigo; Vomiting blood; Vomiting; Wheezing. Suspected of causing Cancer; Genetic mutations; Chromosomal damage. *End-point Targets:* Respiratory system; Eyes; Skin; Central nervous system; Liver; Kidneys; Gastrointestinal tract; Cardiovascular system. *Usage:* Adhesives; Airplane manufacturing glues; Artificial silk; Asphalt; Bactericides; Bookbinding glues; Building materials; Cabinetry; Carbonless paper; Carpet glue; Carpeting; Casein; Cellulose; Chelating agents; Chrome printing; Concrete; Corrosion inhibitor; Cosmetics; Dental disinfectants; Deodorants; Disinfectants; Dry cleaning; Durable-press fabrics; Dyes; Electrical insulation; Embalming fluids; Ethylene glycol; Explosives; Fabric waterproofing, coatings, sizing, and fireproofing; Fats; Fertilizer; Fiberglass; Fingernail polish and remover; Flame retardant; Food preservative and starch; Formica; Fungicide; Fur processing; Furniture; Gelatin; Germicides; Glass etching; Glues; Gold and silver recovery; Grain smut fumigant; Hair conditioners; Hair spray; Hardening agent; Hardwood and vinyl paneling; Herbicide intermediates; Household cleaners and disinfectants; Industrial sterilant; Ink; Insecticide; Insulation; Laminates; Latex; Laundry detergents; Leather; Lime manufacturing; Medicine; Melmac (tn) dinnerware; Methylene dianiline; Mirrors; Mold and mildew cleaners; Nitroparaffin; Oil-well processing; Oils; Paper products; Paper towels; Paper; Particle board; Pesticide inert ingredient; Petroleum-based products; Pharmaceutical aids; Photographic film; Photography; Plaster; Plastics; Plywood; Polishes; Pyridine; Railroad ties; Resins; Rubber; Sewage treatment; Shampoos; Soil sterilant; Sugar and other carbohydrate condensation; Taxidermy; Toilet paper; Toothpaste; Upholstery; Vaccines; Varnish; Vitamins A and E; Waferboard; Wallboard; Wood preservative; Wood veneer; Wool mothproofing; Tissue fixative; Body lotion; Antiperspirant; Mouthwash; Hair setting lotions; Air fresheners; Fabric dyes. Found in Cigarette smoke; Burning trees and other plants; Vehicle/Diesel exhaust; Heated cooking oil. Metabolized as Formic acid. *Note:* Will cross sensitize to formic acid. Comparison of ciliostatic effects showed formaldehyde to be the most toxic of the aldehydes. EPA estimates that 15 people in 1 million will get cancer from lifetime exposure of 1 ppb. Neurotoxin. *References:* 8, 14, 17, 18, 30, 31, 129, 278, 279, 285, 288, 290, 297, 299, 300, 304, 305, 309, 388, 389, 394, 416, 417a, 421, 423, 426, 457.

Formaldehyde dimethylacetal *see* **Methylal.**

Formalin *see* **Formaldehyde.**

Formalith *see* **Formaldehyde.**

Formic acid: *TN/synonyms:* Hydrogencarboxlic acid; Methanoic acid. *OSHA PEL:* 5 ppm or 9 mg/m^3 (8hr/day-40hr/wk). *IDLH:* 30 ppm. *Symptoms:* Eye and throat irritation; Acidosis; Albumin and blood in urine; Bronchitis; Central nervous system depression; Chemical sensitivity; Circulatory collapse; Clammy skin; Conjunctivitis; Corneal inflammation; Cough; Death; Dermatitis; Diarrhea; Dizziness; Epigastric pain; Esophageal, gastric, and pyloric strictures; Excessive salivation; Glottis corrosion and swelling; Inability to swallow; Kidney damage and diseases; Labored or difficult breathing; Mental disturbances; Mucous membrane ulceration; Nasal discharge; Nasal mucosa inflammation; Nausea; Shock; Skin burns; Tearing; Thirst; Throat malaise; Ulcerative stomach inflammation; Vertigo; Visual disturbances; Vomiting; Weak, rapid pulse. *End-point Targets:* Respiratory system; Skin; Kidneys; Liver; Eyes. *Usage:* Animal feed; Antiseptic; Baked goods; Candy; Cellulose; Dehairing hides; Electroplating; Fabric sizing; Food flavor adjunct and preservative; Fumigant; Hydrogen peroxide; Ice cream; Insecticide manufacturing; Lacquers; Latex rubber; Leather tanning; Nickel plating; Non-alcoholic beverages; Paint strippers; Perfumes; Pesticide inert ingredient; Plasticizers; Refrigerant; Silvering glass; Solvent; Textile dyes; Wire stripping compound. *Note:* Chemical sensitivity is rare but may occur if patient is first sensitized to formaldehyde. *References:* 128, 304, 388, 423.

Formic aldehyde *see* **Formaldehyde.**

Formol *see* **Formaldehyde.**

Formontrile *see* **Hydrogen cyanide.**

2-Formylfuran *see* **Furfural.**

Formyl trichloride *see* **Chloroform.**

Fosferno M 50 (tn) *see* **Methyl parathion.**

Freon 10 *see* **Carbon tetrachloride.**

Freon 11 *see* **Fluorotrichloromethane.**

Freon 12 *see* **Dichlorodifluoromethane.**

Freon 13B1 *see* **Trifluorobromomethane.**

Freon 21 *see* **Dichloromonofluoromethane.**

Freon 40 (tn) *see* **Methyl chloride.**

Freon 114 *see* **Dichlorotetrafluoroethane.**

Fumigran *see* **Acrylonitrile.**

Fumogas (tn) *see* **Ethylene dibromide.**

Fural *see* **Furfural.**

Furaldehyde *see* **Furfural.**

Furale *see* **Furfural.**

2-Furanaldehyde *see* **Furfural.**

Furancarbonal *see* **Furfural.**

2-Furancarbonal *see* **Furfural.**

2-Furancarboxaldehyde *see* **Furfural.**

2,5-Furanedione *see* **Maleic anhydride.**

Furfural: *TN/synonyms:* Fural; 2-Furfuraldehyde; 2-Furancarboxaldehyde; Furfuraldehyde; Furfurole; Furole; Furale; Furancarbonal; 2-Furancarbonal; Pyromucic aldehyde; a-Furole; 2-Furanaldehyde; 2-Formylfuran; 2-Furfural; 2-Furylaldehyde; Furfurylaldehyde; Furaldehyde; Artificial ant oil. *NIOSH:* No REL, notified OSHA that documentation doesn't support the worker's safety at established PELs. *OSHA PEL:* 2 ppm or 8 mg/m³ (8hr/day- 40hr/wk-PP/S). *IDLH:* 250 ppm. *Symptoms:* Upper respiratory and eye irritation; Headaches; Dermatitis. *End-point Targets:* Eyes; Respiratory system; skin. *Usage:* Herbicide; Fungicide; Insecticide; Germicide; Food flavoring; Solvent; Lubricating oils; Nitrocellulose; Shoe dye; Chemical intermediate and manufacturing; Road construction; Varnish; Rubber. *References:* 279, 304, 388.

2-Furfural *see* **Furfural.**

Furfuraldehyde *see* **Furfural.**

2-Furfuraldehyde *see* **Furfural.**

Furfurole *see* **Furfural.**

Furfuryl alcohol: *TN/synonyms:* 2-Furylmethanol; 2-Hydroxymethyl-furan. *OSHA PEL:* 10 ppm or 40 mg/m³ (8hr/day-40hr/wk-PP/S); 15 ppm or 60 mg/m³ (exposure not to exceed 15 min). *IDLH:* 250 ppm. *Symptoms:* Eye and mucous membrane irritation; Dizziness; Nausea; Diarrhea; Excess urine formation; Respiratory and body temperature depression; Vomiting; Bronchitis; Cough; Chest pains; Excessive salivation. Suspected of causing Drowsiness. *End-point Targets:* Respiratory system. *Usage:* Solvent; Cellulose; Gums; Dyes; Resins; Leather tanning; Corrosive-resistant sealants and cements; Food flavorings; Missile fuel; Couarone; Liquid propellents. *Classification:* Organic solvent. *References:* 148, 304, 306, 383, 388.

Furfurylaldehyde *see* **Furfural.**

Furole *see* **Furfural.**

a-Furole *see* **Furfural.**

2-Furylaldehyde *see* **Furfural.**

2-Furylmethanol *see* **Furfuryl alcohol.**

Fusel oil *see* **Isoamyl alcohol.**

Fyde *see* **Formaldehyde.**

G 25 (tn) *see* **Chloropicrin.**

Gearphos (tn) *see* **Methyl parathion.**

Gemalgene (tn) *see* **Trichloroethylene.**

Geniphene (tn) *see* **Chlorinated camphene.**

Glacial acetic acid *see* **Acetic acid.**

Glucinium *see* **Beryllium.**

Glucinum *see* **Beryllium.**

Glycerol trichlorohydrin *see* **1,2,3-Trichloropropane.**

Glyceryl trichlorohydrin *see* **1,2,3-Trichloropropane.**

Glycidol *TN/synonyms:* 2,3-Epoxy-1-propanol; Epoxypropyl alcohol; Hydroxymethyl ethylene oxide; 2-Hydroxymethyl oxiran; 3-Hydroxypropylene oxide. *OSHA PEL:* 25 ppm or 75 mg/m³ (8hr/day-40hr/wk-PP/S). *IDLH:* 500 ppm. *Symptoms:* Eye, nasal, throat, and skin irritation; Unconsciousness due to narcotic effects; Central nervous system excitement and then depression. *End-point Targets:* Eyes; Skin; Respiratory system; Central nervous system. *Usage:* Pharmaceuticals; Cosmetics; Glycerin; Detergents; Oils; Dyes. *References:* 147, 304, 388.

Glycidyl phenyl ether *see* **Phenyl glycidyl ether.**

Glycol *see* **Ethylene glycol.**

Glycol alcohol *see* **Ethylene glycol.**

Glycol dibromide *see* **Ethylene dibromide.**

Glycol dinitrate *see* **Ethylene glycol dinitrate.**

Glycol monoethyl ether acetate *see* **2-Ethoxyethyl acetate or Methyl cellosolve acetate.**

Glycol monomethyl ether *see* **Methyl cellosolve.**

Grain alcohol *see* **Ethanol.**

Gray arsenic *see* **Arsenic.**

Gum camphor *see* **Camphor.**

Gumspirits *see* **Turpentine.**

Gum turpentine *see* **Turpentine.**

Guthion *see* **Azinphos-methyl.**

Halane *see* **1,3-Dichloro-5,5-dimethylhydantoin.**

Halcon 242 *see* **Dichlorotetrafluoroethane.**

Halocarbon 13B1 *see* **Trifluorobromomethane.**

Halon 104 *see* **Carbon tetrachloride.**

Halon 112 *see* Dichloromonofluoromethane.

Halon 122 *see* Dichlorodifluoromethane.

Halon 1301 *see* Trifluorobromomethane.

Halowax *see* Tetrachloronaphthalene.

Halowax 1013 *see* Pentachloronaphthalene.

Halowax 1014 *see* Hexachloronaphthalene.

Halowax 1051 (tn) *see* Octachloronaphthalene.

Hastelloy (tn) *see* Nickel.

8056HC (tn) *see* Methyl parathion.

HCH *see* Lindane.

Heavy Oil *see* Creosotes.

Heptane *see* n-Heptane.

n-Heptane *TN/synonyms:* Heptane; Normal-heptane. *NIOSH REL:* 85 ppm or 350 mg/m³ (10hr/day-40hr/wk); 440 ppm (ceiling limit); 1,500 mg/ m³ (exposure not to exceed 15 min). *OSHA PEL:* 400 ppm or 1,600 mg/m³ (8hr/day-40hr/wk-PP/S); 500 ppm or 2,000 mg/ m³ (exposure not to exceed 15 min). *IDLH:* 5,000 ppm. *Symptoms:* Lightheadedness; Giddiness; Stupor; Loss of appetite; Nausea; Dermatitis; Chemical pneumonia; Unconsciousness. *End-point Targets:* Skin; Respiratory system; Peripheral nervous system. *Usage:* Asphalt; Printing ink; Research chemical. *Classification:* Organic solvent (Alkane compound). *Note:* Neurotoxin. *References:* 17, 180, 304, 383, 388, 429.

2-Heptanone *see* Methyl n-amyl ketone.

3-Heptanone *see* Ethyl butyl ketone.

Hercules 3956 (tn) *see* Chlorinated camphene.

Hercules Toxaphene (tn) *see* Chlorinated camphene.

gamma-Hexachlorocyclohexane *see* Lindane.

1,2,3,4,5,6-Hexachlorocyclohexane *see* Lindane.

Hexachlorodiphenyl oxide *see* Chlorinated diphenyl.

Hexachloroethane *TN/synonyms:* Carbon hexachloride; Perchloroethane. *NIOSH:* Carcinogen at any exposure level. *OSHA PEL:* 1 ppm or 10 mg/m³ (8hr/day-40hr/wk-PP/S). *IDLH:* 300 ppm. *Symptoms:* Eye, skin, mucous membrane, and liver irritation; Eye twitching; Eyes become sensitive to light; Eye inflammation; Inability to close eyelids; Tearing; Conjunctiva redness; Central nervous system depression; Liver and kidney damage; Paralysis. Suspected of causing Cancer. *End-point Targets:* Eyes. *Usage:* Solvent; Explosives; Smoke screens; Lubricants; Degreaser; Retards fermentation; Medicines; Celluloid; Anthelmintic drug; Aluminium alloys; Fireworks; Flameproofing; Polymer fibers; Fire extinguisher; Grenades; Plasticizers; Cellulose; Insecticide intermediate; Rubber; Nitrocellulose; Smoke bombs; Veterinary medicine; Paper products; Cleaning products. Formerly used as a moth repellent. **Toxic** by inhalation and ingestion. *Classification:* Chlorinated organic compound. *References:* 146, 304, 388, 399.

6,7,8,9,10,10-Hexachloro-1,5,-5a,6,9,9a-hexahydro-6,9-methano-2,4,3-benzodiaoxathiepin 3-oxide *see* Endosulfan.

Hexachloronaphthalene *TN/synonyms:* Halowax 1014. *OSHA PEL:* 0.2 mg/m³ (8hr/day-40hr/wk-PP/S). *IDLH:* 2 mg/m³. *Symptoms:* Acneform dermatitis; Nausea; Confusion; Jaundice; Coma; Chloracne; Liver tissue death; Drowsiness; Indigestion; Nausea; Enlarged liver; Weakness; Excessive bilirubin in blood; Toxic hepatitis; Skin photosensitivity; Allergic sensitization. *End-point Targets:* Liver,

Skin. *Usage:* Synthetic waxes; Electrical insulation; Resins; Lubricants; Paper; Fire retardant; Waterproofing; Fungicide; Insecticide; Textile coatings. Formerly used as an oil additive, electroplating, and fabric dyes. *References:* 145, 304, 388.

Hexachlorophenyl ether *see* **Chlorinated diphenyl.**

Hexahydrobenzene *see* **Cyclohexane.**

Hexahydrophenol *see* **Cyclohexanol.**

Hexalin *see* **Cyclohexanol.**

Hexamethylene *see* **Cyclohexane.**

Hexanaphthene *see* **Cyclohexane.**

Hexane *see* **n-Hexane.**

n-Hexane *TN/synonyms:* Hexane; Hexyl hydride; Normal-hexane. *OSHA PEL:* 50 ppm or 180 mg/m³ (8hr/day-40hr/wk-PP/S). *IDLH:* 5,000 ppm. *Symptoms:* Eye, nasal, throat, bronchial, and intestinal irritation; Blurred vision; Central nervous system depression; Cerebral dysfunction; Chemical pneumonia; Death; Dermatitis; Dizziness; Facial numbness; Giddiness; Headaches; Impaired speech; Leg spasticity; Lightheadedness; Loss of sensation; Motor and sensory polyneuropathy; Muscle denervation atrophy and degeneration; Muscle cramps, weakness and swelling; Nausea; Nervous system degeneration; Numb extremities; Paralysis; Peripheral neuropathy; Staggering gait; Vertigo; Optic neuropathy; Memory loss; Weight loss; Distal numbness, tingling, or prickling sensation; Fatigue. *End-point Targets:* Skin; Eyes; Respiratory system. *Usage:* Pesticide inert ingredient; Asphalt; Felt-tipped markers; Paint; Extraction of soybean oil, cottonseed oil, flaxseed oil, safflower oil, etc.,; Elastics; Pharmaceuticals; Denatured alcohol; Fabric and leather cleaners; Glues; Rubber cement; Adhesives; Degreasers; Plastics; Petroleum and gasoline based products; Shoes; Shoe cement; Inks; Varnishes; Lacquers; Stains. Found in Gasoline exhaust. *Metabolite:* 2, 5-Hexanedione. *Classification:* Organic solvent (Alkane compound) *Note:* Historically established as a neurotoxin. Metabolite has a greater neurotoxic potential. *References:* 17, 180, 304, 383, 388, 413, 423, 429.

Hexone *TN/synonyms:* Isobutyl methyl ketone; Methyl isobutyl ketone; 4-Methyl 2-pentanone; MIBK. *OSHA PEL:* 50 ppm or 205 mg/m³ (8hr/day-40hr/wk-PP/S); 75 ppm or 300 mg/m³ (exposure not to exceed 15 min). *IDLH:* 3,000 ppm. *Symptoms:* Eye, nasal, throat, and mucus membrane irritation; Headaches; Nausea; Vomiting; Loss of appetite; Diarrhea; Drowsiness; Dizziness; Loss of balance; Weakness; Stomach pain; Sore throat; Fatigue; Insomnia; Intestinal pain; Enlarged liver; Colitis; Unconsciousness due to narcotic effects; Coma; Dermatitis; Central nervous system depression; Lightheadedness; Incoordination; Somnolence; Heartburn; Central nervous system impairment. *End-point Targets:* Respiratory system; Eyes; Skin; Central nervous system. *Usage:* Food flavoring; Perfumes; Paint; Paint thinner; Pesticide inert ingredient; Plastics; Ink; Varnishes; Lacquers; Furniture; Rubbing alcohol; Nitrocellulose; Metal coatings; Medicine; Antibiotics; Dry cleaning; Fruit flavors; Rum; Cheese; Solvent; Metal extraction; Mineral oil; Metallurgy; Methyl amyl alcohol; Methyl isobutyl carbinol. *Note:* Occupational tolerance seems to develop during the work week but is lost over the weekend. Some adverse effects have been noted below OSHA PEL. *Classification:* Organic solvent (Ketone compound). *References:* 144, 304, 305, 383, 388, 423, 432.

sec-Hexyl acetate *TN/synonyms:* 1,3-Dimethylbutyl acetate; Methyl isoamyl acetate. *OSHA PEL:* 50 ppm or 300 mg/m³ (8hr/day-40hr/wk-PP/S).

IDLH: 4,000 ppm. *Symptoms:* Respiratory irritation; Headaches; Dizziness; Nausea. Suspected of causing Eye and nasal irritation; Unconsciousness due to narcotic effects. *End-point Targets:* Central nervous system; Eyes. *Usage:* Solvent; Nitrocellulose; Lacquers. *References:* 273, 304, 388.

Hexyl hydride *see* **n-Hexane.**

HF-A *see* **Hydrogen fluoride.**

High solvent naphtha *see* **Naphtha.**

HI-TRI (tn) *see* **Trichloroethylene.**

HOE 02671 (tn) *see* **Endosulfan.**

Hydralin *see* **Cyclohexanol.**

Hydraulic cement *see* **Portland cement.**

Hydrazine *TN/synonyms:* Diamine; Diamide. *NIOSH:* Carcinogen at any exposure level. *NIOSH REL:* 0.03 ppm or 0.04 mg/m³ (ceiling limit, 2 hr exposure). *OSHA PEL:* 0.1 ppm or 0.1 mg/m³ (8hr/day-40hr/wk-PP/S). *ACGIH:* No threshold value limit will insure prevention of hypersensitive responses. *IDLH:* 80 ppm. *Symptoms:* Eye, nasal, throat, and respiratory irritation; Abdominal pains; Bronchitis; Burns (skin and eyes); Cancer; Cardiac arrhythmias; Central nervous system depression; Chemical hypersensitivity; Conjunctivitis; Contact dermatitis; Convulsions; Dermatitis; Diarrhea; Dizziness; Eczema; Enlarged heart; Enlarged, tender liver; Fever; Fluid in chest cavity; Granular cytoplasmic degeneration; Incoherence; Incoordination; Increase in leukocytes in the blood; Lateral involuntary eye movement; Lethargy; Liver and kidney damage; Muscle fiber degeneration; Nasal congestion; Nausea; Pulmonary edema; Somnolence; Sporadic violence; Temporary blindness; Tissue or bone death; Tracheitis; Tremors; Unconsciousness; Vomiting; Autoimmune disease; Systemic lupus erythematosus. Suspected of causing Cancer. *End-point Targets:* Central nervous system; Respiratory system; Skin; Eyes. *Usage:* Pesticide inert ingredient; Semiconductors; Nickel plating; Wastewater treatment; Photography; Medicine; Pharmaceuticals; Electroplating of metal on glass and plastics; Agricultural chemicals; Explosives; Corrosion inhibitor; Pesticide manufacturing; Solvent; Soldering flux; Rocket propellent; Metallurgy; Urethane; Textile dyes; Experimental medicine. Found in tobacco smoke. *Note:* Dissolves hair. *References:* 143, 280, 304, 306, 388, 389, 423, 429.

Hydrazinobenzene *see* **Phenylhydrazine.**

Hydroacrylic acid *see* **beta-Propiolactone.**

Hydrochloric acid *see* **Hydrogen chloride.**

Hydrochloric ether *see* **Ethyl chloride.**

Hydrocyanic acid *see* **Hydrogen cyanide.**

Hydrofluoric acid *see* **Hydrogen fluoride.**

Hydrogen antimonide *see* **Stibine.**

Hydrogen arsenide *see* **Arsine.**

Hydrogencarboxlic acid *see* **Formic acid.**

Hydrogen chloride *TN/synonyms:* Anhydrous hydrogen chloride; Aqueous hydrogen chloride; Hydrochloric acid; Muriatic acid. *OSHA PEL:* 5 ppm or 7 mg/m³ (ceiling limit-PP/S). *IDLH:* 100 ppm. *Symptoms:* Nasal, throat, and laryngeal inflammation; Cough; Choking; Burns skin, throat, and eyes; Dermatitis. Suspected of causing Laryngeal spasms; Pulmonary edema. *End-point Targets:* Respiratory system; Skin; Eyes. *Usage:* Pesticide inert ingredient; Railroad ties; Cement; Aluminum; Semiconductors; Pharmaceuticals; Synthetic rubber; Glass. *References:* 274, 304, 388, 423, 429.

Hydrogen cyanide *TN/synonyms:* Formontrile; Hydrocyanic acid; Prussic acid; Cyclone B (tn). *OSHA PEL:* 4.7 ppm or 5.0 mg/m³ (exposure not to exceed 15 min). *IDLH:* 50 ppm. *Symptoms:* Eye, skin, and upper respiratory irritation; Abdominal spasms; Altered sense of smell; Asphyxia; Blindness in half the field of vision involving one or both eyes; Bloody expectoration; Cardiac arrhythmias, irregularities, and palpitations; Coma; Confusion; Convulsions; Cough; Death; Depression; Dizziness; Endemic goiter; Enlarged thyroid; Fatigue; Gastric tissue death; Gastrointestinal spasms; Headaches; Hearing disturbances; Heart rate under 60 beats per minute; Hyper-reflexia; Incoordination; Increased hemoglobin and lymphocyte in the blood; Increased respiratory rate; Inhibition of cytochrome oxidase and other metallioenzymes; Insufficient oxygen to cells resulting in a poisonous condition; Labored or difficulty breathing; Leber's hereditary optic atrophy; Low blood pressure; Muscular rigidity; Nasal congestion; Nausea; Neural system degenerative lesions; Nosebleeds; Numbness, tingling, or prickling sensations of extremities; Paralysis on one side of the body; Parkinson-like symptoms; Partial paralysis of lower limbs; Rapid respiration; Respiratory failure; Ringing or tingling in the ear; Shortness of breath; Skin rashes; Slow gasping respiration; Spastic speech impairment; Stupor; T-wave abnormalities in the heart; Temporary cessation of breathing; Thyroid effects; Topical neuropathy; Tremors; Unconsciousness due to inadequate blood flow to the brain; Vision disturbances; Vomiting; Weakness; Weight loss. Suspected of causing behavioral changes; birth defects. *End-point Targets:* Cardiovascular system; Central nervous system; Liver; Kidneys; Skin. *Usage:* Insecticide; Fumigant; Lactic acid; Nylon; Chelating agent; Pharmaceutical; Graphite; Chemical manufacturing;

Pesticide inert ingredient. Found in food, tobacco smoke, vehicle exhaust. *References:* 304, 388, 389, 423, 429, 432, 444.

Hydrogen dioxide *see* **Hydrogen peroxide.**

Hydrogen fluoride *TN/synonyms:* Anhydrous hydrogen fluoride; Aqueous hydrogen fluoride; Hydrofluoric acid; HF-A. *OSHA PEL:* 3.0 ppm (8hr/day-40hr/wk-PP/S); 6.0 ppm (exposure not to exceed 15 min). *ATSDR:* Adverse health effects have been observed in humans who breath 2 to 4 mg/m³ for 10 minutes. *IDLH:* 30 ppm. *Symptoms:* Eye, nasal, and throat irritation; Pulmonary edema; Skin and eye burns; Nasal congestion; Bronchitis; Death; Cardiac arrhythmias; Decreased respiratory function; Nausea; Vomiting; Gastric discomfort; Abnormally low blood calcium; Headaches; Numbness, tingling, or prickling sensation; Vertigo; Chromosomal aberrations. Suspected of causing male reproductive damage; cancer. *End-point Targets:* Eyes; Respiratory system; Skin. *Usages:* Glass etching and polishing; Aluminum. *References:* 304, 363, 388, 429.

Hydrogen nitrate *see* **Nitric acid.**

Hydrogen peroxide *TN/synonyms:* Hydrogen dioxide; Hydroperoxide; Peroxide. *OSHA PEL:* 1.0 ppm or 1.4 mg/m³ (8hr/day-40hr/wk-PP/S). *IDLH:* 75 ppm. *Symptoms:* Eye, nasal, throat, and respiratory irritation; Corneal ulcer; Skin vesiculation and redness; Bleached hair; Mucous membrane congestion; Abdominal distention; Esophagitis; Gastritis; Ruptured colon; Proctitis; Ulcerative colitis; Paralysis of one half of the body; Cerebral embolisms; Vomiting; Collapse; Tonic-clonic seizures. *End-point Targets:* Eyes; Skin; Respiratory system. *Usage:* Rocket propellent; Disinfectant; Antiseptic; Bleach; Hair bleach; Silk; Straw; Ivory; Flour; Gelatin; Fabrics; Dyes; Renovating oil painting; Engraving; Leather; Artificially aged wines and liquors; Oils; Fats; Photography; Fur dyes; Metal cleaning; Pharmaceuticals; Mouthwash; Veterinary medicine; Dentifrices; Sanitary lotions; Food sterilant; Resins; Plastics; Pesticide manufacturing; Plasticizers; Glycerin; Facial creams; Cosmetics; Metallurgy; Paper; Electronics; Textiles; Colonic irrigation agent; Foam resins; Respiratory equipment oxygen source; Wastewater treatment; Dental disinfectant; Metal finishes; Pollution control; Mining. *References:* 142, 304, 385, 456.

Hydrogen phosphide *see* **Phosphine.**

Hydrogen sulfate *see* **Sulfuric acid.**

Hydrogen sulfide *TN/synonyms:* Hydrosulfuric acid; Sewer gas; Sulfuretted hydrogen. *NIOSH REL:* 10 ppm or 15 mg/m^3 (ceiling limit, 10 min exposure). *OSHA PEL:* 10 ppm or 14 mg/m^3 (8hr/day-40hr/wk-PP/S); 15 ppm or 21 mg/m^3 (exposure not to exceed 15 min). *IDLH:* 300 ppm. *Symptoms:* Eye and respiratory irritation; Albumin in urine; Amnesia; Asphyxial convulsions; Brain dysfunction; Bronchial pneumonia; Chemical poisoning; Collapse; Coma; Conjunctivitis; Convulsions; Corneal vesiculation; Cough; Death; Dizziness; Excitement; Eyes become sensitive to light; Fatigue; Gastrointestinal disorders and distress; Headaches; Insomnia; Irritability; Labored or difficult breathing; Nerve inflammation; Nervous system damage; Olfactory nerve paralysis; Peripheral neuropathy; Psychotic disturbances; Pulmonary edema; Respiratory paralysis; Skin redness and pain; Staggering gait; Tearing; Temporary cessation of breathing; Unconsciousness. *End-point Targets:* Respiratory system; Eyes. *Usage:* Plastics; Chemical manufacturing; Metallurgy; Agricultural disinfectant; Lubricants; Rayon. *Note:* Sense of smell will become fatigued and is, therefore, not to be relied upon to

warn of continuous presense. Deaths have been associated with fermenting manure. *References:* 141, 304, 384, 388.

Hydroquinone *TN/synonyms:* 1,4-Benzendiol; Dihydroxybenzene; 1,4-Dihydroxybenzene; Quinol. *NIOSH REL:* 2 mg/m^3 (ceiling limit, 15 min exposure). *OSHA PEL:* 2 mg/m^3 (8hr/day-40hr/wk-PP/S). *IDLH:* Unknown. *Symptoms:* Eye and intestinal irritation; Abdominal cramps; Central nervous system excitement; Collapse; Conjunctivitis; Convulsions; Corneal inflammation and ulceration; Cyanosis; Delirium; Dermatitis; Diarrhea; Dizziness; Eyes become sensitive to light; Gastrointestinal disease; Green or greenish-brown urine; Headaches; Hemoglobin oxides to ferric form; Hemolytic anemia; Inability to utilize oxygen; Labored or difficulty breathing; Muscle twitching; Nausea; Rapid breathing; Respiratory failure; Ringing or tingling in the ear; Feeling of suffocation; Tearing; Vomiting. Suspected of causing Developmental and reproductive effects. *End-point Targets:* Eyes; Respiratory system; Skin; Central nervous system. *Usage:* Pesticide inert ingredient; Photography; Cosmetics; Topical medicine; Fats; Oils; Paints; Varnishes; Motor fuels and oils; Medicine; Acne medicines; Dyes; Rubber. *Note:* Historically established as a neurotoxin. *References:* 167, 304, 306, 388, 413, 423, 435.

Hydroperoxide *see* **Hydrogen peroxide.**

Hydrosulfuric acid *see* **Hydrogen sulfide.**

Hydroxcyclohexane *see* **Cyclohexanol.**

Hydroxybenzene *see* **Phenol.**

1-Hydroxybutane *see* **n-Butyl alcohol.**

2-Hydroxybutane *see* **sec-Butyl alcohol.**

3-Hydroxy-beta-lactone *see* beta-Propiolactone.

(Hydroxymethyl)benzene *see* Benzyl alcohol.

Hydroxymethyl ethylene oxide *see* Glycidol.

2-Hydroxymethylfuran *see* Furfuryl alcohol.

2-Hydroxymethyl oxiran *see* Glycidol.

4-Hydroxy-4-methyl-2-pentanone *see* Diacetone alcohol.

4-Hydroxy-3-(3-oxo-1-phenyl butyl)-2H-1-benzopyran-2-one *see* Warfarin.

3-Hydroxy-propionic acid *see* beta-Propiolactone.

3-Hydroxypropylene oxide *see* Glycidol.

Hydroxytoluene *see* Benzyl alcohol or Cresols.

alpha-Hydroxytoluene *see* Benzyl alcohol.

2-Hydroxytriethylamine *see* 2-Diethylaminoethanol.

2-Hydroyethylamine *see* Ethanolamine.

IBA *see* Isobutyl alcohol.

Icopfume soilbrom-85 (tn) *see* Ethylene dibromide.

Imsol A (tn) *see* Isopropyl alcohol.

Inactive limonene *see* Limonene.

Incoloy (tn) *see* Nickel.

Inconel (tn) *see* Nickel.

Inhibisol (tn) *see* 1,1,1-Trichloroethane.

Iodine: *TN/synonyms:* Iodine crystals; Molecular iodine; Eranol; Iodine colloidol; Actomar (tn); AI3-08544 (tn); Caswell No. 501; Diiodine (tn). *OSHA PEL:* 0.1 ppm or 1.0 mg/m³ (ceiling limit-PP/S). *IDLH:* 10 ppm.

Symptoms: Eye and nasal irritation; Abdominal pain; Bronchitis; Circulatory collapse; Collapse; Conjunctivitis; Cyanosis; Death; Delirium; Diarrhea; Dizziness; Esophageal and pyloric strictures; Excessive salivation; Fecal blood; Glottis swelling; Headaches; Heart rate over 100 beats per minute; Hemorrhagic kidney inflammation; Insufficient oxygen to tissues; Intravascular destruction of red blood cells; Laryngitis; Low blood pressure; Mumps; Nasal inflammation with profuse discharge; Pneumonia; Pulmonary edema; Reduced and absence of urine formation; Shock; Skin burns and rashes; Skin hypersensitivity; Sneezing; Stomach inflammation; Stupor; Tearing; Thyroid disorders; Tight chest; Vomiting. *End-point Targets:* Respiratory system; Eyes; Skin; Central nervous system; Cardiovascular system. *Usage:* Germicides; Antiseptics; Medicine; Disinfectants; Bactericide; Fungicide; Amebicide; Dyes; Soaps; Water disinfectant (drinking and swimming pools); Animal feed supplements; Inks; Aromatic Amines; Iodine isotopes; Stainless steel; Glass; Veterinary medicine; Photography. *Classification:* Halogen. *References:* 63, 304, 388, 432.

Iodine colloidol *see* Iodine.

Iodine crystals *see* Iodine.

Iodomethane *see* Methyl iodide.

IPA (tn) *see* Isopropyl alcohol.

Iscobrome D (tn) *see* Ethylene dibromide.

Isoacetophorone *see* Isophorone.

Isoamyl acetate *TN/synonyms:* Banana oil; Isopentyl acetate; 3-Methyl-1-butanol acetate; 3-Methylbutyl ester of acetic acid; 3-Methylbutyl athanoate. *OSHA PEL:* 100 ppm or 525 mg/m³ (8hr/day-40hr/wk-PP/S). *IDLH:* 3,000 ppm. *Symptoms:* Eye, nasal, throat, and upper respiratory irritation; Unconsciousness due to narcotic effects;

Dermatitis; Sensation of heat; Rapid breathing; Increased pulse rate; Cough; Dry throat; Fatigue; Indigestion; Central nervous system depression; Excess urobilin in urine; Labored or difficult breathing; Headaches; Drowsiness; Cardiac palpitations; Conjunctiva congestion; Weakness; Unconsciousness. *End-point Targets:* Eyes; Skin; Respiratory system. *Usage:* Airplane dopes; Artificial silk, leather, pearls, and glass; Baked goods; Beer; Beverage flavoring; Bronzing liquids; Candies; Chemical manufacturing; Chewing gum; Dry cleaning; Dyes; Fabric finishes and printing ink; Fingernail polish; Fluorescent lamps; Food flavoring; Gelatin; Household cleaning products; Ice Cream; Ices; Lacquers; Leather polishes; Metallic paints; Mineral water; Nitrocellulose; Odor warning agent; Oil colors; Paint; Penicillin extraction; Petroleum based feedstock; Photographic film; Puddings; Resins; Room deodorants; Shoe polish; Smokeless powder; Soft drinks; Solvent; Straw hats; Swelling bath sponges; Syrups; Waterproof varnish; Whiskey. *References:* 140; 304; 388.

Isoamyl alcohol *TN/synonyms:* Fermentation amyl alcohol; Fusel oil; Isobutyl carbinol; Isopentyl alcohol; 3-Methyl-1-butanol; 3-Methyl-2-butanol. *OSHA PEL:* 100 ppm or 360 mg/m^3 (8hr/day-40hr/wk-PP/S); 125 ppm or 450 mg/m^3 (exposure not to exceed 15 min). *IDLH:* 10,000 ppm. *Symptoms:* Eye, nasal, and throat irritation; Amnesia; Birth defects; Cerebellar atrophy; Changes in mood, personality, and behavior; Circulatory collapse; Cirrhosis; Clumsiness; Cold, clammy skin; Coma; Cracking skin; Death; Decreased sense of smell and taste; Diarrhea; Dizziness; Double vision; Euphoria; Headaches; Heavy breathing; Hypothermia; Impaired mental activity; Impaired sensory function; Incoordination; Involuntary eye movement; Labored or difficult breathing; Liver damage; Loss of ability to speak;

Loss of sensation; Mental dullness; Muscular incoordination; Nausea; Pancreatic disorders; Pneumonia; Reduced visual acuity; Respiratory failure; Staggering gait; Stupor; Unconsciousness due to narcotic effects; Vomiting. *End-point Targets:* Eyes; Skin; Respiratory system. *Usage:* Synthetic flavoring; Pharmaceutical; Lubricating oil additive; Hydraulic fluid additive; Solvent; Fats; Oils; Resins; Artificial silk; Lacquers; Smokeless powder; Determining fat in milk. *References:* 139, 304, 388.

Isobutanal *see* **Isobutyl alcohol.**

Isobutenyl methyl ketone *see* **Mesityl oxide.**

Isobutyl acetate *TN/synonyms:* Isobutyl ester of acetic acid; 2-Methylpropyl acetate; 2-Methylpropyl ester of acetic acid; beta-Methylpropyl ethanoate. *OSHA PEL:* 150 ppm or 700 mg/m^3 (8hr/day-40hr/wk-PP/S). *IDLH:* 7,500 ppm. *Symptoms:* Eye, nasal, throat, upper respiratory, and skin irritation; Loss of sensation; Headaches; Drowsiness; Nausea; Vomiting; Dizziness; Unconsciousness; Weakness; Vertigo; Cardiac palpitations; Gastrointestinal disorders; Anemia; Skin lesions; Dermatitis; Liver effects. *End-point Targets:* Skin; Eyes; Respiratory system. *Usage:* Pesticide inert ingredient; Flavoring agent; Nitrocellulose; Paint, lacquer, and varnish thinners; Sealants; Topcoat lacquers; Perfume; Banana, raspberry, strawberry, and butter flavoring. *References:* 166, 304, 388, 423.

Isobutyl alcohol *TN/Synonyms:* IBA; Isobutanal; Isopropylcarbinol; 2-Methyl-1-propanol. *OSHA PEL:* 50 ppm or 150 mg/m^3 (8hr/day-40hr/wk-PP/S). *IDLH:* 8,000 ppm. *Symptoms:* Eye, nasal, throat, and skin irritation; Cardiac arrhythmias and failure; Central nervous system depression; Chemical sensitivity; Coma; Confusion; Cough; Cracking skin; Death; Delirium;

Dermatitis; Diarrhea; Drowsiness; Gastrointestinal hemorrhages; Giddiness; Glucose in urine; Headaches; Impaired performance; Incoordination; Kidney damage; Labored or difficulty breathing; Liver damage; Muscle weakness; Nausea; Pulmonary edema; Respiratory failure; Vertigo; Vomiting. Suspected of causing Cancer. *End-point Targets:* Eyes; Skin; Respiratory system. *Usage:* Pesticide inert ingredient; Lube oil additive; Solvent; Hydraulic fluid; Plasticizers; Perfumes; Flavorings; Rum flavors; Banana flavors; Fruit flavors; Surface coatings; Adhesives; Pharmaceutical; Pesticide manufacture; Fragrances; Sucrose; Paint; Varnish remover; Food additive; Amino resins. *References:* 149, 304, 388, 423, 425.

Isobutyl carbinol *see* **Isoamyl alcohol.**

Isobutyl ester of acetic acid *see* **Isobutyl acetate.**

Isobutylmethylcarbinol *see* **Methyl isobutyl carbinol.**

Isobutyl methyl ketone *see* **Hexone.**

Isohol (tn) *see* **Isopropyl alcohol.**

iso-Nitropropane *see* **2-Nitropropane.**

Isopentyl acetate *see* **Isoamyl acetate.**

Isopentyl alcohol *see* **Isoamyl alcohol.**

Isophorone *TN/Synonyms:* Isoacetophorone; 3,5,5-Trimethyl-2-cyclohexenone; 3,5,5-Trimethyl-2-cyclohexen-1-one. *OSHA PEL:* 4 ppm or 23 mg/m³ (8hr/day-40hr/wk-PP/S). *IDLH:* 800 ppm. *Symptoms:* Eye, nasal, throat, mucous membrane, and respiratory irritation; Pulmonary congestion and degeneration; Liver and kidney damage; Unconsciousness due to narcotic effects; Dermatitis; Nausea; Headaches; Dizziness; Faintness; Inebriation; Feeling of suffocation; Irritability; Central nervous system

depression; Skin burns. Suspected of causing Cancer. *End-point Targets:* Respiratory system; skin. *Usages:* Pesticide inert ingredient; Finishes; Lacquers; Inks; Ink thinner; Polyvinyl; Nitrocellulose; Plastics; Solvent; Oils; Fats; Resins; Gums; Vinyl; Chemical intermediate; Pesticide manufacturing; Acrylics; Epoxy; Polyester; Silicone. *Classification:* Organic solvent (Ketone compound). *Note:* Neurotoxin. *References:* 17, 168, 286, 304, 305, 383, 388, 423, 440.

Isopropanol *see* **Isopropyl alcohol.**

Isopropenyl benzene *see* **alpha-Methyl styrene.**

4-Isopropenyl-1-methylcyclohexene *see* **Limonene.**

4-Isopropenyl-1-methyl-1-cyclohexene *see* **Limonene.**

2-Isopropoxy propane *see* **Isopropyl ether.**

Isopropyl acetate *TN/Synonyms:* Isopropyl ester of acetic acid; 1-Methylethyl ester of acetic acid; 2-Propyl acetate. *NIOSH:* No REL, notified OSHA that documentation doesn't support the worker's safety at established PELs. *OSHA PEL:* 250 ppm or 950 mg/m³ (8hr/day-40hr/wk-PP/S); 310 ppm or 1,185 mg/m³ (exposure not to exceed 15 min). *IDLH:* 16,000 ppm. *Symptoms:* Eye, nasal, conjunctiva, skin, and upper respiratory irritation; Dermatitis; Unconsciousness due to narcotic effects; Chest constriction; Cough; Defatting dermatitis; Central nervous system depression; Weakness; Drowsiness; Cracking skin. *End-point Targets:* Eyes; Skin; Respiratory system. *Usage:* Printing ink; Cellulose; Plastics; Solvent; Oils; Fats; Perfume; Gums; Resins; Shellac; Lacquers; Food flavorings; Insecticide manufacturing; Coatings; Pesticide inert ingredient. *References:* 165, 304, 388, 423.

Isopropyl alcohol *TN/synonyms:* Propan-2-ol; Dimethyl carbinol;

Isopropanol; 2-Propanol; sec-Propyl alcohol; Rubbing alcohol; Visco 1152 (TN); Imsol A (tn); IPA (tn); Isohol (tn); Lutosol (tn); Pro (tn); Petrohol (tn). *OSHA PEL:* 400 ppm or 980 mg/m³ (8hr/day-40hr/wk-PP/S); 500 ppm or 1,225 mg/m³ (exposure not to exceed 15 min). *IDLH:* 12,000 ppm. *Symptoms:* Eye, nasal, throat, and skin irritation; Abdominal pain; Absence of reflexes; Aspirative and bronchial pneumonias; Central nervous system depression; Chemical sensitization to primary and secondary alcohols; Circulatory collapse; Coma; Confusion; Contact dermatitis; Death; Decreased tendon reflexes; Denatured erythrocytes in the blood; Destruction of red blood cells; Dilated pupils; Dizziness; Drowsiness; Dry, cracking skin; Excess urine formation; Fever; Gastrointestinal inflammation; Headaches; Heart rate over 100 beats per minute; Heart rate under 60 beats per minute; Hemolytic anemia; Hemorrhagic pulmonary edema; Hemorrhagic tracheobronchitis; Hypothermia; Impaired speech; Incoordination; Kidney and liver dysfunction; Low blood pressure; Muscle tenderness, hardening of tissue, and swelling; Myoglobin in urine; Nausea; Reduced urine formation; Renal impairment; Respiratory depression and arrest; Stupor; Vomiting blood; Vomiting. *End-point Targets:* Eyes; Skin; Respiratory system. *Usage:* Aerosol insecticides; After-shave; Anesthetic [Avantine (tn)]; Antifreeze; Antiseptic; Baked goods; Candy; Cellulose; Chemical manufacturing; Cosmetics; Disinfectant; Essential oils; Food flavoring adjuvant; Food processing; Gasoline additive; Germicide; Gums; Hair Tonic; Hand lotions; Household cleaning products; Icepacks; Inks; Liniments; Liquid fuels; Liquid soaps; Non-alcoholic beverages; Perfumes; Permanent wave solutions; Pesticide inert ingredient; Pharmaceuticals; Resins; Rubbing alcohol; Shellacs; Solvent; Surgical suture packing; Window cleaners. *Note:* Occupationally acquired sensitivity to isopropyl alcohol also caused reactions to n-propyl alcohol; n-butyl alcohol; 2-Propanol. *Classification:* Organic Solvent; Polar volatile organic compounds. *References:* 164, 304, 383, 388, 423, 452.

Isopropylamine *TN/synonyms:* 2-Aminopropane; Monoisopropylamine; 2-Propylamine; sec-Propylamine. *NIOSH:* No REL, notified OSHA that documentation doesn't support the worker's safety at established PELs. *OSHA PEL:* 5 ppm or 12 mg/m³ (8hr/day-40hr/wk-PP/S); 10 ppm or 24 mg/m³ (exposure not to exceed 15 min). *IDLH:* 4,000 ppm. *Symptoms:* Eye, nasal, throat, and skin irritation; Pulmonary edema; Vision disturbances; Burns skin and eyes; Dermatitis. *End-point Targets:* Respiratory system; Skin; Eyes. *Usage:* Pesticide inert ingredient; Dehairing agent; Leather tanning; Pesticide, herbicide, and bactericide manufacturing; Rubber; Pharmaceuticals; Dyes; Textiles. *References:* 270, 304, 388, 423.

Isopropyl benzene *see* **Cumene.**

Isopropylbenzene *see* **Cumene.**

Isopropylbenzol *see* **Cumene.**

Isopropylcarbinol *see* **Isobutyl alcohol.**

Isopropyl ester of acetic acid *see* **Isopropyl acetate.**

Isopropyl ether *TN/synonyms:* Diisopropyl ether; Diisopropyl oxide; 2-Isopropoxy propane. *OSHA PEL:* 500 ppm or 2,100 mg/m³ (8hr/day-40hr/wk-PP/S). *ACGIH TLV:* 250 ppm or 1,050 mg/m³ (8hr/day-40hr/wk); 310 ppm or 1,320 mg/m³ (exposure not to exceed 15 min). *IDLH:* 10,000 ppm. *Symptoms:* Eye, nasal, skin, mucous membrane, and upper respiratory irritation; Albumin in urine; Bladder inflammation; Bronchial secretions and dilation; Cardiac arrhythmias; Central nervous system depression; Constipation; Convulsions; Cough; Death; Depression; Dermatitis; Dizziness; Drowsiness; Dry, cracked skin; Excess of red blood cells; Excessive salivation; Excitement; Exhaustion; Fatigue; Headaches; Hyperglycemia; Increased heart rate; Irregular respiration; Kidney damage and inflammation; Laryngeal spasm; Loss of appetite; Loss of sensation; Mania; Mental disorders; Metabolic acidosis; Myocardial depression of the heart; Nausea; Painful or difficult urination; Pallor; Profuse sweating; Psychotic disturbances; Respiratory discomfort and paralysis; Sleepiness; Unconsciousness due to narcotic effects; Vomiting. *End-point Targets:* Respiratory system; Skin. *Usage:* Solvent; Oil extraction from animals, vegetables, and minerals; Waxes; Resins; Dyes; Spot cleaner; Metallurgy; Oven cleaners. *References:* 163, 304, 388.

Isopropylideneacetone *see* **Mesityl oxide.**

Isovalerone *see* **Diisobutyl ketone.**

Ivalon *see* **Formaldehyde.**

Ivoir (tn) *see* **Benzyl acetate.**

Jasmolin I or II *see* **Pyrethrum.**

Jaysol S (tn) *see* **Ethanol.**

Jeffersol EB (tn) *see* **2-Butoxyethanol.**

Kanechlor (tn) *see* **Polychlorinated biphenyls.**

Kautschin *see* **Limonene.**

Ketene *TN/synonyms:* Carbomethene; Ethenone; Keto-ethylene. *OSHA PEL:* 0.5 ppm or 0.9 mg/m³ (8hr/day-40hr/wk); 1.5 ppm or 3.0 mg/m³ (exposure not to exceed 15 min). *IDLH:* Unknown. *Symptoms:* Eye, nasal, throat, skin, and lung irritation; Pulmonary edema. *End-point Targets:* Respiratory system; Eyes; Skin. *Usage:* Converting acids into anhydrides; Cellulose acetate; Aspirin; Medicine;

Acrylic acid. *Note:* Respiratory reactions may be delayed. *References:* 162, 304, 388.

Keto-ethylene *see* **Ketene.**

Ketone propane *see* **Acetone.**

beta-Ketopropane *see* **Acetone.**

Killmaster (tn) *see* **Chlorpyrifos.**

beta-Lactone *see* **beta-Propiolactone.**

Lanadin (tn) *see* **Trichloroethylene.**

Larvacide (tn) *see* **Chloropicrin.**

Larvacide 100 (tn) *see* **Chloropicrin.**

Laurel camphor *see* **Camphor.**

Lead *TN/synonyms:* Plumbum; Olow; Pigment metal; CI77575 (tn). *Compounds:* Lead acetate; Lead chloride; Lead chromate; Lead nitrate; Lead oxide; Lead phosphate; Lead sulfate. *NIOSH REL:* 0.1 mg/m³-[Air concentration to be maintained so that worker's blood lead remains 0.060 mg/100 g of whole blood]. *OSHA PEL:* 0.05 mg/m³ (8hr/day-40hr/wk-PP/S). *CDC:* 10 µg/dl in blood is considered poisoned. Irreversible neurological damage can occur between 9 & 15 µg/dl, especially in children. *ATSDR MRL:* No MRLs have been developed because it doesn't appear there is a safe threshold for the most sensitive effects of lead. *IDLH:* 700 mg/m³. *Symptoms:* Eye irritation; Abdominal pain and cramps; Abnormal amounts of sugar or uric acid in the blood; Abnormal liver function; Alters enzyme activity; Anemia; Behavioral abnormalities; Brain dysfunction; Cardiac lesions; Colic; Constipation; Convulsions; Death; Decrease in or excessive phosphorus in urine; Decrease in the enzyme cytochrome P-450; Delusions; Destruction of erythrocytes in the blood; Diarrhea; Depression; Electrocardiogram abnormalities; Excess amino acids in the blood; Facial pallor;

Female infertility; Gingival lead lined gums; Growth retardation; Hearing loss; Hypochromic, normocytic anemia; Increase in reticulocytes in the blood and nitrogenous bodies (esp. urea) in blood; Insomnia; Interstitial fibrosis; Joint pains; Kidney diseases; Lassitude; Learning disabilities; Loss of appetite; Low blood pressure; Lowered IQ; Malnutrition; Menstrual disorders; Metal fume fever; Metallic taste; Mitochondrial changes; Muscle weakness and cramps; Nausea; Neurobehavorial impairment; Pale eyes; Paralysis of wrists and/or ankles; Protein in urine; Psychosis; Reduced hemoglobin in the blood; Sperm damage; Spontaneous abortions; Testicular damage; Thirst; Toxic delirium; Tremors; Vomiting; Weakness; Weight loss; Polyneuropathy; Loss of vision; Neurochemistry changes; Central nervous system pathology; Impaired psychomotor functions; Impaired memory; Fatigue; Irritablitiy; Nervousness; Anxiety; Sexual disorders; Headaches. Suspected of causing Sudden Infant Death Syndrome; Pulmonary irritation, edema, and hemorrhage; Decreased thyroid function; Immune system damage; Neonate lethality; Chromosomal aberrations; DNA damage; Cancer. *End-point Targets:* Gastrointestinal tract; Central nervous system; Kidneys; Blood; Gingival tissue. *Usage:* Lead crystal; Pesticide inert ingredient; Batteries; Sheet lead; Solder; Pipes; Roofing materials; Caulking; Buckles; Petroleum refining; Tetraethyl lead and Tetramethyl lead; X-ray and radiation protection; Pigments; Paints; Plastics; Ceramics; Electrical devices; Ballast; TV glass; Brass; Bronze; Gasoline additive. *Note:* Historically established as a neurotoxin. Lead has been shown to affect all organs and/or systems in the body. Lead from lead crystal will leach into liquids. *References:* 17, 37, 299, 304, 306, 346, 387, 388, 413, 423, 429, 432, 449.

Lead tetraethyl *see* **Tetraethyl lead.**

Lead tetramethyl *see* **Tetramethyl lead.**

Lethurin (tn) *see* **Trichloroethylene.**

Lime *see* **Calcium oxide.**

Limonen *see* **Limonene.**

Limonene *TN/Synonyms:* 1,8(9)-p-Menthadiene; 1,8-p-Methadiene; 1- Methyl-4-(1-methylethenyl)Cyclohexene; 1-Methyl-4-Isopropenyl-1-cyclohexene; 4-Isopropenyl-1-methyl- 1-cyclohexene; 4-Isopropenyl-1-methylcyclohexene; Acintene DP; Dipentene; alpha-Limonene; Cajeputen; Cajeputene; Cinen; Cinene; delta-1, 8-Terpodiene; Dipenten; Dipentene; Dipentene 200; dl-Limonene; Eulimen; Inactive limonene; Kautschin; Limonen; Nesol; p-Mentha-1,8-diene; dl-Mentha-1,8-diene; Unitene. *OSHA PEL:* None. *Symptoms:* Stomach irritation; Skin and eye irritation and burns; Abdominal pain; Albumin in urine; Blood in urine; Burning pain in mouth and throat; Coma; Contact dermatitis; Convulsions; Cyanosis; Death; Delirium; Dizziness; Excessive salivation; Excitement; Feeling of suffocation; Fever; Heart rate over 100 beats per minute; Hypothermia; Incoordination; Kidney damage and lesions; Nausea; Painful urination; Pneumonia; Pulmonary edema; Respiratory failure; Skin sensitization; Somnolence; Stupor; Swollen tongue, lips, or gingival mucosa; Vomiting. Suspected of causing Cancer; Birth defects. *End-point Targets:* Kidneys; Respiratory system; Skin; Eyes. *Usage:* Air fresheners; Baked goods; Candy; Chewing gum; Cologne; Deodorant; Detergent; Dishwashing liquid; Fabric softeners; Facial cream; Fingernail polish remover; Food flavoring; Gallstone treatment; Gelatin; Hand lotion; Herbal medicine; Ice cream; Medicine; Non-alcoholic beverages; Paint brush cleaners; Perfume; Pesticide inert ingredient; Preservatives; Pudding; Shampoo; Shaving cream; Soap; Solvent; Terpene resins. Found in cigarette smoke, citrus fruit, wood. *Contaminates* breast milk. *Classification:* Polar volatile organic compounds. *References:* 39, 423, 452.

alpha-Limonene *see* **Limonene.**

dl-Limonene *see* **Limonene.**

Linalol *see* **Linalyl alcohol.**

Linalool *see* **Linalyl alcohol.**

beta-Linalool *see* **Linalyl alcohol.**

Linalyl alcohol *TN/synonyms:* Linalool; Linalol; 3,7-Dimethyl-1, 6-octadien-3-ol; 2,6-Dimethyl-2,7-octadiene-6-ol; 2,6-Dimethylocta-2,7-doen-6-ol; 3,7-Dimethylocta-1,6-dien-3-ol; Allo-ocimenol; beta-Linalool. *OSHA PEL:* None. *Symptoms:* Skin irritation; Contact dermatitis; Psoriasis; Respiratory depression; Vasodilation; Decrease in blood pressure; Central nervous system depression. Suspected of causing Unconsciousness due to narcotic effects; Incoordination. *Endpoint Targets:* Central nervous system; Skin; Respiratory system. *Usage:* Food flavoring; Mace; Perfume; Cologne; Bar soap; Shampoo; Deodorant; Hand lotion; Fingernail polish remover; Detergent; Powdered bleach; Fabric softeners; Air fresheners; Non-alcoholic beverages; Ice cream; Candy; Baked goods; Gelatins; Puddings; Chewing gum; Condiments; Aftershave. Found in more than 200 oils from spices, herbs, leaves, flowers, and wood. *Classification:* Polar volatile organic compounds. *References:* 40, 452.

Lindane *TN/synonyms:* BHC; gamma-Hexachlorocyclohexane; HCH; 1,2,3,4,5,6-Hexachlorocyclohexane. *OSHA PEL:* 0.5 mg/m³ (8hr/day-40hr/wk-PP/S). *IDLH:* 1,000 mg/m³. *Symptoms:* Eye, nasal, throat, and skin irritation; Headaches; Nausea; Clonic convulsions; Respiratory difficulty; Cyanosis; Aplastic anemia; Muscle spasms; Central nervous system stimulant; Death; Irritability; Grand mal convulsions; Dermatitis; Blood disorders; Mental and motor retardation in children; Vomiting; Hyperactivity; Muscle and kidney tissue death; Coma; Gastrointestinal inflammation. Suspected of causing Liver damage. *Endpoint Targets:* Eyes; Central Nervous system; Blood; Liver; Kidneys; Skin. *Usage:* Pesticide; Insecticide; Rodenticide; Medicine; Veterinary medicine. *References:* 161, 304, 388.

Liquid Pitch Oil *see* **Creosotes.**

Lorsban (tn) *see* **Chlorpyrifos.**

Lutosol (tn) *see* **Isopropyl alcohol.**

Lutrol-9 (tn) *see* **Ethylene glycol.**

Lye *see* **Sodium hydroxide.**

Lysoform *see* **Formaldehyde.**

M40 (tn) *see* **Methyl parathion.**

M80 (tn) *see* **Methyl parathion.**

MA *see* **Monomethyl aniline.**

Mace *see* **alpha-Chloroacetophenone.**

Macrogol 400 BPC (tn) *see* **Ethylene glycol.**

Magnesia fume *see* **Magnesium oxide.**

Magnesium oxide *TN/synonyms:* Magnesia fume. *NIOSH:* No REL, notified OSHA that documentation doesn't support the worker's safety at established PELs. *OSHA PEL:* 10 mg/m³ (8hr/day-40hr/wk). *IDLH:* NE. *Symptoms:* Eye and nasal irritation; Metal fume fever; Cough; Chest pains; Flu-like fever; Increase in leukocytes in the blood; Nausea; Malaise; Depression; Respiratory, cardiovascular, and central nervous system paralysis; Low blood pressure; Skin vasodilation; Cardiac arrest; Insufficient oxygen; Loss of sensation. *End-point Targets:* Respiratory system; Eyes. *Usage:* Pesticide inert ingredient; Medicine; Animal feed; Fertilizers; Insulation; Wallboard; Petroleum additive; Cement; Paper; Food additive; Rubber; Fire bricks; Antacids; Casein; Glue; Optical instruments; Laxative; Aircraft windshields; Cosmetics. *References:* 160, 299, 304, 388, 423.

Malathion *TN/synonyms:* S-[1,2-bis (ethoxycarbonyl)ethyl]0,0-demethylphosphorodithioate; Diethyl (dimethoxyphosphinothioylthio) succinate; Fifanon (tn). *OSHA PEL:* 10 mg/m³ (8hr/day-40hr/wk-PP/S). *IDLH:* 5,000 mg/m³. *Symptoms:* Eye and skin irritation; Abdominal cramps; Aching eyes; Anxiety; Blurred vision; Bronchial secretions and constriction; Coma; Confusion; Constricted pupils; Convulsions; Cyanosis; Death; Diarrhea; Dizziness; Drowsiness; Excessive salivation; Giddiness; Headaches; Heart damage; Immune complex kidney diseases; Incoordination; Inhibits cholinesterase enzymes; Intestinal swelling; Irregular or slow heartbeat; Kidney dysfunction; Laryngeal spasms; Loss of appetite; Loss of reflexes; Muscular involuntary contractions; Nasal discharge; Nausea; Paralysis; Profuse sweating; Protein in urine; Restlessness; Slurred speech; Staggering gait; Tearing; Tight chest; Tremors; Twitching; Vomiting; Weakness; Wheezing. Suspected of causing Chromosomal aberrations. *End-point Targets:* Respiratory system; Liver; Blood cholinesterase; Central nervous system; Cardiovascular system; Gastrointestinal tract. *Usage:* Insecticide; Pesticide inert ingredient; Medicine; Veterinary medicine; Livestock/Poultry dip and sprays. *Classification:* Organophosphate. *Note:* Historically established as a neurotoxin. *References:* 17, 159, 304, 388, 413, 423.

Maleic acid anhydride *see* **Maleic anhydride.**

Maleic anhydride *TN/synonyms:* cis-Butenedioic anhydride; 2,5-Fur-

anedione; Maleic acid anhydride; Toxilic anhydride. *OSHA PEL:* 1 mg/m³ or 0.25 ppm (8hr/day-40hr/wk-PP/S). *IDLH:* Unknown. *Symptoms:* Eye, nasal, throat, skin, and upper respiratory irritation; Conjunctivitis; Eyes become sensitive to light; Double vision; Bronchial asthma; Dermatitis; Cough; Chemical sensitization; Bronchitis; Corneal inflammation; Occupational asthma; Headaches; Nosebleeds; Nausea. *End-point Targets:* Eyes; Respiratory system; Skin. *Usage:* Pesticide inert ingredient; Resins; Dyes; Polyester; Pharmaceuticals; Pesticides manufacturing; Oil and fat preservative; Permanent-press fabrics; Corrosion inhibitors; Lubricant additive; Food acidulants; Chemical intermediate; Plastics; Lacquers. *References:* 158, 304, 388, 423.

Malix (tn) *see* **Endosulfan.**

Manganese *TN/synonyms:* Elemental manganese; Colloidal manganese; Manganese-55. *Compounds:* Manganese chloride; Manganese sulfate; Manganese tetroxide; Manganese dioxide; Potassium permangante. *OSHA PEL:* 5 mg/m³ (ceiling limit); *fumes:* 1 mg/m³ (8hr/day-40hr/wk); 3 mg/m³ (exposure not to exceed 15 min). *ATSDR MRL:* .002 mg/m³ (Inhalation, more than 1 year). *IDLH:* NE. *Symptoms:* Abnormal tension of arteries or muscles; Anxiety; Bronchitis; Confusion; Cough; Decreased pulmonary function; Decreased libido; Depression; Dry throat; Emotional lability; Fatigue; Flu-like fever; Hallucinations; Headaches; Impotence; Increased pulmonary infections; Impaired memory; Insomnia; Irritability; Labored or difficulty breathing; Lassitude; Lethargy; Low-back pains; Malaise; Metal fume fever; Muscle rigidity; Nervousness; Parkinson's-like symptoms; Pneumonia; Psychosis; Pulmonary inflammation and injury; Rales; Slow and clumsy gait; Speech disturbances; Staggering gait; Sexual disorders; Tight chest; Tremors; Vomiting; Weakness. Suspected of causing Immune system activation; Birth defects; Testicular damage; Decreased sperm count. *End-point Targets:* Respiratory system; Central nervous system; Blood; Kidneys. *Usage:* Steel; Stainless-steel; Dry-cell batteries; Matches; Fireworks; Glass-bonding materials (adhesive); Amethyst glass; Ceramics; Pesticides; Fertilizers; Nutritional supplements; Glazes; Varnishes; Fungicide; Disinfectant; Anti-algae agent; Metal cleaning; Leather tanning and bleaching; Preservative; Gasoline anti-knock additive; Pesticide inert ingredient; Asphalt; Lime manufacturing. *Note:* Historically established as a neurotoxin. *References:* 17, 299, 304, 364, 388, 413, 423, 429.

Manganese-55 *see* **Manganese.**

Mar M (tn) *see* **Nickel.**

MCB *see* **Chlorobenzene.**

MDI *see* **Methylene bisphenyl isocyanate.**

MEK *see* **2-Butanone.**

MENCS (tn) *see* **1,3-Dichloropropene.**

dl-Mentha-1,8-diene *see* **Limonene.**

p-Mentha-1,8-diene *see* **Limonene.**

1,8(9)-p-Menthadiene *see* **Limonene.**

ME-Parathion (tn) *see* **Methyl parathion.**

Meptox (tn) *see* **Methyl parathion.**

Mercaptoethane *see* **Ethyl mercaptan.**

Mercaptomethane *see* **Methyl mercaptan.**

Mercury *TN/synonyms:* Colloidal mercury; Metallic mercury; Quicksilver. *OSHA PEL:* Organic: 0.01 mg/m³ or 0.03 mg/m³ (8hr/day-40hr/wk-PP/S);

Vapors: 0.05 mg/m³ (8hr/day-40hr/wk-PP/S). *IDLH:* Organic: 10 mg/m³; Vapors: 28 mg/m³. *Symptoms:* Eye and skin irritation; Altered libido; Birth defects; Bronchial pneumonia; Chest pain; Constipation; Cough; Diarrhea; Dizziness; Emotional disturbances; Excessive salivation; Fatigue; Fetal brain damage; Gastrointestinal disturbance; Headaches; Impaired speech; Incoordination; Indecision; Insomnia; Irreversible brain damage; Irritability; Labored or difficulty breathing; Loss of appetite; Menstrual disorders; Metal fume fever; Nausea; Numbness, tingling, or prickling sensation; Protein in urine; Skin burns; Spastic or jerky muscle movement; Spontaneous abortions; Stomach inflammation; Tearing; Tremors; Vision and hearing disturbances; Vomiting; Weakness; Weight-loss; Autoimmune disease; Immune-complex glomerulonephritis; Personality changes; Polyneuropathy; Loss of field of vision. Suspected of altering sperm production. *End-point Targets:* Central nervous system; Kidneys; Eyes; Skin; Respiratory system. *Usage:* Pigments; Bactericides; Antiseptics; Fireworks; Dental amalgam; Pesticide inert ingredient; Asphalt; Agricultural chemical; Photography; Taxidermy; Electrical equipment; Electroplating; Felt making; Textiles. Banned in interior paint in 1990; however, existing stocks were not recalled. *Note:* Historically established as a neurotoxin. *References:* 17, 280, 299, 304, 388, 413, 423, 429, 432, 449.

Mesityl oxide *TN/synonyms:* Isobutenyl methyl ketone; Isopropylideneacetone; Methyl isobutenyl ketone; 4-Methyl-3-penten-2-one. *NIOSH REL:* 10 ppm or 40 mg/m³ (10hr/day-40hr/wk). *OSHA PEL:* 15 ppm or 60 mg/m³ (8hr/day-40hr/wk-PP/S); 25 ppm or 100 mg/m³ (exposure not to exceed 15 min). *IDLH:* 5,000 ppm. *Symptoms:* Eye, skin, and mucus membrane irritation; Unconsciousness due to narcotic effects; Coma; Dermatitis; Central nervous system depression; Liver, lung, and kidney injuries. *End-point Targets:* Eyes; Skin; Respiratory system. *Usage:* Food flavoring; Perfumes; Plastics; Pesticide inert ingredient; Chemical intermediate; Solvent; Gums; Resins; Lacquers; Varnishes; Enamels; Leather; Rubber; Cellulose; Inks; Paint; Varnish removers; Insect repellent. *Classification:* Organic solvent (Ketone compound). *References:* 157, 304, 305, 383, 388, 423, 437.

Metacid 50 (tn) *see* **Methyl parathion.**

Metacide (tn) *see* **Methyl parathion.**

Metafos (tn) *see* **Methyl parathion.**

Metallic mercury *see* **Mercury.**

Metallic tin *see* **Tin.**

Metallum problematum *see* **Tellurium.**

Metaphos (tn) *see* **Methyl parathion.**

Metaphosphoric acid *see* **Phosphoric acid.**

Metapon (tn) *see* **Methyl parathion.**

Methacrylate monomer *see* **Methyl metacrylate.**

1,8-p-Methadiene *see* **Limonene.**

Methanal *see* **Formaldehyde.**

Methanecarboxlic acid *see* **Acetic acid.**

Methanethiol *see* **Methyl mercaptan.**

Methane trichloride *see* **Chloroform.**

Methanoic acid *see* **Formic acid.**

Methanol *see* **Methyl alcohol.**

Methenyl chloride *see* **Chloroform.**

Methoxycarbonylethylene *see* **Methyl acrylate.**

Methoxychloromethyl ether *see* **Chloromethyl methyl ether.**

2-Methoxyethanol *see* **Methyl cellosolve.**

2-Methoxyethyl acetate *see* **Methyl cellosolve acetate.**

Methoxymethyl methyl ether *see* **Methylal.**

Methyl acetate *TN/synonyms:* Methyl ester of acetic acid; Methyl ethanoate. *OSHA PEL:* 200 ppm or 610 mg/m³ (8hr/day-40hr/wk-PP/S); 250 ppm or 750 mg/m³ (exposure not to exceed 15 min). *IDLH:* 10,000 ppm. *Symptoms:* Eye, nasal, throat, and upper respiratory irritation; Headaches; Drowsiness; Vertigo; Eye burns; Tearing; Cardiac palpitations; Chest constriction; Labored or difficulty breathing; Blindness; Unconsciousness; Vision disturbances; Nervousness; Optic nerve atrophy. Suspected of causing Unconsciousness due to narcotic effects; Death; Pulmonary edema; Liver, kidney, and myocardium effects. *End-point Targets:* Respiratory system; Skin; Eyes. *Usage:* Solvent; Nitrocellulose; Resins; Oils; Artificial leather; Pesticide; Alcoholic beverages; Rum; Brandy; Whiskey; Fruit flavors; Paint remover; Lacquer. *Synergistic effects:* Reacts slowly with water to form acetic acid and methanol. *Note:* Neurotoxin. *References:* 17, 155, 304, 388.

Methyl acetone *see* **2-Butanone.**

beta-Methylacrolein *see* **Crotonaldehyde.**

Methyl acrylate *TN/synonyms:* Methoxycarbonylethylene; Methyl ester of acrylic acid; Methyl propenoate. *OSHA PEL:* 10 ppm or 35 mg/m³ (8hr/day-40hr/wk-PP/S). *IDLH:* 1,000 ppm. *Symptoms:* Eye, upper respiratory, and skin irritation; Lethargy; Convulsions; Rapid respiration; Eye burns; Dermatitis; Contact dermatitis; Chemical sensitivity. *Target Organs:* Respiratory system; Eyes; Skin. *Usage:* Acrylic fibers; Dental applications;

Medicine; Pharmaceuticals; Microencapsulation; Time-released pesticides; Leather finishes; Textiles; Paper; Plastic films; Vitamin B1; Coatings; Polishes; Adhesives; Chemical manufacturing. *Additive/Contaminants:* Usually contains an inhibitor such as hydroquinone. *Note:* Repetitious testing or exposure may induce allergic reactions. *References:* 154, 304, 388.

Methylal *TN/synonyms:* Dimethoxymethane; Formal; Formaldehyde dimethylacetal; Methoxymethyl methyl ether; Methylene dimethyl ether. *OSHA PEL:* 1,000 ppm or 3,100 mg/m³ (8hr/day-40hr/wk-PP/S). *IDLH:* 15,000 ppm. *Symptoms:* Eye, skin, and upper respiratory irritation; Respiratory and central nervous system depression; Loss of sensation. *End-point Targets:* Skin; Respiratory system; Central nervous system. *Usage:* Perfume; External ointments; Solvent; Fuels; Adhesives; Coatings; Artificial resins; Oven cleaners. *References:* 170, 304, 388.

Methyl alcohol *TN/synonyms:* Carbinol; Columbian spirits; Methanol; Wood alcohol; Wood spirits. *OSHA PEL:* 200 ppm or 260 mg/m³ (8hr/day-40hr/wk-PP/S); 250 ppm or 325 mg/m³ (exposure not to exceed 15 min). *IDLH:* 25,000 ppm. *Symptoms:* Eye irritation; Acidosis; Apathy; Blindness; Blurred vision; Central blind spots in vision; Central nervous system depression; Circulatory collapse; Cold and clammy extremities; Coma; Conjunctivitis; Convulsions; Death; Delirium; Diarrhea; Diminished visual acuity; Dimness of vision; Drowsiness; Excitement; Fatigue; Gastric disturbances; Giddiness; Headaches; Heart rate below 60 beats per minute; Heart rate over 100 beats per minute; Insomnia; Labored or difficulty breathing; Leg cramps and pain; Lightheadedness; Loss of appetite; Mania; Motor dysfunction and restlessness; Nausea; Numbness, tingling, or prickling sensation; Optic congestion; Respiratory

failure; Restlessness; Slow pulse; Temporary cessation of breathing; Upper abdominal and back pains; Vertigo; Vision disturbances; Vomiting; Weakness. *End-point Targets:* Eyes; Skin; Central nervous system; Gastrointestinal tract. *Usage:* Pesticide inert ingredient; Inks; Solvent; Antifreeze; Fuel; Extraction of animal and vegetable oils; Pharmaceuticals; Vitamins; Hormones; Plastics; De-icing agent; Aspartame; Chemical manufacturing; Liniments; Embalming fluid; Control onion smut; Pesticides; Slimicide; Wood preservative; Household cleaners; Bactericide; Disinfectants; Detergents. *Note:* Historically established as a neurotoxin. *References:* 17, 153, 304, 388, 413, 423, 429.

Methyl aldehyde *see* **Formaldehyde.**

Methylamine *TN/synonyms:* Aminomethane; Anhydrous methylamine; Aqueous methylamine; Monomethylamine. *OSHA PEL:* 10 ppm or 12 mg/m³ (8hr/day-40hr/wk-PP/S). *IDLH:* 100 ppm. *Symptoms:* Eye, nasal, throat, skin, and respiratory system irritation; Cough; Skin and mucus membrane burns; Dermatitis; Conjunctivitis; Allergic or chemical bronchitis; Olfactory fatigue; Irritability. *End-point Targets:* Respiratory system; Eyes; Skin. *Usage:* Leather tanning; Dyes; Pharmaceuticals; Insecticide, pesticide, and fungicide intermediate; Fuel additive; Paint remover; Solvent; Photography; Rocket propellent; Textiles. *References:* 178, 304, 388.

(Methylamino) benzene *see* **Monomethyl aniline.**

1-Methyl-2-aminobenzene: o-Toluidine.

Methyl amyl alcohol *see* **Methyl isobutyl carbinol.**

Methyl n-amyl ketone *TN/synonyms:* Amyl methyl ketone; n-Amyl methyl ketone; 2-Heptanone. *OSHA*

PEL: 100 ppm or 465 mg/m³ (8hr/day-40hr/wk-PP/S). *ACGIH TLV:* 50 ppm or 235 mg/m³ (8hr/day-40hr/wk-PP/S). *IDLH:* 4,000 ppm. *Symptoms:* Eye, mucus membrane, and skin irritation; Headaches; Unconsciousness due to narcotic effects; Coma; Dermatitis; Central nervous system depression. *End-point Targets:* Eyes; Skin; Respiratory system; Central nervous system; Peripheral nervous system. *Usage:* Food flavoring; Perfumes; Plastics; Pesticide inert ingredient; Printing ink; Fragrances; Cosmetic creams and lotions; Hand and body lotions; Soaps; Detergent; Solvent. *Classification:* Organic solvent (Ketone compound). *Note:* Dissolves some forms of plastic. *References:* 156, 304, 305, 383, 388, 423.

Methyl aniline *see* **Monomethyl aniline.**

o-Methylaniline: *see* **o-Toluidine.**

N-Methyl aniline *see* **Monomethyl aniline.**

2-Methylaniline: *see* **o-Toluidine.**

Methyl azinphos *see* **Azinphos-methyl.**

2-Methylaziridine *see* **Propylene imine.**

Methyl benzene *see* **Toluene.**

Methyl benzol *see* **Toluene.**

Methyl bromide *TN/synonyms:* Bromomethane; Monobromomethane; Methyl fumes; Embafume (r); Terabol (r). *NIOSH:* Carcinogen at any exposure level. Reduce exposure to lowest feasible concentration. *OSHA PEL:* 5 ppm or 20 mg/m³ (8hr/day-40hr/wk-PP/S). *ATSDR MRL:* 0.2 ppm (Inhalation, less than 15 days); 0.005 ppm (Inhalation, more than 14 days); 0.3 ppm (Ingestion, more than 14 days). *IDLH:* 2,000 ppm. *Symptoms:* Eye, skin, and lung irritation; Abdominal cramps; Absence of urine formation; Blurred vision; Brain damage; Bron-

chial pneumonia; Central nervous system injury; Clonic convulsions; Coma; Convulsions; Death; Dizziness; Double vision; Fatigue; Hand tremors; Headaches; Impaired respiratory function; Incoordination; Kidney and respiratory failure; Labored or difficulty breathing; Liver congestion and focal hemorrhage; Loss of appetite; Loss of sensation; Malaise; Muscle aches; Nausea; Polyneuropathy; Protein in urine; Pulmonary edema; Skin vesiculation, lesions, redness, itching, and blisters; Vertigo; Vision disturbances; Vomiting; Weakness. Suspected of causing Paralysis; Testicular degeneration and atrophy; Methylates DNA; Chromosomal aberrations; Genetic mutation; Birth defects; Cancer. *End-point Targets:* Central nervous system; Respiratory system; Kidneys; Skin; Eyes. *Usages:* Insecticide; Fungicide; Rodenticide; Disinfectant; Wool degreaser; Extraction solvent for oils from nuts, seeds, and wool; Pesticide inert ingredient; Fire extinguisher; Aerosol propellents; Refrigerants. Found in automobile exhaust. *Synergistic effect:* Attacks aluminum to form aluminum trimethyl which is spontaneously flammable. *Classification:* Organic solvent. *Note:* Historically established as a neurotoxin. Adverse health effects are generally delayed. *References:* 286, 304, 316, 371, 383, 388, 413, 423.

3-Methyl-1-butanol *see* **Isoamyl alcohol.**

3-Methyl-2-butanol *see* **Isoamyl alcohol.**

3-Methyl-1-butanol acetate *see* **Isoamyl acetate.**

1-Methylbutyl acetate *see* **sec-Amyl acetate.**

3-Methylbutyl athanoate *see* **Isoamyl acetate.**

3-Methylbutyl ester of acetic acid *see* **Isoamyl acetate.**

Methylcarbinol *see* **Ethanol.**

Methyl cellosolve *TN/synonyms:* EGME; Ethylene glycol monomethyl ether; Glycol monomethyl ether; 2-Methoxyethanol. *NIOSH REL:* Reduce exposure to lowest feasible level. *OSHA PEL:* 25 ppm or 80 mg/m³ (8hr/day-40hr/wk-PP/S). *IDLH:* 2,000 ppm. *Symptoms:* Eye, nasal, and throat irritation; Headaches; Drowsiness; Weakness; Incoordination; Death; Fatigue; Staggering gait; Personality changes; Decreased mental ability; Brain dysfunction; Bone marrow depression; Reduction of cellular elements in blood; Tremors; Somnolence; Anemic pallor. Suspected of causing Cancer; Birth defects; Testicular atrophy; Embryo death; Liver, kidney, and lung damage; Anemia. *End-point Targets:* Central nervous system; Blood; Skin; Eyes. *Usage:* Lacquers; Metal coatings; Baking enamels; Varnish; Epoxy resin coatings; Printing inks; Textile dyes and pigments; Leather; Anti-icing additive for brakes and aviation fuel; Gasoline additive; Pesticide inert ingredient. *References:* 275, 304, 313, 388, 423, 449.

Methyl cellosolve acetate *TN/synonyms:* EGMEA; Ethylene glycol monomethyl ether acetate; Glycol monomethyl ether acetate; 2-Methoxyethyl acetate. *NIOSH REL:* Reduce exposure to lowest feasible level. *OSHA PEL:* 25 ppm or 120 mg/m³ (8hr/day-40hr/wk-PP/S). *IDLH:* 4,000 ppm. *Symptoms:* Eye irritation; Kidney and brain damage; Nausea; Vomiting; Diarrhea; Headaches; Abdominal and lumbar pain; Frequent, excess urination; Reduced and absence of urine formation; Kidney failure; Renal insufficiency resulting in a toxic condition; Pulmonary edema; Drowsiness; Cyanosis; Coma; Death; Brain, lung, liver, meninges, and heart lesions. *End-point Targets:* Kidneys; Brain; Central nervous system; Peripheral nervous system. *Usage:* Solvent; Lacquer; Airplane dopes; Nitrocellulose; Cellulose; Gums; Resins; Waxes; Oils; Textile printing; Photographic films; Silkscreening inks; Oven cleaners. *Note:* Patients may be misdiagnosed with Schizophrenia or Narcolepsy. *References:* 152, 304, 388.

Methyl chloride *TN/synonyms:* Chloromethane; Monochloromethane; Artic (tn); R 40 (tn); Freon 40 (tn). *NIOSH:* Carcinogen at any exposure level. Reduce exposure to the lowest feasible level. *OSHA PEL:* 50 ppm or 105 mg/m³ (8hr/day-40hr/wk-PP/S); 100 ppm or 210 mg/m³ (exposure not to exceed 15 min). *ATSDR MRL:* 0.46 ppm (Inhalation, less than 15 days); 0.40 ppm (Inhalation, more than 14 days). *IDLH:* 10,000 ppm. *Symptoms:* Absence of urine formation; Albumin and protein in urine; Central nervous system depression; Cirrhosis; Coma; Convulsions; Death; Decreased blood pressure; Dizziness; Electrocardiogram abnormalities; Fatigue; Frostbite; Heart rate over 100 beats per minute; Impaired balance; Increased pulse rate; Jaundice; Liver and kidney damage; Nausea; Partial or complete loss of sensation; Personality changes; Slurred speech; Staggering or abnormal gait; Tremors; Vertigo; Vision disturbances; Vomiting. Suspected of causing Cancer; Genetic mutations; Immune system damage; DNA damage; Birth defects; Testicular lesions; Dominant lethal mutations; Decreased fertility. *End-point Targets:* Central nervous system; Liver; Kidneys; Skin. *Usage:* Silicones; Pesticide; Fumigants; Pesticide and fumigant intermediate; Fire-extinguishers; Aerosol propellants; Plastics; Chlorinated water (swimming pools); Polystyrene insulation; Refrigerant; Pesticide inert ingredient; Synthetic rubber; Methyl cellulose; Tetramethyl lead; Triptane; Quaternary amines; Methyl mercaptan; Methionine. *Synergistic effects:* Reacts with water (hydrolyzes) to form hydrochloric acid. Natural product when wood, grass, charcoal, cigarettes, and coal are burned. *Classification:* Organic solvent. *Note:* Historically established as a neurotoxin. *References:* 304, 316, 331, 383, 388, 413, 423, 429.

Methyl chloroform *see* **1,1,1-Trichloroethane.**

Methyl cyanide *see* **Acetonitrile.**

Methyldinitrobenzene *see* **Dinitrotoluenes.**

Methyl-E 605 (tn) *see* **Methyl parathion.**

Methylene bisphenyl isocyanate *TN/synonyms:* 4,4'-Diphenylmethane diisocyanate; MDI; Methylene bis(4-phenyl) isocyanate; Methylene di-p-phenylene ester of isocyanic acid; Polyisocyanates. *NIOSH REL:* 0.05 mg/m^3 or 0.005 ppm (10hr/day-40hr/wk); 0.2 mg/m^3 0.02 ppm (Ceiling limit, 10 min exposure). *OSHA PEL:* 0.2 mg/m^3 or 0.02 ppm (Ceiling limit-PP/S). *EPA/ OTS:* >0.001 ppm (Pulmonary hypersensitivity; Substantial lung dysfunction). *IDLH:* 100 mg/m^3. *Symptoms:* Eye, nasal, and throat irritation; Cough; Chest pains; Pulmonary secretions; Labored or difficult breathing; Asthma; Dermatitis; Pulmonary and dermal sensitization; Allergic-type reactions. Suspected of causing Genetic mutations; Cancer. *End-point Targets:* Respiratory system; Eyes. *Usage:* Plastics; Adhesives; Particle board; Plywood; Elastic; Foam (cushions); Flexible foam; Paints; Automotive paint; Coatings; Foam blown insulation; Foam caulking; Hardwood floor sealants; Waterproofing agents; Automobile products; Furniture finishes; Polyurethane; Fiberglass (bathtubs); Waferboard; Fabric coating. *Note:* 13–17% of the general population and about 20% of the workers to experience allergic-type reactions. *References:* 304, 388, 445.

Methylene bis(4-phenyl) isocyanate *see* **Methylene bisphenyl isocyanate.**

Methylene chloride *TN/synonyms:* Dichloromethane; Methylene dichlo-

ride; Narkotil (tn); Salaesthin (tn); Solmethine (tn). *NIOSH:* Carcinogen at any exposure level. Reduce exposure to lowest possible level. *OSHA PEL:* 500 ppm (8hr/day-40hr/wk-PP/S); 1,000 ppm (ceiling limit); 2,000 ppm (5 min max peak in any 2 hrs). *ACGIH:* Suspected human carcinogen. *ACGIH TLV:* 50 ppm or 175 mg/m^3 (8hr/day-40hr/wk). *ATSDR MRL:* 1.0 ppm (Inhalation, less than 15 days); 0.4 ppm (Inhalation, more than 14 days). *IDLH:* 5,000 ppm. *Symptoms:* Eye, nasal, throat, skin irritation; Fatigue; Weakness; Sleepiness; Lightheadedness; Dizziness; Reduced coordination; Limbs numb and/or tingling; Nausea; Death; Loss of consciousness; Liver and kidney damage; Increase in serum bilirubin; Partial or complete loss of sensation; Decrease in psychomotor skills and behavioral performance. Suspected of causing Cancer (lung); Low birth weight; Low sperm count; DNA damage; Genetic mutations; Chromosomal aberrations; Brain damage. *End-point Targets:* Skin; Cardiovascular system; Central nervous system. *Usage:* Paint strippers and removers; Aerosol propellant; Automotive products; Insecticides; Pesticide; Pesticide inert ingredient; Photographic film; Medicine; Pharmaceuticals; Metal cleaning; Urethane foams; Extraction solvent for spice oleoresins, hops, and for removing caffeine from coffee; Grain fumigant; Hair spray; Room deodorants; Plastics; Adhesives; Foam blowing of polyurethane; Flame retardant coatings; Perfumes; Oven cleaners. *Note:* Does not easily burn. *Classification:* Halogenated organic compound; Polar volatile organic compounds. *Note:* Neurotoxin. *References:* 8, 17, 304, 345, 388, 423, 432, 452.

Methylene dichloride *see* **Methylene chloride.**

Methylene dimethyl ether *see* **Methylal.**

Methylene di-p-phenylene ester

of isocyanic acid: *see* **Methylene bisphenyl isocyanate.**

Methylene oxide *see* **Formaldehyde.**

Methyl ester of acetic acid *see* **Methyl acetate.**

Methyl ester of acrylic acid *see* **Methyl acrylate.**

Methyl ester of formic acid *see* **Methyl formate.**

Methyl ester of methacrylic acid *see* **Methyl methacrylate.**

Methyl ethanoate *see* **Methyl acetate.**

Methyl ethyl carbinol *see* **sec-Butyl alcohol.**

2-Methylethyleneimine *see* **Propylene imine.**

Methyl ethylene oxide *see* **Propylene oxide.**

1-Methylethyl ester of acetic acid *see* **Isopropyl acetate.**

Methyl ethyl ketone *see* **2-Butanone.**

N-(1-Methylethyl)-2-propanamine *see* **Diisopropylamine.**

Methyl formaldehyde *see* **Acetaldehyde.**

Methyl formate *TN/synonyms:* Methyl ester of formic acid; Methyl methanoate. *OSHA PEL:* 100 ppm or 250 mg/m³ (8hr/day-40hr/wk-PP/S); 150 ppm or 375 mg/m³ (exposure not to exceed 15 min). *IDLH:* 5,000 ppm. *Symptoms:* Eye and nasal irritation; Chest oppression; Labored or difficulty breathing; Vision disturbances; Central nervous system depression; Headaches; Dizziness; Vomiting; Nausea; Temporary blindness; Euphoria; Depression; Tearing. Suspected of causing Pulmonary edema. *End-point Targets:* Eyes; Respiratory system; Central nervous system. *Usage:* Refrigerant; Solvent; Fumigant; Larvicide; Insecticide; Anti-

leukemia drugs; Military poison gas; Chemical intermediate. *Synergistic effects:* Reacts slowly with water to form methanol and formic acid. *References:* 151, 304, 388.

Methyl Fosferno (tn) *see* **Methyl parathion.**

Methyl fumes *see* **Methyl bromide.**

5-Methyl-3-heptanone *TN/synonyms:* Amyl ethyl ketone; Ethyl amyl ketone. *OSHA PEL:* 25 ppm or 130 mg/m³ (8hr/day-40hr/wk-PP/S). *IDLH:* 3,000 ppm. *Symptoms:* Eye and mucous membrane irritation; Headaches; Unconsciousness due to narcotic effects; Coma; Dermatitis. *End-point Targets:* Eye; Skin; Respiratory system; Central nervous system. *Usage:* Food flavoring; Perfumes; Pesticide inert ingredient; Plastics; Printing inks. *References:* 276, 304, 388, 423.

Methyl hydrazine *TN/synonyms:* Monomethyl hydrazine; MMH. *NIOSH:* Carcinogen at any exposure level. *NIOSH REL:* 0.04 ppm or 0.08 mg/m³ (ceiling limit, 2 hr exposure). *OSHA PEL:* 0.2 ppm or 0.35 mg/m³ (ceiling limit-PP/S). *IDLH:* 50 ppm. *ACGIH:* Suspected human carcinogen. *Symptoms:* Eye and respiratory irritation; Vomiting; Tremors; Diarrhea; Incoordination; Inability to utilize oxygen; Cyanosis; Convulsions; Liver and kidney damage; Methemogolbin in urine; Changes in heart muscle; Nausea; Blood in urine; Granules in red blood cells; Malaise; Vomiting; Eye and skin burns; Destruction of red blood cells. Suspected of causing Cancer. *End-point Targets:* Central nervous system; Respiratory system; Liver; Blood; Cardiovascular system; Eyes. *Usage:* Solvent; Chemical intermediate; Antibiotic (Ceftriaxone); Medicine; Missile propellent. Found in toxic mushrooms. *References:* 258, 304, 306, 388.

Methyl iodide *TN/synonyms:* Iodomethane; Monoiodomethane.

NIOSH: Carcinogen at any exposure level. *OSHA PEL:* 2 ppm or 10 mg/m³ (8hr/day-40hr/wk-PP/S). *IDLH:* 800 ppm. *ACGIH:* Suspected human carcinogen. *Symptoms:* Eye, lung, and skin irritation; Central nervous system depression; Cerebellar neurologic symptoms; Coma; Convulsions; Death; Dermatitis; Diarrhea; Dizziness; Double vision; Drowsiness; Incoordination; Irritability; Kidney failure; Nausea; Parkinson-like symptoms; Partial or complete loss of sensation; Psychiatric disturbances; Shaking; Skin blistering; Slurred speech; Staggering gait; Vertigo; Visual disturbances; Vomiting; Weakness. Suspected of causing Cancer; Birth defects; Genetic mutations. *End-point Targets:* Central nervous system; Skin; Eyes. *Usage:* Refrigerants; Aerosol propellants; Pesticides; Fumigants; Fire extinguishers; Degreasers; Chemical intermediate. *Classification:* Organic solvent. *References:* 150, 304, 316, 383, 388.

Methyl isoamyl acetate *see* sec-**Hexyl acetate.**

Methyl isobutenyl ketone *see* **Mesityl oxide.**

Methyl isobutyl carbinol *TN/ synonyms:* Isobutylmethylcarbinol; Methyl amyl alcohol; 4-Methyl-2-pentanol; MIBC. *OSHA PEL:* 25 ppm or 100 mg/m³ (8hr/day-40hr/wk-PP/S); 40 ppm or 165 mg/m³ (exposure not to exceed 15 min). *IDLH:* 2,000 ppm. *Symptoms:* Eye irritation; Headaches; Drowsiness; Dermatitis. *End-point Targets:* Skin; Eyes. *Usage:* Solvent; Metallurgy; Coatings; Plastics; Petroleum and gas processing. *References:* 277, 304, 388.

Methyl isobutyl ketone *see* **Hexone.**

1-Methyl-4-Isopropenyl-1-cyclohexene *see* **Limonene.**

Methyl ketone *see* **Acetone.**

Methyl mercaptan *TN/synonyms:*
Mercaptomethane; Methanethiol; Methyl sulfhydrate; Thiomethyl alcohol; Thiomethanol. *NIOSH REL:* 0.5 ppm or 1 mg/m³ (ceiling limit, 15 min exposure). *OSHA PEL:* 0.5 ppm or 1 mg/m³ (8hr/day-40hr/wk-PP/S). *IDLH:* 400 ppm. *Symptoms:* Unconsciousness due to narcotic effects; Cyanosis; Convulsions; Pulmonary irritation; Hemolytic anemia; Hemoglobin oxidizes to ferric form; Coma. Suspected of causing Lethargy. *End-point Targets:* Respiratory system; Central nervous system. *Usages:* Pesticides; Jet fuel additive; Plastics; Poultry feed; Food additive; Synthesis of the amino acid methionine; Odor additive for odorless gases. (Not considered acceptable for use in natural gas.) Found in filbert nuts, beaufort cheese, decaying organic matter in marshes, coal tar, some natural gas, some crude oils, and decaying wood products in pulp mills; and is a natural substance in human blood, brain, and other tissue, and is expelled in urine and feces. *Classification:* Organic solvent (Thiol compound). *References:* 304, 306, 376, 383, 388.

Methyl methacrylate *TN/synonyms:* Methacrylate monomer; Methyl ester of methacrylic acid; Methyl-2-methyl-2-propenoate. *OSHA PEL:* 100 ppm or 410 mg/m³ (8hr/day-40hr/wk-PP/S). *IDLH:* 4,000 ppm. *Symptoms:* Eye, nasal, and throat irritation; Dermatitis; Central nervous system depression; Kidney and liver lesions; Low blood pressure; Death; Skin redness; Pulmonary edema; Cardiac arrest; Pain in extremities; Memory loss; Irritability; Weakness; Autonomic impaired muscle tone; Brain dysfunction; Chemical sensitivity. *End-point Targets:* Eyes; Respiratory system; Skin. *Usage:* Pesticide inert ingredient; Cultured marble; Water-repellent for concrete; Chemical intermediate; Resins; Plastics; Plexiglass (tn); Lucite (tn); Dentures; Bone cement; Medicinal spray adhesive; Bandages; Dental cement;

Hard contact lenses; Acrylics; Coatings; Molding powders and resins; Highway coating; Glue; Photocopier developer. *Additive:* Usually contains hydroquinone as an inhibitor. *References:* 169, 304, 388, 423.

Methyl methanoate *see* **Methyl formate.**

1-Methyl-4-(1-methylethenyl)Cyclohexene *see* **Limonene.**

Methyl-2-methyl-2-propenoate *see* **Methyl methacrylate.**

Methyl Niran (tn) *see* **Methyl parathion.**

N-Methyl-N-nitrosomethanamine *see* **N-Nitrosodimethylamine.**

Methyloxirane *see* **Propylene oxide.**

Methyl parathion *TN/synonyms:* Dimethyl 4-nitrophenyl phosphorothioate; Dimethyl p-nitrophenyl phosphorothioate; Dimethyl p-nitrophenyl thiophosphate; Dimethyl parathion; o,o-dimethyl o-(p-nitrophenyl) phosphorothioate; Parathion methyl homolog; Parathion-methyl; Phosphorothioc acid; A-Gro (tn); Azofos (tn); Azophos (tn); Bay E-601 (tn); Bay 11405 (tn); Bladan-M (tn); Cekumethion (tn); Dalf (tn); Devithion (tn); Drexel Methyl Parathion 4E (tn); E 601 (tn); ENT 17,292 (tn); Folodol-80/M (tn); Fosferno M 50 (tn); Gearphos (tn); 8056HC (tn); M40 (tn); M80 (tn); ME-Parathion (tn); Metapon (tn); Meptox (tn); Metacid 50 (tn); Metacide (tn); Metafos (tn); Metaphos (tn); Methyl-E 605 (tn); Methyl Fosferno (tn); Methyl Niran (tn); Methylthiophos (tn); Nitros 80 (tn); Metron (tn); Nitorx (tn); Oleovofotox (tn); Parafest M-50 Parataf (tn); M-Parathion (tn); Paratox (tn); Parton-M (tn); Partron-M (tn); Penncap-M (tn); Sinafid M-49 (tn); Sixty-Three Special E.C. Insecticide (tn); Tekwaisa (tn); Thiophenit (tn); Thylpar M-50 (tn); Vofatox (tn); Wofatos (tn); Wofatox (tn); Wofotox (tn). *OSHA PEL:* 0.2 mg/m^3 (8hr/day-40hr/wk). *ATSDR MRL:* 0.05 ppm (Ingestion, less than 14 days). *Symptoms:* Upper gastrointestinal irritation; Abdominal cramps; Acute myocardial degeneration; Allergic dermatitis; Anxiety; Blurred vision; Bronchial constriction; Cardiovascular failure; Chest tightness; Confusion; Death; Depression; Diarrhea; Dizziness; Erythrocyte and plasma depression in the blood; Excessive salivation; Headaches; Heart rate under 60 beats per minute; Impaired concentration; Impaired memory; Incontinence; Incoordination; Inhibited cholinesterase enzymes; Insufficient oxygen to the myocardial; Liver and kidney degeneration; Loss of appetite; Low blood pressure; Memory loss; Mental illness; Muscle involuntary contraction; Nausea; Pulmonary edema; Respiratory paralysis; Schizophrenic manifestations; Slurred speech; Sweating; Tearing; Tremors; Unconsciousness; Vascular congestion, hemorrhage, and endothelial damage; Vomiting; Weakness; Wheezing. Suspected of causing Immunosuppression; Neurological effects on fetuses; Birth defects. *Usage:* Insecticide; Restricted-use pesticide; Rodenticide. *Note:* Highly poisonous, related to nerve gas chemicals. *References:* 365, 388.

4-Methyl-2-pentanol *see* **Methyl isobutyl carbinol.**

2-Methyl-2-pentanol-4-one *see* **Diacetone alcohol.**

4-Methyl 2-pentanone *see* **Hexone.**

4-Methyl-3-penten-2-one *see* **Mesityl oxide.**

Methylphenol *see* **Cresols.**

Methylphenyl amine *see* **Monomethyl aniline.**

1-Methyl-1-phenyl-ethylene *see* **alpha-Methyl styrene.**

2-Methyl-1-propanol *see* **Isobutyl alcohol.**

Methyl propenoate *see* Methyl acrylate.

1-Methylpropyl acetate *see* sec-Butyl acetate.

2-Methylpropyl acetate *see* Isobutyl acetate.

2-Methylpropyl ester of acetic acid *see* Isobutyl acetate.

beta-Methylpropyl ethanoate *see* Isobutyl acetate.

Methyl propyl ketone *see* 2-Pentanone.

Methyl n-propyl ketone *see* 2-Pentanone.

3-(1-Methyl-2-pyrrolidyl) pyridine *see* Nicotine.

Methylstyrene *see* Vinyl toluene.

alpha-Methyl styrene *TN/synonyms:* AMS; Isopropenyl benzene; 1-Methyl-1-phenyl-ethylene; 2-Phenyl propylene. *OSHA PEL:* 50 ppm or 240 mg/m³ (8hr/day-40hr/wk-PP/S); 100 ppm or 485 mg/m³ (exposure not to exceed 15 min). *IDLH:* 5,000 ppm. *Symptoms:* Eye, nasal, and throat irritation; Drowsiness; Dermatitis; Central nervous system depression; Occupational hepatitis; Antibody response; Eyes become sensitive to light; Narrowing of field of vision. *End-point Targets:* Eyes; Respiratory system; Skin. *Usage:* Plastics; Resins; Polyesters; Surface coatings; Adhesives; Waxes; Synthetic rubber; Pesticide inert ingredient. *Additive:* Usually contains tert-butyl catechol as an inhibitor. *References:* 126, 304, 388, 423.

Methyl sulfate *see* Dimethyl sulfate.

Methyl sulfate salt *see* Paraquat.

Methyl sulfhydrate *see* Methyl mercaptan.

Methylthiophos (tn) *see* Methyl parathion.

Methyl toluene *see* Xylenes.

Methyl trichloride *see* Chloroform.

Methyltrichloromethane *see* 1,1,1-Trichloroethane.

1-Methyl-2,4,6-trinitrobenzene *see* 2,4,6-Trinitrotoluene.

Metron (tn) *see* Methyl parathion.

Mevinphos *see* Phosdrin.

MIBC *see* Methyl isobutyl carbinol.

MIBK *see* Hexone.

MIC (tn) *see* 1,3-Dichloropropene.

Mica *TN/synonyms:* Silicate mica. *OSHA PEL:* 3 mg/m³ (8hr/day-40hr/wk [respiration]). *IDLH:* NE. *Symptoms:* Respiratory irritation; Pneumoconiosis; Cough; Labored or difficulty breathing; Weakness; Weight loss; Pulmonary damage; Liver granulomas. *End-point Targets:* Lungs. *Usage:* Pesticide inert ingredient; Heat-resistant glass; Aircraft construction; Electric cables; Pneumatic tires; Welding rods; Cardboard; Plastics; Dry lubricants; Paper; Paint; Insulation; Glass; Ceramics; Dusting agent; Incandescent lamps; Cosmetics; Roofing materials; Wallpaper and wallboard joint cement; Rubber; Capacitors; Textiles. *References:* 171, 304, 388, 423.

Microlysin (tn) *see* Chloropicrin.

Mineral spirits *see* Stoddard solvent.

MITC (tn) *see* 1,3-Dichloropropene.

MMH *see* Methyl hydrazine.

Molasses alcohol *see* Ethanol.

Molecular bromine *see* Bromine.

Molecular chlorine *see* Chlorine.

Molecular iodine *see* Iodine.

Molybdenum *NIOSH:* No REL, notified OSHA that documentation doesn't support the worker's safety at established PELs. *OSHA PEL:* Insoluble: 10 mg/m³ (8hr/day-40hr/wk-PP/S); Soluble: 05 mg/m³ (8hr/day-40hr/wk). IDLH: NE. *Symptoms:* Pneumoconiosis; Gout-like symptoms; Increased blood uric acid; Anemia. Suspected of causing Eye, nasal, and throat irritation; Loss of appetite; Diarrhea; Weight loss; Listlessness; Liver and kidney damage; Incoordination; Labored or difficult breathing. *End-point Targets:* Respiratory system. *Usage:* Electrical components; Steel alloy; Tools; Rifle barrels; Spark plugs; Tungsten steel; Glass to metal seals; Lubricant additive; Aircraft and automobile parts; Pigments; Paint; Lacquers; Inks; Rubber; Leather; Fertilizer; Ammonia. *References:* 172, 304, 388.

Monel (tn) *see* **Nickel.**

Monoammonium salt of sulfamic acid *see* **Ammonium sulfamate.**

Monobromomethane *see* **Methyl bromide.**

Monobromotrifluoromethane *see* **Trifluorobromomethane.**

Monochlorobenzene *see* **Chlorobenzene.**

Monochlorodimethyl ether *see* **Chloromethyl methyl ether.**

Monochloroethane *see* **Ethyl chloride.**

Monochloroethylene *see* **Vinyl chloride.**

Monochloromethane *see* **Methyl chloride.**

Monochloromethyl methyl ether *see* **Chloromethyl methyl ether.**

Monoethanolamine *see* **Ethanolamine.**

Monoethylamine *see* **Ethylamine.**

Monoethylene glycol *see* **Ethylene glycol.**

Monofluorotrichloromethane *see* **Fluorotrichloromethane.**

Monohydroxy benzene *see* **Phenol.**

Monoiodomethane *see* **Methyl iodide.**

Monoisopropylamine *see* **Isopropylamine.**

Monomethylamine *see* **Methylamine.**

Monomethyl aniline *TN/synonyms:* MA; Methyl aniline; N-Methyl aniline; (Methylamino) benzene; Methylphenyl amine. *OSHA PEL:* 0.5 ppm or 2 mg/m³ (8hr/day-40hr/wk-PP/S). *IDLH:* 100 ppm. *Symptoms:* Blood and hemoglobin in urine; Cardiac arrhythmias; Cardiovascular collapse; Coma; Confusion; Convulsions; Cyanosis; Death; Diminished urine formation; Disorientation; Dizziness; Drowsiness; Dry throat; Headaches; Hemoglobin oxidizes to ferric form; Incoordination; Labored or difficult breathing; Lethargy; Liver and kidney damage; Nausea; Painful urination; Pulmonary edema; Renal insufficiency; Respiratory paralysis; Ringing or tingling in the ear; Shock; Vertigo; Weakness. *End-point Targets:* Respiratory system; Liver; Kidneys; Blood. *Usage:* Acid formulations; Solvent; Nitrocellulose. *References:* 173, 304, 388.

Monomethyl hydrazine *see* **Methyl hydrazine.**

Mononitrogen monoxide *see* **Nitric oxide.**

Monophenylhydrazine *see* **Phenylhydrazine.**

Monoxide *see* **Carbon monoxide.**

Morbicid *see* **Formaldehyde.**

Morpholine *TN/synonyms:* Diethylene imidoxide; Diethylene oximide; Tetrahydro-1,4-oxazine; Tetrahydro-p-oxazine. *OSHA PEL:* 20 ppm or 70 mg/m³ (8hr/day-40hr/wk-PP/S); 30 ppm or 105 mg/m³ (exposure not to exceed 15 min). *IDLH:* 8,000 ppm. *Symptoms:* Eye, nasal, respiratory, and skin irritation; Cough; Liver and kidney damage; Vision disturbance; Corneal swelling; Foggy vision. *End-point Targets:* Respiratory system; Eyes; Skin. *Usage:* Pesticide inert ingredient; Solvent; Resins; Waxes; Casein; Dyes; Paper; Paperboard; Cardboard; Adhesives; Corrosion inhibitor; Plasticizers; Lubricant additive; Insecticides; Fungicides; Herbicides; Local anesthetics; Antiseptic; Rubber; Pharmaceuticals; Fabric softener; Fabric whitening; Photography; Household cleaners. *References:* 8, 174, 304, 388, 423.

Motox (tn) *see* **Chlorinated camphene.**

MPK *see* **2-Pentanone.**

Muriatic acid *see* **Hydrogen chloride.**

Muriatic ether *see* **Ethyl chloride.**

Naled *TN/synonyms:* Dimethyl-1, 2-dibromo-2,2-dichloroethyl phosphate; Dibrom; 1,2-Dibromo-2,2-dichloroethyl dimethyl phosphate. *OSHA PEL:* 3 mg/m³ (8hr/day-40hr/wk-PP/S). *IDLH:* 1,800 mg/m³. *Symptoms:* Eye and skin irritation; Abdominal cramps; Anxiety; Apathy; Blurred or dimness of vision; Bronchial constriction; Cardiac irregularities; Coma; Confusion; Constricted pupils; Convulsions; Cough; Cyanosis; Death; Depression; Diarrhea; Difficulty breathing; Dilated pupils; Disorientation; Drowsiness; Emotional instability; Excessive dreaming; Excessive salivation; Eye pain; Giddiness; Headaches; Heart rate below 30 beats per minute; Heart rate over 100 beats per minute; Hypothermia; Incontinence; Incoordination; Inhibits cholinesterase enzymes; Insomnia; Laryngeal spasms; Loss of appetite; Low blood pressure; Muscle involuntary contractions, spasms, and twitching; Nasal discharge; Nausea; Neurosis; Nightmares; Paralysis; Profuse sweating; Pulmonary rales; Respiratory arrest; Restlessness; Slurred speech; Spontaneous horizontal involuntary eye movement; Tearing; Tension; Tight chest; Vertigo; Vomiting; Weakness; Wheezing. *End-point Targets:* Respiratory system; Central nervous system; Cardiovascular system; Skin; Eyes; Blood cholinesterase. *Usage:* Acaricide; Insecticide; Veterinary medicine; Animal insect repellents; Water-based paints; Floor polishes; Pesticide; Mosquito control. *References:* 81, 304, 388.

Naphtha *TN/synonyms:* Crude solvent coal tar naphtha; High solvent naphtha. *OSHA PEL:* 100 ppm or 400 mg/m³ (8hr/day-40hr/wk-PP/S). *IDLH:* 10,000 ppm. *Symptoms:* Eye, nasal, throat, and skin irritation; Dermatitis; Lightheadedness; Headaches; Loss of appetite; Dizziness; Indigestion; Nausea; Insomnia. *End-point Targets:* Respiratory system; Eyes; Skin. *Usage:* Soap; Detergent; Rubber cement; Aspirin; Varnishes; Antiseptics; Sulfa drugs; Plastics; Paints; Plexiglass; Clothing; Construction material; Film; Toys; Kitchen utensils; Furniture; Cosmetics; Food flavoring; Solvents; Aspartame; Saccharin; Sorbitol; Perfumes; Explosives; Dyes; Fertilizers; Pesticide inert ingredient; Household cleaners and disinfectants; Furniture polish; Glass cleaners; Metal cleaners; Spot remover. *Component:* Cumene. *Classification:* Organic solvent (Refined petroleum). *Reference:* 8, 271, 295, 304, 383, 388, 423.

Naphthalene *TN/synonyms:* Naphthalin; Tar camphor; White tar. *OSHA PEL:* 10 ppm or 50 mg/m³ (8hr/day-40hr/wk-PP/S); 15 ppm or 75 mg/m³ (exposure not to exceed 15 min). *IDLH:* 500 ppm. *Symptoms:* Eye and bladder irritation; Headaches; Confusion; Excitement; Lethargy; Listlessness; Vertigo; Malaise; Nausea; Vomiting; Abdominal pains; Profuse sweating; Jaundice; Blood, protein, and hemoglobin in urine; Granules in red blood cells; Decrease serum bilirubin; Increased reticulocyte count; Neonate jaundice; Neonate hemolytic anemia; Kidney failure; Dermatitis; Hemolytic anemia; Diarrhea; Cataracts; Lethargy; Listlessness; Vertigo; Death. *End-point Targets:* Eyes; Blood; Liver; Kidneys; Skin; Red blood cells; Central nervous system. *Usage:* Dyes; Resins; Mothballs; Ink; Wood preservative; Coaltar production; Synthetic tanning; Insecticides; Lotions; Topical antiseptics; Medicine; Rug, carpet, and upholstery shampoo; Phthalic anhydride; Carbamate insecticides; Antiseptics; Lubricants; Scintillation counting fluid; Chemical manufacturing; Pesticide inert ingredient; Air fresheners/deodorizers; Glass cleaners. Found in burning fossil fuels and tobacco smoke. *References:* 8, 304, 336, 388, 423, 429.

Naphthalin *see* **Naphthalene.**

alpha-Naphthyl-N-methylcarbamate *see* **Carbaryl.**

1-Naphthyl N-Methylcarbamate *see* **Carbaryl.**

Narcogen (tn) *see* **Trichloroethylene.**

Narkogen (tn) *see* **Trichloroethylene.**

Narkosoid (tn) *see* **Trichloroethylene.**

Narkotil (tn) *see* **Methylene chloride.**

Naxol *see* **Cyclohexanol.**

NCI-C00533 (tn) *see* **Chloropicrin.**

NDMA *see* **N-Nitrosodimethylamine.**

Nema (tn) *see* **Tetrachloroethylene.**

Nesol *see* **Limonene.**

Netis (tn) *see* **Ethylene dibromide.**

NEU-TRI (tn) *see* **Trichloroethylene.**

Nialk (tn) *see* **Trichloroethylene.**

Nibren wax *see* **Tetrachloronaphthalene.**

Nickel *TN/synonyms:* CI77775; Nickel 200; Nickel 201; Nickel 205; Nickel 270; Alnico, NP 2; Monel (tn); Inconel (tn); Incoloy (tn); Nimonic (tn); Hastelloy (tn); Udimet (tn); Mar M (tn); Rene 41 (tn); Waspaloy (tn); Raney nickel (tn). *Compounds:* Nickel oxide; Nickel sulfate; Nickel chloride; Nickel subsulfide; Nickel acetate; Nickel nitrate. *NIOSH:* Carcinogen at any exposure level. *NIOSH REL:* 0.015 mg/m³ (10hr/day-40hr/wk). *OSHA PEL:* Soluble: 0.1 mg/m³ (8hr/day-40hr/wk); Insoluble 1.0 mg/m³ (8hr/day-40hr/wk). *ATSDR MRL:* 0.00005 mg/m³ (Inhalation, more than 14 days [This MRL may not protect sensitive individuals.]) *IDLH:* NE. *Symptoms:* Abdominal cramps; Allergic contact dermatitis; Bronchitis; Cancer (nasal, lung); Cardiac arrest; Chromosomal aberrations; Convulsions; Cool body temperature; Cough; Cyanosis; Death; Delirium; Diarrhea; Emphysema; Epigastric pain; Excessive salivation; Fatigue; Giddiness; Headaches; Incoordination; Increase in blood reticulocytes; Increase in leukocytes in the blood; Increase in serum bilirubin; Increased rate or depth of respiration; Interacts with DNA; Irregular breathing; Lethargy; Metal fume fever; Muscle pain; Nausea; Pneumonia; Substernal pain; Vertigo; Vision loss; Vomiting; Weakness. Suspected of causing Coronary constriction; Myocardial depression; Liver atrophy; Kidney damage; Hypoglycemia; Low birth weight; Testicular degeneration; Sperm abnormalities. *End-point Targets:* Respiratory system; Paranasal sinus; Central nervous system. *Usage:* Jewelry; Coins; Stainless-steel; Ceramics; Pigments; Cast iron; Batteries; Electroplating; Aluminum; Electrical circuits; Dyes; Pesticide inert ingredient; Chemical intermediate; Lime manufacturing;

Asphalt; Alloy in copper, gold, chromium, iron, molybdenum, silver, zinc. Found in tobacco smoke. *Note:* The average latency period for cancer appears to be about 25 years (range 4 to 51 years). *References:* 187, 299, 304, 344, 388, 389, 423, 429, 432.

Nickel 200 *see* **Nickel.**

Nickel 201 *see* **Nickel.**

Nickel 205 *see* **Nickel.**

Nickel 270 *see* **Nickel.**

Nickel carbonyl *TN/synonyms:* Nickel tetracarbonyl. *NIOSH:* Carcinogen at any exposure level. *OSHA PEL:* 0.001 ppm or 0.007 mg/m³ (8hr/day-40hr/wk-PP/S). *IDLH:* 7 ppm. *Symptoms:* Contact dermatitis; Allergic asthma; Pneumonia; Pulmonary congestion, tissue death, and edema; Vertigo; Headaches; Chest tightness; Weakness; Profuse sweating; Cough; Vomiting; Labored or difficulty breathing; Brain hemorrhage; Giddiness; Myocardial infraction; Stroke; Epigastric pain; Fever; Increase in leukocytes in the blood; Respiratory failure; Death; Cerebral swelling; Chemical pneumonia; Electroencephalogram abnormalities; Cancer; Tremors; Involuntary muscle twitching. *End-point Targets:* Nasal cavities; Lungs; Skin. *Usage:* Nickel refining; Acrylics; Glass plating; Metallurgy; Electronic components; Chemical manufacturing; Paint; Inks; Metal alloy; Coinage; Electroplating. *Note:* Nickel carbonyl is the most toxic of the nickel compounds and is has been historically established as a neurotoxin. The average latency period for cancer appears to be about 25 years (range 4 to 51 years). *References:* 187, 304, 388, 413, 432.

Nickel tetracarbonyl *see* **Nickel carbonyl.**

Nicotine *TN/synonyms:* 3-(1-Methyl-2-pyrrolidyl) pyridine; Black leaf 40 (tn). *OSHA PEL:* 0.5 mg/m³ (8hr/day-40hr/wk-PP/S). *IDLH:* 35 mg/m³. *Symptoms:* Abdominal pain; Absolute exhaustion; Agitation; Burning sensation in mouth and throat; Cardiovascular constriction; Central nervous system excitement followed by central nervous system depression; Cold sweats; Collapse; Confusion; Convulsions; Cyanosis; Death; Diarrhea; Dizziness; Elevated blood pressure; Excessive salivation; Faintness; Headaches; Heart rate over 100 beats per minute; In severe poisoning blood pressure decreases; Incoordination; Labored or difficulty breathing; Nausea; Paroxysmal atrial fibrosis; Profuse sweating; Respiratory paralysis; Tremors; Vision and auditory disturbances; Vomiting; Weakness; Suspected of causing Low birth weight; Birth defects. *End-point Targets:* Central nervous system; Cardiovascular system; Lungs; Gastrointestinal tract. *Usage:* Insecticide; Leather tanning; Veterinary medicine; Greenhouse fumigant. Found in Tobacco and Tobacco smoke. *Note:* Nicotine is one of the most lethal poisons known. *References:* 193, 304, 388, 389, 449.

Nimonic (tn) *see* **Nickel.**

Ni-Par S-20TM (tn) *see* **2-Nitropropane.**

Ni-Par S-30TM (tn) *see* **2-Nitropropane.**

Nitorx (tn) *see* **Methyl parathion.**

Nitric acid *TN/synonyms:* Aqua fortis; Engravers acid; Hydrogen nitrate; Red fuming nitric acid; RFNA; White fuming nitric acid; WFNA. *OSHA PEL:* 2 ppm or 5 mg/m³ (8hr/day-40hr/wk-PP/S); 4 ppm or 10 mg/m³ (exposure not to exceed 15 min). *IDLH:* 100 ppm. *Symptoms:* Eye, mucous membrane, and skin irritation; Delayed pulmonary edema; Pneumonia; Bronchitis; Dental erosion; Labored or difficult breating; Mouth, throat, and esophagus corrosion and pain; Inability or difficulty swallowing; Inhibited blood clotting; Nausea; Vomiting; Gastric hemorrhage; Thirst; Circulatory collapse; Clammy skin; Weak, rapid pulse; Shallow respiration; Esophageal, gastric and pyloric strictures; Death; Glottis swelling; Kidney failure and ischemic lesions. *End-point Targets:* Eyes; Respiratory system; Skin; Teeth. *Usage:* Nitrates; Dyes; Wart remover; Pharmaceuticals; Photoengraving; Veterinary medicine; Jewelry; Engineering industry; Cauterizing agent; Explosives; Nitrocellulose lacquers; Fertilizers; Ammonium nitrate; Adipic acid; Isocyanates; Potassium nitrate; Aromatic nitrogen products; Nuclear fuel; Sodium nitrates; Steel pickling; Nitroparaffins; Aniline; Dinitrobenzenes. *Note:* Fumes contain dissolved nitrogen. *References:* 192, 304, 388.

Nitric oxide *TN/synonyms:* Mononitrogen monoxide; Nitrogen monoxide. *OSHA PEL:* 25 ppm or 30 mg/m³ (8hr/day-40hr/wk). *IDLH:* 100 ppm. *Symptoms:* Eye, nasal, and throat irritation; Drowsiness; Unconsciousness; Cough; Fatigue; Nausea; Choking; Headaches; Abdominal pain; Uneasiness; Restlessness; Increased rate or depth of respiration; Labored or difficulty breathing; Pulmonary edema; Rapid and shallow respiration; Cyanosis; Frothy expectoration; Anxiety; Confusion; Lethargy; Unconsciousness; Inability to utilize oxygen; Pneumonia; Weakness; Dental corrosion. *End-point Targets:* Respiratory system. *Usage:* Rayon bleaching; Propylene; Methyl ether; Nitrosyl carbonyls. Found in Diesel exhaust. *Synergistic effects:* Reacts with water to form nitric acid and contact with air converts it to nitrogen dioxide, nitrogen tetroxide, or both. *Note:* Symptoms are generally delayed, except for slight cough, fatigue, and nausea. *References:* 191, 304, 388, 394.

p-Nitroaniline *TN/synonyms:* para-Aminonitrobenzene; 4-Nitroaniline; 4-Nitrobenzenamine; p-Nitrophenyl-amine; PNA. *OSHA PEL:* 3 mg/m³ (10hr/day-40hr/wk-PP/S). *IDLH:* 300 mg/m³. *Symptoms:* Anemia; Blood and hemoglobin in urine; Cardiac arrhythmias; Cardiovascular collapse; Confusion; Convulsions; Cyanosis; Death; Diarrhea; Disorientation; Drowsiness; Dryness of throat; Granules in red blood cells; Headaches; Heart rate over 100 beats per minute; Hemoglobin oxidizes to ferric form; Incoordination; Increase in leukocytes in the blood; Irritability; Jaundice; Labored or difficult breathing; Lethargy; Liver damage; Nausea; Navy blue or black lips, tongue, and mucous membranes; Painful urination; Rapid respiration; Renal insufficiency; Respiratory distress and arrest; Ringing or tingling in the ear; Shock; Slate grey skin; Sleepiness; Vertigo; Vomiting. *End-point Targets:* Blood; Heart; Lungs; Liver. *Usage:* Dyes; Pigments; Gasoline additive; Veterinary medicine; Pharmaceuticals; Crayons. *Note:* Child fatalities have been associated with eating crayons. *References:* 261, 304, 388.

4-Nitroaniline *see* **p-Nitroaniline.**

4-Nitrobenzenamine *see* **p-Nitroaniline.**

Nitrobenzene *TN/synonyms:* Essence of mirbane; Nitrobenzol; Oil of mirbane; Caswell No. 600 (tn). *OSHA PEL:* 1 ppm or 5 mg/m³ (8hr/day-40hr/wk-PP/S). *IDLH:* 200 ppm. *Symptoms:* Eye irritation; Inability to utilize oxygen; Dermatitis; Anemia; Death; Methemoglobin in urine; Enlarged, tender liver; Jaundice; Altered serum chemistry of the liver; Headaches; Confusion; Vertigo; Nausea; Vomiting; Paralysis; Tremors; Impaired balance; Coma. Suspected of causing Brainstem damage; Cerebellum damage; Testicular degeneration; Decreased sperm levels; Birth defects; Low birth weight; Cancer. *End-point Targets:*

Blood; Liver; Kidneys; Central nervous system; Skin. *Usage:* Lubricating oils; Dyes; Food flavoring; Soap perfume; Shoe dyes; Pesticides; Medication; Synthetic rubber; Toilet deodorant; Furniture polish; Solvent in Petroleum refining; Cellulose ethers and acetates; Aniline; Acetaminophen. *References:* 304, 326, 388.

Nitrobenzol *see* **Nitrobenzene.**

Nitrocarbol *see* **Nitromethane.**

p-Nitrochlorobenzene *TN/synonyms:* p-Chloronitrobenzene; 4-Chloronitrobenzene; 1-Chloro-4-nitrobenzene; PCNB; PNCB. *NIOSH:* Carcinogen at any exposure level. Reduce exposure to lowest possible concentration. *OSHA PEL:* 1 mg/m³ (8hr/day-40hr/wk-PP/S). *IDLH:* 1,000 mg/m³. *Symptoms:* Inability to utilize oxygen; Unpleasant taste; Mild anemia; Hemoglobin oxidizes to ferric form; Cyanosis; Headaches; Weakness; Anemia; Granules in red blood cells; Vertigo; Allergic dermatitis; Cardiac disorder. Suspected of causing Cancer (skin); Blood in urine; Hemoglobin in urine. *Endpoint Targets:* Blood; Liver; Kidneys; Cardiovascular system. *Usage:* Agricultural chemicals; Methyl parathion; Medicine; Acetaminophen; Bacteriostat; Rubber. *References:* 262, 305, 388.

Nitrochloroform *see* **Chloropicrin.**

Nitroethane *OSHA PEL:* 100 ppm or 310 mg/m³ (8hr/day-40hr/wk-PP/S). *IDLH:* 1,000 ppm. *Symptoms:* Eye, nasal, throat, respiratory, and mucous membrane irritation; Dermatitis; Cough; Labored or difficulty breathing; Nausea; Vomiting. Suspected of causing Tearing; Pulmonary rales and edema; Liver and kidney injury; Unconsciousness due to narcotic effects. *End-point Targets:* Skin. *Usage:* Solvent; Cellulose; Vinyl; Resins; Waxes; Plasticizers; Solid propellant; Fats;

Dyes; Pesticide inert ingredient. *References:* 190, 304, 388, 423.

Nitrogen dioxide *TN/synonyms:* Dinitrogen tetroxide; Nitrogen peroxide; Nitrogen tetroxide; NTO. *OSHA PEL:* 1.0 ppm or 1.8 mg/m³ (exposure not to exceed 15 min) *IDLH:* 50 ppm. *Symptoms:* Eye irritation; Cough; Mucoid frothy sputum; Labored or difficulty breathing; Chest pain; Cyanosis; Rapid respiration; Heart rate over 100 beats per minute; Methemoglobin in urine; Fatigue; Nausea; Pulmonary inflammation and edema; Bronchial inflammatory destruction; Silo-fillers disease. *End-point Targets:* Respiratory system; Cardiovascular system. *Usage:* Flour bleach; Explosives; Cellulose; Hemostatic cotton; Acrylates; Nitric acid; Sulfuric acid; Rocket fuel; Calibration gas; Agricultural chemicals. Found in Smog; Gas fires; Paraffin heaters; Drying clothes; and Diesel exhaust. *Synergistic effects:* Reacts with water to form nitric acid. *Note:* Symptoms are generally delayed. *References:* 189, 304, 388, 394.

Nitrogen monoxide *see* **Nitric oxide.**

Nitrogen peroxide *see* **Nitrogen dioxide.**

Nitrogen tetroxide *see* **Nitrogen dioxide.**

Nitroglycol *see* **Ethylene glycol dinitrate.**

Nitroisopropane *see* **2-Nitropropane.**

Nitromethane *TN/synonyms:* Nitrocarbol. *NIOSH:* No REL, notified OSHA that documentation doesn't support the worker's safety at established PELs. *OSHA PEL:* 100 ppm or 250 mg/m³ (8hr/day-40hr/wk-PP/S). *IDLH:* 1,000 ppm. *Symptoms:* Skin and mucous membrane irritation; Dermatitis; Central nervous system depression. *End-point Targets:* Skin. *Usage:* Pesticide inert ingredient; Propellents; Fuel additive; Rocket fuel; Solvent;

Cellulose; Polymers; Waxes; Racing fuel additive. *References:* 188, 304, 388, 423.

Nitrophenols *Compounds: 2-Nitrophenol:* 2-Hydroxynitrobenzene; o-nitrophenol; Atonik (tn). *4-Nitrophenol:* 4-Hydroxynitrobene; p-Nitrophenol; PNP. *OSHA PEL:* None. *ATSDR MRL:* 0.03 mg/m^3 (Inhalation, less than 14 days). *Symptoms:* Abdominal pain; Bloody diarrhea; Burning pain in mouth and throat; Cataracts; Chemical smell on breath; Convulsions; Cyanosis; Death; Decreased body temperature; Delirium; Dizziness; Excessive bilirubin in blood; Excitement; Frothing at nose and mouth; Granules in red blood cells; Headaches; Hemoglobin oxidizes to ferric form; Hemolytic anemia; Low blood pressure; Mouth, esophagus, and stomach necrotic lesions; Mucous rales; Profuse sweating; Pulmonary edema; Renal insufficiency; Respiratory, circulatory, and cardiac failure; Ringing or tingling in the ear; Scanty, dark-colored or smokey urine; Shallow respiration; Shock-like symptoms; Shock; Skin redness and itching; Stertorous breathing; Unconsciousness; Vomiting; Weak, irregular pulse; Weakness. Suspected of causing Protein in urine; Corneal opacity; Birth defects. *End-point Targets:* Blood. *Usage:* Dyes; Pigments; Rubber; Fungicides; Glucose; Leather tanning; Insecticides; Methyl parathion; N-acetyl- 4-aminophenol; Pesticide inert ingredient; Pharmaceuticals; Wood preservative; Photography; Plant growth stimulators. *References:* 194, 366, 423.

p-Nitrophenylamine *see* **p-Nitroaniline.**

Nitropropane *see* **1-Nitropropane.**

sec-Nitropropane *see* **2-Nitropropane.**

1-Nitropropane *TN/synonyms:* Nitropropane; 1-NP. *OSHA PEL:* 25 ppm or 90 mg/m^3 (8hr/day-40hr/wk).

IDLH: 2,300 ppm. *Symptoms:* Eye and respiratory irritation; Headaches; Nausea; Vomiting; Diarrhea; Gastrointestinal distress; Liver and kidney injury; Loss of appetite; Hemoglobin oxidizes to ferric form; Cyanosis. *End-point Targets:* Eyes; Central nervous system. *Usage:* Solvent; Cellulose; Vinyl resins; Lacquers; Synthetic rubber; Fats; Oils; Dyes; Chemical intermediate; Waxes; Gasoline additive. *References:* 123, 304, 388.

2-Nitropropane *TN/synonyms:* Dimethylnitromethane; sec-Nitropropane; iso-Nitropropane; Nitroisopropane; 2-NP; Ni-Par S-20TM (tn); Ni-Par S-30TM (tn). *NIOSH:* Carcinogen at any exposure level. Reduce exposure to lowest feasible concentration. *OSHA PEL:* 10 ppm or 35 mg/m^3 (8hr/day-40hr/wk). *ACGIH:* Suspected human carcinogen. *ACGIH TLV:* 10 ppm or 35 mg/m^3 (ceiling limit). *IDLH:* 2,300 ppm. *Symptoms:* Respiratory irritation; Headaches; Loss of appetite; Nausea; Vomiting; Diarrhea; Death; Liver damage; Destruction of parenchymal liver cells; Cancer (liver). *End-point Targets:* Respiratory system; Central nervous system. *Usage:* Pesticide inert ingredient; Saturated vegetable oil; Vinyl coatings; Epoxy paints; Nitrocellulose lacquer; Chlorinated rubber; Printing ink; Adhesives; Construction materials; Furniture; Plastics; Marine coatings; Polyesters; Resins. *Classification:* Organic solvent. *References:* 304, 305, 383, 388, 411, 417, 423, 443.

Nitros 80 (tn) *see* **Methyl parathion.**

N-Nitrosodimethylamine *TN/synonyms:* Dimethylnitrosamine; N, N,-Dimethylnitrosamine; DMNA; N-Methyl-N-nitrosomethanamine; NDMA. *NIOSH:* Carcinogen at any exposure level. Reduce exposure to lowest feasible concentration. *OSHA:* No PEL, 1 of 13 chemicals recognized as an occupational carcinogen. Exposure of workers is to be controlled through required engineering controls, work practices, and personal protective equipment. *ACGIH:* Suspected human carcinogen [skin]. *IDLH:* Carcinogen. *Symptoms:* Nausea; Vomiting; Diarrhea; Abdominal cramps; Headaches; Fever; Enlarged liver; Jaundice; Reduced function in liver, kidneys, and lungs; Cancer; Liver tissue death; Cirrhosis; Death; Liver ascites (accumulation of serous fluid); Malaise; Generalized hemorrhaging; Low platelet count; Abdominal cramps; Weakness. Suspected of causing DNA damage. *End-point Targets:* Liver; Kidneys; Lungs. *Usage:* Solvent; Plastics; Lubricants; Research chemical; Rubber; Plasticizers; High-energy batteries. No longer added to beverages. Found in Tobacco smoke. *Note:* Plastic components from dialysis units may leach NDMA into the blood. *References:* 182, 304, 306, 388, 389.

Nitrotrichloromethane *see* **Chloropicrin.**

5-Norbornene-2,3-di-methanol-1,4,5,6,7,7-hexachlorocyclic sulfite *see* **Endosulfan.**

Normal-heptane *see* **n-Heptane.**

Normal-hexane *see* **n-Hexane.**

Normal-octane *see* **Octane.**

Normal pentane *see* **n-Pentane**

NP 2 *see* **Nickel.**

1-NP *see* **1-Nitropropane.**

2-NP *see* **2-Nitropropane.**

NSC 8819 *see* **Acrolein.**

NTO *see* **Nitrogen dioxide.**

OCBM *see* **o-Chlorobenzylidene malononitrile.**

Octachlorocamphene *see* **Chlorinated camphene.**

Octachloronaphthalene *TN/synonyms:* Halowax 1051 (tn); 1,2,3,4,5,6,7,8-Octachloronaphthalene; Perchloronaphthalene. *OSHA PEL:* 0.1 mg/m^3 (8hr/day-40hr/wk-PP/S); 0.3 mg/m^3 (exposure not to exceed 15 min). *IDLH:* Unknown. *Symptoms:* Acne-form dermatitis; Liver damage; Jaundice. *End-point Targets:* Skin; Liver. *Usage:* Fireproofing; Waterproofing additive; Lubricant additive. *References:* 198, 304, 388.

1,2,3,4,5,6,7,8-Octachloronaphthalene: see Octachloronaphthalene.

Octane *TN/synonyms:* n-Octane; Normal-octane. *NIOSH REL:* 75 ppm or 350 mg/m^3 (10hr/day-40hr/wk); 385 ppm or 1,800 mg/m^3 (ceiling limit, 15 min exposure). *OSHA PEL:* 300 ppm or 1,450 mg/m^3 (8hr/day-40hr/wk-PP/S); 375 ppm or 1,800 mg/m^3 (exposure not to exceed 15 min). *IDLH:* 5,000 ppm. *Symptoms:* Eye, nasal, respiratory, and brain irritation; Drowsiness; Dermatitis; Chemical pneumonia; Giddiness; Vertigo; Headaches; Stupor; Convulsions; Inability to utilize oxygen in the upper airways; Widespread internal hemorrhaging; Pulmonary edema and hemorrhage; Central nervous system depression; Dry, cracked skin. *End-point Targets:* Skin; Eyes; Respiratory system. *Usage:* Asphalt; Gasoline additive; Solvent; Lacquers; Polymers; Rocket propellent. *Classification:* Organic solvent (Alkane compound). *Note:* Neurotoxin. *References:* 17, 199, 304, 383, 388, 429.

n-Octane *see* **Octane:**

Octoil (tn) *see* **Di-sec octyl phthalate.**

Octyl phthalate *see* **Di-sec octyl phthalate.**

Oil of mirbane *see* **Nitrobenzene.**

Oil of vitriol *see* **Sulfuric acid.**

Oleovofotox (tn) *see* **Methyl parathion.**

Olow *see* **Lead.**

Omal (tn) *see* **2,4,6-Trichlorophenol.**

Orthophosphoric acid *see* **Phosphoric acid.**

Oxalic acid *TN/synonyms:* Ethanedioic acid; Oxalic acid (aqueous); Oxalic acid dihydrate. *OSHA PEL:* 1 mg/m³ (ceiling limit-PP/S); 2 mg/m³ (exposure not to exceed 15 min). *IDLH:* 500 mg/m³. *Symptoms:* Eye, mucus membrane, and skin irritation; Eye burns; Localized pain; Cyanosis; Shock; Collapse; Convulsions; Throat, esophagus, and stomach pain; Low blood pressure; Vomiting; Headaches; Stupor; Coma; Death; Kidney damage; Reduced urine formation; Albumin and blood in urine. *End-point Targets:* Respiratory system; Skin; Kidneys; Eyes. *Usage:* Pesticide inert ingredient; Textile finishes; Bleach; Stain removers; Metal cleaning; Dyes; Straw hats; Leathers; Ink; Paint and varnish removers; Wood cleaning; Metal polishes; Ceramics; Pigments; Paper; Photography; Engraving; Rubber; Glucose; Automobile radiator cleaners; Spot remover. *References:* 8, 200, 304, 388, 423.

Oxalic acid (aqueous) *see* **Oxalic acid.**

Oxalic acid dihydrate *see* **Oxalic acid.**

2-Oxetanone *see* **beta-Propiolactone.**

1-Oxindene *see* **2,3-Benzofuran.**

Oxirane *see* **Ethylene oxide.**

Oxomethane *see* **Formaldehyde.**

Oxyfume (tn) *see* **Ethylene oxide.**

Oxymethylene *see* **Formaldehyde.**

PAN *see* **Phthalic anhydride.**

Paraactaldehyde *see* **Paraldehyde.**

Paracetaldehyde *see* **Paraldehyde.**

Paracide (tn) *see* **p-Dichlorobenzene.**

Paradichlorobenzene *see* **p-Dichlorobenzene.**

Parafest M-50 Parataf (tn) *see* **Methyl parathion.**

Paral *see* **Paraldehyde.**

Paraldehyde *TN/Synonyms:* Trimmer of acetaldehyde; 2,4,6-Trimethyl-1,3,5-Trioxane; p-Acetaldehyde; Elaldehyde; Paraactaldehyde; Paracetaldehyde; Paral; Paraldehyde Draught; Paraldehyde Enema. *OSHA PEL:* None, meets OSHA criteria for medical records rule. *Symptoms:* Acidosis; Albumin in urine; Amnesia; Cardiac failure; Collapse; Coma; Constricted pupils; Cyanosis; Delirium; Delusions; Dilated pupils; Dizziness; Drowsiness; Excitement; Gastritis hemorrhage; Impaired memory, intelligence, and speech; Increase in leukocytes in the blood; Increased nitrogenous bodies (esp. urea) in blood; Kidney degeneration; Labored respiration; Loss of appetite; Low blood pressure; Muscular irritability; Partial or complete loss of sensation; Pulmonary edema and hemorrhage; Reduced urine formation; Respiratory depression; Toxic hepatitis; Tremors; Unsteady Gait; Vein inflammation in conjunction with the formation of a blood clot; Visual and auditory hallucinations; Weight loss. *End-point Targets:* Insufficient data. *Usage:* Rubber; Dyes; Medicine; Solvent; Fats; Oils; Waxes; Gums; Resins; Leather; Cellulose; Sedatives; Concrete. *References:* 202, 279, 299.

Paraldehyde Draught *see* **Paraldehyde.**

Paraldehyde Enema *see* **Paraldehyde.**

Parathion-methyl *see* **Methyl parathion.**

Parathion methyl homolog *see* **Methyl parathion.**

Paraquat *TN/synonyms:* 1,1'-Dimethyl-4-4'-bipyridium dichloride; N,

N'-Dimethyl-4,4'-bipyridinium dichloride; Paraquat chloride; Paraquat dichloride; Methyl sulfate salt. *OSHA PEL:* 0.1 mg/m^3 (8hr/day-40hr/wk-PP/S). *IDLH:* 1.5 mg/m^3. *Symptoms:* Eye, nasal, and gastrointestinal irritation; Nosebleeds; Dermatitis; Fingernail damage; Heart, liver, and kidney damage; Acute pulmonary inflammation; Nervous system effects. *End-point Targets:* Eyes; Respiratory system; Heart; Liver; Kidneys; Gastrointestinal tract. *Usage:* Herbicide; Pesticide inert ingredient; Desiccant. *Note:* Historically established as a neurotoxin. *References:* 264, 304, 388, 413, 423.

Paraquat chloride *see* **Paraquat.**

Paraquat dichloride *see* **Paraquat.**

M-Parathion (tn) *see* **Methyl parathion.**

Paratox (tn) *see* **Methyl parathion.**

Parton-M (tn) *see* **Methyl parathion.**

Partron-M (tn) *see* **Methyl parathion.**

PCBs *see* **Polychlorinated biphenyls.**

PCE *see* **Tetrachloroethylene.**

PCNB *see* **p-Nitrochlorobenzene.**

PCP *see* **Pentachlorophenol.**

Pebble lime *see* **Calcium oxide.**

Penncap-M (tn) *see* **Methyl parathion.**

Penphene (tn) *see* **Chlorinated camphene.**

Penta *see* **Pentachlorophenol.**

Pentaborane *TN/synonyms:* Pentaboron nonahydride; Stable pentaborane. *OSHA PEL:* 0.005 ppm or 0.1 mg/m^3 (8hr/day-40hr/wk-PP/S); 0.015 ppm or 0.03 mg/m^3 (exposure not to exceed 15 min). *IDLH:* 3 ppm. *Symptoms:* Eye, mucous membrane, and skin irritation; Anemia; Behavioral changes; Brain degeneration and dysfunction; Conjunctivitis; Convulsions; Corneal ulceration and opacity; Deficiency of lymphocytes in blood; Destruction of nerve cells; Diarrhea; Disorientation; Dizziness; Drowsiness; Hair loss; Headaches; Impaired (poor) judgment; Incoordination; Increase in leukocytes in blood; Lightheadedness; Loss of appetite, concentration, and recent memory; Metabolic acidosis; Muscle cramps and pain; Nausea; Nervous excitement; Profuse sweating; Rhabdomyolsis (a disease characterized by destruction of skeletal muscles); Semi-coma; Skin flushing and rashes; Tonic spasms of the face, neck, abdomen, and limbs; Tremors; Visual disturbances; Vomiting; Weight loss. Suspected of causing Liver and kidney damage; Sterility. *End-point Targets:* Central nervous system; Skin. *Usage:* Corrosion inhibitor; Fuel (Air breathing engines); Glass; Soaps; Detergents. *References:* 203, 304, 388.

Pentaboron nonahydride *see* **Pentaboron.**

Pentachloronaphthalene *TN/synonyms:* Halowax 1013; 1,2,4,5,6-Pentachloronaphthalene. *OSHA PEL:* 0.5 mg/m^3 (8hr/day-40hr/wk-PP/S). *IDLH:* Unknown. *Symptoms:* Headaches; Fatigue; Vertigo; Loss of appetite; Sever itching; Acne-form dermatitis; Jaundice; Liver and adrenal gland tissue death; Toxic hepatitis; Chloracne; Heart and kidney swelling; Drowsiness; Indigestion; Nausea; Enlarged liver; Weakness; Coma; Diminished bilirubin in blood; Excessive bilirubin in blood. *End-point Targets:* Skin; Liver; Central nervous system. *Usage:* Waxes; Electrical insulation; Lubricants; Batteries; Wood; Paper; Textiles. *References:* 204, 304, 388.

1,2,4,5,6-Pentachloronaphthalene: *see* **Pentachloronaphthalene.**

Pentachlorophenol *TN/synonyms:* PCP; Penta; 2,3,4,5,6-Pentachlorophenol. *OSHA PEL:* 0.5 mg/m³ (8hr/day-40hr/wk-PP/S). *IDLH:* 150 mg/m³. *Symptoms:* Eye, nasal, throat, and upper respiratory irritation; Abdominal pain; Aplastic anemia; Cardiac failure; Chest pain; Collapse; Contact dermatitis; Convulsions; Corneal opacity and numbness; Cough; Death; Decreased blood pressure; Dilated pupils; Dizziness; Fever above 106 degrees; Headaches; Heart rate over 100 beats per minute; High fever; Labored or difficult breathing; Loss of appetite; Lung, liver, and kidney damage; Microscopic blood in urine; Muscle weakness; Nausea; Nervous system disorders; Profuse sweating; Rapid respiration; Renal insufficiency; Sneezing; Vomiting; Weakness; Weight loss. Suspected of causing Cancer (Hodgkin's disease, leukemia). *End-point Targets:* Cardiovascular system; Respiratory system; Eyes; Liver; Kidneys; Skin; Central nervous system. *Usage:* Fungicide; Pesticide; Termiticide; Paint; Pesticide inert ingredient; Mold and Mildew cleaners; Antiseptic cleaners; Starch preservative; Glues; Dextrins; Molluscicide; Fermentation inhibitors; Paper; Hardwoods; Particle board; Wood preservative; Fumigant; Herbicide; Slimicide; Algicide; Disinfectants; Defoliant. *Contaminants:* A hexachlorodibenzo-p-dioxin; A hexachlorodibenzofuran; Hexachlorobenzene; A tetra-chlorophenol. *Synergistic effects:* Impurities increase toxic effects. *References:* 205, 304, 388, 423.

2,3,4,5,6-Pentachlorophenol *see* **Pentachlorophenol.**

Pentane *see* **n-Pentane.**

n-Pentane *TN/synonyms:* Pentane; Normal pentane. *NIOSH REL:* 120 ppm or 350 mg/m³ (10hr/day-40hr/wk); 610 ppm or 1,800 mg/m³ (ceiling limit 15 min exposure). *OSHA PEL:* 600 ppm or 1,800 mg/m³ (8hr/day-40hr/wk-PP/S); 750 ppm or 2,250 mg/m³ (exposure not to exceed 15 min).

IDLH: 15,000 ppm. *Symptoms:* Eye and skin irritation; Dermatitis; Chemical pneumonia; Drowsiness; Unconsciousness; Death; Defatting dermatitis; Dry skin; Central nervous system depression; Exhilaration; Dizziness; Headaches; Nausea; Gasoline taste in mouth; Confusion; Loss of manual dexterity to do fine work; Polyneuropathy; Loss of appetite; Weakness; Numbness, tingling, or prickling sensation; Fatigue; Muscle failure. *End-point Targets:* Skin; Eyes; Respiratory system. *Usage:* Pesticide inert ingredient; Aerosol propellant; Liquid grain fumigants; Gasoline, aviation, and farm fuel additive; Artificial ice; Ammonia; Blowing agent for plastics; Lighter fluid; Blowtorch fuel; Solvent; Belts; Chemical manufacturing. *Classification:* Organic solvent (Alkane compound). *Note:* Neurotoxin. *References:* 17, 183, 304, 383, 388, 423.

1-Pentanol acetate *see* **n-Amyl acetate.**

2-Pentanol acetate *see* **sec-Amyl acetate.**

2-Pentanone *TN/synonyms:* Ethyl acetone; Methyl propyl ketone; MPK; Methyl n-propyl ketone. *NIOSH REL:* 150 ppm or 530 mg/m³ (10hr/day-40hr/wk). *OSHA PEL:* 200 ppm or 700 mg/m³ (8hr/day-40hr/wk-PP/S); 250 ppm or 875 mg/m³ (exposure not to exceed 15 min). *IDLH:* 5,000 ppm. *Symptoms:* Eye and mucous membrane irritation; Headaches; Dermatitis; Unconsciousness due to narcotic effects; Coma. *End-point Targets:* Respiratory system; Eyes; Skin; Central nervous system. *Usage:* Food flavoring; Perfumes; Plastics; Printing ink; Cosmetics; Pharmaceuticals; Diethyl ketone; Surface coatings; Lacquers; Lacquer removers. *Classification:* Organic solvent. *References:* 231, 304, 306, 383, 388.

2-Pentyl acetate *see* **sec-Amyl acetate.**

Pentyl ester of acetic acid *see* n-Amyl acetate.

2-Pentyl ester of acetic acid *see* sec-Amyl acetate.

Per *see* Tetrachloroethylene.

Perawin (tn) *see* Tetrachloroethylene.

Perc *see* Tetrachloroethylene.

Perchlor *see* Tetrachloroethylene.

Perchlorethylene *see* Tetrachloroethylene.

Perchloroethane *see* Hexachloroethane.

Perchloroethylene *see* Tetrachloroethylene.

Perchloronaphthalene *see* Octachloronaphthalene.

Perclene (tn) *see* Tetrachloroethylene.

Percosolv (tn) *see* Tetrachloroethylene.

Perk *see* Tetrachloroethylene.

Perklone (tn) *see* Tetrachloroethylene.

Perm-A-Chor (tn) *see* Trichloroethylene.

Perma-A-Chlor (tn) *see* Trichloroethylene.

Peroxide *see* Hydrogen peroxide.

PerSec (tn) *see* Tetrachloroethylene.

Pestmaster EDB-85 (tn) *see* Ethylene dibromide.

Petrohol (tn) *see* Isopropyl alcohol.

Petroleum distillates *TN/synonyms:* Aliphatic petroleum naphtha; Petroleum naphtha. *NIOSH REL:* 350 mg/m³ (10hr/day-40hr/wk); 1,800 mg/m³ (ceiling limit, 15 min exposure). *OSHA PEL:* 400 ppm or 1,600 mg/m³ (8hr/day-40hr/wk-PP/S). *IDLH:* 10,000 ppm. *Symptoms:* Eye, nasal, and throat irritation; Dizziness; Headaches; Nausea; Dry, cracked skin; Drowsiness; Death. *End-point Targets:* Skin; Eyes; Respiratory system; Central nervous system. *Usage:* Water proofing; Paint rust proofing; Paint thinner; Silver polish; Metal cleaners; Room deodorizers; Furniture polish; Oven cleaners; Pesticide inert ingredient. *Note:* Neurotoxin. *References:* 8, 17, 271, 304, 388, 423.

Petroleum ether *see* Stoddard solvent.

Petroleum naphthta *see* Petroleum distillates.

Petroleum solvent *see* Stoddard solvent.

Petzinol (tn) *see* Trichloroethylene.

PGE *see* Phenyl glycidyl ether.

Phenacyl chloride *see* alpha-Chloroacetophenone.

Phenatox (tn) *see* Chlorinated camphene.

Phenchlor (tn) *see* 2,4,6-Trichlorophenol.

Phene *see* Benzene.

Phenicide (tn) *see* Chlorinated camphene.

Phenoclor (tn) *see* Polychlorinated biphenyls.

Phenol *TN/synonyms:* Carbolic acid; Hydroxybenzene; Monohydroxy benzene; Phenyl alcohol; Phenyl hydroxide. *NIOSH REL:* 5 ppm or 19 mg/m³ (10hr/day-40hr/wk); 15.6 ppm or 60 mg/m³ (ceiling limit, 15 min exposure). *OSHA PEL:* 5 ppm or 19 mg/m³ (8hr/day-40hr/wk-PP/S). *HSDB TOXS:* Some individuals may be hypersensitive with lethal or serious effects at very low exposures. *IDLH:* 250 ppm. *Symptoms:* Eye, nasal, and throat irritation; Abdominal pain; Cardiac arrhythmias and failure; Cardiovascular collapse; Chemical odor on breath;

Chromosomal aberrations and damage; Cold sweats; Collapse; Coma; Confusion; Convulsions; Cyanosis; Dark pigmentation of the ligaments, cartilage, and fibrous tissue; Dark urine; Dermatitis; Diarrhea; Difficulty swallowing; Dizziness; Excessive bilirubin in blood; Excitement; Fainting; Frothing at nose and mouth; Genetic mutations; Granules in red blood cells; Headaches; Hemoglobin oxidizes to ferric form; Hemolytic anemia; Hypothermia; Liver, kidney, and heart damage; Loss of appetite; Low blood pressure; Muscle aches, pain, and twitching; Nausea; Pallor; Profuse sweating; Pulmonary edema; Renal insufficiency; Ringing or tingling in the ear; Shallow respiration; Shock; Skin burns; Spontaneous abortions; Tremors; Unconsciousness; Vomiting; Weak, irregular pulse; Weakness; Weight loss. *End-point Targets:* Liver; Kidneys; Skin. *Usage:* Disinfectants; Pesticide inert ingredient; Furniture and floor polishes; Mold and mildew cleaners; Air fresheners; Railroad ties; Waferboard; Chemical intermediate; Toilet bowl cleaners; Cesspool cleaners; Drain cleaners; Resins; Dyes; Antiseptics; Plasticizers; Petroleum refining; Solvent; Vaccine preservative; Pharmaceutical aids; Glue; Veterinary medicine; Adhesives; Plastics; Household cleaning products; Bandages; Chemxfoliation (skin peeling); Embalming fluid; Aspirin; Nylon; Toys; Detergents; Polyurethane; Photography; Immunotherapy solution. Found in Tobacco smoke. Derivative of Benzene. *Note:* Historically established as a neurotoxin. *References:* 207, 286, 299, 304, 388, 389, 413, 423, 429, 457.

Phenolcarinol *see* **Benzyl alcohol.**

Phenol trinitrate *see* **Picric acid.**

Phenoxy benzene *see* **Phenyl ether.**

Phenyl alcohol *see* **Phenol.**

Phenylamine *see* **Aniline.**

Phenyl chloride *see* **Chlorobenzene.**

Phenyl chloromethyl ketone *see* **alpha-Chloroacetophenone.**

p-Phenylene diamine *TN/synonyms:* 4-Amino aniline; 1,4-Benzenediamine; p-Diaminobenzene; 1,4-Diaminobenzene. *OSHA PEL:* 0.1 mg/m³ (8hr/day-40hr/wk-PP/S). *ACGIH:* No threshold value limit will insure prevention of hypersensitive responses. *IDLH:* Unknown. *Symptoms:* Pharynx and larynx irritation; Bronchial and allergic asthma; Sensitive dermatitis; Vertigo; Anemia; Gastritis; Death; Tremors; Convulsions; Coma; Chemical hypersensitivity. *End-point Targets:* Respiratory system; Skin. *Usage:* Fur dyes; Photography; Rubber; Gasoline additive; Hair dye. *References:* 201, 304, 388.

Phenyl 2,3-epoxypropyl ether *see* **Phenyl glycidyl ether.**

Phenylethane *see* **Ethyl benzene.**

Phenyl ether *TN/synonyms:* Diphenyl ether; Diphenyl oxide; Phenoxy benzene; Phenyl oxide. *OSHA PEL:* 1 ppm or 7 mg/m³ (8hr/day-40hr/wk-PP/S). *IDLH:* NE. *Symptoms:* Eye, nasal, skin, and respiratory irritation; Nausea; Liver and kidney degenerative lesions. *End-point Targets:* Eyes; Skin; Respiratory system. *Usage:* Pesticide inert ingredient; Perfumes; Fragrances; Soaps; Lubricants; Detergents; Resins; Laminated electrical insulation. *References:* 208, 304, 388, 423.

Phenyl ether-biphenyl mixture *TN/synonyms:* Diphenyl oxide-diphenyl mixture; Dowtherm A (tn). *OSHA PEL:* 1 ppm or 7 mg/m³ (8hr/day-40hr/wk-PP/S). *IDLH:* NE. *Symptoms:* Eye, nasal, and skin irritation; Nausea; Corneal burns; Liver and kidney degenerative lesions. *End-point Targets:* Eyes; Skin; Respiratory system. *Usage:* Pesticide inert ingredient; Industrial heat transfer medium. *Note:* Typical mixture contains 75% phenyl ether and

25% biphenyl. *References:* 263, 304, 388, 423.

Phenylethylene *see* **Styrene.**

Phenyl glycidyl ether *TN/synonyms:* 1,2-Epoxy-3-phenoxy propane; Glycidyl phenyl ether; PGE; Phenyl 2,3-epoxypropyl ether. *NIOSH:* Carcinogen at any exposure level. *NIOSH REL:* 1 ppm or 6 mg/m³ (ceiling limit, 15 min exposure). *OSHA PEL:* 1 ppm or 6 mg/m³ (8hr/day-40hr/wk-PP/S). *IDLH:* Unknown. *Symptoms:* Eye, skin, and upper respiratory irritation; Sensitive dermatitis; Unconsciousness due to narcotic effects. Suspected of causing Cancer. *End-point Targets:* Skin; Eyes; Central nervous system. *Usage:* Plasticizer; Resins; Adhesives; Lamination. *References:* 209, 304, 305, 388, 401.

Phenylhydrazine *TN/synonyms:* Hydrazinobenzene; Monophenylhydrazine. *NIOSH:* Carcinogen at any exposure level. *NIOSH REL:* 0.14 ppm or 0.6 mg/m³ (ceiling limit, 2 hr exposure). *OSHA PEL:* 5 ppm or 20 mg/m³ (8hr/day-40hr/wk-PP/S); 10 ppm or 45 mg/m³ (exposure not to exceed 15 min). *ACGIH:* Suspected human carcinogen. *IDLH:* 295 ppm. *Symptoms:* Contact dermatitis; Cyanosis; Dark urine; Decrease in hemoglobin; Diarrhea; Enlarged liver; Excess urobilin in urine; Excessive bilirubin in blood; Fatigue; Giddiness; Granules in red blood cells; Hemoglobin oxidizes to ferric form; Hemolytic anemia; Increase in leukocytes in the blood; Jaundice; Kidney damage; Labored or difficulty breathing; Liver damage; Loss of appetite; Low blood pressure; Nausea; Vascular blood clotting. Suspected of causing Cancer. *End-point Targets:* Blood; Respiratory system; Liver; Kidneys; Skin. *Usage:* Dyes; Antipyrine; Sugar reagent; Aldehydes; Ketones; Pharmaceuticals. *References:* 206, 304, 306, 388.

Phenyl hydride *see* **Benzene.**

Phenyl hydroxide *see* **Phenol.**

Phenyl methane *see* **Toluene.**

Phenylmethanol *see* **Benzyl alcohol.**

Phenylmethyl alcohol *see* **Benzyl alcohol.**

Phenyl oxide *see* **Phenyl ether.**

Phenyl phosphate *see* **Triphenyl phosphate.**

2-Phenyl propane *see* **Cumene.**

2-Phenyl propylene *see* **alpha-Methyl styrene.**

Philex (tn) *see* **Trichloroethylene.**

Phosdrin *TN/Synonyms:* 2-Carbomethoxy-1-methylvinyl dimethyl phosphate; Mevinphos. *OSHA PEL:* 0.01 ppm or 0.10 mg/m³ (8hr/day-40hr/wk-PP/S); 0.03 ppm or 0.30 mg/m³ (exposure not to exceed 15 min). *IDLH:* 4 ppm. *Symptoms:* Eye and skin irritation; Constricted pupils; Nasal discharge; Headaches; Tight chest; Wheezing; Laryngeal spasm; Excessive salivation; Cyanosis; Loss of appetite; Nausea; Vomiting; Abdominal cramps; Diarrhea; Paralysis; Incoordination; Convulsions; Low blood pressure; Cardiac irregularities. *End-point Targets:* Respiratory system; Central nervous system; Cardiovascular system; Skin; Blood cholinesterase. *Usage:* Insecticide. *References:* 35, 304, 388.

Phosgene *TN/synonyms:* Carbon oxychloride; Carbonyl chloride; Chloroformyl chloride. *NIOSH REL:* 0.1 ppm or 0.4 mg/m³ (10hr/day-40hr/wk); 0.2 ppm or 0.8 mg/m³ (ceiling limit, 15 min exposure). *OSHA PEL:* 0.1 ppm or 0.4 mg/m³ (8hr/day-40hr/wk-PP/S). *IDLH:* 2 ppm. *Symptoms:* Eye, throat, and respiratory irritation; Alveolar swelling; Capillary leakage; Cardiac failure; Chest constriction and pain; Choking; Circulatory failure; Cough; Cyanosis; Death; Dry land drowning from accumulation of blood plasma in lungs; Dry, burning throat;

Eyelid spasms; Feeling of oppression; Foamy, bloody sputum; Headaches; Hemoconcentration; Inability to utilize oxygen; Increase in leukocytes in the blood; Labored or difficult breathing; Malaise; Nausea; Painful breathing; Peribronchial swelling; Pneumonia; Pulmonary congestion, edema, and hemorrhage; Skin burns; Tearing; Trachea, bronchi, and bronchioli degeneration; Vomiting. Suspected of causing Conjunctiva congestion. *End-point Targets:* Respiratory system; Skin; Eyes. *Usage:* Military warfare gas; Dyes; Coal tar; Urea resins; Isocyanates; Toluene Diisocyanate; Polycarbonate Resins; Insecticide manufacturing; Pharmaceuticals. *Synergistic effects:* Reacts slowly with water to form hydrochloric acid and carbon dioxide. Solvents, paint removers, and nonflammable dry cleaning fluids (chlorinated hydrocarbons, especially carbon tetrachloride, chloroform, and methylene chloride) will decompose into phosgene in the presence of fire or heat. *Note:* A burning cigarette is sufficient heat to decompose trichloroethylene into phosgene gas. Symptoms may be delayed for up to 24 hours. *References:* 210, 304, 388.

Phosphine *TN/synonyms:* Hydrogen phosphide; Phosphorated hydrogen; Phosphorus hydride; Phosphorus trihydride. *OSHA PEL:* 0.3 ppm or 0.4 mg/m^3 (8hr/day-40hr/wk); 1 ppm or 1 mg/m^3 (exposure not to exceed 15 min. *IDLH:* 200 ppm. *Symptoms:* Gastrointestinal and pulmonary irritation; Abdominal pains; Absent ankle reflex; Bilateral diffuse rales; Bronchitis; Cerebral difficulties; Chest pressure or tightness; Chills; Cough; Death; Diarrhea; Dizziness; Double vision; Epigastric pain; Fainting; Fatigue; Fluorescent green sputum; Giddiness; Headaches; Incoordination; Jaundice; Labored or difficult breathing; Lethargy; Liver injury; Loss of appetite; Muscle pains; Myocardial injury; Nausea; Numbness; Osteomyelitis of the jaw bones; Partial or complete loss of sensation; Petechial hemorrhages on the surface of the liver and brain; Pulmonary edema; Stupor; Substernal burning and pain; Thirst; Tonic convulsions; Tremors; Unconsciousness due to inadequate blood flow to the brain; Vertigo; Vomiting; Weakness; Widespread small-vessel injuries. Suspected of causing Chromosomal aberrations. *End-point Targets:* Respiratory system. *Usage:* Pesticide; Plastics; Insecticide; Animal feed and tobacco leaf fumigant; Rodenticide; N-type semiconductors; Flame retardant manufacturing. *References:* 211, 304, 388, 429.

Phosphorated hydrogen *see* **Phosphine.**

Phosphoric acid *TN/synonyms:* Metaphosphoric acid; Orthophosphoric acid; Phosphoric acid (aqueous); White phosphoric acid. *OSHA PEL:* 1 mg/m^3 (8hr/day-40hr/wk-PP/S); 3 mg/m^3 (exposure not to exceed 15 min). *IDLH:* 10,000 mg/m^3. *Symptoms:* Upper respiratory, eye, throat, and skin irritation; Burns skin and eyes; Dermatitis; Gastric hemorrhage; Stomach, duodenum, jejunum, and pancreas tissue death; Coughing; Tearing; Nausea; Vomiting; Labored or difficult breathing; Elevated lactic dehydrogenase (an enzyme); Decreased pulmonary functions; Mucous membrane corrosion and pain; Difficulty swallowing; Inhibited blood clotting; Epigastric pain; Thirst; Circulatory collapse; Clammy skin; Weak, rapid pulse; Shallow respiration; Death; Circulatory shock; Glottis swelling; Delayed esophageal, gastric, and pyloric strictures; Kidney failure; Heart and liver ischemic lesions. *End-point Targets:* Respiratory system; Eyes; Skin. *Usage:* Pesticide inert ingredient; Dental cement; Engraving; Food acidulant and flavoring; Beverage acidulant; Soft drinks; Rust proofing metals; Rubber latex; Veterinary medicine; Sugar-bearing juices; Gelatin; Electro-polishing; Gasoline additive; Dyes; Yeast; Waxes; Polishes; Ceramics; Activated carbon; Fertilizers; Dentifrices; Water treatments; Chelating agent for lead poisoning; Medicine; Electrolyte fuel cells; Soaps; Detergents; Jellies and preserves; Bricks; Lithography; Photoengraving; Opal glass; Electric lights; Penicillin extraction; Fabric finishes; Food preservative; Animal feed; Presoak cleaners; Cleaners; Pet food; Fire control agent; Antifreeze; Textiles; Diammonium phosphate; Monoammonium phosphate; Shampoo; Disinfectant inactive ingredient. *References:* 8, 212, 290, 304, 388, 423, 456.

Phosphoric acid (aqueous) *see* **Phosphoric acid.**

Phosphorothioc acid *see* **Methyl parathion.**

Phosphorus *TN/synonyms:* Elemental white phosphorus; White phosphorus. *OSHA PEL:* 0.1 mg/m³ (8hr/day-40hr/wk-PP/S). *IDLH:* NE. *Symptoms:* Eye, gastrointestinal, respiratory irritation; Abdominal pain; Absent or reduced urine formation; Anemia; Belching; Blood and albumin in urine; Bone death; Burns skin and eyes; Cardiovascular collapse; Central nervous system damage; Coma; Convulsions; Corneal opacity; Death; Delirium; Dental pain; Diarrhea; Enlarged, tender liver; Excessive salivation; Eyelid spasms; Eyes become sensitive to light; Garlic breath; Hemorrhaging; Inhibits blood clotting; Jaundice; Jaw pain and swelling; Kidney damage; Liver failure; Malnutrition and wasting away; Nausea; Osteomyelitis of the jaw bone; Renal insufficiency; Severe itching; Shock; Spontaneous bone fractures; Tearing; Vomiting blood; Vomiting; Weight loss. *End-point Targets:* Respiratory system; Liver; Kidneys; Jaw; Teeth; Blood; Eyes; Skin. *Usage:* Plasticizers; Gasoline and oil additives; Flame retardants; Insecticide paste; Rodenticide; Smoke screens; Fireworks; Matches;

Phosphoric acid; Phosphine; Phosphoric anhydride; Phosphorus trichloride; Phosphorus pentachloride; Fertilizers; Pesticide manufacturing; Smoke bombs; Tracer bullets. *References:* 214, 304, 388.

Phosphorus hydride *see* **Phosphine.**

Phosphorus pentasulfide *TN/synonyms:* Phosphorus persulfide; Phosphorus sulfide. *OSHA PEL:* 1 mg/m³ (10hr/day-40hr/wk-PP/S); 3 mg/m³ (exposure not to exceed 15 min). *IDLH:* 750 mg/m³. *Symptoms:* Eye and respiratory irritation; Albumin in urine; Amnesia; Asphyxial convulsions; Bronchial pneumonia; Cardiac dilatation, palpitations, and arrhythmias; Collapse; Coma; Confusion; Conjunctiva pain; Conjunctivitis; Contact skin redness and pain; Convulsions; Corneal opacity and vesiculation; Cough; Death; Diarrhea; Dizziness; Excessive salivation; Eyes become sensitive to light; Fatigue; Gastrointestinal distress; Giddiness; Headaches; Insomnia; Irritability; Labored or difficult breathing; Loss of smell; Muscle cramps; Nasal mucosa inflammation; Nausea; Osteomyelitis of the jaw bones; Peripheral neuropathy; Profuse sweating; Psychotic disturbances; Pulmonary edema; Rapid respiration; Respiratory paralysis; Tearing; Temporary cessation of breathing; Tracheobronchitis; Unconsciousness; Vertigo; Vomiting; Weakness. *End-point Targets:* Respiratory system; Central nervous system; Eyes; Skin. *Usage:* Matches; Ignition compounds; Lube oil additives; Organophosphate pesticide and insecticide manufacturing; Malathion; Chlorpyrifos; Terubphos. *Synergistic effects:* Reacts with water to form hydrogen sulfide and sulfur dioxide. *References:* 213, 304, 388.

Phosphorus persulfide *see* **Phosphorus pentasulfide.**

Phosphorus sulfide *see* **Phosphorus pentasulfide.**

Phosphorus trihydride *see* **Phosphine.**

Phthalic acid anhydride *see* **Phthalic anhydride.**

Phthalic anhydride *TN/synonyms:* 1,2-Benzenedicarboxylic anhydride; PAN; Phthalic acid anhydride. *OSHA PEL:* 6 mg/m³ or 1 ppm (8hr/day-40hr/wk-PP/S). *IDLH:* 10,000 mg/m³. *Symptoms:* Eye, mucous membrane, and upper respiratory irritation; Conjunctivitis; Nasal ulcer bleeding; Bronchitis; Bronchial asthma; Dermatitis; Bloody sputum; Emphysema; Decreased blood pressure; Central nervous system excitement; Hives; Nasal discharge; Tearing; Wheezing; Chemical hypersensitivity; Occupational asthma. *End-point Targets:* Respiratory system; Eyes; Skin; Liver; Kidneys. *Usage:* Pesticide inert ingredient; Synthetic indigo; Resins; Pharmaceutical intermediate; Insecticides; Diethyl phthalate; Dimethyl phthalate; Insect repellents; Polyester; Dyes; Pigments; Rubber; Synthetic rubber; Epoxy resins; Plasticizers. *Synergistic effects:* Converts to phthalic acid in hot water. *References:* 215, 304, 388, 423.

Pic-Chlor (tn) *see* **Chloropicrin.**

Picfume (tn) *see* **Chloropicrin.**

Picric acid *TN/synonyms:* Phenol trinitrate; 2,4,6-Trinitrophenol. *NIOSH REL:* 0.1 mg/m³ (10hr/day-40hr/wk); 0.3 mg/m³ (exposure not to exceed 15 min). *OSHA PEL:* 0.1 mg/m³ (8hr/day-40hr/wk-PP/S). *IDLH:* 100 mg/m³. *Symptoms:* Eye irritation; Abdominal pain; Reduced or absence of urine formation; Agranulocytic anemia; Anxiety; Bitter taste; Blood and albumin in urine; Cataracts; Central nervous system dysfunction; Chemical hypersensitivity; Coma; Contact dermatitis; Convulsions; Cyanosis; Dark or port-wine colored urine; Death; Decreased urine output; Destruction of erythrocytes in the blood; Diarrhea; Excitement; Fatigue; Fever above 106 degrees; Fever; Flushed face; Frequent, excessive urination; Gastrointestinal inflammation; Headaches; Heart rate over 100 beats per minute; Hemorrhagic kidney inflammation; Hepatitis; Increased rate or depth of respiration; Jaundice; Kidney lesions; Labored or difficult breathing; Muscle cramps; Nausea; Peripheral nerve inflammation; Respiratory failure; Restlessness; Severe itching; Skin eruptions; Skin rashes; Stupor; Sweating; Tender liver; Tender, painful muscles; Thirst; Unconsciousness; Vertigo; Vomiting; Weakness; Yellow-stained hair and skin. *End-point Targets:* Kidneys; Liver; Blood; Skin; Eyes. *Usage:* Explosives; Wool and silk dyes; Germicide; Fungicide; Leather; Electric batteries; Etching copper; Colored glass; Textiles; Antiseptics; Astringents; Rocket fuel; Photography; Pesticide inert ingredient. No longer used as an antiseptic on surgical dressings because of adverse central nervous system effects. *References:* 216, 304, 388, 423.

Picride (tn) *see* **Chloropicrin.**

Pigment metal *see* **Lead.**

Pimelic ketone *see* **Cyclohexanone.**

Pindone *TN/synonyms:* tert-Butyl valone; 1,3-Dioxo-2-pivaloylindane; Pival; Pivalyl; 2-Pivalyl-1,3-indandione. *OSHA PEL:* 0.1 mg/m³ (8hr/day-40hr/wk-PP/S). *IDLH:* 200 mg/m³. *Symptoms:* Nosebleeds; Inhibits blood clotting; Smokey urine; Black tarry stools; Abdominal and back pains; Bleeding gums; Pallor; Petechial rash; Massive bruising; Blood in urine; Fecal bleeding; Paralysis; Cerebral hemorrhage; Hemorrhagic shock; Death; Loss of appetite; Nausea; Vomiting; Diarrhea; Chemical sensitivity. *End-point Targets:* Blood; Prothrombin. *Usage:* Insecticide; Rodenticide; Medicine. *Note:* Symptoms may be delayed from a few days to a few weeks. *References:* 217, 304, 388.

Pival *see* **Pindone.**

Pivalyl *see* **Pindone.**

2-Pivalyl-1,3-indandione *see* **Pindone.**

Platinol AH (tn) *see* **Di-sec octyl phthalate.**

Plumbum *see* **Lead.**

PNA *see* **p-Nitroaniline.**

PNCB *see* **p-Nitrochlorobenzene.**

Polychlorinated biphenyls *TN/ synonyms:* Aroclor (tn); Fenclor (tn); Kanechlor (tn); Phenoclor (tn); Chlorodiphenyl; PCBs. *NIOSH:* Carcinogen at any exposure level. *NIOSH REL:* 0.001 mg/m^3 (10hr/day-40hr/wk). *OSHA PEL:* 42% chlorine: 1.0 mg/m^3 (8hr/day-40/wk-PP/S); 54% chlorine: 0.5 mg/m^3 (8hr/day-40/wk-PP/S). *ATSDR MRL:* 0.005 ug/kg/day (Ingestion, more than 365 days). *IDLH:* 42% chlorine: 10 mg/m^3; 54% chlorine: 5 mg/m^3. *Symptoms:* Eye and skin irritation; Acne-form dermatitis; Altered menstrual cycles; Cancer (liver, blood, skin, and gastrointestinal); Chest tightness; Chloracne; Decreased fertility; Depression; Dizziness; Epigastric distress and pain; Fatigue; Fatty food intolerance; Fetal neurobehavioral deficits; Headaches; High blood pressure; Impaired lung function; Joint pain; Liver damage; Loss of appetite; Low birth weight; Nausea; Premature births; Stomach inflammation; Autoimmune disease; Autoimmune thyroid disease. Suspected of causing Pericardial swelling; Gastric ulcers, cysts, and hemorrhages; Increased erythrocyte and hemoglobin counts; Anemia; Kidney damage; Antibody production; Immunosuppression. *End-point Targets:* Respiratory system; Skin; Eyes; Liver. *Usage:* Plasticizer; Surface coatings; Inks; Adhesives; Pesticide extenders; Carbonless paper; Capacitors; Transformers; Asphalt; Waterproofing;

Coatings; Lubricants; Rubber; Resins; Waxes; Pesticide manufacture. *Synergistic effects:* When burned, fumes contain polychlorinated dibenzofurans and chlorinated dibenzo-p-dioxins. **Contaminates** breast milk. *Classification:* Organochlorine. *Note:* Historically established as a neurotoxin. *References:* 280, 318, 343, 388, 408, 413, 429, 449.

Polychlorocamphene *see* **Chlorinated camphene.**

Polycizer DBP (tn) *see* **Dibutylphthalate.**

Polycyclic aromatic hydrocarbons *Compounds:* Acenaphthene; Acenaphthylene; Anthracene; Benzo(a)anthracene; Benzo(a)pyrene; Benzo(b)fluoran-thene; Benzo(g,h,i)perylene; Benzo(k)fluoranthene; Chrysene; Dibenzo(a,h)anthracene; Fluoranthene; Fluorene; Indeno(1,2,3-cd)pyrene; Phenanthrene; Pyrene. *NIOSH REL:* 0.1 mg/m^3 (10hr/day-40hr/wk). *OSHA PEL*: 0.2 mg/m^3 (8hr/day-40hr/wk). *IDHL:* 400 mg/m^3. *Symptoms:* Atherosclerosis; Diarrhea; Pigment metabolism disorder; Inhibits bone marrow function; Abnormal decrease in blood platelets; Toxic production and development of blood cells; Gene mutations; Binds to DNA; Skin lesions; Cancer (scrotal, lungs, and skin). Suspected of causing Birth defects; Low birth weight; Neonate lethality; Decreased fertility; Sterility. *End-point Targets:* Blood; Skin. Usages: *Anthracene:* Laxatives; Chemotherapeutic agent; Intermediate in dye production; Smoke screens; Scintillation counter crystals; Organic semiconductor research. *Acenaphthene:* Dye intermediate in Plastics; Insecticides; and Fungicide. *Fluorene:* Chemical intermediate. *Phenanthrene:* Dyes; Explosives; Biological Research. *Fluoranthene:* Lining material to protect the interior of steel and ductible-iron drinking water pipes and storage tanks. *Benzo(a)pyrene:* Asphalt. Benzo(a)-

anthracene; Benzo(b)fluoranthene; Benzo(k)fluoranthene; Benzo(g,h,i)-perylene; Dibenzo(a,h)anthracene; Indeno(1,2,3-(cd)pyrene; and Pyrene have no known commerical use, but are used as research chemicals. *PAHs:* Crude oil; Coal tar pitch; Creosote; Asphalt; Roofing tar; Cigarette smoke; Coal; Oil; Gas; Garbage; Organic substances; Vehicle exhaust; Agricultural and wood burning. Found in cigarette smoke. *Note:* PAHs generally don't burn easily and they last in the environment for months to years. *References:* 337, 388, 389.

Polyisocyanates *see* **Methylene bisphenyl isocyanate or Toluene-2, 4-diisocyanate.**

Polystream (tn) *see* **Benzene.**

Portland cement *TN/synonyms:* Cement; Hydraulic cement; Portland cement silicate. *OSHA PEL:* 5 mg/m³ (8hr/day-40hr/wk-PP/S); 10 mg/m³ (Total). *IDLH:* NE. *Symptoms:* Eye and nasal irritation; Cough; Expectoration; Labored or difficult breathing on exertion; Wheezing; Chronic bronchitis; Dermatitis. *End-point Targets:* Respiratory system; Eyes; Skin. *Usage:* Concrete; Cement. *References:* 304, 388.

Portland cement silicate *see* **Portland cement.**

Potassium chromate *see* **Chromic acid.**

Potato alcohol *see* **Ethanol.**

Preserv-O-Sote (tn) *see* **Creosotes.**

Primary amyl acetate *see* **n-Amyl acetate.**

Pro (tn) *see* **Isopropyl alcohol.**

Profume A (tn) *see* **Chloropicrin.**

Propane *TN/synonyms:* Bottled gas; Dimethyl methane; n-Propane; Propyl hydride. *OSHA PEL:* 1,000 ppm or 1,800 mg (8hr/day-40hr/wk-PP/S). *IDLH:* 20,000 ppm. *Symptoms:*

Dizziness; Disorientation; Excitement; Colic; Frostbite; Stupor; Excessive salivation; Retrograde amnesia; Headaches; Numbness; Chills; Vomiting; Shortness of breath; Unconsciousness; Insufficient blood oxygenation; Death; Skin burns; Central nervous system depression. *End-point Targets:* Central nervous system. *Usage:* Residential, welding, commercial and industrial fuels; Refrigerant; Solvent; Aerosol propellant; Hair spray; Deodorant; Antiperspirants; Pesticide inert ingredient; Shave cream; Topical medication. *References:* 14, 15, 22, 219, 304, 388, 423.

n-Propane *see* **Propane.**

n-Propanol *see* **n-Propyl alcohol.**

Propan-2-ol *see* **Isopropyl alcohol.**

1-Propanol *see* **n-Propyl alcohol.**

2-Propanol *see* **Isopropyl alcohol.**

Propanone *see* **Acetone.**

2-Propanone *see* **Acetone.**

Propellent 12 *see* **Dichlorodifluoromethane.**

Propenal *see* **Acrolein.**

Prop-2-en-1-al *see* **Acrolein.**

2-Propenal *see* **Acrolein.**

Propenamide *see* **Acrylamide.**

2-Propenamide *see* **Acrylamide.**

Propenenitrile *see* **Acrylonitrile.**

2-Propenenitrile *see* **Acrylonitrile.**

1-Propene-3-ol *see* **Allyl alcohol.**

Propene oxide *see* **Propylene oxide.**

2-Propenic acid *see* **Ethyl methacrylate.**

Propenol *see* **Allyl alcohol.**

2-Propenol *see* **Allyl alcohol.**

2-Propen-1-one *see* **Acrolein.**

beta-Propiolactone *TN/synonyms:* BPL; Hydroacrylic acid; 3-Hydroxy-beta-lactone; 3-Hydroxy-propionic acid; beta-Lactone; 2-Oxetanone; 3-Propiolactone. *NIOSH:* Carcinogen at any exposure level. Reduce exposure to lowest feasible level. *OSHA:* No PEL, 1 of 13 chemicals recognized as an occupational carcinogen. Exposure of workers is to be controlled through required engineering controls, work practices, and personal protective equipment. *ACGIH:* Suspected human carcinogen. *ACGIH TLV:* 0.5 ppm or 1.5 mg/m³ (8hr/day-40hr/wk). *IDLH:* Carcinogen. *Symptoms:* Skin irritation, blistering, and burns; Corneal opacity; Frequent urination; Painful or difficult urination; Blood in urine; Cancer. *End-point Target:* Kidneys; Skin; Lungs; Eyes. *Usage:* Disinfectants; Blood plasma sterilant; Vaccine sterilant; Milk sterilant; Surgical instrument sterilization; Water sterilant; Chemical intermediate. *References:* 124, 304, 306, 388.

3-Propiolactone *see* **beta-Propiolactone.**

Propylacetate *see* **n-Propyl acetate.**

n-Propyl acetate *TN/synonyms:* Propylacetate; n-Propyl ester of acetic acid. *OSHA PEL:* 200 ppm or 840 mg/m³ (8hr/day-40hr/wk-PP/S); 250 ppm or 1,050 mg/m³ (exposure not to exceed 15 min). *IDLH:* 8,000 ppm. *Symptoms:* Eye, nasal, throat, mucous membrane, and skin irritation; Unconsciousness due to narcotic effects; Dermatitis; Chest constriction; Cough; Defatting dermatitis; Nausea; Vomiting; Dizziness. *End-point Targets:* Respiratory system; Eyes; Skin; Central nervous system. *Usage:* Plastics; Food flavoring; Perfumes; Nitrocellulose; Cellulose; Lacquers; Solvent; Inks; Waxes; Insecticide manufacturing. *References:* 184, 304, 388, 429.

2-Propyl acetate *see* **Isopropyl acetate.**

Propyl alcohol *see* **n-Propyl alcohol.**

n-Propyl alcohol *TN/synonyms:* Ethyl carbinol; 1-Propanol; n-Propanol; Propyl alcohol. *OSHA PEL:* 200 ppm or 500 mg/m³ (8hr/day-40hr/wk-PP/S); 250 ppm or 625 mg/m³ (exposure not to exceed 15 min). *IDLH:* 4,000 ppm. *Symptoms:* Eye, nasal, and throat irritation; Abdominal cramps; Absence of reflexes; Central nervous system depression; Chemical hypersensitivity; Circulatory collapse; Coma; Confusion; Death; Depressed respiration; Destruction of red blood cells; Diarrhea; Dizziness; Drowsiness; Dry, cracking skin; Excess urine formation; Gastrointestinal inflammation and pain; Headaches; Hypothermia; Incoordination; Kidney and liver dysfunction; Kidney impairment; Low blood pressure; Muscle tenderness, tissue hardening, and swelling; Nausea; Pneumonia; Reduced urine formation; Respiratory arrest; Slow pulse and heart rate; Stupor; Vomiting blood; Vomiting. *End-point Targets:* Skin; Eyes; Respiratory system; Gastrointestinal tract. *Usage:* Antiseptic; Baked goods; Brake fluids; Candy; Cattle feed additive; Cellulose; Chemical intermediate; Cleaners; Contact lenses; Cosmetics; Degreasers; Dental lotions; Disinfectant; Food flavoring; Gums; Ice cream; Ices; Lacquers; Non-alcoholic beverages; Pesticide inert ingredient; Pharmaceuticals; Polishes; Printing inks; Resins; Solvent; Vegetable oils. *Note:* Occupationally acquired sensitivity to isopropyl alcohol also caused reactions to n-propyl alcohol; n-butyl alcohol; 2-Propanol. Neurotoxin. *References:* 17, 185, 304, 388, 423, 429.

sec-Propyl alcohol *see* **Isopropyl alcohol.**

sec-Propylamine *see* **Isopropylamine.**

2-Propylamine *see* **Isopropylamine.**

n-Propyl carbinol *see* **n-Butyl alcohol.**

Propylene aldehyde *see* **Crotonaldehyde.**

Propylene dichloride *TN/synonyms:* Dichloro-1,2-propane; 1,2-Dichloropropane. *NIOSH:* Carcinogen at any exposure level. Reduce exposure to lowest feasible concentration. *OSHA PEL:* 75 ppm or 350 mg/m^3 (8hr/day-40hr/wk-PP/S); 110 ppm or 510 mg/m^3 (exposure not to exceed 15 min). *IDLH:* 2,000 ppm. *Symptoms:* Eye, mucous membrane, and skin irritation; Abdominal pains; Anemia; Blood in urine; Bronchial pneumonia; Central nervous system damage; Choking; Coma; Conjunctiva hemorrhages; Cough; Defatting dermatitis; Dermatitis; Disorientation; Dizziness; Drowsiness; Emphysema; Headaches; Heart rate over 100 beats per minute; Hemolytic anemia; Kidney damage and failure; Lightheadedness; Liver damage; Nausea; Night sweats; Nosebleed; Reduced urine formation; Unexpanded fetal lungs at birth; Vertigo; Vomiting. Suspected of causing Liver and kidney disease; Cancer. *End-point Targets:* Skin; Eyes; Respiratory system; Liver; Kidneys. *Usage:* Pesticide; Pesticide inert ingredient; Petrochloroethylene; Carbon tetrachloride; Insecticide; Solvent; Plastics; Resins; Rubber; Oils; Fats; Dry cleaning; Gasoline additive; Waxes; Gums; Cellulose; Scouring compounds; Spot removers; Metal degreasing; Soil fumigant; Toluene Diisocyanate; Paper; Livestock insecticide. *References:* 220, 286, 304, 388, 423, 442.

Propylene imine *TN/synonyms:* 2-Methylaziridine; 2-Methylethyleneimine; Propylene imine (inhibited); Propylenimine. *NIOSH:* Carcinogen at any exposure level. *OSHA PEL:* 2 ppm or 5 mg/m^3 (8hr/day-40hr/wk-PP/S). *ACGIH:* Suspected human carcinogen. *IDLH:* 500 ppm. *Symptoms:* Skin irritation, inflammation, burns, and tissue death; Eye and upper respiratory irritation; Bronchial pneumonia; Bronchitis; Conjunctivitis; Corneal inflammation; Dermatitis; Diphtheria-like mutations of trachea and bronchi; Dizziness; Eye burns; Headaches; Laryngeal swelling; Mental dullness; Nasal secretions; Nausea; Pulmonary edema; Retching; Septum and vocal cord ulcerations; Shortness of breath; Temple pain; Vomiting. Suspected of causing Cancer. *End-point Targets:* Eyes; Skin; Respiratory system; Liver; Kidneys. *Usage:* Latex paints; Textiles; Paper; Photography; Gelatins; Oil additives; Polymers; Rubber; Pharmaceuticals; Adhesives; Cellulose derivatives; Petroleum refining; Rocket fuels; Agricultural chemicals; Medicine; Inks. *Synergistic effects:* Hydrolyzes in water to form methylethanolamine. *Note:* Symptoms may be delayed for several days. *References:* 219, 304, 388.

Propylene imine (inhibited) *see* **Propylene imine.**

Propylene oxide *TN/synonyms:* 1,2-Epoxy propane; Methyl ethylene oxide; Methyloxirane; Propene oxide; 1,2-Propylene oxide. *NIOSH:* Carcinogen at any exposure level. Reduce exposure to lowest feasible concentration. *OSHA PEL:* 20 ppm or 50 mg/m^3 (8hr/day-40hr/wk-PP/S). *IDLH:* 2,000 ppm. *Symptoms:* Eye, skin, upper respiratory, and lung irritation; Blisters and burns skin; Central nervous system depression; Skin tissue death; Incoordination; Depression; Corneal burns; Nausea; Vomiting; Inebriation; Contact dermatitis; Chromosomal aberrations; Elevated blood alkylhistidine; DNA damage. Suspected of causing Cancer. *End-point Targets:* Eyes; Skin; Respiratory system. *Usage:* Pesticide inert ingredient; Packaged food sterilization; Herbicide; Lubricants; Detergents; Solvent; Soil steriIant; Polyurethane; Propylene glycol; Glycerol; Food additive; Modified food starch; Brake fluids; Disinfectants;

Insecticides; Miticides; Bacteriostat; Fungicide; Cocoa; Flexible and rigid foams; Coatings; Adhesives. *Additives/Contaminants:* Alkalis; Aqueous acids; Amines; and Acidic alcohols. *References:* 221, 304, 388, 393, 423, 429.

1,2-Propylene oxide *see* **Propylene oxide.**

Propylenimine *see* **Propylene imine.**

n-Propyl ester of acetic acid *see* **n-Propyl acetate.**

Propyl hydride *see* **Propane.**

Prussic acid *see* **Hydrogen cyanide.**

PS (tn) *see* **Chloropicrin.**

Pyrethrin I or II *see* **Pyrethrum.**

Pyrethrum *TN/synonyms:* Cinerin I or II; Jasmolin I or II; Pyrethrin I or II; Pyrethrum I or II. *OSHA PEL:* 5 mg/m³ (8hr/day-40hr/wk-PP/S). *IDLH:* 5,000 mg/m³. *Symptoms:* Absolute exhaustion; Allergic reactions; Asthma; Chemical sensitivity; Chest pains; Clonic convulsions; Collapse; Conjunctivitis; Contact dermatitis; Cough; Death; Dermatitis; Diarrhea; Excitement; Facial swelling; Fatigue; Fever; Headaches; Heart rate over 100 beats per minute; Incoordination; Labored or difficult breathing; Muscular fibrillation; Nasal discharge and congestion; Nasal mucosa inflammation; Nausea; Numbness of lips and tongue; Pallor; Paralysis; Pneumonia; Profuse sweating; Pulmonary damage; Respiratory paralysis and failure; Restlessness; Ringing or tingling in the ear; Severe itching; Shortness of breath; Skin redness; Skin sensitivity to light; Sneezing; Stupor; Unusual amount of eosinophils in blood; Vomiting. *End-point Targets:* Respiratory system; Skin; Central nervous system. *Usage:* Insecticide; Pesticide inert ingredient; Livestock, pet, and household insect sprays; Paper finish for food packaging. No longer used in human or veterinary

medicines. *Note:* Neurotoxin. *References:* 17, 222, 304, 388, 423.

Pyrethrum I or II *see* **Pyrethrum.**

Pyridine *TN/synonyms:* Azabenzene; Azine. *OSHA PEL:* 5 ppm or 15 mg/m³ (8hr/day-40hr/wk-PP/S). *NIOSH IDLH:* 3,600 ppm. *Symptoms:* Eye and skin irritation; Headaches; Giddiness; Nervousness; Dizziness; Insomnia; Central nervous system depression; Slurred speech; Nausea; Loss of appetite; Frequent urination; Dermatitis; Liver and kidney damage; Slow reflexes; Stupor; Sleepiness; Increased pulse and respiration. *End-point Targets:* Central nervous system; Liver; Kidneys; Skin; Gastrointestinal tract. *Usage:* Medicines; Antihistamines; Steroids; Sulfa-type drugs; Antibacterial agents; Vitamins; Food flavorings; Pesticides; Dyes; Adhesives (polycarbonate resins); Rubber products; Paints; Waterproofing for fabrics; Denaturation of alcohol; Intermediate in making insecticides and herbicides. *References:* 304, 377, 388.

alpha-Pyridylamine *see* **2-Aminopyridine.**

Pyrinex (tn) *see* **Chlorpyrifos.**

Pyrobenzol *see* **Benzene.**

Pyrobenzole *see* **Benzene.**

Pyromucic aldehyde *see* **Furfural.**

Pyrrolylene *see* **1,3-Butadiene.**

Quartz *see* **Silica.**

Quaternium-15 *see* **Formaldehyde.**

Quick lime *see* **Calcium oxide.**

Quicksilver *see* **Mercury.**

Quinol *see* **Hydroquinone.**

Quinone *TN/synonyms:* 1,4-Benzoquinone; p-Benzoquinone; 1,4-Cyclohexadiene dioxide; p-Quinone. *OSHA PEL:* 0.4 mg/m³ or 0.1 ppm (8hr/day-40hr/wk-PP/S). *IDLH:* 300 mg/m³.

Symptoms: Eye and skin irritation; Corneal inflammation; Corneal and skin ulceration; Dermatitis; Skin redness and tissue death; Visual disturbances. *End-point Targets:* Eyes; Skin. *Usage:* Leather tanning; Making gelatin insoluble; Fur coats to strengthen animal fibers; Rubber; Dyes; Cosmetics; p-Benzoquinonedioxime; Hydroquinone; Fungicide manufacturing; Oxidizing agent; Photography; Adhesives; Pharmaceuticals; Cortisone; Barbiturates; Polymers; Resins. *References:* 223, 304, 388.

p-Quinone *see* **Quinone.**

R 40 (tn) *see* **Methyl chloride.**

Ramor *see* **Thallium.**

Raney nickel (tn) *see* **Nickel.**

Red fuming nitric acid *see* **Nitric acid.**

Refrigerant 11 *see* **Fluorotrichloromethane.**

Refrigerant 12 *see* **Dichlorodifluoromethane.**

Refrigerant 13B1 *see* **Trifluorobromomethane.**

Refrigerant 21 *see* **Dichloromonofluoromethane.**

Refrigerant 114 *see* **Dichlorotetrafluoroethane.**

Rene 41 (tn) *see* **Nickel.**

RFNA *see* **Nitric acid.**

Rhoplex AC-33 (tn) *see* **Ethyl methacrylate.**

Rubbing alcohol *see* **Isopropyl alcohol.**

Rutile: *see* **Titanium dioxide.**

S 1 (tn) *see* **Chloropicrin.**

Salaesthin (tn) *see* **Methylene chloride.**

Santryuum (tn) *see* **Ethylene dibromide.**

Seekay wax *see* **Tetrachloronaphthalene.**

Selenium *TN/synonyms:* Elemental selenium; Selenium alloy. *Compounds:* Sodium selenite; Sodium selenate; Selenium dioxide. *OSHA PEL:* 0.2 mg/m^3-PP/S. *IDLH:* Unknown. *Symptoms:* Eye, nasal, throat, bronchial, and mucous membrane irritation; Bronchitis; Chills; Coated tongue; Cough; Dermatitis; Eye redness; Fatigue; Fever; Fingernail changes; Garlic breath; Gastrointestinal distress; Headaches; Irritability; Labored or difficult breathing; Loss of smell; Metallic taste; Nausea; Nervousness; Nosebleeds; Pallor; Skin and eye burns; Sneezing; Vision disturbances; Vomiting. Suspected of causing Anemia; Liver and kidney damage. *End-point Targets:* Upper respiratory system; Eyes; Skin; Liver; Kidneys; Blood. *Usage:* Glass; Photography; Pigments; Electrical instruments and apparatus; Radios; Televisions; Selenium photocells; Semiconductors; Telephotographic apparatus; Rubber; Steel; Copper; Metal alloys; Textiles; Petroleum; Medical therapeutic agents; Photocopiers. *Note:* Occurs as an impurity in most sulfide ores. Historically established as a neurotoxin. *References:* 17, 227, 304, 388, 413.

Selenium alloy *see* **Selenium.**

Sevin *see* **Carbaryl.**

Sewer gas *see* **Hydrogen sulfide.**

SFA *see* **Sodium fluoroacetate.**

Shell silver *see* **Silver.**

Sicol 150 (tn) *see* **Di-sec octyl phthalate.**

Silber *see* **Silver.**

Silflake *see* **Silver.**

Silica *TN/synonyms:* Silica flour; Crystalline silica; Cristobalite; Quartz; Tridymite; Tripoli. *NIOSH:* Carcinogen at any exposure level. *NIOSH REL:* 0.05 mg/m^3 (10hr/day-40hr/wk). *OSHA PEL:* cristobalite, tridymite: 0.05 mg/m^3 (10hr/day-40hr/wk); quartz, Tripoli: 0.10 mg/m^3 (10hr/day-

40hr/wk). *IDLH:* NE. *Symptoms:* Cough; Labored or difficult breathing; Wheezing; Impaired pulmonary function; Silicosis; Progressive massive fibrosis; Autoimmune disease; Systemic sclerosis; Scleroderma. Suspected of causing Cancer (lung). *End-point Targets:* Respiratory system. *Usage:* Inert filler in flour; Toothpaste; Scouring powder; Metal polishes; Sandblasting; Clay; Glazing. *Note:* A component of many mineral dusts. *References:* 280, 292, 304, 311, 388, 423.

Silica flour *see* **Silica.**

Silica gel *see* **Amorphous silica.**

Silicate mica *see* **Mica.**

Silicon dioxide (amorphous) *see* **Amorphous silica.**

Silpowder *see* **Silver.**

Silver *TN/synonyms:* Argentum; Argentum crede; CI77820 (tn); Shell silver; Silver atom; Silver colloidal; Silflake; Silpowder; Silber. *Compounds:* Silver nitrate; Silver (I) oxide; Silver (II) oxide; Silver sulfide; Silver chloride. *OSHA PEL:* 0.01 mg/m³ (8hr/day-40hr/wk-PP/S). *IDLH:* NE. *Symptoms:* Upper respiratory irritation; Blue-gray eyes, nasal septum, throat, and skin (irreversible aygyria); Skin irritation and ulcerations; Gastrointestinal distress; Contact dermatitis; Silver deposits in neurons in the central nervous system. Suspected of causing Listlessness; Loss of appetite; Malaise; Memory loss. *End-point Targets:* Nasal septum; Skin; Eyes. *Usage:* Jewelry; Photography; Electrical and electronic components; Paints; Batteries; Brazing alloys and solders; Sterling ware; Mirrors; Dental amalgam; Medicine (treatment of burns); Formaldehyde; Ethylene oxide; Water purification and disinfection (swimming pools); Cloud seeding; Antibacterial agent; Metal cleaners. *References:* 304, 320, 388.

Silver atom *see* **Silver.**

Silver colloidal *see* **Silver.**

Sinafid M-49 (tn) *see* **Methyl parathion.**

Sixty-Three Special E.C. Insecticide (tn) *see* **Methyl parathion.**

Soda lye *see* **Sodium hydroxide.**

Sodium borates (borax) *see* **Boron.**

Sodium fluoroacetate *TN/synonyms:* SFA; Sodium monofluoroacetate. *OSHA PEL:* 0.05 mg/m³ (8hr/day-40hr/wk); 0.15 mg/m³ (exposure not to exceed 15 min). *IDLH:* 5 mg/m³. *Symptoms:* Alternating weak and strong pulse; Apprehension; Auditory hallucinations; Blurred vision; Brain damage and atrophy; Cardiac arrest; Cerebellar dysfunction; Coma; Convulsions; Death; Ectopic heartbeat; Excessive salivation; Facial numbness, tingling, or prickling sensation; Heart rate over 100 beats per minute; Incoordination; Involuntary eye movement; Kidney failure; Kidney, liver, neurologic, and thyroid dysfunction; Loss of speech; Muscle twitching; Neurologic impairment; Psychomotor agitation; Pulmonary edema; Ventricular fibrillation; Vomiting. *End-point Targets:* Cardiovascular system; Lungs; Kidneys; Central nervous system. *Usage:* Rodenticide; Predator elimination (coyotes). *References:* 228, 304, 388.

Sodium hydrate *see* **Sodium hydroxide.**

Sodium hydroxide *TN/synonyms:* Caustic soda; Lye; Soda lye; Sodium hydrate. *OSHA PEL:* 2 mg/m³ (ceiling limit). *IDLH:* 250 mg/m³. *Symptoms:* Eye, nasal, skin, and upper respiratory irritation; Burns (eyes and skin); Cold, clammy skin; Collapse; Corneal swelling, ulceration, and opacity; Death; Esophageal perforation and strictures; Excessive salivation; Eyes become sensitive to light; Glottis, pharyngeal, esophageal, and intracellular swelling; Mucous membrane tissue death; Nasal passage ulceration; Pneumonia; Shock; Temporary hair loss; Tissue corrosion;

Vomiting. Suspected of causing Cancer. *End-point Targets:* Eyes; Respiratory system. *Usage:* Aluminum processing; Bleaches; Cellophane; Disinfectant; Dissolving casein and rubber; Dyes; Electroplating; Etching glass; Explosives; Fats; Fluorocarbons; Food industry (peeling fruits and vegetables); Household anti-mildew agent and fungicide; Laundry detergents; Metal processing; Oxide coatings; Paper; Petroleum refining; Plastics; Rayon; Resins; Soaps; Stain remover; Textiles; Tin plating; Vegetable oil refining; Veterinary medicine; Water treatment; Oven cleaners. *References:* 8, 229, 304, 388.

Sodium monofluoroacetate *see* **Sodium fluoroacetate.**

Soilfume (tn) *see* **Ethylene dibromide.**

Solmethine (tn) *see* **Methylene chloride.**

Solvent ether *see* **Ethyl ether.**

Spirits of hartshorn *see* **Ammonia.**

Spirits of turpentine *see* **Turpentine.**

Spirits of wine *see* **Ethanol.**

Spotting naphtha *see* **Stoddard solvent.**

Stable pentaborane *see* **Pentaborane.**

Steam distilled turpentine *see* **Turpentine.**

Stibine *TN/synonyms:* Antimony hydride; Antimony trihydride; Hydrogen antimonide. *OSHA PEL:* 0.1 ppm or 0.5 mg/m³ (8hr/day-40hr/wk). *IDLH:* 40 mg/m³. *Symptoms:* Pulmonary irritation; Abdominal and lumbar pain; Absence of urine formation; Capillary engorgement; Conjunctivitis; Corneal inflammation; Death; Decreased leukocytes in blood; Dermatitis; Destruction of red blood cells; Diarrhea; Excessive proliferation of normal cells in spleen; Glomerular kidney inflammation; Hair loss; Headaches; Heart, kidney, and liver damage; Hemoglobin, albumin, and blood in urine; Hemolytic anemia; Increase in erythrocytes in blood; Jaundice; Labored or difficult breathing; Myocardial swelling; Nasal septum ulceration; Nausea; Pneumoconiosis; Shock; Silicosis; Vomiting; Weak, irregular pulse; Weakness; Weight loss. *End-point Targets:* Blood; Liver; Kidneys; Lungs; Central nervous system. *Usage:* Fumigant; Silicone; Semi-conductors. *Synergistic effects:* Forms when alloys containing certain forms of antimony compounds are treated with steam or any source of fresh hydrogen. *References:* 230, 304, 388.

Stibium *see* **Antimony.**

Stoddard solvent *TN/synonyms:* Dry cleaning safety solvent; Mineral spirits; Petroleum solvent; Spotting naphtha; Petroleum ether. *NIOSH REL:* 350 mg/m³ (10hr/day-40hr/wk); 1,800 mg/m³ (ceiling limit, 15 min exposure). *OSHA PEL:* 100 ppm or 525 mg/m³ (8hr/day-40hr/wk-PP/S). *IDLH:* 29,500 mg/m³. *Symptoms:* Eye, nasal, and throat irritation; Dizziness; Dermatitis. *End-point Targets:* Skin; Eyes; Respiratory system; Central nervous system. *Usage:* Dry cleaning; Enamel and oil based paints; Wood stains and finishes; Varnishes; Pesticide inert ingredient; Pearl glue; Household cleaners; Furniture polish; Oven cleaners. *Classification:* Organic solvent (Refined Petroleum). *References:* 8, 186, 304, 383, 388, 423.

Strobane-T (tn) *see* **Chlorinated camphene.**

Styrene *TN/synonyms:* Ethenyl benzene; Phenylethylene; Styrene monomer; Styrol; Vinyl benzene; Cinnamene. *OSHA PEL:* 50 ppm or 215 mg/m³ (8hr/day-40hr/wk-PP/S); 100 ppm or 425 mg/m³ (exposure not to exceed 15 min). *ATSDR MRL:* 70 ppm

(Ingestion, more than 14 days). *ATSDR NOAEL:* 1 ppm (Inhalation, more than 365 days). *IDLH:* 5,000 ppm. *Symptoms:* Eye, nasal, and throat irritation; Anxiety; Central nervous system depression; Decreased ability to concentrate; Defatting dermatitis; Depression; Drowsiness; Electroencephalogram changes; Fatigue; Headaches; Immune system sensitization; Impaired balance and coordination; Insomnia; Irritability; Kidney damage; Lassitude; Listlessness; Malaise; Memory changes; Nausea; Nervousness; Sexual disorders; Unconsciousness due to narcotic effects; Unsteady gait; Vomiting; Weakness. Suspected of causing Granules in red blood cells; Decrease in hemoglobin and erythrocytes; Chromosomal aberrations; Spontaneous abortions; Low birth weight; Cancer (leukemia and lymphoma). *End-point Targets:* Central nervous system; Respiratory system; Eyes; Skin. *Usage:* Adhesives; Appliances; Audio and video tape cassettes; Automobile parts; Battery cases; Brushes; Car bumpers; Carpet backing; Carpeting; Cements; Combs; Conveyer belts; Cultured marble; Dishwashing liquid; Disposable dinnerware; Drinking cups; Eyeglasses; Fiberglass laminating; Fiberglass; Food containers; Food flavoring; Furniture; Games; Hobby kits; Ink; Insulators; Insulation boards; Latex paint; Loose-fill packaging; Luggage; Molded shutters; Packaging; Paper coatings; Pesticide inert ingredient; Photocopier toner and ink; Picnic coolers; Pipes; Plastics; Polystyrene; Polyesters; Resins; Refrigerator doorliners; Room dividers; Rubber; Shower drains; Shower stalls; Soap dishes; Telephones; Television cabinets; Tires; Toys; Upholstery backcoatings; Vinyl floor tiles; Wall panels; Weatherstriping. Found in Cigarette smoke; Automobile exhaust. *Additives:* Usually contains an inhibitor such as tert-butylcatechol. *Classification:* Organic solvent. *Note:* Historically established as a neurotoxin.

The styrene in food packaging will leach into food. *References:* 17, 299, 304, 367, 383, 388, 413, 423, 429, 430, 459, 460.

Styrene monomer *see* **Styrene.**

Styrol *see* **Styrene.**

Sulfamate *see* **Ammonium sulfamate.**

Sulfate wood turpentine *see* **Turpentine.**

Sulfotepp *see* **TEDP.**

Sulfuretted hydrogen *see* **Hydrogen sulfide.**

Sulfur chloride *see* **Sulfur monochloride.**

Sulfur difluoride dioxide *see* **Sulfur fluoride.**

Sulfur dioxide *TN/synonyms:* Sulfurous acid anhydride; Sulfurous oxide; Sulfur oxide. *OSHA PEL:* 2 ppm or 5 mg/m³ (8hr/day-40hr/wk-PP/S); 5 ppm or 10 mg/m³ (exposure not to exceed 15 min). *IDLH:* 100 ppm. *Symptoms:* Eye, nasal, throat, and skin irritation; Abdominal pain; Agitation; Alters sense of taste and smell; Asphyxia; Blindness; Bronchial asthma; Bronchial spasms; Bronchitis; Chemical bronchial pneumonia; Chemical sensitivity; Chest pains and constriction; Choking; Convulsions; Corneal damage; Cough; Cyanosis; Death; Dental caries (tooth decay); Diarrhea; Difficulty swallowing; Emphysema; Eye and skin burns; Fatigue; Fever; Hives; Inflammation of the iris; Inhibits thyroid function; Labored or difficult breathing; Laryngeal swelling; Loss of smell; Menstrual disorders; Metabolic acidosis; Mouth and pharyngeal redness; Nasal discharge; Nasal septum ulceration; Nausea; Nervous system disorders; Neurotic disorders; Olfactory fatigue; Periodontal and gingival disorders; Peripheral nerve inflammation; Pulmonary edema and impaired function; Reflex bronchial constriction; Respiratory paralysis and arrest; Skin lesions; Sneezing; Tearing; Tooth sensitivity to temperature changes; Tracheitis; Tremors; Vertigo; Vomiting. *End-point Targets:* Respiratory system; Skin; Eyes. *Usage:* Acetyl chloride; Antiseptics; Beer; Beet sugars; Bleaching agent; Chlorine dioxide; Corn syrups; Disinfectant; Flour bleaching; Food processing; Fruit and vegetable preservative; Gelatin; Glass; Glue; Insect fumigant; Leather tanning; Liquors; Mineral processing; Molasses; Oil refining; Oils; Paper; Pesticide inert ingredient; Petroleum refining; Refrigerant; Sodium sulfate; Solvent; Sufuryl chloride; Textiles; Thionyl chloride; Tile drain cleaning agent; Veterinary medicine; Warning agent in grain fumigants; Water treatment; Wicker products; Wine. Found in diesel exhaust. *Synergistic effects:* Reacts with water to form sulfuric acid. *Note:* About 10 to 20% of the adult population is estimated to be hypersensitive to the adverse respiratory effects. Historically established as a neurotoxin. *References:* 232, 304, 388, 394, 413, 423.

Sulfuric acid *TN/synonyms:* Battery acid; Hydrogen sulfate; Oil of vitriol. *OSHA PEL:* 1 mg/m³ (8hr/day-40hr/wk-PP/S). *IDLH:* 80 mg/m³. *Symptoms:* Eye, nasal, and throat irritation; Pulmonary edema; Bronchitis; Emphysema; Conjunctivitis; Stomach inflammation; Dental erosion; Tracheobronchitis; Skin and eye burns; Dermatitis. *End-point Targets:* Respiratory system; Eyes; Skin; Teeth. *Usage:* Vehicle batteries; Pesticide inert ingredient; Fiberglass. *References:* 304, 388, 423, 429.

Sulfur monochloride *TN/synonyms:* Sulfur chloride; Sulfur subchloride; Thiosulfurous dichloride. *OSHA PEL:* 1 ppm or 6 mg/m³ (Ceiling limit-PP/S). *IDLH:* 10 ppm. *Symptoms:* Eye, nasal, throat, and respiratory irritation; Circulatory collapse and shock; Clammy skin; Cough; Death; Diarrhea;

Epigastric pain; Esophageal, gastric, and pyloric strictures; Eye and skin burns; Gastric hemorrhage; Glottis swelling; Difficulty swallowing; Inhibited blood clotting; Kidney failure; Mucous membrane corrosion, pain, and tissue death; Nausea; Pulmonary edema; Tearing; Thirst; Vomiting; Weak, rapid pulse. *End-point Targets:* Respiratory system; Skin; Eyes. *Usage:* Textiles; Rubber; Synthetic rubbers; Rubber goods; Lubricants; Varnishes; Inks; Paints; Cements; Dyes; Vegetable oils; Hardening soft woods; Sugar juices; Military poisonous gas; Pharmaceutical; Gold extraction; Rubber-coated fabrics; Pesticide inert ingredient. *Synergistic effects:* Decomposes violently in water to form Hydrochloric acid; Sulfur dioxide; Sulfur; Sulfite; Thiosulfate; and hydrogen sulfide. *References:* 233, 304, 388, 423.

Sulfurous acid anhydride *see* **Sulfur dioxide.**

Sulfurous oxide *see* **Sulfur dioxide.**

Sulfur oxide *see* **Sulfur dioxide.**

Sulfur subchloride *see* **Sulfur monochloride.**

Sulfuryl fluoride *TN/synonyms:* Sulfur difluoride dioxide. *OSHA PEL:* 5 ppm or 20 mg/m³ (8hr/day-40hr/wk); 10 ppm or 40 mg/m³ (exposure not to exceed 15 min). *IDLH:* 1,000 ppm. *Symptoms:* Respiratory irritation; Conjunctivitis; Nasal discharge; Numbness, tingling, or prickling sensation; Central nervous system depression. Suspected of causing Unconsciousness due to narcotic effects; Tremors; Convulsions; Pulmonary edema; Kidney injury. *End-point Targets:* Respiratory system; Central nervous system. *Usage:* Insecticide; Fumigant. *References:* 234, 304, 388.

Sulphocarbonic anhydride *see* **Carbon disulfide.**

Sulphuret of carbon *see* **Carbon disulfide.**

Superlysoform *see* **Formaldehyde.**

Suscon (tn) *see* **Chlorpyrifos.**

Symmetrical tetrabromoethane *see* **Acetylene tetrabromide.**

Symmetrical tetrachloroethane *see* **1,1,2,2-Tetrachloroethane.**

Synthetic 3956 (tn) *see* **Chlorinated camphene.**

Synthetic camphor *see* **Camphor.**

Systox *see* **Demeton.**

2,4,6-T *see* **2,4,6-Trichlorophenol.**

Tar camphor *see* **Naphthalene.**

TBE *see* **Acetylene tetrabromide.**

TBP *see* **Tributyl phosphate.**

TCE *see* **Trichloroethylene.**

TCP *see* **Triorthocresyl phosphate.**

TDI *see* **Toluene-2,4-diisocyanate.**

2,4-TDI *see* **Toluene-2,4-diisocyanate.**

TEA *see* **Triethylamine.**

Tear gas *see* **alpha-Chloroacetophenone.**

Tecsol (tn) *see* **Ethanol.**

Tecsol C (tn) *see* **Ethanol.**

TEDP *TN/synonyms:* Dithion; Sulfotepp; Tetraethyl dithionopyrophospha'e; Tetraethyl dithiopyro-phosphate. *OSHA PEL:* 0.2 mg/m³ (8hr/day-40hr/wk-PP/S). *IDLH:* 35 mg/m³. *Symptoms:* Eye and skin irritation; Abdominal cramps; Blurred vision; Bronchial constriction; Cardiac irregularities; Chest tightness; Cheyne-Stokes respiration; Ciliary muscle spasms; Constricted pupils; Convulsions; Cyanosis; Death; Diarrhea; Disorientation; Drowsiness; Excessive salivation; Eye pains; Giddiness; Headaches; Heart rate below 60 beats per minute; Heart rate over 100 beats per minute; High blood pressure; Incontinence; Incoordination; Inhibited cholinesterase; Labored or difficult breathing; Localized sweating; Loss of appetite; Mental confusion; Muscle twitching and involuntary contractions; Nasal discharge; Nausea; Paralysis; Pulmonary rales; Respiratory arrest; Slurred speech; Tearing; Vertigo; Vomiting; Weakness. Suspected of causing Hypothermia. *End-point Targets:* Central nervous system; Respiratory system; Cardiovascular system. *Usage:* Pesticide; Insecticide; Acaricide; Greenhouse fumigant. *References:* 235, 304, 388.

Tekwaisa (tn) *see* **Methyl parathion.**

TEL *see* **Tetraethyl lead.**

Tellurium *TN/synonyms:* Aurum paradoxum; Metallum problematum. *OSHA PEL:* 0.1 mg/m³ (8hr/day-40hr/wk-PP/S). *IDLH:* NE. *Symptoms:* Garlic breath; Profuse sweating; Dry mouth; Metallic taste; Somnolence; Loss of appetite; Nausea; Inability to sweat; Dermatitis; Skin lesions; Liver injury. *End-point Targets:* Skin; Central nervous system. *Usage:* Pigments; Chinaware; Porcelains; Enamels; Glass; Black finish silverware; Semiconductors; Blasting caps; Rubber; Cast iron. *References:* 235, 304, 388.

Telone (r) *see* **1,3-Dichloropropene.**

Telone C-17 (r) *see* **1,3-Dichloropropene.**

Telone II (r) (M-3993) *see* **1,3-Dichloropropene.**

TEPP *TN/synonyms:* Ethyl pyrophosphate; Tetraethyl pyrophosphate. *OSHA PEL:* 0.05 mg/m³ (8hr/day-40hr/wk). *IDLH:* 10 mg/m³. *Symptoms:* Blurred vision; Cardiac irregularities; Cheyne-Stokes respiration; Convulsions; Cyanosis; Diarrhea; Eye pain; Headaches; Localized sweating;

Loss of appetite; Low blood pressure; Muscle twitching; Nasal discharge; Nausea; Paralysis; Tearing; Tight chest; Vomiting; Weakness. *End-point Targets:* Central nervous system; Respiratory system; Cardiovascular system; Gastrointestinal tract. *Usage:* Insecticide. *References:* 265, 304, 388.

Terabol (r) *see* **Methyl bromide.**

delta-1,8-Terpodiene *see* **Limonene.**

Terr-O-Cide 15-D (tn) *see* **1,3-Dichloropropene.**

Terr-O-Cide 30-D (tn) *see* **1,3-Dichloropropene.**

Terr-O-Gas 57/43T (tn) *see* **1,3-Dichloropropene.**

Tetlen (tn) *see* **Tetrachloroethylene.**

Tetrabromoacetylene *see* **Acetylene tetrabromide.**

Tetrabromoethane *see* **Acetylene tetrabromide.**

1,1,2,2-Tetrabromoethane *see* **Acetylene tetrabromide.**

Tetracap (tn) *see* **Tetrachloroethylene.**

Tetrachlorethylene *see* **Tetrachloroethylene.**

1,1,2,2-Tetrachloroethane *TN/ synonyms:* Acetylene tetrachloride; Symmetrical tetrachloroethane. *NIOSH:* Carcinogen at any exposure level. *OSHA PEL:* 1 ppm or 7 mg/m^3 (8hr/ day-40hr/wk-PP/S). *IDLH:* 150 ppm. *Symptoms:* Eye irritation; Abdominal pains; Absence of reflex; Burning or prickling sensation in hands and or feet; Cancer; Cardiac arrhythmias; Central nervous system depression; Cellular damage; Changes in blood clotting; Cirrhosis; Coma; Constipation; Death; Decrease in white blood cells; Decrease in heart rate; Dermatitis; Diarrhea; Drowsiness; Enlarged and tender liver; Excessive monocytes

in the blood; Excessive sweating; Fatigue; Hand tremors; Headaches; Impaired mental processes, perception, manual dexterity, and equilibrium; Increased reaction time; Incoordination; Inebriation; Insomnia; Irritability; Jaundice; Kidney damage and inflammation; Lightheadedness; Liver diseases; Loss of appetite; Loss of gag reflexes; Low blood pressure; Malaise; Nausea; Nervousness; Neurological disturbances; Numbness in limbs; Paralysis; Respiratory failure; Ringing sound in ears; Skin dryness, crackling, scaling, and inflammation; Toxic hepatitis; Tremors; Unconsciousness; Unsteady gait; Vertigo; Vomiting; Weight loss. *End-point Targets:* Liver; Kidneys; Central nervous system. *Usage:* Adhesives; Artificial leather, pearls, and silk; Bleach; Cellulose; Cement; Copal; Crystallography; Denatured alcohol; Dichloroethylenes; Fats; Fur coats; Herbicide; Insecticide manufacturing; Lacquers; Metal cleaning and degreasing; Moth-proofing; Oils; Paint removers; Paints; Phosphorus; Photographic film; Phthalic anhydride; Polyesters; Resins; Rubber; Rust removers; Soil sterilization; Solvent; Sulfur; Tetrachloroethylene; Textiles; Trichloroethylene; Varnish; Waxes; Pesticide inert ingredient. *Classification:* Organic solvent; Chlorinated organic compounds. *References:* 254, 304, 383, 388, 399, 423.

Tetrachloroethene *see* **Tetrachloroethylene.**

Tetrachloroethylene *TN/synonyms:* Perchlorethylene; Perchloroethylene; Perk; Tetrachlorethylene; Perchlor; Carbon bichloride; Carbon dichloride; Per; Perc; 1,1,2,2-Tetrachloroethane; Tetrachloroethene; PCE; Ankilostin (tn); Antisal 1 (tn); Dee-Solv (tn); Didakene (tn); Dowper (tn); ENT 1860 (tn); Fedal-Un (tn); Nema (tn); Perclene (tn); Percosolv (tn); Perklone (tn); PerSec (tn); Tetlen (tn); Tetracap (tn); Tetraleno (tn);

Tetravee (tn); Tetroguer (tn); Tetropil (tn); Perawin (tn); Tetralex (tn); Dowclene EC (tn). *NIOSH:* Carcinogen at any exposure level. Minimize workplace exposure concentrations; limit number of workers exposed. *OSHA PEL:* 25 ppm or 170 mg/m³ (8hr/day-40hr/wk-PP/S). *ATSDR MRL:* 1 ppm (Inhalation, less than 15 days); 0.01 ppm (Inhalation, more than 14 days). *IDLH:* 500 ppm. *Symptoms:* Eye, nasal, throat, and upper respiratory irritation; Collapse; Coma; Death; Disorientation; Dizziness; Drowsiness; Flushed face and neck; Headaches; Incoordination; Lightheadedness; Liver and kidney damage; Loss of appetite; Loss of consciousness; Nausea; Neuropsychologic disturbances; Organic affective syndrome; Skin redness and burns; Somnolence; Toxic brain dysfunction; Tremors; Vertigo. Suspected of causing Cancer; Low birth weight; Menstrual disorders; Spontaneous abortions. *End-point Targets:* Brain; Liver; Kidneys; Eyes; Upper Respiratory system; Central Nervous system. *Usage:* Adhesives; Aerosol cleaners; Auto brake quieters and cleaners; Belt lubricants; Chemical intermediate; Detergents; Dry cleaning; Fabric finishes; Glues; Intermediate for Fluorocarbon 113, 114, 115, and 116; Lubricants; Metal cleaning; Pesticide inert ingredient; Pesticide intermediate; Pharmaceuticals; Polishes; Printing ink; Production of trichloroacetic acid; Rubber coatings; Rug, carpet, and upholstery shampoo; Sealants; Silicone lubricants; Silicone; Soap; Soot remover; Spot remover; Suede protectors; Textile processing; Used to dissolve fats, greases, waxes, and oils; Water repellents; Wood cleaner. Metabolizes as oxiranes and acryl chlorides which are highly cytotoxic. **Contaminates** breast milk. *Classification:* Organic solvent; Halogenated organic compound. *Note:* Neurotoxin. *References:* 8, 17, 304, 342, 383, 388, 395, 423, 429, 432.

1,1,2,2-Tetrachloroethylene *see* **Tetrachloroethylene.**

Tetrachloromethane *see* **Carbon tetrachloride.**

Tetrachloronaphthalene *TN/ synonyms:* Halowax; Nibren wax; Seekay wax. *OSHA PEL:* 2 mg/m³ (8hr/day-40hr/wk-PP/S). *IDLH:* Unknown. *Symptoms:* Acne-form dermatitis; Headaches; Fatigue; Loss of appetite; Vertigo; Jaundice; Liver injury; Kidney and heart swelling; Adrenal tissue death; Drowsiness; Indigestion; Nausea; Enlarged liver; Weakness; Coma. *End-point Targets:* Liver; Skin. *Usage:* Synthetic waxes; Electrical insulation; Lubricants; Batteries; Wood coatings; Paper; Textiles. No longer used as a pesticide. *References:* 238, 304, 388.

Tetraethoxysilane *see* **Ethyl silicate.**

Tetraethyl dithionopyrophosphate *see* **TEDP.**

Tetraethyl dithiopyro-phosphate *see* **TEDP.**

Tetraethyl lead *TN/synonyms:* Lead tetraethyl; TEL. *OSHA PEL:* 0.075 mg/m³ (8hr/day-40hr/wk-PP/S). *IDLH:* 40 mg/m³. *Symptoms:* Eye irritation; Abdominal pain; Albumin, cylindroids, and hemoglobin in urine; Anemia; Anxiety; Brain dysfunction; Colic; Coma; Constipation; Convulsions; Death; Delirium; Delusions; Depression; Diarrhea; Disorientation; Emotional instability; Fatigue; Hallucinations; Headaches; Heart rate below 60 beats per minutes; Hyper-reflexia; Hypothermia; Incoordination; Insomnia; Intracranial pressure; Irritability; Kidney lesions; Lassitude; Loss of appetite; Low blood pressure; Mania; Metallic taste; Muscle pains; Muscle weakness, pain, and cramps; Nausea; Nightmares; Numbness, tingling, or prickling sensations; Pallor; Psychosis;

Reduced urine formation; Respiratory failure; Restlessness; Spastic movements; Tremors; Visual disturbances; Vomiting; Weakness; Weight loss. *Endpoint Targets:* Central nervous system; Cardiovascular system; Kidneys; Eyes. *Usage:* Anti-knock gasoline additive. No longer used as a fungicide. *Note:* Historically established as a neurotoxin. *References:* 239, 304, 388, 413.

Tetraethyl pyrophosphate *see* **TEPP.**

Tetraethyl silicate *see* **Ethyl silicate.**

Tetrahydrofuran *TN/synonyms:* Diethylene oxide; 1,4-Epoxybutane; Tetramethylene; THF. *OSHA PEL:* 200 ppm or 590 mg/m³ (8hr/day-40hr/wk-PP/S); 250 ppm or 735 mg/m³ (exposure not to exceed 15 min). *IDLH:* 20,000 ppm. *Symptoms:* Eye and upper respiratory system irritation; Nausea; Dizziness; Headaches. *End-point Targets:* Eyes; Skin; Respiratory system; Central nervous system. *Usage:* Food packaging; Solvent; Oils; Rubber; Adipic acid; Indirect food additive; Food adjuvant; Resins; Plastics; Magnetic tapes; Cleaners; Printing ink; Adhesives; Lacquers; Motor fuels; Vitamins; Hormones; Perfumes; Pharmaceuticals; Insecticide manufacturing; Tetraethyl and trimethyl lead; Coatings. *References:* 240, 304, 388.

Tetrahydro-p-oxazine *see* **Morpholine.**

Tetrahydro-1,4-oxazine *see* **Morpholine.**

Tetraleno (tn) *see* **Tetrachloroethylene.**

Tetralex (tn) *see* **Tetrachloroethylene.**

Tetramethylene *see* **Tetrahydrofuran.**

Tetramethyl lead *TN/synonyms:* Lead tetramethyl; TML. *OSHA PEL:* 0.075 mg/m³ (8hr/day-40hr/wk-PP/S). *IDLH:* 40 mg/m³. *Symptoms:*

Abdominal pains; Albumin, cylindroids, and hemoglobin in urine; Anemia; Anxiety; Brain dysfunction; Colic; Coma; Constipation; Convulsions; Death; Delirium; Depression; Diarrhea; Dry throat; Fecal blood; Hallucinations; Heart muscle degeneration and swelling; Insomnia; Irritability; Loss of appetite; Low blood pressure; Mania; Metallic taste; Muscle weakness, pains, and cramps; Myocardial fragmentation; Nausea; Nightmares; Numbness, tingling, or prickling sensations; Peripheral circulatory collapse; Reduced urine formation; Restlessness; Thirst; Visual disturbances; Vomiting. *End-point Targets:* Central nervous system; Cardiovascular system; Kidneys. *Usage:* Anti-knock gasoline additive. *References:* 241, 304, 388.

Tetramethyl succinodinitrile *see* **Tetramethyl succinonitrile.**

Tetramethyl succinonitrile *TN/synonyms:* Tetramethyl succinodinitrile; TMSN. *OSHA PEL:* 3 mg/m³ or 0.5 ppm (8hr/day-40hr/wk-PP/S). *IDLH:* 5 ppm. *Symptoms:* Eye, nasal, throat, and respiratory irritation; Headaches; Nausea; Convulsions; Coma; Pulmonary edema; Liver damage; Hemoglobin oxidizes to ferric form; Liver and kidney fatty degeneration; Respiratory distress; Fatigue; Pneumonia. *End-point Targets:* Central nervous system. *Usage:* Rocket propellents; Explosives; Diesel fuel additive; Military warfare gas. *Classification:* Organic solvent (Nitrile compound). *References:* 304, 306, 383, 388.

Tetramethylthiuram disulfide *see* **Thiram.**

Tetravee (tn) *see* **Tetrachloroethylene.**

Tetroguer (tn) *see* **Tetrachloroethylene.**

Tetropil (tn) *see* **Tetrachloroethylene.**

T-Gas (tn) *see* **Ethylene oxide.**

Thallium *TN/synonyms:* Ramor. *Compounds:* Thallium acetate; Thallium chloride; Thallium nitrate; Thallium oxide; Thallium sulfate; Thallium carbonate; Thallium bromide; Thallium iodine; Thallium fluoride. *OSHA PEL:* 0.1 mg/m^3 (8hr/day-40hr/wk-PP/S). *ATSDR MRL:* 0.00008 ug/kg/day (Ingestion, less than 14 days). *IDLH:* 20 mg/m^3. *Symptoms:* Abdominal pains; Axonal neuron degeneration; Burning feet phenomenon; Cardiac and respiratory failure; Chest pains; Convulsions; Death; Delerium; Diarrhea; Dropping or drooping of a body part or organ; Electrocardiogram abnormalities; Eye disorder which prevents both eyes from focusing on the same object; Hair loss; Incoordination; Kidney tubular tissue death; Liver and kidney damage; Liver tissue death, fatty changes, and altered serum levels; Mitochondria degeneration; Multiple cranial palsies; Muscle cramps and twitching; Muscle fiber death, splitting, and central nucleation; Myelin loss; Myocardial damage to the heart; Nausea; Numbness of toes and fingers; Paralysis of the legs; Peripheral nerve inflammation; Polyneuropathy; Psychosis; Pulmonary edema; Retrosternal tightness; Tremors; Vomiting. Suspected of causing Birth defects; Structural alterations in the brains of fetuses; Fetal growth retardation; Embryo lethality; Decreased fertility; DNA damage; Dominant lethal mutations in males. *End-point Targets:* Eyes; Central nervous system; Lungs; Liver; Kidneys; Gastrointestinal tract; Body hair. *Usage:* Semiconductor switches and closures; Cardiac imaging; Refractive optical glass and artificial gems; Fireworks; Photocells; Rodenticide; Fungicides; Mercury and silver alloy. Found in Cigarette smoke; Power plants; Cement plants; and Smelters. *Note:* Historically established as a neurotoxin. *References:* 299, 304, 378, 388, 413.

THF *see* **Tetrahydrofuran.**

Thifor (tn) *see* **Endosulfan.**

Thiodan (tn) *see* **Endosulfan.**

Thiomethanol *see* **Methyl mercaptan.**

Thiomethyl alcohol *see* **Methyl mercaptan.**

Thionax (tn) *see* **Endosulfan.**

Thionex (tn) *see* **Endosulfan.**

Thiophenit (tn) *see* **Methyl parathion.**

Thiosulfurous dichloride *see* **Sulfur monochloride.**

Thiram *TN/synonyms:* bis(Dimethylthiocarbamoyl) disulfide; Tetramethylthiuram disulfide. *OSHA PEL:* 5 mg/m^3 (8hr/day-40hr/wk-PP/S varies). *IDLH:* 1,500 mg/m^3. *Symptoms:* Eye and mucous membrane irritation; Alcohol intolerance; Allergic dermatitis; Catatonia; Chest pain; Coma; Confusion; Cough; Death; Delirium; Dermatitis; Diarrhea; Dizziness; Drowsiness; Emotional liability; Enlarged thyroid gland; Flaccid paralysis; Hallucinations; Headaches; Heart rate over 100 beats per minute; Hepatitis; Incoordination; Inhibited DNA synthesis; Lethargy; Liver dysfunction; Loss of appetite; Loss of muscle tone; Myocardial disorders caused by defective metabolism; Nausea; Nosebleeds; Peripheral neuropathy; Respiratory paralysis; Skin lesions; Suppression of tendon reflexes; Tremors; Vomiting; Weakness; Weight loss. *End-point Targets:* Respiratory system; Skin. *Usage:* Pesticide; Wood preservative; Mushroom disinfectant; Synthetic rubber; Bacteriostat soap; Medicine; Antifungal agents; Lube-oil additive; Antiseptic sprays; Fats; Oils. *Note:* Alcohol intolerance may produce Flushed face; Cardiac palpitations; Rapid pulse; Dizziness; and Low blood pressure. *References:* 242, 299, 304, 388.

Threthylen (tn) *see* **Trichloroethylene.**

Threthylene (tn) *see* **Trichloro-ethylene.**

Thylpar M-50 (tn) *see* **Methyl parathion.**

Tin *Inorganic:* Metallic tin; Tin flake; Tin powder. *Organic:* Stannous chloride; Stannous oxide; Dibutyltin chloride; Tin salt; Tin crystals; Tin protochloride; Stannic anhydride; Tin peroxide; Stannic acid; Dichlorodibutyltin; Dichlorodibutyl-stannane; Organotin compounds; Tributyltin oxide; Methyltins. *OSHA PEL: Inorganic:* 2.0 mg/m^3 (8hr/day-40hr/wk-PP/S); *Organic:* 0.1 mg/m^3 (8hr/day-40hr/wk-PP/S). *IDLH: Inorganic*-400 mg/m^3; *Organic*-Unknown. *Symptoms:* Eye, skin, upper respiratory, stomach, and intestinal irritation; Abdominal pains; Aggressiveness; Benign form of pneumoconiosis (stannosis); Convulsions; Cough; Death; Dermatitis; Disorientation; Swelling of the white matter of the central nervous system; Eyes become sensitive to light; Headaches; Impaired memory; Kidney damage; Liver fatty degeneration; Loss of concentration; Loss of sensation; Memory loss; Metal fume fever; Partial paralysis; Proximal tubule epithelial degeneration; Psychotic behavior; Psychoneurologic disturbances; Respiratory depression; Sensory disturbances; Severe itching; Skin burns; Tremors; Unconsciousness due to inadequate blood flow to the brain; Urine retention; Vertigo; Visual impairment; Vomiting; Weakness. Suspected of causing Anemia; Destruction of red blood cells; Liver tissue death; Immune system impairment; Birth defects; Low birth weight; DNA damage; Genetic mutations. *End-point Targets:* Central nervous system; Eyes; Liver; Urinary tract; Skin; Blood. *Usage:* Aircraft components; Anthelmintic drugs; Bactericides; Brass; Bronze; Coated wire; Colored glass; Containers; Dental materials; Dyes; Electronics; Fabrics; Fencing; Fingernail polish; Flooring; Food canning; Fungicide; Glass; Leather; Mining; Nuclear reactor components; Paints; Paper; Perfumes; Pesticides; Pewter; Pharmaceuticals; Pipes; Polyurethane foams; Rodent repellents; Ropes; Silicone; Silverware; Soaps; Soft plastics; Soldering material; Wood preservative. *Classification:* Organotin. *Note:* Historically established as a neurotoxin. *References:* 299, 304, 368, 388, 413.

Tin flake *see* **Tin.**

Tin powder *see* **Tin.**

Titanium dioxide *TN/synonyms:* Rutile; Titanium oxide; Titanium peroxide. *NIOSH:* Carcinogen at any exposure level. Reduce exposure to lowest feasible concentration. *OSHA PEL:* 10 mg/m^3 (8hr/day-40hr/wk). *IDLH:* NE. *Symptoms:* Pulmonary fibrosis, lesions, and irritation; Contact dermatitis; Allergic sensitization; Bronchitis. Suspected of causing Cancer. *End-point Targets:* Lungs. *Usage:* Ceramic pigments; Enamels; Paints; Lacquers; Inks; Plastics; Paper; Water-based paints; Leather finishes; Confectionery panned goods; Sunscreens; Icings; Cosmetics; Porcelain; Floor coverings; Fabrics; Upholstery; Nylon; Rayon; Semiconductors; Adhesives; Glass fibers; Tablet coatings; Rubbers; Sugar syrups; Roofing; Dry beverage mixtures; Tobacco wrappings; Ointments; Lotions; Body dusting powders; White cheese; Food additive; Varnishes; Porcelain glazing; Tires; Paperboard; White shoe polish; Dyes; Pesticide inert ingredient. *References:* 243, 299, 304, 388, 423.

Titanium oxide *see* **Titanium dioxide.**

Titanium peroxide *see* **Titanium dioxide.**

TMA *see* **Trimellitic anhydride.**

TMAN *see* **Trimellitic anhydride.**

TML *see* **Tetramethyl lead.**

TMSN *see* **Tetramethyl succinonitrile.**

TNT *see* **2,4,6-Trinitrotoluene.**

TOCP *see* **Triorthocresyl phosphate.**

Toluene *TN/synonyms:* Methyl benzene; Methyl benzol; Phenyl methane; Toluol. *OSHA PEL:* 100 ppm or 375 mg/m³ (8hr/day-40hr/wk-PP/S); 150 ppm or 560 mg/m³ (exposure not to exceed 15 min). *ATSDR MRL:* 4 ppm (Inhalation, less than 15 days); 1 ppm (Inhalation, more than 14 days). *IDLH:* 2,000 ppm. *Symptoms:* Eye, skin, and respiratory irritation; Abdominal pain; Anemia; Birth defects; Central nervous system dysfunction and depression; Coma; Confusion; Death; Delirium; Dermatitis; Dilated pupils; Dizziness; Drowsiness; Dry skin; Emotional instability; Enlarged liver; Euphoria; Fatigue; Fetal anomalies and developmental delay; Fetal central nervous system dysfunction; Hallucinations; Headaches; Impaired reaction time, perception, and motor control; Incoordination; Insomnia; Liver disorders and injury; Mild to severe toxic brain dysfunction; Muscle fatigue; Nausea; Nervousness; Neurobehavioral changes; Numbness, tingling, or prickling sensation; Organic affective syndrome; Psychosis; Tearing; Vertigo; Vision disturbances; Vomiting; Weakness. Suspected of causing Blurred vision; Involuntary eye movement; Tremors; Staggering gait; Abnormal electroencephalogram. *End-point Targets:* Central nervous system; Liver; Skin. *Usage:* Paint; Paint rust proofing; Paint remover and thinners; Pesticide inert ingredient; Plastics; Printing ink; Gasoline and Gasoline additive; Cosmetics; Stain remover; Leather; Detergents; Cleaning agents; Pharmaceuticals; Medicine; Paper; Asphalt; Explosives; Coatings; Resins; Gums; Rubber; Lacquer; Adhesive; Fingernail polish; Furniture; Fabric coatings; Fiberglass; Solvent; Fiberglass bathtubs; Porcelain enameling of steel (bathtubs/appliances); Magnetic tapes; Perfumes; Rubber cement; Paint brush cleaner; Glue; Dye; Shoes; Benzene; Caprolactam; Polyurethane; Dental adhesive. Found in Automobile exhaust; Cigarette smoke. *Classification:* Organic solvent; Polar volatile organic compounds. *Note:* Historically established as a neurotoxin. *References:* 17, 19, 144, 286, 304, 383, 388, 413, 423, 429, 432, 449, 451, 452.

Toluene-2,4-diisocyanate *TN/synonyms:* TDI; 2,4-TDI; 2,4-Toluene diisocyanate; Polyisocyanates. *NIOSH:* Carcinogen at any exposure level. *OSHA PEL:* 0.005 ppm or 0.040 mg/m³ (8hr/day-40hr/wk-PP/S); 0.020 ppm or 0.150 mg/m³ (exposure not to exceed 15 min). *EPA/OTS:* > 0.001 ppm (Pulmonary hypersensitivity; substantial lung dysfunction). *IDLH:* 10 ppm. *Symptoms:* Nasal and throat irritation; Choking; Paroxysmal cough; Chest pains; Retrosternal soreness; Nausea; Vomiting; Abdominal pains; Bronchial spasms; Pulmonary edema; Labored or difficult breathing; Asthma; Conjunctivitis; Tearing; Dermatitis; Pulmonary and skin sensitizer; Allergic-type symptoms. Suspected of causing Cancer; Genetic mutations; Cerebral dysfunction; Blurred vision; Involuntary eye movement; Tremors; Abnormal electroencephalogram; Staggering gait. *End-point Targets:* Respiratory system; Skin. *Usage:* Plastics; Adhesives; Particle board; Plywood; Elastic; Foam cushions; Flexible foam; Paints; Automotive paint; Coatings; Foam blown insulation; Foam caulking; Hardwood floor sealants; Waterproofing agents; Automobile products; Furniture finishes; Polyurethane; Printing inks. *Synergistic effects:* Reacts slowly with water to form carbon dioxide and polyureas. *Note:* 13-17% of the general population and about 20% of the workers to experience allergic-type reactions. *References:* 144, 304, 306, 388, 391, 429, 445.

2,4-Toluene diisocyanate *see* **Toluene-2,4-diisocyanate.**

alpha-Toluenol *see* **Benzyl alcohol.**

o-Toluidine *TN/synonyms:* o-Aminotoluene; 2-Aminotoluene; 1-Methyl-2-aminobenzene; o-Methylaniline; 2-Methylaniline; ortho-Toluidine. *NIOSH:* Carcinogen at any exposure level. *NIOSH REL:* 2 ppm or 9 mg/m^3 (10hr/day-40hr/wk). *OSHA PEL:* 5 ppm or 22 mg/m^3 (8hr/day-40hr/wk). *ACGIH:* Suspected human carcinogen. *IDLH:* 100 ppm. *Symptoms:* Anemia; Blood and hemoglobin in urine; Cardiac arrhythmias; Cardiovascular collapse; Confusion; Convulsions; Cyanosis; Death; Dermatitis; Disorientation; Dizziness; Drowsiness; Dry throat; Eye burns; Headaches; Hemoglobin oxidizes to ferric form; Inability to utilize oxygen; Incoordination; Lethargy; Loss of appetite; Nausea; Navy blue to black lips, tongue, and mucous membranes; Painful urination; Renal insufficiency; Respiratory paralysis; Ringing or tingling in the ear; Shock; Skin lesions; Slate gray skin; Vertigo; Vomiting; Weakness; Weight loss. Suspected of causing Cancer (bladder); Genetic mutations; Cerebral dysfunction; Blurred vision; Involuntary eye movement; Tremors; Staggering gait; Abnormal electroencephalogram. *End-point Targets:* Blood; Kidneys; Liver; Cardiovascular system; Skin; Eyes. *Usage:* Textile printing; Dyes; Resins; Rubber; Glucose; Rodine based products; Pharmaceuticals; Pesticide intermediate. Found in Tobacco smoke. *Classification:* Aromatic amines. *References:* 144, 197, 304, 385, 388, 389, 418.

ortho-Toluidine *see* **o-Toluidine.**

Toluol *see* **Toluene.**

Tolyethylene *see* **Vinyl toluene.**

Toxakil (tn) *see* **Chlorinated camphene.**

Toxaphene *see* **Chlorinated camphene.**

Toxilic anhydride *see* **Maleic anhydride.**

TPP *see* **Triphenyl phosphate.**

Tremolite *see* **Asbestos.**

Tretylene (tn) *see* **Trichloroethylene.**

Triad (tn) *see* **Trichloroethylene.**

Trial (tn) *see* **Trichloroethylene.**

Triasol (tn) *see* **Trichloroethylene.**

Tributyl ester of phosphoric acid *see* **Tributyl phosphate.**

Tributyl phosphate *TN/synonyms:* Butyl phosphate; TBP; Tributyl ester of phosphoric acid; tri-n-Butyl phosphate. *OSHA PEL:* 0.2 ppm or 2.5 mg/m^3 (8hr/day-40hr/wk-PP/S). *IDLH:* 125 ppm. *Symptoms:* Eye, throat, mucous membrane, respiratory, and skin irritation; Headaches; Nausea; Paralysis; Convulsions; Muscle twitching; Weakness; Pulmonary edema; Death. Suspected of inhibiting red blood cells and plasma cholinesterase enzymes. *End-point Targets:* Respiratory system; Skin; Eyes. *Usage:* Pesticide inert ingredient; Antifoaming agent; Plasticizer; Cellulose; Lacquers; Plastics; Vinyl resins; Heavy metal extraction; Aircraft hydraulic fluids; Pigments. *References:* 244, 304, 388, 423.

Tricalcium arsenate *see* **Calcium arsenate.**

Tricalcium ortho-arsenate *see* **Calcium arsenate.**

Tri-Chlor (tn) *see* **Chloropicrin.**

Trichloran (tn) *see* **Trichloroethylene.**

1,1,1-Trichloroethane *TN/synonyms:* Methyl chloroform; Methyltrichloromethane; Trichloromethylmethane; a-Trichloromethane; Chlorothene (tn); Aerothene TT (tn); Inhibisol (tn). *NIOSH REL:* 350 ppm (Ceiling limit). *OSHA PEL:* 350 ppm (8hr/day-40hr/wk); 450 ppm (exposure not to exceed 15 minutes). *ATSDR MRL:* 0.225 ppm (Inhalation, less than 15 days). *IDLH:* 1,000 ppm. *Symptoms:* Eye and skin irritation; Low blood pressure; Diarrhea; Vomiting; Central nervous system depression; Nausea; Dizziness; Cardiac arrhythmia; Respiratory failure; Mild liver damage; Skin red, dry, cracking, scaling, or swelling; Mental dullness; Lightheadedness; Loss of sensation; Incoordination; Headaches; Fatigue; Unconsciousness; Inebriation; Impaired perception, manual dexterity, and equilibrium; Increased reaction time; Drowsiness; Sleepiness; Weakness; Ringing sound in ears; Unsteady gait; Burning or prickling sensation in hands and or feet; Cellular damage; Decrease in heart rate; Changes in blood clotting; Death. Suspected of causing Low birth weight; Birth defects; Chromosomal aberrations. *End-point Targets:* Central nervous system. *Usage:* Adhesive cleaner; Adhesives; Aerosol spray paint; Aerosols; Battery terminal protectors; Belt lubricants; Brake cleaners; Carburetor cleaners; Carpet glue; Carpeting; Chlorine bleach scouring powder; Circuit board cleaners; Door spray lubricants; Drain cleaners; Dry cleaning; Electric shaver cleaners; Electronic component cleaners; Engine degreaser; Fabric finishes; Gasket remover and adhesive; Liquid cleaners and detergent; Lubricants; Oven cleaners; Paint primers; Paint remover and stripper; Paint; Pesticide inert ingredient; Pesticides intermediate; Photographic film; Printing inks; Rust remover; Shoe polish; Silicone lubricants; Solid rodenticides; Spot remover; Spray and solid insecticides; Spray degreasers; Stain repellents; Suede protectors; Textiles; Tire cleaners; Typewriter correction fluid; Varnishes; Wallpaper glue; Water repel-lents; Wigs; Wood cleaner, finishes, and stains. *Classification:* Organic solvent; Halogenated organic compound; Chlorinated organic compound. *References:* 328, 383, 388, 399, 423, 429, 432.

beta-Trichloroethane *see* **1,1, 2-Trichloroethane.**

1,1,2-Trichloroethane *TN/synonyms:* beta-Trichloroethane; Vinyl trichloride. *NIOSH:* Carcinogen at any exposure level. *OSHA PEL:* 10 ppm or 45 mg/m^3 (8hr/day-40hr/wk-PP/S). *IDLH:* 500 ppm. *Symptoms:* Nasal and eye irritation; Central nervous system depression; Dizziness; Headaches; Nausea; Fatigue; Liver and kidney damage; Gastrointestinal inflammation and congestion; Immune system disorders; Lightheadedness; Impaired coordination and balance; Drowsiness; Coma; Convulsions; Staggering gait; Stupor; Death. Suspected of causing Cancer. *End-point Targets:* Central nervous system; Eyes; Nose; Liver; Kidneys. *Usage:* Pesticide inert ingredient; Adhesives; Teflon tubing; Lacquers; Coatings; Solvent; Rubbers; Polyesters; Fats; Oils; Waxes; Resins; Medicine; Decongestant aerosols; Glues. *Classification:* Organic solvent. *References:* 255, 286, 304, 383, 388, 423, 429.

Trichloroethylene *TN/synonyms:* Acetylene trichloride; 1-Chloro-2,2-dichloroethylene; 1,1-Dichloro-2-chloroethylene; Ethinyl trichloride; TCE; 1,1, 2-Trichloroethylene; Algylen (tn); Anamenth (tn); Benzinol (tn); Blacosolv (tn); Blancosolv (tn); Cecolene (tn); Chlorilen (tn); Chlorylea (tn); Chlorylen (tn); Chorylen (tn); Circosolv (tn); Crawhaspol (tn); Densinfluat (tn); Dow-Tri (tn); Dukeron (tn); Fleck-Flip (tn); Flock Flip (tn); Fluate (tn); Gemalgene (tn); HI-TRI (tn); Lanadin (tn); Lethurin (tn); Narcogen (tn); Narkogen (tn); Narkosoid (tn); NEU-TRI (tn); Nialk (tn); Perma-A-Chlor (tn); Perm-A-Chor (tn); Petzinol (tn); Philex (tn);

Threthylen (tn); Threthylene (tn); Tretylene (tn); Triad (tn); Trial (tn); Triasol (tn); Trichloran (tn); Trochloren (tn); Triclene (tn); Trielene (tn); Trielin (tn); Triklone (tn); Trilen (tn); Trilene (tn); Triline (tn); Trimar (tn); Troil (tn); TRI-plus(tn); TRI-plus M (tn); Vestrol (tn); Vitran; Westrosol (tn). *NIOSH:* Carcinogen at any exposure level. *NIOSH REL:* 25 ppm (10hr/day-40hr/wk). *OSHA PEL:* 50 ppm or 270 mg/m³ (8hr/day-40hr/wk-PP/S); 200 ppm or 1,080 mg/m³ (exposure not to exceed 15 min). *ATSDR MRL:* 0.1 ppm (Inhalation; more than 15 days). *IDLH:* 1,000 ppm. *Symptoms:* Eye, nasal, and throat irritation; Alters immune function; Anxiety; Behavioral problems; Blindness; Blood disorders; Cardiac arrhythmias and failure; Central nervous system depression; Chromosomal abnormalities; Confusion; Cranial and peripheral neuropathy; Decreased feelings in hands; Dermatitis; Diarrhea; Dizziness; Drowsiness; Dry throat; Excessive fatigue; Headaches; Immune system abnormalities; Insomnia; Kidney failure; Lack of muscular coordination; Liver damage and failure; Loss of appetite; Loss of consciousness; Loss of sensation; Nausea; Nervous system damage; Numbness, tingling, or prickling sensation; Paralysis; Peripheral nerve damage; Pulmonary hemorrhaging; Sensitivity and allergy to chemical; Skin burns and rashes; Slowed heart rate; Somnolence; Tremors; Vertigo; Vision disturbances; Vomiting. Suspected of causing Cancer. *End-point Targets:* Respiratory system; Heart; Liver; Kidneys; Central nervous system; Skin. *Usage:* Metal degreaser; Textiles; Waterless dyes; Adhesives; Lubricants; Paints; Varnishes; Paint Stripper; Pesticides; Polyvinyl chloride; Dry cleaning; Pharmaceuticals; Polychlorinated aliphatics; Flame retardants; Insecticides; Refrigerant; Typewriter correction fluid; Spot removers; Rug-cleaners; Pesticide inert ingredient; Degreasers; Shoe adhesives; Lacquers; Caffeine extraction; Pain relievers; Anesthetic agent. *Classification:* Organic solvent; Polar volatile organic compounds; Halogenated organic compound. *Note:* Historically established as a neurotoxin. *References:* 17, 286, 299, 304, 306, 341, 383, 388, 404, 413, 423, 429, 432, 452.

1,1,2-Trichloroethylene *see* **Trichloroethylene.**

1,4,6-Trichlorofenol *see* **2,4,6-Trichlorophenol.**

Trichlorofluoromethane *see* **Fluorotrichloromethane.**

Trichlorohydrin *see* **1,2,3-Trichloropropane.**

Trichloromethane *see* **Chloroform.**

a-Trichloromethane *see* **1,1,1-Trichloroethane.**

Trichloromethylmethane *see* **1,1,1-Trichloroethane.**

Trichloromonofluoromethane *see* **Fluorotrichloromethane.**

Trichloronitromethane *see* **Chloropicrin.**

2,4,6-Trichlorophenol *TN/synonyms:* 2,4,6-T; 1,4,6-Trichlorofenol; Caswell No. 880C (tn); Dowicide 2S(tn); Omal (tn); Phenchlor (tn). *OSHA PEL:* None. *ATSDR MRL:* 1.5 ppm (Ingestion, more than 14 days). *Symptoms:* None confirmed. Suspected of causing Liver damage; Blood effects; Spleen damage; Development and reproductive effects; Sperm death; Cancer (leukemia and liver); Labored breathing; Excessive proliferation of normal cells in bone marrow. *Usage:* Preservative for wood, leather, and glue; Anti-mildew for fabric/textiles; Pesticides; Antiseptic; Disinfectant; Sanitizer; Bactericide; Germicide; Fungicide; Herbicide; Defoliant; Pentachlorophenol; 2,3,4,6-Tetrachlorophenol; Feedstock. *References:* 304, 338, 388.

1,2,3-Trichloropropane *TN/synonyms:* Allyl trichloride; Glycerol trichlorohydrin; Glyceryl trichlorohydrin; Trichlorohydrin. *NIOSH:* Carcinogen at any exposure level. *OSHA PEL:* 10 ppm or 60 mg/m³ (8hr/day-40hr/wk-PP/S). *ATSDR MRL:* 0.0003 ppm (Inhalation, less than 15 days). *IDLH:* 1,000 ppm. *Symptoms:* Eye, throat, and skin irritation; Central nervous system depression; Dizziness; Headaches; Nausea; Fatigue; Liver injury. Suspected of causing Kidney and blood damage; Genetic mutations. *End-point Targets:* Eyes; Respiratory system; Skin; Central nervous system; Liver. *Usage:* Paint and varnish remover; Cleaning and degreasing agents; Extractive agent; Intermediate in polysulfone liquid polymers and dichloropropene, synthesis of hexafluoropropylene; Crosslinking agent in the synthesis of polysulfides. *Contaminants:* Chlorohexene; Chlorohexadienes. *References:* 256, 304, 379, 388.

Triclene (tn) *see* **Trichloroethylene.**

Tridymite *see* **Silica.**

Trielene (tn) *see* **Trichloroethylene.**

Trielin (tn) *see* **Trichloroethylene.**

Triethylamine *TN/synonyms:* TEA. *NIOSH:* No REL; notified OSHA that documentation doesn't support the worker's safety at established PELs. *OSHA PEL:* 10 ppm or 40 mg/m³ (8hr/day-40hr/wk-PP/S); 15 ppm or 60 mg/m³ (exposure not to exceed 15 min). *IDLH:* 1,000 ppm. *Symptoms:* Eye, nasal, throat, respiratory, and skin irritation; Corneal swelling and inflammation; Visual disturbances; Blurred vision; Death. *End-point Targets:* Respiratory system; Skin; Eyes. *Usage:* Pesticide inert ingredient; Enamels; Paint; Polyurethane foams; Copper soldering; Solvent; Rubber; Propellants; Waterproofing; Epoxy resins; Dyes; Amino resins; Antibiotics;

2,4,5-T; Herbicide and pesticide manufacturing; Artificial sweeteners; Ketenes; Photography; Printing inks; Carpet cleaners. *Note:* Capable of causing death or permanent injury from exposures from normal use. *References:* 245, 304, 388, 423.

Trifluoroborane *see* **Boron trifluoride.**

Trifluorobromomethane *TN/synonyms:* Bromotrifluoromethane; Fluorocarbon 1301; Freon 13B1; Halocarbon 13B1; Halon 1301; Monobromotrifluoromethane; Refrigerant 13B1; Trifluoromonobromethane. *OSHA PEL:* 1,000 ppm or 6,100 mg/m³ (8hr/day-40hr/wk). *IDLH:* 50,000 ppm. *Symptoms:* Pulmonary irritation; Lightheadedness; Cardiac arrhythmias; Decreased psychomotor performance; Tremors; Numbness, tingling, or prickling sensation; Confusion; Coma (rarely); Death; Freezing of airway soft tissues; Defatting dermatitis; Euphoria; Mental dullness; Heart and nervous system effects. *End-point Targets:* Heart; Central nervous system. *Usage:* Refrigerant; Aerosol sprays; Fire extinguisher; Pharmaceutical processing; Foam blowing agent; Food freezant; Solvents; Metal processing; Hair spray; Cosmetics; Household cleaning sprays; Medical sprays. *References:* 246, 304, 388.

Trifluoromonobromethane *see* **Trifluorobromomethane.**

Triklone (tn) *see* **Trichloroethylene.**

Trilen (tn) *see* **Trichloroethylene.**

Trilene (tn) *see* **Trichloroethylene.**

Triline (tn) *see* **Trichloroethylene.**

Trimar (tn) *see* **Trichloroethylene.**

Trimellitic acid anhydride *see* **Trimellitic anhydride.**

Trimellitic acid 1,2-anhydride *see* **Trimellitic anhydride.**

Trimellitic acid cyclic 1,2-anhydride see **Trimellitic anhydride.**

Trimellitic anhydride *TN/synonyms:* Anhydrotrimellitic acid; 1,2,4-Benezenetricarboxlic acid anhydride; 1,2,4-Benezenetricarboxlic acid; cyclic 1,2-anhydride; Benezenetricarboxlic anhydride; 4-Carboxyphthalic anhydride; 1,3-Dihydro-1,3-dioxo- 5-isobenzofurancarboxylic acid; 1, 3-Dioxo-5-Phthalacarboxylic acid; Diphenylmethane-4,4'-diisocyanate-trimellic anhydride-ethomid ht polymer; TMA; TMAN; Trimellitic acid anhydride; Trimellitic acid 1,2-anhydride; and Trimellitic acid cyclic 1,2-anhydride. *OSHA PEL:* .005 ppm (8hr/day-40hr/wk-PP/S). > *EPA/OTS:* 0.001 ppm (Pulmonary hypersensitivity; substantial lung dysfunction). *Symptoms:* Respiratory tract, eye, nasal, throat, and skin irritation; Noncardiac pulmonary edema; Immune system sensitization; Nasal mucosa inflammation; Asthma; TMA-flu; Cough; Wheezing; Labored breathing; Malaise; Chills; Fever; Muscle and joint pain; Runny nose; Sneezing; Nosebleeds; Shortness of breath; Heartburn; Nausea; Headaches; Antibody response; Hemolytic anemia; Blood expectoration. *Endpoint Targets:* Respiratory system; Immune system. *Usage:* Resins; Adhesives; Polymers; Dyes; Printing inks; Plastics; Plasticizer; Wire insulation; Gaskets; Automobile upholstery; Foamed vinyl flooring; Epoxy resins; Paints; Coatings; Polyesters; Agricultural chemicals; Pigments; Pharmaceuticals; Fiberglass; Wire enamel; Pesticide inert ingredient. *Note:* 13–17% of the general population and about 20% of the workers to experience allergic-type reactions. *References:* 20, 64, 388, 415, 423, 445.

3,5,5-Trimethyl-2-cyclohexenone see **Isophorone.**

3,5,5-Trimethyl-2-cyclohexen-1-one see **Isophorone.**

2,4,6-Trimethyl-1,3,5-Trioxane see **Paraldehyde.**

Trimmer of acetaldehyde see **Paraldehyde.**

2,4,6-Trinitrophenol see **Picric acid.**

Trinitrotoluene see **2,4,6-Trinitrotoluene.**

sym-Trinitrotoluene see **2,4, 6-Trinitroltoluene.**

2,4,6-Trinitrotoluene *TN/synonyms:* 1-Methyl-2,4,6-trinitrobenzene; TNT; Trinitrotoluene; sym-Trinitrotoluene; Trinitrotoluol. *OSHA PEL:* 0.5 mg/m^3 (8hr/day-40hr/wk-PP/S). *IDLH:* NE. *Symptoms:* Eye irritation; Anemia; Aplastic anemia; Cardiac irregularities; Cataracts; Coma; Cough; Cyanosis; Death; Dermatitis; Dizziness; Fatigue; Hemoglobin oxidizes to ferric form; Hemorrhaging; Increases in glutamic oxalacetic transaminase, lactic dehydrogenase, serum alamine aminotransferase, reticulocytes in the blood of the bone marrow, leukocytes, and bilirubin; Jaundice; Kidney damage; Labored or difficult breathing; Liver damage, diseases, tissue death, and failure; Loss of appetite; Muscle pain; Nausea; Neurotic symptoms; Peripheral neuropathy; Sneezing; Sore throat; Toxic hepatitis; Weakness. Suspected of causing Cerebral dysfunction; Blurred vision; Involuntary eye movement; Tremors; Staggering gait; Abnormal electroencephalogram. *Endpoint Targets:* Blood; Liver; Eyes; Cardiovascular system; Central nervous system; Kidneys; Skin. *Usage:* Explosive; Grenades; Dyes; Photography. *Note:* Symptoms may be delayed 4 months or longer. *References:* 144, 257, 304, 388.

Trinitrotoluol see **2,4,6-Trinitrotoluene.**

o-Trinitrotoluol see **Triorthocresyl phosphate.**

Tri-o-cresyl ester of phosphoric acid *see* **Triorthocresyl phosphate.**

Tri-o-cresyl phosphate *see* **Triorthocresyl phosphate.**

Triorthocresyl phosphate *TN/synonyms:* TCP; TOCP; Tri-o-cresyl ester of phosphoric acid; Tri-o-cresyl phosphate; o-Trinitrotoluol. *OSHA PEL:* 0.1 mg/m³ (8hr/day-40hr/wk-PP/S). *IDLH:* 40 mg/m³. *Symptoms:* Cramps in calves; Death; Destruction of myelin sheathing; Gastrointestinal distress; Headache; Hypothalamic syndrome; Inhibition of plasma cholinesterase enzymes; Leg aches; Loss of appetite; Multi-nerve inflammation; Nausea; Numbness, tingling, or prickling in feet or hands; Paralysis; Peripheral neuropathy; Respiratory paralysis; Stomach inflammation; Toxic brain dysfunction; Vertigo; Weak feet; Wrist drops. *End-point Targets:* Peripheral nervous system; Central nervous system. *Usage:* Plasticizer; Lacquers; Varnishes; Lubricating oil additive; Shoe cement; Adhesives. *Note:* Historically established as a neurotoxin. *References:* 266, 304, 388, 413.

Triphenyl ester of phosphoric acid *see* **Triphenyl phosphate.**

Triphenyl phosphate *TN/synonyms:* Phenyl phosphate; TPP; Triphenyl ester of phosphoric acid. *OSHA PEL:* 3 mg/m³ (8hr/day-40hr/wk). *IDLH:* Unknown. *Symptoms:* Minor changes in blood enzymes; Inhibition of cholinesterase enzymes; Weakness in hands; Absence of deep tendon reflexes; Reduced motor skills. Suspected of causing Muscle weakness; Paralysis. *End-point Targets:* Blood. *Usage:* Celluloid; Roofing paper; Nitrocellulose; Airplane dopes; Flame retardant; Plasticizers; Lacquers; Varnishes; Cellulose; Adhesives; Upholstery; Hydraulic fluid. *Note:* Humans are more susceptible to changes in cholinesterase than rodents. *References:* 247, 304, 388.

TRI-plus (tn) *see* **Trichloroethylene.**

TRI-plus M (tn) *see* **Trichloroethylene.**

Tripoli *see* **Silica.**

Trochloren (tn) *see* **Trichloroethylene.**

Troil (tn) *see* **Trichloroethylene.**

Turpentine *TN/synonyms:* Gumspirits; Gum turpentine; Spirits of turpentine; Steam distilled turpentine; Sulfate wood turpentine; Turps; Wood turpentine. *OSHA PEL:* 100 ppm or 560 mg/m³ (8hr/day-40hr/wk-PP/S). *IDLH:* 1,500 ppm. *Symptoms:* Skin, eye, nasal, throat, gastric, and bladder irritation; Abdominal pain; Blood and albumin in urine; Burning pain in mouth and throat; Chemical sensitization; Chest pains; Choking; Coma; Conjunctiva congestion; Contact dermatitis; Convulsions; Coughing; Cyanosis; Death; Delirium; Diarrhea; Dizziness; Excessive salivation; Excitement; Eyelid spasms; Feeling of suffocation; Fever; Headaches; Heart rate over 100 beats per minute; Hypothermia; Incoordination; Kidney damage and lesions; Labored or difficult breathing; Nausea; Painful urination; Pneumonia; Pulmonary edema; Respiratory failure; Sensitive dermatitis; Skin and eye burns; Somnolence; Stupor; Swollen tongue, lips, or gingival mucosa; Turpentine odor in breath; Vertigo; Visual disturbances; Vomiting. Suspected of causing Cancer; Birth defects. *End-point Targets:* Skin; Eyes; Kidneys; Respiratory system. *Usage:* Paint thinner and remover; Solvent; Oils; Resins; Varnishes; Automotive paints; Perfume; Aerosols; Deodorizers; Candy; Baked goods; Chewing gum; Synthetic pine oil; Terpenes; Polishes; Inks; Expectorants; Medicine; Ointments; Insecticide; Synthetic camphor; Cleaning products; Putty; Mastics; Cutting and grinding fluids; Pinene based perfumes and food flavors;

Pesticide inert ingredient. *Note:* Neurotoxin. *References:* 17, 248, 299, 304, 388, 423.

Turps *see* **Turpentine.**

Udimet (tn) *see* **Nickel.**

UDMH *see* **1,1-Dimethylhydrazine.**

Uniflex DBP (tn) *see* **Dibutylphthalate.**

Unifume (tn) *see* **Ethylene dibromide.**

Unitene *see* **Limonene.**

Unslaked lime *see* **Calcium oxide.**

Unsymmetrical dimethylhydrazine *see* **1,1-Dimethylhydrazine.**

VAC (tn) *see* **Vinyl acetate.**

Valerone *see* **Diisobutyl ketone.**

Vanadic anhydride *see* **Vanadium pentoxide.**

Vanadium pentaoxide *see* **Vanadium pentoxide.**

Vanadium pentoxide *TN/synonyms:* Divanadium pentoxide; Vanadic anhydride; Vanaium oxide; Vanadium pentaoxide. *NIOSH REL:* 0.05 mg/m³ (ceiling limit, 15 min exposure). *OSHA PEL:* 0.05 mg/m³ (8hr/day-40hr/wk-PP/S). *ATSDR MRL:* 0.003 ug/kg/day (Ingestion); 0.01 mg/m³ (Inhalation, less than 15 days); 0.006 mg/m³ (Inhalation, more than 14 days). *IDLH:* 70 mg/m³. *Symptoms:* Eye and throat irritation; Abnormal decrease in blood platelets; Allergic dermatitis; Asthenoautonomic syndrome; Bronchitis; Cancer (brain, liver, lung); Chromosomal aberrations; Cough; Death; Decrease in physical strength; Dizziness; DNA damage; Drowsiness; Eczema; Enlarged spleen; Epigastric pain; Euphoria; Fine rales; Green tongue; Headaches; High blood pressure; Inebriation; Labored or difficult breathing; Liver damage, enlargement, and failure; Loss of appetite; Loss of sensation; Memory loss; Metallic taste; Nervousness; Numbness, tingling, or prickling sensations; Occupational acroosteolysis (dissolution of the finger tips); Peripheral-vegetative syndrome; Pyramidal syndrome; Raynaud's syndrome; Respiratory diseases; Scleroderma; Sleeping disturbances; Somnolence; Staggering gait; Unconsciousness due to narcotic effects; Vasomotor disturbances; Visual disturbances; Wheezing. Suspected of causing Birth defects; Low birth weight; Ovarian dysfunction; Decline in libido; Increase hemoglobin levels. *End-point Targets:* Respiratory system; Skin; Eyes. *Usage:* Steel industry; Rubber; Plastic; Ceramics; Black dyes; Inks; Pigments; Textiles; Paints; Varnishes; Pesticides; Methyl chloroform; Chloroacetaldehyde; Ethylene oxide; Construction materials; Automotive parts; Electrical wire insulation; Household equipment; Medical supplies; Paper; Glass; Adhesive for plastics; Floor tiles. No longer used as an extraction solvent, refrigerant, aerosol propellent or ingredient in medicine and cosmetics. *References:* 304, 369, 388.

Vanaium oxide *see* **Vanadium pentoxide.**

VC *see* **Vinyl chloride.**

VCM *see* **Vinyl chloride.**

VCN *see* **Acrylonitrile.**

Ventox *see* **Acrylonitrile.**

Vestrol (tn) *see* **Trichloroethylene.**

Vinyl acetate *TN/synonyms:* Acetic acid; ethenyl ester; Ethylene ester; Acetic acid; vinyl ester; 1-Acetoxyethylene; Ethanoic acid; Ethenyl ester; Ethenyl acetate; Ethenyl ethanoate; Vinyl A monomer; Vinyl ethanoate; VAC (tn); Vinyl Acetate HQ (tn); VYAC ZESET T (tn). *NIOSH REL:* 4 ppm or 15 mg/m³ (Ceiling limit, 15 min exposure). *OSHA PEL:* 10 ppm or 30 mg/m³ (8hr/day-40hr/wk); 20 ppm or 60 mg/m³ (exposure not to exceed 15 min). *ATSDR MRL:* 0.6 ppm (Inhalation, more than 14 days). *Symptoms:*

Eye, nasal, throat, and respiratory irritation; Gasping; Labored breathing; Pulmonary congestion, hemorrhage, and edema; Skin blisters. Suspected of causing Death; Immunosuppression; Sperm abnormalities. *End-point Targets:* Respiratory system. *Usage:* Adhesives; Glues; Paint; Textile fibers; Textile sizings and finishes; Paper coating; Ink; Laminated safety glass; Plastic floor coverings; Phonograph records; Flexible coatings and sheeting; Acrylic fibers; Polyvinyl alcohol; Ethylene/vinyl acetate; Polyvinyl butyral; Polyvinyl chloride; Pesticide inert ingredient; Hair spray. *Classification:* Organic solvent. *References:* 13, 14, 380, 383, 388, 423, 436.

Vinyl Acetate HQ (tn) *see* **Vinyl acetate.**

Vinyl A monomer *see* **Vinyl acetate.**

Vinyl benzene *see* **Styrene.**

Vinyl cabinol *see* **Allyl alcohol.**

Vinyl chloride *TN/synonyms:* Chloroethene; Chloroethylene; Ethylene monochloride; Monochloroethylene; VC; Vinyl chloride monomer; VCM; 1-Chloroethylene. *NIOSH:* Carcinogen at any exposure level. Reduce exposure to lowest reliably detectable concentration. *OSHA PEL:* 1 ppm (8hr/day-40hr/wk); 5 ppm (Ceiling limit, 15 min exposure). *ATSDR MRL:* 0.006 ppm (Inhalation, more than 14 days). *ACGIH:* Confirmed human carcinogen. *IDLH:* NIOSH-Carcinogen. *Symptoms:* Pulmonary and kidney irritation; Abdominal pains; Abnormal chest x-rays; Abnormal decrease in blood platelets; Acroosteolysis (dissolution of the finger tips); Autoimmune responses similar to sclerosis; Benign uterine growths; Binds to IgG protein; Blockage of blood vessels; Cancer (central nervous system, respiratory tract, lymphatic, and blood); Cyanosis of extremities; Death; Decreased libido; Decreased respiratory function; Dis-

comfort upon exposure to cold; Dizziness; Drowsiness; Emphysema; Euphoria; Gastrointestinal bleeding; Headaches; Impotency; Inhibits blood clotting; Joint and muscle pain; Liver damage and enlargement; Loss of consciousness; Menstrual disturbances; Nausea; Numbness; Ovarian dysfunction; Pallor; Peripheral neuropathy; Pregnant toxemia; Prolapsed genital organs; Pulmonary fibrosis; Raynaud's phenomenon symptoms (aka Vinyl chloride disease); Scleroderma-like skin changes; Systemic sclerosis; Scleroderma; Spontaneous abortions; Stiff hands; Thickening of blood vessel walls and skin; Weakness; Autoimmune disease. Suspected of causing Birth defects; Testicular damage. *End-point Targets:* Liver; Central nervous system; Blood; Lymphatic system. *Usage:* PVC pipes; Automobile and furniture upholstery; Packaging materials; Wall coverings; Wire Coatings; Photographic film; Plastics; Glass; Paper; Pesticide inert ingredient. Found in Tobacco smoke. *Additives/Contaminants:* Stabilized with inhibitors such as phenol. *Note:* Occupational exposure of males has been associated with increased rates of spontaneous abortions in their spouses. Neurotoxin. *References:* 17, 249, 280, 304, 306, 381, 388, 400, 423, 429, 449.

Vinyl chloride monomer *see* **Vinyl chloride.**

Vinyl cyanide *see* **Acrylonitrile.**

Vinyl ethanoate *see* **Vinyl acetate.**

Vinylethylene *see* **1,3-Butadiene.**

Vinyl toluene *TN/synonyms:* Ethenylmethylbenzene; Methylstyrene; Tolyethylene. *OSHA PEL:* 100 ppm or 480 mg/m³ (8hr/day-40hr/wk-PP/S). *ACGIH TLV:* 50 ppm or 240 mg/m³ (8hr/day-40hr/wk-PP/S). *IDLH:* 5,000 ppm. *Symptoms:* Eye, skin, and upper respiratory irritation; Drowsiness; Loss of sensation; Chromosomal aberrations. Suspected of causing Cerebral dysfunction; Blurred vision; Involuntary eye movement; Tremors; Staggering gait; Abnormal electroencephalogram. *End-point Targets:* Eyes; Skin; Respiratory system. *Usage:* Plastics; Polyester resins; Surface coatings; Quick-drying oils. *Additives/Contaminants:* Usually inhibited with tert-butyl catechol. *References:* 144, 251, 304, 388.

Vinyl trichloride *see* **1,1,2-Trichloroethane.**

Visco 1152 (TN) *see* **Isopropyl alcohol.**

Vitran (tn) *see* **Trichloroethylene.**

Vofatox (tn) *see* **Methyl parathion.**

Voilet 3 *see* **Xylenes.**

Vorlex (tn) *see* **1,3-Dichloropropene.**

VYAC ZESET T (tn) *see* **Vinyl acetate.**

WARF *see* **Warfarin.**

Warfarin *TN/synonyms:* 3-(alpha-Acetonyl)-benzyl-4-hydroxycoumarin; 4-Hydroxy-3-(3-oxo-1-phenyl butyl)-2H-1-benzopyran-2-one; WARF. *OSHA PEL:* 0.1 mg/m³ (8hr/day-40hr/wk-PP/S). *IDLH:* 350 mg/m³. *Symptoms:* Blood in urine; Back pain; Bruising of arms and legs; Nosebleeds; Bleeding lips and gums; Muscle membrane hemorrhaging; Pallor; Cerebral hemorrhage; Hemorrhagic shock; Death; Retina hemorrhages; Skin tissue death; Abdominal pain; Vomiting; Fecal blood; Petechial rashes; Abnormal blood indices; Loss of appetite; Nausea; Diarrhea; Skin lesions; Birth defects; Stillbirths. *End-point Targets:* Blood; Cardiovascular system. *Usage:* Pesticide; Rodenticide; Medicine. *References:* 251, 304, 388, 449.

Wash oil *see* **Creosotes.**

Waspaloy (tn) *see* **Nickel.**

Weeviltox (tn) *see* **Carbon disulfide.**

Westrosol (tn) *see* **Trichloroethylene.**

WFNA *see* **Nitric acid.**

White fuming nitric acid *see* **Nitric acid.**

White phosphoric acid *see* **Phosphoric acid.**

White phosphorus *see* **Phosphorus.**

White tar *see* **Naphthalene.**

Wofatos (tn) *see* **Methyl parathion.**

Wofatox (tn) *see* **Methyl parathion.**

Wofotox (tn) *see* **Methyl parathion.**

Wood alcohol *see* **Methyl alcohol.**

Wood creosote *see* **Creosotes.**

Wood spirits *see* **Methyl alcohol.**

Wood turpentine *see* **Turpentine.**

Xylenes *TN/synonyms:* Dimethylbenzene; Xylol; Methyl toluene; Voilet 3 (tn). *Isomers m-Xylene*: 1,3-Dimethylbenzene; 1,3-Xylene; m-Dimethylbenzene; m-Xylol; m-Methyltoluene; meta-Xylene; *o-Xylene*: 1,2-Dimethylbenzene; 1,2-Xylene; o-Dimethylbenzene; o-Xylol; o-Methyltoluene; ortho-Xylene; *p-Xylene*: 1,4-Dimethylbenzene; 1,4-Xylene; p-Dimethylbenzene; p-Xylol; p-Methyltoluene; para-Xylene; Scintillar (tn). *OSHA PEL:* 100 ppm or 435 mg/m³ (8hr/day-40hr/wk-PP/S); 150 ppm or 655 mg/m³ (exposure not to exceed 15 min). *IDLH:* 1,000 ppm. *Symptoms:* Eye, nasal, throat, and respiratory irritation; Abdominal pain; Abnormal electrocardiograms; Amnesia; Brain hemorrhage; Cardiac palpitations; Confusion; Corneal vacuolization; Death; Dermatitis; Dizziness; Drowsiness; Epileptic convulsions; Excitement; Fatigue; Gastric discomfort; Headaches; Impaired mathematical ability, balance, pulmonary function, and reaction time;

Labored breathing; Lightheadedness; Liver and kidney damage; Loss of appetite and patience; Nausea; Pulmonary congestion, hemorrhaging, edema, and damage; Reduced coordination; Respiratory failure; Short-term memory loss; Staggering gait; Tremors; Unconsciousness due to narcotic effects; Ventricular fibrillation; Vomiting. Suspected of causing Birth defects; Spontaneous abortions; Cerebral dysfunction; Blurred vision; Involuntary eye movement. *End-point Targets:* Central nervous system; Eyes; Blood; Skin; Gastrointestinal tract; Liver; Kidneys. *Usages:* Gasoline additive; Paint; Varnish; Shellac; Rust preventives; Printing; Rubber; Leather; Cleaning agents; Airplane fuel; Plastic (soft drink bottles); Polyester fabrics; Photography; Coating for paper and fabrics; Vitamins; Insecticide; Pharmaceuticals; Construction materials; Pesticide inert ingredient; Air fresheners; Fiberglass; Fiberglass bathtubs; Porcelain enamelling of steel (bathtubs and appliances); Adhesives. Found in Cigarette smoke; petroleum; coal tar; smoke from forest fires; automobile exhaust. Mixed Xylenes usually contain the three forms of xylenes and 6% to 15% ethylbenzene. *Classification:* Organic solvent; Polar volatile organic compounds. *Note:* Neurotoxin. *References:* 17, 144, 304, 339, 383, 388, 423, 429, 432, 452.

Xylidine *TN/synonyms:* Aminodimethylbenzene; Aminoxylene; Dimethylaminobenzene. *Isomers:* o-Xylidine; m-Xylidine; p-Xylidine. *OSHA PEL:* 2 ppm or 10 mg/m³ (8hr/day-40hr/wk-PP/S). *IDLH:* 150 ppm. *Symptoms:* Inability to utilize oxygen; Cyanosis; Lung, liver, and kidney damage; Hemoglobin oxidizes to ferric form; Headaches; Dizziness. *End-point Targets:* Blood; Lungs; Liver; Kidneys; Cardiovascular system. *Usage:* Dyes; Pharmaceuticals; Gasoline additive; Wood preservatives; Textiles; Lacquers; Shampoo. *References:* 84, 288, 304, 306, 388.

Xyolol *see* **Xylenes.**

Zinc chloride *OSHA PEL:* 1 mg/m³ (8hr/day-40hr/wk); 2 mg/m³ (exposure not to exceed 15 min). *IDLH:* 4,800 mg/m³. *Symptoms:* Eye, nasal, throat, and skin irritation; Abdominal pain; Abnormally low blood calcium; Bronchial pneumonia; Chest pains and constriction; Chromosomal aberrations; Conjunctivitis; Copious sputum; Cough; Cyanosis; Death; Dermatosis; Diarrhea; Esophagus and pyloric strictures; Fever; Increased blood amylase; Labored or difficult breathing; Nasal passage ulceration; Nausea; Nutrition malabsorbtion syndrome; Pancreas inflammation; Pulmonary edema and fibrosis; Rapid pulse and respiration; Respiratory insufficiency; Retrosternal and epigastric pain; Right ventricular hypertrophy; Skin burns; Vomiting. *End-point Targets:* Respiratory system; Skin; Eyes. *Usage:* Activated carbon; Animal feed; Artificial silk; Asphalt; Astringent; Bacteriostat; Benzyl chloride; Carbonizing woolen goods; Cellulose; Chemosurgery for skin cancer; Corrosion inhibitor; Cosmetics; Cotton; Crepe; Denatured alcohol; Dental cement; Dentifrices; Dialysis additive; Dimethyl zinc; Dry cell batteries; Drying agent; Dyes; Electroplating; Eye drops; Fabric sizing; Feather pillows; Food additive; Glass etching; Golf balls; Herbicide; Magnesia and metal cements; Medicine; Mouthwash; Oil refining; Paint; Parchment paper; Pesticides; Plumbing pipe solder; Preservatives; Railroad ties; Rubber; Skin fresheners; Smoke bombs; Soldering fluxes; Solvent; Sterilizing feathers; Textiles; Toilet bowl cleaner; Vaginal douches; Veterinary medicine; Water treatment; Wood flame retardant and preservative. *References:* 252, 304, 388.

Zinc oxide *OSHA PEL:* 5 mg/m³ (8hr/day-40hr/wk) 10 mg/m³ (exposure not to exceed 15 min). *IDLH:* NE.

Symptoms: Sweet or metallic taste; Dry throat; Cough; Chills; Fever; Tight chest; Labored or difficult breathing; Rales; Reduced pulmonary function; Blurred vision; Muscle cramps and pain; Lower back pain; Nausea; Vomiting; Fatigue; Lassitude; Malaise; Metal fume fever; Dermatitis; Boils; Conjunctivitis; Gastrointestinal disturbances; Pneumonia; Increase in leukocytes in the blood; Liver dysfunction; Gastrointestinal inflammation; Yawning; Weakness; Body aches; Headaches. *End-point Targets:* Respiratory system; Skin. *Usage:* Anticaking agent; Antiseptics; Astringents; Body dusting powder; Carpeting; Ceramics; Copy paper; Cosmetics; Dental cement, disclosing waxes, and impression paste; Dietary supplements; Elastic; Electrical insulation; Enamels; Fabrics; Fax machines; Flame retardant; Floor tiles; Insecticidal adjuvant in animal feed; Lubricants; Matches; Medicine; Mildew control; Office copying machines; Ointments; Opaque and transparent glass; Paints; Pesticide inert ingredient; Photography; Pigments; Plastics; Porcelains; Quicksetting cements; Rayon; Rubber; Semiconductors; Tires; Topical protectorates; White glues; White inks. *Note:* In one report, symptoms didn't appear until after 6 months of occupational exposure. *References:* 253, 304, 388, 423.

6

Environmentally Concerned Health and Public Interest Organizations and Publications and Other Resources

International Organizations

Arts, Crafts and Theater Safety, Inc. (A.C.T.S.) 181 Thompson St., #23, New York NY 10012-2586, (212) 777-0062; Hours: 9 a.m. to 5 p.m. *Contact:* Nonona Rossol. *Type of Organization:* Educational. *Services:* Answers inquiries about health science referrals, speakers bureau, educational courses, OSHA compliance assistance. *Publication:* ACTS FACTS. *Subscription fees:* $10 for U.S. residence; $12 U.S. for Canadian residence, and $16 U.S. for other countries.

Candida Research and Information Foundation, PO Box 2719, Castro Valley CA 94546, (510) 582-2179; Hours: 10 a.m. to 2 p.m. (Mon–Fri). *Type of Organization:* Educational public service agency with emphasis on chronic illness and environmental illness research. *Services:* Counseling, nationwide support groups, referral services, educational materials, and public research library. *Publication:* CRIF Newsletter. *Membership/Subscription Fees:* U.S.–$20 per year; Outside the

U.S.–$30 per year.

Center for Safety in the Arts 5 Bechman Street, Suite 1030, New York NY 10038, (212) 227-6220; Hours: 9 a.m. to 5 p.m. (Mon–Fri). *Contact:* Angela Bubin. *Type of Organization:* Research clearinghouse for health and safety information for the visual, performing, and museum arts as well as art education. *Services:* Information center, Public library, Consultations, Training, Lecture programs, and various Publications. *Publication:* Art Hazards News. *Subscription:* $21 per year.

The Lavender Mask, PO Box 191, Shutesbury MA 01072, (413) 367-9213, please, no late night calls). *Contact:* Shemaya Laurel. *Type of Organization:* Lesbians with environmental illness network. *Services:* Informal contact. *Publication:* The Lavender Mask. *Membership:* By donation.

Parents Against Cancer Plus, PO Box 99724, Troy MI 48099-9724, (313)

649-5134; Hours: 9 a.m. to 4 p.m. *Contact:* Phyllis R. Gorski. *Type of Organization:* Environmental Health organization seeking prevention of disease through pollution prevention. An organization for parents and others. *Services:* Community education programs; Networking for parents of children with cancer and other diseases or conditions; Lobbying for environmental cancer and other disease research seeking prevention. *Publication:* None though one is being planned. *Membership dues:* None. *Subscription fees:* $10 per year.

Pesticide Action Network — North America Regional Center, 965 Mission Street, #514, San Francisco CA 94103, (415) 541-9140; Hours: 9 a.m. to 5 p.m. *Contact:* Monica Moore, Regional Coordinator. *Type of Organization:* Center for international grassroots networks working to limit the use of hazardous pesticides and working towards safe, sustainable alternatives. *Services:* Low cost access to reports, books, articles, and documents on pesticides, integrated pest management, organic agriculture, developmental studies and public health activities. *Publication:* Global Pesticide Campaign. *Subscription:* $25 per year. $15 for low income.

Protect All Children's Environment, P.O. Box 482, Marble Falls, TX 78654, (512) 693-6311; Hours: 9 a.m. to 5 p.m. (Mon-Fri) 24 hours for poison victims. *Contact:* E.M.T. O'Nan de Iglesios. *Type of Organization:* Poison victim's organization. *Services:* Legal and medical referrals and periodic position papers. *Membership fees:* $35 per year suggested membership dues.

National Organizations

Action on Smoking and Health (ASH), 2013 H Street NW, Washington DC 20006, (202) 659-4310; Hours 9 a.m. to 5 p.m. (Mon-Fri). *Type of Organization:* Legal action arm of the nonsmoker's rights movement. *Services:* Education and legal action. *Publication:* Smoking & Health Review. *Membership/Subscription Fees:* $15 per year.

Association of Birth Defect Children, 5400 Diplomat Circle, Suite 270, Orlando FL 32810, (407) 629-1466; Hours: 9 a.m. to 4 p.m. (Mon-Fri). *Contact:* Betty Mekdeci. *Type of Organization:* Birth defect information clearinghouse. Reports and researches environmental causes for birth defects. *Services:* Parent matching, birth defect information and fact sheets, and maintaining the National Environmental Birth Defect Registry. *Publication:* ABDC Newsletter. *Membership (including newsletter):* $25 to $50 per year. *Newsletter only:* $12 per year, Low Income $5 per year.

The Center for Neighborhood Technology, 2125 W. North Ave., Chicago IL 60657, (312) 278-4800; Hours: 9 a.m. to 5 p.m. *Contact:* Scott Bernstein. *Type of Organization:* Research, public policy, and technical assistance organization working on energy and environmental issues affecting urban neighborhoods. *Service:* Energy efficiency audits, community development information services. *Publication:* The Neighborhood Works. *Subscription Fee:* $30 per year for individuals and $40 per year for institutions.

Center for Science in the Public Interest, 1875 Connecticut Ave. NW, #300, Washington DC 20009-5728, (202) 332-9110; Hours: 9 a.m. to 5 p.m. (Mon-Fri). *Type of Organization:* Consumer group that addresses food and nutrition issues, alcohol policy, and organic and sustainable agriculture. *Services:* Provides a membership kit, discount on products, publishes literature, books, posters, and other materials; Lobbies government and industry; and will answer nutrition-related questions from individuals. *Publication:* Nutrition Action Healthletter. *Subscription:* $19.95 per year.

Chemical Injury Information Network, P.O. Box 301, White Sulphur Springs MT 59645. *Type of Organization:* Support/advocacy organization for the chemically injured. *Services:* Membership package, resource literature, physician and attorney referrals, medical/governmental research for documenting chemically related health problems. *Publication:* Our Toxic Times. *Membership/Subscription Fees:* None, donation accepted.

Ecology Center for Southern California, P.O. Box 35559, Los Angeles CA 90035, (310) 559-9160. *Type of Organization:* Environmental media. *Services:* Newspaper, radio and television series and documentaries; environmental directory; speaker's bureau; and public service announcements. *Publications:* The Compendium. *Membership/Subscription Fees:* $20 per year regular, $15 per year low income.

Household Hazardous Waste Project, 1031 E. Battlefield, Suite 214, Springfield MO 65807, (417) 889-5000; Hours: 1 p.m. to 5 p.m. (Mon-Fri). *Contact:* Marie Steinwachs. *Type of Organization:* Programs of University Extension. *Services:* Training, consultation, educational materials and publications, information referral service.

National Toxic Campaign Fund 1168 Commonwealth Ave., Boston MA 02135, (617) 232-0327; Hours 9 a.m. to 5 p.m. *Type of Organization:* An environmental organization working to implement citizen-based preventative solutions to national toxic and environmental problems. *Publication:* Toxic Times. *Membership/Subscription Fees:* $15 to $100 per year for individuals to receive publication and consumer toxics protection information. $25 to $100 per year for an Organizational Membership to receive access to staff, publication, testing lab services, organizing and technical reports.

Share, Care and Prayer, Inc., P.O. Box 2080, Frazier Park CA 93225. *Contact:* Janet Dauble. *Type of Organization:* Christian ministry encouraging, educating, and equipping the environmentally ill (includes those with multiple food, chemical, and inhalant allergies; candidiasis; and CFIDS). *Services:* Tape library, correspondence directory, educational materials, encouragement, and prayer. *Publication:* Share, Care and Prayer Newsletter. *Membership/Subscription Fees:* Supported by contributions.

Working Group on Community Right-to-Know, 215 Pennsylvania Ave. SE, Washington DC 20003-1155, (202) 546-9707; Hours: 9 a.m. to 6 p.m. *Contact:* Paul Orum, Coordinator. *Type of Organization:* Represents more than a dozen environmental and public interest organizations and serves as a nationwide network for activists working to protect and promote the right to know about toxic pollution. *Publication:* Working Notes on Community Right-to-Know. *Subscription:* Common subscription starts at $15 per year.

City, State, and Regional Organizations

Alabama

Allergy and E.I. Support Group of Alabama — HEAL, P.O. Box 913, Pell City AL 35125, (205) 338-9780 or (205) 763-2709. *Contact:* Gail Benefield or Vikki Blalock. *Area Covered:* State of Alabama. *Type of Organization:* Support Group. *Services:* Support and research. *Publication:* Allergy and E.I. Support Group of Alabama — HEAL Newsletter. *Membership/Subscription Fee:* Individuals-$7.50 per year; Family-$10 per year.

Arizona

Yauapai Association for the Chemically Sensitive, 425 S. Alarcon, #1, Prescott AZ 86303, (602) 445-6186 anytime. *Contact:* Sallie Bones. *Area Covered:* Yauapai, Prescott Valley, Dewey, Cottonwood, Sedona, and Verde Valley Counties. *Type of Organization:* Support group for people with MCS. *Services:* Informal picnic meetings, scheduled irregularly and information exchange. *Membership Fees:* None.

Arkansas

Friends United for a Safe Environment (FUSE Inc.), 1313 Hazel St., Texarkana AR 75501, (903) 793-3736 Hours: 9 a.m. to 5 p.m. (Mon-Fri) or (903) 838-4114 All hours. *Area Covered:* Miller County AR, and Bowie County TX. *Contact:* Donald Preston. *Type of Organization:* Grassroots environmental. *Services:* Environmental watch, information, and speakers bureau. *Publication:* FUSE (published irregularly). *Membership:* $10 per year.

California

Environmental Health Association, 1800 S. Robertson Blvd., Suite 380, Los Angeles CA 90035, (213) 837-2048; Hours: 9 a.m. to 7 p.m. (Mon-Fri). *Contact:* Anne Jackson, Director. *Area Covered:* Los Angeles, Orange, Riverside, and Ventura Counties. *Type of Organization:* Self-help network for people with chronic immune dysfunction including the chemically sensitive, chronic fatigue, and candida. *Services:* Monthly meetings and educational resources. *Publication:* Human Ecology Resources. *Membership/Subscription Fees:* $5, $10 for membership, $12 for the newsletter.

Environmental Health Association, P.O. Box 86505, San Diego CA 92138, (619) 588-7509. *Contact:* Giovanna De Santi-Medina. *Area Covered:* City of San Diego. *Type of Organization:* Support group for the chemically sensitive and allergic patient. *Services:* Quarterly meetings, periodic publications, and referrals. *Publication:* EnviroNews. *Membership/Subscription Fees:* $15 per year and $7.50 for the disabled.

Environmental Health Coalition, 1717 Kettner Blvd., Suite 100, San Diego CA 92101, (619) 235-0281; Hours: 9 a.m. to 6 p.m. *Contact:* Diane Takvirian, Executive Director. *Area Covered:* San Diego County, but model programs for national action. *Type of Organization:* Community-based education and advocacy organization dedicated to preventing illnesses resulting from exposure to toxic chemicals in the home, work place, and the community. *Service:* Publications offered on safe use, disposal, and safe substitutes for toxic household products. Community and youth educational slide shows and videotapes. *Publication:* Toxinformer. *Membership/Subscription Fees:* $25 per year.

Environmental Health Network

of California, P.O. Box 1155, Larkspur CA 94939, (415) 331-9804. *Contact:* Susan Molloy. *Area Covered:* San Francisco Bay Area, national networking. *Type of Organization:* Support group for people with environmental illness and or multiple chemical sensitivity. Networking with other disability/environmental groups. *Services:* Information and referral, monthly meetings with guest speakers, special focus groups of various topics, and peer counselor training sessions. *Publication:* The New Reactor. *Membership/Subscription Fees:* $10 for people on fixed income/disability benefits, $20 for employed people.

Morongo Basin Human Ecology Action League, 7880 Wesley Rd., Joshua Tree CA 92252, (619) 228-2970. *Contact:* Connie Sacks. *Area Covered:* Morongo Basin area. *Type of Organization:* Referral, education, and support. *Membership Fees:* None.

Northwest Coalition for Alternatives to Pesticides: Regional organization *see* **Oregon for detailed listing.**

Response Team for the Chemically Injured, P.O. Box 0608, Atascadero CA 93423, (805) 461-3662; Hours 9 a.m. to 4 p.m. *Type of Organization:* Emergency response team for toxic exposures. *Services:* Provides on-site help in the form of resources and referrals.

Stop-Styro Clearinghouse, Administration of Toxics Program, City of Berkeley, 2180 Milvia Street, Berkeley CA 94704, (415) 644-6510, TDD (415) 644-6915; Hours: 9 a.m. to 5 p.m. *Contact;* Cheri A. EIR, Administrator. *Area Covered:* City of Berkeley.

Colorado

Colorado Pesticide Network, 2205 Meade St., Denver CO 80211, (303) 333-8258. *Contact:* Dot Kivett. *Area Covered:* State of Colorado.

Type of Organization: All volunteer. *Services:* Aids people with pesticide complaints, network with like-minded individuals and organizations, education on alternatives to pesticide use, and provides information on local and state ordinances and laws. *Publication:* Colorado Pesticide Network News. *Membership/Subscription Fees:* $5 per year.

Rocky Mountain Environmental Health Association, 575 South Dale Court, Denver CO 80219, (303) 922-0090; Hours: 9 a.m. to 5 p.m. (Mon-Fri). *Contact:* David Foster. *Area Covered:* Rocky Mountain Region. *Type of Organization:* A volunteer support group for all persons whose lifestyle and or health has been adversely affected by the environment. *Services:* Meetings, lending library, resource guide for less toxic living, and educational tapes. *Publication:* RMEHA Newsletter. *Membership/Subscription Fees:* $20 per year.

Florida

Arise Foundation, 4001 Edmund F. Benson Blvd., Miami FL 33178-2384, (305) 59-ARISE; Hours: 7:30 a.m.-5 p.m. *Contact:* Edmund F. Benson. *Area Covered:* Dade County, national networking. *Type of Organization:* Environmental education. *Services:* Works with public schools, county governments, and public hospitals on environmental issues. *Membership Fees:* None.

Citizens Reaction Against Pollution, 6356 Sundown Dr., Jacksonville FL 32244, (904) 771-3098. *Contact:* John N. Austin. *Area Covered:* Duval County, state and national networking. *Type of Organization:* Grassroot environmental group concentrating on military and incinerator pollution. *Services:* Primarily investigations with reports provided to the media. *Membership Fees:* None.

Georgia

H.E.A.L. Atlanta Chapter, P.O. Box 28116, Atlanta GA 30358, (404) 221-3079. *Area Covered:* State of Georgia. *Type of Organization:* Support group for food and chemically sensitive people. *Services:* Monthly support meetings and telephone support services. *Publication:* Healing News & Views. *Membership/Subscription Fee:* $6 per year disabled, $12 per year regular, $24 per year corporate.

Idaho

Idaho Citizen's Network, P.O. Box 362, Kellogg ID 83837, (208) 682-4387; Hours 9 a.m. to 5 p.m. *Contact:* Barbara Miller. *Area Covered:* State of Idaho. *Type of Organization:* Grassroot organization working to resolve issues of social injustice, homelessness, and Hazardous Waste clean up and related health care issues. *Services:* Provide office space and technical assistance in putting together strategies for utilizing strength in numbers and creating new leadership in resolving issues. *Publication:* Citizen Networker. *Membership/Subscription Fees:* Low or Fixed Income—$12 per year, Individual—$18 per year, and Family—$25 per year.

Northwest Coalition for Alternatives to Pesticides: Regional organization *see* **Oregon for detailed listing.**

Illinois

Chicago Area EI/MCS Study Groups, 616 S. Newbury Pl, Arlington Heights IL 60006, (708) 945-7429. *Area Covered:* northern Illinois and Chicago metropolitan area. *Type of Organization:* Environmental illness and multiple chemical sensitivity support group. *Services:* Monthly meetings from September through June. *Publication:* CanaryNews. *Membership/Subscrip-*

tion Fees: $18 per family; sliding scale for special needs.

The Human Ecology Study Group, 3217 N Peoria, Peoria IL 61603, (309) 688-2059. *Contact:* Vilma Kinney. *Area Covered:* Chicago metropolitan area. *Type of Organization:* Human ecology study group. *Services:* Help for the MCS person. *Publication:* Human Ecology Study Group Newsletter. *Membership/Subscription Fees:* $10 per year.

Indiana

Central Indiana H.E.A.L., 1940 S 925 E, Zionsville IN 46077; (317) 769-6261. *Contact:* Lew Bartlet. *Area Covered:* State of Indiana and bordering states. *Type of Organization:* Support for persons with environmental illness and complex allergies. *Services:* Food sources, physician referral, book and video tape library, co-op buying programs, meetings with guest speakers. *Publication:* Central Indiana H.E.A.L. Newsletter. *Membership/Subscription Fees:* $10 per year.

Chemical Injury Information Network, 52145 Farmington Square Rd., Granger IN 46530, (219) 271-8990. *Contact:* Irene Wilkenfeld, President. *Area Covered:* State of Indiana. *Type of Organization:* Support/advocacy organization for the chemically injured. *Services:* Membership package, resource literature, physician and attorney referrals, medical/governmental research for documenting chemically related health problems. *Publication:* Our Toxic Times. *Membership/Subscription Fees:* None, donation accepted.

Iowa

Des Moines Allergy Support Group, 2620 64th, Des Moines IA 50322, (515) 276-2784. *Contact:* Coleen Stanger. *Area Covered:* Des Moines metropolitan area. *Type of Organiza-*

tion: Support group for allergies, candida overgrowth, and chemical sensitivities. *Services:* Monthly meetings providing support, education, idea exchanges, and some advocacy for health issues. *Membership fees:* None.

Louisiana

Injured Workers Union, P.O. Box 1029, Baton Rouge LA 70821, (504) 344-7416 or 800-228-6942; Hours: 9 a.m. to 5 p.m. *Contact:* Allen Bernard. *Type of Organization:* It is part of the Louisiana Consumers League and works primarily on Worker's Compensation Insurance problems. It also works on other insurance/financial problems related to job injuries. It fights to change compensation and workplace safety practices and laws. *Membership Fees:* $5 per month.

LA W.A.T.C.H., Loyola University, Box 12, New Orleans LA 70118, (504) 861-5830 or 800-228-6942; Hours: 9 a.m. to 5 p.m. *Contact:* Bill Temmink. *Area Covered:* State of Louisiana. *Type of Organization:* Workplace safety and chemical awareness. *Services:* Geared towards helping workers and unions assess risks at work and finding ways to lessen those risks. *Membership Fee:* $25 per year.

Massachusetts

Chemical Injury Information Network, P.O. Box 1186, Andover MA 01810, (508) 686-7103. *Contact:* Theo Fournier, President. *Area Covered:* State of Massachusetts. *Type of Organization:* Support/advocacy organization for the chemically injured. *Services:* Membership package, resource literature, physician and attorney referrals, medical/governmental research for documenting chemically related health problems. *Publication:* Our Toxic Times. *Membership/Subscription Fees:* None, donation accepted.

Michigan

Chemical Injury Information Network, 1602 Lyons, Mt. Pleasant MI 48858, (517) 773-1373. *Contact:* Mary Lou Reed, President. *Area Covered:* State of Michigan. *Type of Organization:* Support/advocacy organization for the chemically injured. *Services:* Membership package, resource literature, physician and attorney referrals, medical/governmental research for documenting chemically related health problems. *Publication:* Our Toxic Times. *Membership/Subscription Fees:* None, donation accepted.

Environmental Illness Support Group, 1020 E. Thomas L Parkway, Lansing MI 48917, (517) 321-1409 or 2607 Marion, Lansing MI 48910, (517) 372-0637. *Contacts:* Dorothy Skilling or Barnara Herman. *Area Covered:* Lansing metropolitan area. *Type of Organization:* Support group for the chemically hypersensitive. *Services:* Meetings providing information and support. *Membership fees:* Donations.

Toxics Reduction Project, Ecology Center of Ann Arbor, 417 Detroit St., Ann Arbor MI 48104, (313) 663-2400; Hours: 9:30 a.m. to 5 p.m. *Contact:* Tracey Easthope or Charles Griffith. *Area Covered:* State of Michigan. *Type of Organization:* Community-based environmental education and advocacy and assistance to grassroot groups on toxics. *Publication:* Eco-Reports and Michigan Toxic Watch. *Subscriptions:* Eco-Reports — $15 to $25 per year. Michigan Toxic Watch — $5 per year.

Montana

Chemical Injury Information Network, P.O. Box 301, White Sulphur Springs, MT 59645, (406) 547-2255

Area Covered: State of Montana. *Type of Organization:* Support/advocacy organization for the chemically injured. *Services:* Membership package, resource literature, physician and attorney referrals, medical/governmental research for documenting chemically related health problems. *Publication:* Our Toxic Times. *Membership/Subscription Fees:* None, donation accepted.

New Hampshire

New Hampshire Toxic Hazards Campaign, 26 Wilders Grove, Newton NH 03858, (603) 382-6963; Hours: 8 a.m. to 8 p.m. *Contact:* Martha Railey. *Area Covered:* State of New Hampshire. *Type of Organization:* Environmental group concerned with superfund sites, landspills, incinerators, ash dumps, health issues, air quality, right-to-know laws, RCRA, and pesticides. *Services:* Organizing grassroot support to toxic clean up. *Membership Fees:* None.

Nebraska

Citizen Action of Nebraska, 941 "O" Street, Suite 600, Lincoln NE 68508, (402) 477-8689; Hours: 9 a.m. to 5 p.m. *Contact:* Mary Harding, Executive Director. *Area Covered:* State of Nebraska. *Type of Organization:* Citizen's lobbying group working to pass environmental, health, and consumer legislation. *Publication:* Citizen Action News. *Membership/Subscription Fees:* $5 per year membership/$15 per year newsletter.

New York

Human Ecology League of Central New York, 3773 Dorothy Drive, Syracuse NY 13215, (315) 492-0091; Hours: 9 a.m. to 9 p.m. *Contact:* Eleanor Hathaway. *Area Covered:* Central

New York and national networking. *Type of Organization:* Support group for those with allergies, multiple chemical sensitivities (MCS), and environmental illness (EI). *Services:* Meeting, "Resource for Recovery" bulletin, cassette tape lending library, telephone support services. *Publications:* The Healer Newsletter. *Membership/Subscription Fee:* $15 per year.

New York City H.E.A.L., c/o Sandy Anello, 506 E. 84th Street, New York NY 10028, (212) 517-5937. *Contact:* Sandy Anello. *Area Covered:* New York City. *Type of Organization:* Support group for allergies, candida, and environmental illness. *Services:* Monthly meetings with guest speakers. *Publication:* NYC H.E.A.L. Newsletter. *Membership/Subscription Fees:* $20 per year for singles, $25 per year for families, $5 for non-members to attend meetings.

New York Coalition for Alternatives to Pesticides, 33 Central Avenue, Albany NY 12210, (518) 426-8246. *Contact:* Tracy Frisch. *Area Covered:* State of New York, national networking. *Type of Organization:* Citizens organization working to reduce pesticide use, promote alternatives, and support protective policies. Also works on various aspects of environmental health issues, including chemical sensitivities. *Services:* Information and referral organizational support publications, speakers bureau, workshops, and other advocacy projects. *Publication:* NYCAP News Quarterly. *Membership/Subscription Fees:* $15 per year individuals, $25 for organizations, and $50 per year for businesses.

Ohio

Citizen Action, 1406 W. 6th Street, Cleveland OH 44113, (216) 861-5200; Hours: 9 a.m. to 5 p.m. *Contact:* Sandy Buchanan. *Area Covered:* State of Ohio. *Type of Organization:* Consumer and environmental organization.

Services: Community organizing lobbying effort working on ballot initiative requiring companies to warn people when they expose them to chemicals that cause cancer or birth defects. *Publication:* Toxic Watch. *Membership/Subscription Fees:* $5 per year for membership; $15 for year for membership and subscription.

Oklahoma

Earth Concerns of Oklahoma, P.O. Box 1373, Tulsa OK 74101-1372, (918) 744-1827. *Contact:* Tim Collins. *Area Covered:* Oklahoma, northwest Arkansas, southwest Missouri, and southern Kansas. *Type of Organization:* Broad scope of environmental issues with a strong sub-group concerning multiple chemical sensitivities, environmental illness, etc. *Services:* Informational publications, self-help assistance, lobbying, environmental activism, and humor in the face of crisis. *Publication:* The Ecological. *Subscription fees:* $10 per year.

Oregon

Northwest Coalition for Alternatives to Pesticides, P.O. Box 1393, Eugene OR 97440, (503) 344-5044; Hours: 11 a.m. to 5 p.m. (Mon-Fri). *Contact:* Norma Greer. *Area Covered:* Oregon, Washington, Idaho, Eastern Montana, and Northern California. *Type of Organization:* Pesticide reform. *Services:* Promotes sustainable resource management, prevention of pest problems, use of alternatives to pesticides and protection of an individuals rights to be free from pesticide exposure. *Publication:* Journal of Pesticide Reform. *Membership/Subscription Fees:* Basic membership $25 per year.

Pennsylvania

Delaware Valley Toxics Coalition, 125 S. 9th St., 7th Flr., Philadelphia PA 19107, (215) 627-5300; Hours: 9 a.m. to 5 p.m. *Contact:* Greg Schrim. *Area Covered:* Philadelphia metropolitan area. *Type of Organization:* Provides information and assistance to individuals and local community groups in identifying environmental health hazards and works to mitigate or eliminate these problems. *Services:* Provides information about toxic chemicals, including health effects, environmental standards, sources of toxic chemical pollution, strategies for mitigating or eliminating hazards. *Membership:* Not a membership organization.

South Carolina

Chemical Injury Information Network, HC 60 Box 53, Due West SC 29639, (803) 379-8494. *Contact:* Lynn Wegener, President. *Area Covered:* State of South Carolina. *Type of Organization:* Support/advocacy organization for the chemical injured. *Services:* Membership package, resource literature, physician and attorney referrals, medical/governmental research for documenting chemically related health problems. *Publication:* Our Toxic Times. *Membership/Subscription Fees:* None, donation accepted.

Texas

The Chemical Connection, RR 1 Box 276A65, Wimberly TX 78676, (512) 847-9245. *Contact:* Susan Pitman. *Area Covered:* State of Texas. *Type of Organization:* Public health network of Texans sensitive to chemicals. *Services:* Connecting people who understand that chemical exposure affects their health with others who share experiences and solutions. Its ultimate goal is to secure a healthy environment and economy for Texas. *Publication:* The Chemical Connection (not published on a regular basis). *Membership/Subscriptions Fee:* None, small donations to help with printing and postage are appreciated.

Texans United Education Fund, 3400 Montrose, Suite 225, Houston TX 77006, (713) 453-0857; Hours 8 a.m. to 5 p.m. *Contact:* Richard Abraham, Executive Director. *Area Covered:* State of Texas. *Type of Organization:* Environmental. *Services:* Advocacy and organizing assistance. *Publication:* Texas Report. *Membership/Subscription Fees:* $15 per year.

Texas Coalition on Occupational Safety and Health (TexCOSH), 5735 Regina, Beaumont TX 77706, (409) 898-1427; Hours: 8 a.m. to 9 p.m. *Contact:* Karyl Dunson. *Area Covered: State of Texas. Type of Organization:* Health and safety information for workers who have become injured or ill from workplace exposures. *Services:* Information and referral services. Classes on safety information, tracking occupational diseases. Plans pro-active support. *Membership Fees:* Information not yet available.

Utah

Utah Environment Center, 637 East 400 South, Suite F, Salt Lake City UT 84102, (801) 332-0220; Hours: 9 a.m. to 5 p.m., but irregular. *Contact:* Alan Miller. *Area Covered:* State of Texas. *Type of Organization:* Environmental health group specializing in air and water quality and waste management. *Services:* Community organizing, coalition building, lobbying, public policy formulation. *Membership Fees:* None.

Virginia

H.E.A.L. of Richmond, 12350 Natural Bark Dr., Chesterfield VA 23832, (000) 288-0161; Hours 9 a.m. to 6 p.m. *Contact:* Linda Schonfeld. *Area Covered:* Richmond and surrounding area. *Type of Organization:* Self-help support group for environmental illness, chemical allergies, and candida. *Services:* Support meetings. *Publication:* Today's Alternatives Toward Health. *Membership/Subscription Fees:* $12 per year.

Washington

Washington Toxics Coalition, 4516 University Way NE, Seattle WA 98105, (206) 632-1545; Hours: 9 a.m. to 5 p.m. *Area Covered:* State of Washington. *Type of Organization:* Environmental. *Services:* Information on health and environmental effects of pesticides and other toxic chemicals. *Publication:* Alternatives. *Membership Fees:* $20 per year.

Wyoming

Northwest Coalition for Alternatives to Pesticides: Regional organization *see* **Oregon for detailed listing.**

Chemical Injury Information Network — Wyoming, P.O. Box 130, Sheridan Wy 82801, (307) 672-3619. *Contact:* E.J. Hando, President. *Area Covered:* State of Wyoming. *Type of Organization:* Support/advocacy organization for the chemically injured. *Services:* Membership package, resource literature, physician and attorney referrals, medical/governmental research and publications for documenting chemically related health problems. *Publication:* Our Toxic Times. *Membership/Subscription Fees:* None, donation accepted.

Publications

Allergy Connections, P.O. Box 154, Pewaukee WI 53072, *Publisher/Editor:* Angela McCormick. *Type of* *Publication:* Offers support, information, and inspiration for people with allergies, environmental illness, and candidiasis. *Subscription:* $8 per year. Free sample with self addressed, stamped envelope. $52 postage required.

Environment & Health, P.O. Box 41057, Santa Barbara CA 93140. *Editor:* Joanne Bahura. *Type of Publication:* Environmental health issues. *Publication:* Environment and Health. *Membership/Subscription Fees:* $20 individuals; $45 business, organizations, clinics, $15 students/low income for 6 issues.

Green Alternatives, Box 28, An-nandale NY 12504, (914) 246-6948. *Publisher/ Editor:* Annie Berthold-Bond. *Type of Publication:* Consumer's guide to safe, effective, globally responsible products and practices. *Subscription:* $22.50 per year.

New Health Standard Journal, Burgandy Court Publishers, P.O. Box 8182, Fort Collins CO 80526, (303) 229-8484. *Publisher/Editor:* Nancy Watson. *Type of Publications:* Environmental health journal. *Subscription:* $18 per year for 6 issues.

Research Services

See previous listing for Chemical Injury Information Network under National Organizations.

Environmental Access Research Network, Route 1, Box 16-G, Epping ND 58843. *Contact:* Cindy Duehring, Research Director. *Type of Organization:* Medical and Governmental literature research and library regarding chemical, health, and environmental issues.

Minnesota Pesticide Coalition—Health Alternative, 22 Garden Drive, Silver Bay MN 55614, (218) 226-4043. *Contact:* Mary Pacholke. *Area Covered:* State of Minnesota. *Type of Organization:* Researches and dispenses information on pesticides. Consults with environmental organization and individuals on health issues and provides educational material.

Speakers

Arts, Crafts and Theater Safety, Inc. (A.C.T.S.), 181 Thompson St., #23, New York NY 10012-2586, (212) 777-0062; Hours 9 a.m. to 5 p.m. *Contact:* Nonona Rossol. *Topic/Issues:* Health and safety issues in the arts and OSHA compliance.

Edmund F. Benson, 4001 Edmund F. Benson Blvd., Miami FL 33178-2384, (305) 59-ARISE; Hours: 7:30 a.m. to 5 p.m. *Topic/Issues:* Environmental Education.

Center for Safety in the Arts, 5 Bechman Street, Suite 1030, New York NY 10038, (212) 227-6220; Hours: 9 a.m. to 5 p.m. (Mon-Fri). *Contact:* Angela Bubin. *Topics/Issues:* Health and safety relating to the arts.

Edmund Fitzgerald, 1200 Old Dump Road, Bigfork MT 59911, (406) 537-5548. *Topics/Issues:* Recycling.

Irene Wilkenfeld, 52145 Farmington Square Road, Granger IN 46530, (219) 271-8990; Hours: 9 a.m. to 9 p.m. *Topics/Issues:* The sick school syndrome/detoxifying our contaminated classrooms, how to prevent environmental illness environmental awareness lectures, workshops, seminars, and consultations.

Bibliography

1. Aatron Medical Services, Service Information Package, Hawthorne, CA.
2. Accu-Chem Laboratories, Service Schedule, Richardson, TX.
3. American Lung Association of Washington, press release for brochure, *Indoor Air Pollution in the Office,* Seattle, WA, 1992 (undated).
4. Antibody Assay Laboratories, Service Information Package, Santa Ana, CA.
5. Ashford, N.A., and C.S. Miller, *Chemical Exposures: Low Levels and High Stakes,* New York: Van Nostrand Reinhold, 1991.
6. Ashford, N.A., and C.S. Miller, "Chemical Sensitivity: A Report to the New Jersey State Department of Health," New Jersey State Department of Health, December 1989.
7. Bardana, E.J., and A. Monanaro, "Common Medical Conditions Often Present as 'Toxicity'; 'Chemical Sensitive' Patients: Avoiding the Pitfalls," *The Journal of Respiratory Diseases,* 10(1) (Jan. 1989): 32–45.
8. Berthold-Bond, A., *Clean & Green,* Woodstock, NY: Ceres Press, 1990.
9. Broughton, A., et al; "Chronic Health Effects and Immunological Alterations Associated with Exposure to Pesticides," *Comment Toxicology,* 4(1) (1990): 59–71.
10. "California: Air Board Lists Formaldehyde as Air Toxic: Control Program Could Take Year to Develop," *Environmental Reporter,* March 20, 1992, p. 2575.
11. California Senate Office of Research, Elisabeth Kersten, director, and Bruce Jennings, "Pesticides and Regulation: The Myth of Safety," Senate Reprographics, April 1991.
12. Castleman, B.I., and G.E. Ziem "Corporate Influence on Threshold Limit Values," *American Journal of Industrial Medicine* 13 (1988): 531–559.
13. Chesebrough-Ponds USA Co., product label for Rave All in One hair spray, ca. 1992.
14. Chesebrough-Ponds USA Co., product label for Super-hold Aqua Net Professional hair spray, SDA-34-782, ca. 1992.
15. Colgate-Palmolive Company, product label for Extra Protection Formula shave cream, ca. 1992.
16. Combe Incorporated, product label for Lanacane, ca. 1992.
17. Concrete Facts, "99.99 Percent?" March 1991, Vol. 1. no. 1 and/or Rachel's Hazardous Waste News #207, "Hazardous Waste Incineration—Part 4; Real Alternatives to Incinerations," November 14, 1990.
18. "Congress: HR 1066 Needed to Turn Heat Up on Employers, Regulators, Congress Told," *Indoor Pollution News,* Washington, DC: Buraff, August 22, 1991.
19. ESPE GmbH & Co., KG, Material Safety Data Sheet for IMPREGUM F Adhesive, January 27, 1988.
20. Fielder, R.J., et al, *Toxicity Review: Trimellitic Anhydride,* London: Crown, 1983.
21. Gard, Z., *American Academy of Environmental Medicine Newsletter,* Winter 1990.
22. The Gillette Company, product label for Right Guard deodorant, ca. 1992.
23. Grier, N., NCAP (Northwest Coalition for Alternatives to Pesticides) member letter, Winter 1991.
24. Hileman, B., "Multiple Chemical Sensitivity," *Chemical and Engineering News,* July 22, 1991.
25. "Household Waste Need Not Trash the Environment," *ChemEcology* July/August 1991.
26. Lum, M., Dept. of Health and Human Services, letter to Dr. Grace Ziem, Oct. 29, 1991.
27. Institute of Medicine, Division of Health Promotion and Disease Prevention, *Role of the*

Primary Care Physician in Occupational and Environmental Medicine, Washington, DC: National Academy Press, 1988.

28. Institute of Medicine, Division of Health Promotion and Disease Prevention, *Addressing the Physician Shortage in Occupational and Environmental Medicine,* Washington, DC: National Academy Press, 1991.

29. K-mart Corporation, product label for Baby Lotion, ca. 1992.

30. Lander Co., product label for Rose Scented Skin Cream, ca. 1992.

31. Lander Co., product label for Vitamin E Lotion, ca. 1992.

31a. McCullough, M., "Study Raises Worries of Illness from Carpet," *Philadelphia Inquirer,* August 26, 1992.

32. Meggs, W.J., "Multiple Chemical Sensitivities and the Immune System," prepared for the invited workshop on Multiple Chemical Sensitivities (MCS) sponsored by the Association of Occupational and Environmental Clinics (AOEC), Washington, DC, September 19–20, 1991.

33. Morrow, L.A., et al, "PET and Neurobehavioral Evidence of Tetrabromoethane Encephalopathy," *Journal of Neuropsychiatry,* 2(4) (Fall 1990).

34. National Library of Medicine's Toxicology Information Program, Agency for Toxic Substances and Disease Registry, Hazardous Substances Data Bank, "Methylacrylate Acid, Ethyl Ester," as of January 12, 1992.

35. National Library of Medicine's Toxicology Information Program, Agency for Toxic Substances and Disease Registry, Hazardous Substances Data Bank, "Phosdine," as of January 14, 1992.

36. National Library of Medicine's Toxicology Information Program, Agency for Toxic Substances and Disease Registry, Hazardous Substances Data Bank, "1,4-Dinitrobenzene," as of February 9, 1992.

37. National Library of Medicine's Toxicology Information Program, Agency for Toxic Substances and Disease Registry, Hazardous Substances Data Bank, "Lead," as of November 7, 1991.

38. National Library of Medicine's Toxicology Information Program, Agency for Toxic Substances and Disease Registry, Hazardous Substances Data Bank, "1,3-Dichloropropene," as of January 10, 1992.

39. National Library of Medicine's Toxicology Information Program, Agency for Toxic Substances and Disease Registry, Hazardous Substances Data Bank, "Linonene," as of January 10, 1992.

40. National Library of Medicine's Toxicology Information Program, Agency for Toxic Substances and Disease Registry, Hazardous Substances Data Bank, "Linalyl Alcohol," as of January 10, 1992.

41. National Library of Medicine's Toxicology Information Program, Agency for Toxic Substances and Disease Registry, Hazardous Substances Data Bank, "2,4-D," as of January 10, 1992.

42. National Library of Medicine's Toxicology Information Program, Agency for Toxic Substances and Disease Registry, Hazardous Substances Data Bank, "1,3-Dichloro-5,5-dimethylhydantoin," as of January 10, 1992.

43. National Library of Medicine's Toxicology Information Program, Agency for Toxic Substances and Disease Registry, Hazardous Substances Data Bank, "2-Butoxyethanol," as of January 11, 1992.

44. National Library of Medicine's Toxicology Information Program, Agency for Toxic Substances and Disease Registry, Hazardous Substances Data Bank, "2-Aminopyridine," as of January 11, 1992.

45. National Library of Medicine's Toxicology Information Program, Agency for Toxic Substances and Disease Registry, Hazardous Substances Data Bank, "2-Diethylaminoethanol," as of January 11, 1992.

46. National Library of Medicine's Toxicology Information Program, Agency for Toxic Substances and Disease Registry, Hazardous Substances Data Bank, "Acetic Acid," as of January 12, 1992.

47. National Library of Medicine's Toxicology Information Program, Agency for Toxic Substances and Disease Registry, Hazardous Substances Data Bank, "Allyl Chloride," as of January 12, 1992.

48. National Library of Medicine's Toxicology Information Program, Agency for Toxic Substances and Disease Registry, Hazardous Substances Data Bank, "Azinphosmethyl," as of January 12, 1992.
49. National Library of Medicine's Toxicology Information Program, Agency for Toxic Substances and Disease Registry, Hazardous Substances Data Bank, "Benzoyl Peroxide," as of January 12, 1992.
50. National Library of Medicine's Toxicology Information Program, Agency for Toxic Substances and Disease Registry, Hazardous Substances Data Bank, "Benzyl Chloride," as of January 12, 1992.
51. National Library of Medicine's Toxicology Information Program, Agency for Toxic Substances and Disease Registry, Hazardous Substances Data Bank, "Allyl Alcohol," as of January 12, 1992.
52. National Library of Medicine's Toxicology Information Program, Agency for Toxic Substances and Disease Registry, Hazardous Substances Data Bank, "Calcium Arsenate," as of January 12, 1992.
53. National Library of Medicine's Toxicology Information Program, Agency for Toxic Substances and Disease Registry, Hazardous Substances Data Bank, "Calcium Oxide," as of January 12, 1992.
54. National Library of Medicine's Toxicology Information Program, Agency for Toxic Substances and Disease Registry, Hazardous Substances Data Bank, "Camphor," as of January 12, 1992.
55. National Library of Medicine's Toxicology Information Program, Agency for Toxic Substances and Disease Registry, Hazardous Substances Data Bank, "Carbaryl," as of January 14, 1992.
56. National Library of Medicine's Toxicology Information Program, Agency for Toxic Substances and Disease Registry, Hazardous Substances Data Bank, "Carbon Dioxide," as of January 12, 1992.
57. National Library of Medicine's Toxicology Information Program, Agency for Toxic Substances and Disease Registry, Hazardous Substances Data Bank, "Carbon Monoxide," as of January 12, 1992.
58. National Library of Medicine's Toxicology Information Program, Agency for Toxic Substances and Disease Registry, Hazardous Substances Data Bank, "Chlorinated Camphene," as of January 12, 1992.
59. National Library of Medicine's Toxicology Information Program, Agency for Toxic Substances and Disease Registry, Hazardous Substances Data Bank, "Polychlorinated Biphenyls," as of January 12, 1992.
60. National Library of Medicine's Toxicology Information Program, Agency for Toxic Substances and Disease Registry, Hazardous Substances Data Bank, "Chlorine Dioxide," as of January 12, 1992.
61. National Library of Medicine's Toxicology Information Program, Agency for Toxic Substances and Disease Registry, Hazardous Substances Data Bank, "Acetone," as of January 13, 1992.
62. National Library of Medicine's Toxicology Information Program, Agency for Toxic Substances and Disease Registry, Hazardous Substances Data Bank, "Ethanol," as of January 13, 1992.
63. National Library of Medicine's Toxicology Information Program, Agency for Toxic Substances and Disease Registry, Hazardous Substances Data Bank, "Iodine," as of January 13, 1992.
64. National Library of Medicine's Toxicology Information Program, Agency for Toxic Substances and Disease Registry, Hazardous Substances Data Bank, "Trimellitic Anhydride," as of January 13, 1992.
65. National Library of Medicine's Toxicology Information Program, Agency for Toxic Substances and Disease Registry, Hazardous Substances Data Bank, "Chlorpyrifos," as of January 13, 1992.
66. National Library of Medicine's Toxicology Information Program, Agency for Toxic Substances and Disease Registry, Hazardous Substances Data Bank, "Cyclohexanol," as of January 14, 1992.

67. National Library of Medicine's Toxicology Information Program, Agency for Toxic Substances and Disease Registry, Hazardous Substances Data Bank, "Cyclohexane," as of January 14, 1992.

68. National Library of Medicine's Toxicology Information Program, Agency for Toxic Substances and Disease Registry, Hazardous Substances Data Bank, "Chlorobenzene," as of January 14, 1992.

69. National Library of Medicine's Toxicology Information Program, Agency for Toxic Substances and Disease Registry, Hazardous Substances Data Bank, "Crotonaldehyde," as of January 14, 1992.

70. National Library of Medicine's Toxicology Information Program, Agency for Toxic Substances and Disease Registry, Hazardous Substances Data Bank, "Cumeme," as of January 14, 1992.

71. National Library of Medicine's Toxicology Information Program, Agency for Toxic Substances and Disease Registry, Hazardous Substances Data Bank, "Chloromethyl Methyl Ether," as of January 14, 1992.

72. National Library of Medicine's Toxicology Information Program, Agency for Toxic Substances and Disease Registry, Hazardous Substances Data Bank, "Chloropicrin," as of January 14, 1992.

73. National Library of Medicine's Toxicology Information Program, Agency for Toxic Substances and Disease Registry, Hazardous Substances Data Bank, "Creosote, Wood," as of January 14, 1992.

74. National Library of Medicine's Toxicology Information Program, Agency for Toxic Substances and Disease Registry, Hazardous Substances Data Bank, "Coal Tar Creosote," as of January 14, 1992.

75. National Library of Medicine's Toxicology Information Program, Agency for Toxic Substances and Disease Registry, Hazardous Substances Data Bank, "Benzene," as of January 14, 1992.

76. National Library of Medicine's Toxicology Information Program, Agency for Toxic Substances and Disease Registry, Hazardous Substances Data Bank, "Diethylamine," as of January 14, 1992.

77. National Library of Medicine's Toxicology Information Program, Agency for Toxic Substances and Disease Registry, Hazardous Substances Data Bank, "Diglycidyl Ether," as of January 14, 1992.

78. National Library of Medicine's Toxicology Information Program, Agency for Toxic Substances and Disease Registry, Hazardous Substances Data Bank, "Diisobutyl Ketone," as of January 14, 1992.

79. National Library of Medicine's Toxicology Information Program, Agency for Toxic Substances and Disease Registry, Hazardous Substances Data Bank, "Diisopropylamine," as of January 14, 1992.

80. National Library of Medicine's Toxicology Information Program, Agency for Toxic Substances and Disease Registry, Hazardous Substances Data Bank, "N,N-Dimethylacetamide," as of January 14, 1992.

81. National Library of Medicine's Toxicology Information Program, Agency for Toxic Substances and Disease Registry, Hazardous Substances Data Bank, "Naled," as of January 14, 1992.

82. National Library of Medicine's Toxicology Information Program, Agency for Toxic Substances and Disease Registry, Hazardous Substances Data Bank, "Dimethylamine," as of January 14, 1992.

83. National Library of Medicine's Toxicology Information Program, Agency for Toxic Substances and Disease Registry, Hazardous Substances Data Bank, "Dimethylaniline," as of January 14, 1992.

84. National Library of Medicine's Toxicology Information Program, Agency for Toxic Substances and Disease Registry, Hazardous Substances Data Bank, "Xylidine," as of January 14, 1992.

85. National Library of Medicine's Toxicology Information Program, Agency for Toxic Substances and Disease Registry, Hazardous Substances Data Bank, "N,N-Dimethylformamide," as of January 14, 1992.

86. National Library of Medicine's Toxicology Information Program, Agency for Toxic Substances and Disease Registry, Hazardous Substances Data Bank, "Dimethylphthalate," as of January 14, 1992.
87. National Library of Medicine's Toxicology Information Program, Agency for Toxic Substances and Disease Registry, Hazardous Substances Data Bank, "Dinitrobenzene," as of January 14, 1992.
88. National Library of Medicine's Toxicology Information Program, Agency for Toxic Substances and Disease Registry, Hazardous Substances Data Bank, "4,6-Dinitro-o-cresol," as of January 14, 1992.
89. National Library of Medicine's Toxicology Information Program, Agency for Toxic Substances and Disease Registry, Hazardous Substances Data Bank, "Benzyl acetate," as of January 14, 1992.
90. National Library of Medicine's Toxicology Information Program, Agency for Toxic Substances and Disease Registry, Hazardous Substances Data Bank, "Benzyl alcohol," as of January 14, 1992.
91. National Library of Medicine's Toxicology Information Program, Agency for Toxic Substances and Disease Registry, Hazardous Substances Data Bank, "1,1,2,2-Tetrabromoethane," as of January 14, 1992.
92. National Library of Medicine's Toxicology Information Program, Agency for Toxic Substances and Disease Registry, Hazardous Substances Data Bank, "Ammonium Sulfamate," as of January 14, 1992.
93. National Library of Medicine's Toxicology Information Program, Agency for Toxic Substances and Disease Registry, Hazardous Substances Data Bank, "Dimethyl sulfate," as of January 14, 1992.
94. National Library of Medicine's Toxicology Information Program, Agency for Toxic Substances and Disease Registry, Hazardous Substances Data Bank, "Acetaldehyde," as of January 14, 1992.
95. National Library of Medicine's Toxicology Information Program, Agency for Toxic Substances and Disease Registry, Hazardous Substances Data Bank, "Acetonitrile," as of January 14, 1992.
96. National Library of Medicine's Toxicology Information Program, Agency for Toxic Substances and Disease Registry, Hazardous Substances Data Bank, "Acrolein," as of January 14, 1992.
97. National Library of Medicine's Toxicology Information Program, Agency for Toxic Substances and Disease Registry, Hazardous Substances Data Bank, "2-Chloro-1,3-Butadiene," as of January 14, 1992.
98. National Library of Medicine's Toxicology Information Program, Agency for Toxic Substances and Disease Registry, Hazardous Substances Data Bank, "Bromine," as of January 14, 1992.
99. National Library of Medicine's Toxicology Information Program, Agency for Toxic Substances and Disease Registry, Hazardous Substances Data Bank, "N-Butylamine," as of January 14, 1992.
100. National Library of Medicine's Toxicology Information Program, Agency for Toxic Substances and Disease Registry, Hazardous Substances Data Bank, "Chlorine," as of January 14, 1992.
101. National Library of Medicine's Toxicology Information Program, Agency for Toxic Substances and Disease Registry, Hazardous Substances Data Bank, "Chloroacetaldehyde," as of January 14, 1992.
102. National Library of Medicine's Toxicology Information Program, Agency for Toxic Substances and Disease Registry, Hazardous Substances Data Bank, "Decaborane," as of January 14, 1992.
103. National Library of Medicine's Toxicology Information Program, Agency for Toxic Substances and Disease Registry, Hazardous Substances Data Bank, "4-Hydroxy-4-Methyl-2-Pentanone," as of January 14, 1992.
104. National Library of Medicine's Toxicology Information Program, Agency for Toxic Substances and Disease Registry, Hazardous Substances Data Bank, "Dichlorodifluoromethane," as of January 14, 1992.

105. National Library of Medicine's Toxicology Information Program, Agency for Toxic Substances and Disease Registry, Hazardous Substances Data Bank, "bis(2-Chloroethyl) Ether," as of January 14, 1992.

106. National Library of Medicine's Toxicology Information Program, Agency for Toxic Substances and Disease Registry, Hazardous Substances Data Bank, "1,2-Dichloroethylene," as of January 14, 1992.

107. National Library of Medicine's Toxicology Information Program, Agency for Toxic Substances and Disease Registry, Hazardous Substances Data Bank, "Freon 21," as of January 14, 1992.

108. National Library of Medicine's Toxicology Information Program, Agency for Toxic Substances and Disease Registry, Hazardous Substances Data Bank, "Freon 114," as of January 14, 1992.

109. National Library of Medicine's Toxicology Information Program, Agency for Toxic Substances and Disease Registry, Hazardous Substances Data Bank, "Aniline," as of January 14, 1992.

110. National Library of Medicine's Toxicology Information Program, Agency for Toxic Substances and Disease Registry, Hazardous Substances Data Bank, "Ethyl Silicate," as of January 16, 1992.

111. National Library of Medicine's Toxicology Information Program, Agency for Toxic Substances and Disease Registry, Hazardous Substances Data Bank, "Acetic Anhydride," as of January 16, 1992.

112. National Library of Medicine's Toxicology Information Program, Agency for Toxic Substances and Disease Registry, Hazardous Substances Data Bank, "EPN," as of January 14, 1992.

113. National Library of Medicine's Toxicology Information Program, Agency for Toxic Substances and Disease Registry, Hazardous Substances Data Bank, "Ethyl Acetate," as of January 16, 1992.

114. National Library of Medicine's Toxicology Information Program, Agency for Toxic Substances and Disease Registry, Hazardous Substances Data Bank, "2-Aminoethanol," as of January 16, 1992.

115. National Library of Medicine's Toxicology Information Program, Agency for Toxic Substances and Disease Registry, Hazardous Substances Data Bank, "Ethyl Bromide," as of January 16, 1992.

116. National Library of Medicine's Toxicology Information Program, Agency for Toxic Substances and Disease Registry, Hazardous Substances Data Bank, "Ethyl Acrylate," as of January 16, 1992.

117. National Library of Medicine's Toxicology Information Program, Agency for Toxic Substances and Disease Registry, Hazardous Substances Data Bank, "Ethyl Butyl Ketone," as of January 16, 1992.

118. National Library of Medicine's Toxicology Information Program, Agency for Toxic Substances and Disease Registry, Hazardous Substances Data Bank, "Diethyl Ether," as of January 16, 1992.

119. National Library of Medicine's Toxicology Information Program, Agency for Toxic Substances and Disease Registry, Hazardous Substances Data Bank, "Ethyl Chloride," as of January 16, 1992.

120. National Library of Medicine's Toxicology Information Program, Agency for Toxic Substances and Disease Registry, Hazardous Substances Data Bank, "Ethylene Glycol Monoethyl Ether Acetate," as of January 16, 1992.

121. National Library of Medicine's Toxicology Information Program, Agency for Toxic Substances and Disease Registry, Hazardous Substances Data Bank, "Ethyl Mercaptan," as of January 16, 1992.

122. National Library of Medicine's Toxicology Information Program, Agency for Toxic Substances and Disease Registry, Hazardous Substances Data Bank, "Ethyl Formate," as of Jnauary 16, 1992.

123. National Library of Medicine's Toxicology Information Program, Agency for Toxic Substances and Disease Registry, Hazardous Substances Data Bank, "1Nitropropane," as of January 16, 1992.

124. National Library of Medicine's Toxicology Information Program, Agency for Toxic Substances and Disease Registry, Hazardous Substances Data Bank, "beta-Propiolactone," as of January 16, 1992.

125. National Library of Medicine's Toxicology Information Program, Agency for Toxic Substances and Disease Registry, Hazardous Substances Data Bank, "Dinitrotoluene," as of January 16, 1992.

126. National Library of Medicine's Toxicology Information Program, Agency for Toxic Substances and Disease Registry, Hazardous Substances Data Bank, "alpha-Methyl Styrene," as of January 16, 1992.

127. National Library of Medicine's Toxicology Information Program, Agency for Toxic Substances and Disease Registry, Hazardous Substances Data Bank, "Epichlorohydrin," as of January 16, 1992.

128. National Library of Medicine's Toxicology Information Program, Agency for Toxic Substances and Disease Registry, Hazardous Substances Data Bank, "Formic Acid," as of January 17, 1992.

129. National Library of Medicine's Toxicology Information Program, Agency for Toxic Substances and Disease Registry, Hazardous Substances Data Bank, "Formaldehyde," as of January 17, 1992.

130. National Library of Medicine's Toxicology Information Program, Agency for Toxic Substances and Disease Registry, Hazardous Substances Data Bank, "Freon 11," as of January 17, 1992.

131. National Library of Medicine's Toxicology Information Program, Agency for Toxic Substances and Disease Registry, Hazardous Substances Data Bank, "Ferbam," as of January 17, 1992.

132. National Library of Medicine's Toxicology Information Program, Agency for Toxic Substances and Disease Registry, Hazardous Substances Data Bank, "Ethyleneimine," as of January 17, 1992.

133. National Library of Medicine's Toxicology Information Program, Agency for Toxic Substances and Disease Registry, Hazardous Substances Data Bank, "Ethylenediamine," as of January 17, 1992.

134. National Library of Medicine's Toxicology Information Program, Agency for Toxic Substances and Disease Registry, Hazardous Substances Data Bank, "Ethylene Glycol Dinitrate," as of January 17, 1992.

135. National Library of Medicine's Toxicology Information Program, Agency for Toxic Substances and Disease Registry, Hazardous Substances Data Bank, "1,2-Dichloroethane," as of January 17, 1992.

136. National Library of Medicine's Toxicology Information Program, Agency for Toxic Substances and Disease Registry, Hazardous Substances Data Bank, "Ethylene Dibromide," as of January 17, 1992.

137. National Library of Medicine's Toxicology Information Program, Agency for Toxic Substances and Disease Registry, Hazardous Substances Data Bank, "Ethylamine," as of January 17, 1992.

138. National Library of Medicine's Toxicology Information Program, Agency for Toxic Substances and Disease Registry, Hazardous Substances Data Bank, "Systox," as of January 17, 1992.

139. National Library of Medicine's Toxicology Information Program, Agency for Toxic Substances and Disease Registry, Hazardous Substances Data Bank, "Isoamyl Alcohol," as of January 18, 1992.

140. National Library of Medicine's Toxicology Information Program, Agency for Toxic Substances and Disease Registry, Hazardous Substances Data Bank, "Isoamyl Acetate," as of January 18, 1992.

141. National Library of Medicine's Toxicology Information Program, Agency for Toxic Substances and Disease Registry, Hazardous Substances Data Bank, "Hydrogen Sulfide," as of January 18, 1992.

142. National Library of Medicine's Toxicology Information Program, Agency for Toxic Substances and Disease Registry, Hazardous Substances Data Bank, "Hydrogen Peroxide," as of January 18, 1992.

143. National Library of Medicine's Toxicology Information Program, Agency for Toxic Substances and Disease Registry, Hazardous Substances Data Bank, "Hydrazine," as of January 18, 1992.

144. National Library of Medicine's Toxicology Information Program, Agency for Toxic Substances and Disease Registry, Hazardous Substances Data Bank, "Methyl Isobutyl Ketone," as of January 18, 1992.

145. National Library of Medicine's Toxicology Information Program, Agency for Toxic Substances and Disease Registry, Hazardous Substances Data Bank, "Hexachloro-naphthalene," as of January 18, 1992.

146. National Library of Medicine's Toxicology Information Program, Agency for Toxic Substances and Disease Registry, Hazardous Substances Data Bank, "Hexachloroethane," as of January 18, 1992.

147. National Library of Medicine's Toxicology Information Program, Agency for Toxic Substances and Disease Registry, Hazardous Substances Data Bank, "Glycidol," as of January 18, 1992.

148. National Library of Medicine's Toxicology Information Program, Agency for Toxic Substances and Disease Registry, Hazardous Substances Data Bank, "Furfuryl Alcohol," as of January 18, 1992.

149. National Library of Medicine's Toxicology Information Program, Agency for Toxic Substances and Disease Registry, Hazardous Substances Data Bank, "2-Methyl-1-Pentanol," as of January 18, 1992.

150. National Library of Medicine's Toxicology Information Program, Agency for Toxic Substances and Disease Registry, Hazardous Substances Data Bank, "Iodomethane," as of January 18, 1992.

151. National Library of Medicine's Toxicology Information Program, Agency for Toxic Substances and Disease Registry, Hazardous Substances Data Bank, "Methyl Formate," as of January 18, 1992.

152. National Library of Medicine's Toxicology Information Program, Agency for Toxic Substances and Disease Registry, Hazardous Substances Data Bank, "Methyl Cellosolve Acetate," as of January 18, 1992.

153. National Library of Medicine's Toxicology Information Program, Agency for Toxic Substances and Disease Registry, Hazardous Substances Data Bank, "Methanol," as of January 18, 1992.

154. National Library of Medicine's Toxicology Information Program, Agency for Toxic Substances and Disease Registry, Hazardous Substances Data Bank, "Methyl Acrylate," as of January 18, 1992.

155. National Library of Medicine's Toxicology Information Program, Agency for Toxic Substances and Disease Registry, Hazardous Substances Data Bank, "Methyl Acetate," as of January 18, 1992.

156. National Library of Medicine's Toxicology Information Program, Agency for Toxic Substances and Disease Registry, Hazardous Substances Data Bank, "2-Heptanone," as of January 18, 1992.

157. National Library of Medicine's Toxicology Information Program, Agency for Toxic Substances and Disease Registry, Hazardous Substances Data Bank, "Mesityl Oxide," as of January 18, 1992.

158. National Library of Medicine's Toxicology Information Program, Agency for Toxic Substances and Disease Registry, Hazardous Substances Data Bank, "Maleic Anhydride," as of January 18, 1992.

159. National Library of Medicine's Toxicology Information Program, Agency for Toxic Substances and Disease Registry, Hazardous Substances Data Bank, "Malathion," as of January 18, 1992.

160. National Library of Medicine's Toxicology Information Program, Agency for Toxic Substances and Disease Registry, Hazardous Substances Data Bank, "Magnesium Oxide," as of January 18, 1992.

161. National Library of Medicine's Toxicology Information Program, Agency for Toxic Substances and Disease Registry, Hazardous Substances Data Bank, "Lindane," as of January 18, 1992.

162. National Library of Medicine's Toxicology Information Program, Agency for Toxic Substances and Disease Registry, Hazardous Substances Data Bank, "Ketene," as of January 18, 1992.

163. National Library of Medicine's Toxicology Information Program, Agency for Toxic Substances and Disease Registry, Hazardous Substances Data Bank, "Isopropyl Ether," as of January 18, 1992.

164. National Library of Medicine's Toxicology Information Program, Agency for Toxic Substances and Disease Registry, Hazardous Substances Data Bank, "Isopropanol," as of January 24, 1992.

165. National Library of Medicine's Toxicology Information Program, Agency for Toxic Substances and Disease Registry, Hazardous Substances Data Bank, "Isopropyl Acetate," as of January 18, 1992.

166. National Library of Medicine's Toxicology Information Program, Agency for Toxic Substances and Disease Registry, Hazardous Substances Data Bank, "Isobutyl Acetate," as of January 18, 1992.

167. National Library of Medicine's Toxicology Information Program, Agency for Toxic Substances and Disease Registry, Hazardous Substances Data Bank, "Hydroquinone," as of January 18, 1992.

168. National Library of Medicine's Toxicology Information Program, Agency for Toxic Substances and Disease Registry, Hazardous Substances Data Bank, "Isophorone," as of January 19, 1992.

169. National Library of Medicine's Toxicology Information Program, Agency for Toxic Substances and Disease Registry, Hazardous Substances Data Bank, "Methyl Methacrylate," as of January 19, 1992.

170. National Library of Medicine's Toxicology Information Program, Agency for Toxic Substances and Disease Registry, Hazardous Substances Data Bank, "Methylal," as of January 19, 1992.

171. National Library of Medicine's Toxicology Information Program, Agency for Toxic Substances and Disease Registry, Hazardous Substances Data Bank, "Mica," as of January 19, 1992.

172. National Library of Medicine's Toxicology Information Program, Agency for Toxic Substances and Disease Registry, Hazardous Substances Data Bank, "Molybdenum," as of January 19, 1992.

173. National Library of Medicine's Toxicology Information Program, Agency for Toxic Substances and Disease Registry, Hazardous Substances Data Bank, "N-Methylaniline," as of January 19, 1992.

174. National Library of Medicine's Toxicology Information Program, Agency for Toxic Substances and Disease Registry, Hazardous Substances Data Bank, "Morpholine," as of January 19, 1992.

175. National Library of Medicine's Toxicology Information Program, Agency for Toxic Substances and Disease Registry, Hazardous Substances Data Bank, "n-Amyl Acetate," as of January 19, 1992.

176. National Library of Medicine's Toxicology Information Program, Agency for Toxic Substances and Disease Registry, Hazardous Substances Data Bank, "n-Butyl Acetate," as of January 19, 1992.

177. National Library of Medicine's Toxicology Information Program, Agency for Toxic Substances and Disease Registry, Hazardous Substances Data Bank, "n-Butyl Alcohol," as of January 19, 1992.

178. National Library of Medicine's Toxicology Information Program, Agency for Toxic Substances and Disease Registry, Hazardous Substances Data Bank, "Methylamine," as of January 19, 1992.

179. National Library of Medicine's Toxicology Information Program, Agency for Toxic Substances and Disease Registry, Hazardous Substances Data Bank, "n-Ethylmorpholine," as of January 19, 1992.

180. National Library of Medicine's Toxicology Information Program, Agency for Toxic Substances and Disease Registry, Hazardous Substances Data Bank, "Heptane," as of January 19, 1992.

181. National Library of Medicine's Toxicology Information Program, Agency for Toxic Substances and Disease Registry, Hazardous Substances Data Bank, "n-Hexane," as of January 19, 1992.

182. National Library of Medicine's Toxicology Information Program, Agency for Toxic Substances and Disease Registry, Hazardous Substances Data Bank, "n-Nitrosodimethyla-mine," as of January 19, 1992.

183. National Library of Medicine's Toxicology Information Program, Agency for Toxic Substances and Disease Registry, Hazardous Substances Data Bank, "Pentane," as of January 19, 1992.

184. National Library of Medicine's Toxicology Information Program, Agency for Toxic Substances and Disease Registry, Hazardous Substances Data Bank, "n-Propyl Acetate," as of January 19, 1992.

185. National Library of Medicine's Toxicology Information Program, Agency for Toxic Substances and Disease Registry, Hazardous Substances Data Bank, "n-Propanol," as of January 19, 1992.

186. National Library of Medicine's Toxicology Information Program, Agency for Toxic Substances and Disease Registry, Hazardous Substances Data Bank, "Petroleum Ether," as of January 19, 1992.

187. National Library of Medicine's Toxicology Information Program, Agency for Toxic Substances and Disease Registry, Hazardous Substances Data Bank, "Nickel Carbonyl," as of January 19, 1992.

188. National Library of Medicine's Toxicology Information Program, Agency for Toxic Substances and Disease Registry, Hazardous Substances Data Bank, "Nitromethane," as of January 19, 1992.

189. National Library of Medicine's Toxicology Information Program, Agency for Toxic Substances and Disease Registry, Hazardous Substances Data Bank, "Nitrogen Dioxide," as of January 19, 1992.

190. National Library of Medicine's Toxicology Information Program, Agency for Toxic Substances and Disease Registry, Hazardous Substances Data Bank, "Nitroethane," as of January 19, 1992.

191. National Library of Medicine's Toxicology Information Program, Agency for Toxic Substances and Disease Registry, Hazardous Substances Data Bank, "Nitric Oxide," as of January 19, 1992.

192. National Library of Medicine's Toxicology Information Program, Agency for Toxic Substances and Disease Registry, Hazardous Substances Data Bank, "Nitric Acid," as of January 19, 1992.

193. National Library of Medicine's Toxicology Information Program, Agency for Toxic Substances and Disease Registry, Hazardous Substances Data Bank, "Nicotine," as of January 19, 1992.

194. National Library of Medicine's Toxicology Information Program, Agency for Toxic Substances and Disease Registry, Hazardous Substances Data Bank, "Nitrophenols," as of January 22, 1992.

195. National Library of Medicine's Toxicology Information Program, Agency for Toxic Substances and Disease Registry, Hazardous Substances Data Bank, "2-Chlorobenzalmalo-nonitrile," as of January 22, 1992.

196. National Library of Medicine's Toxicology Information Program, Agency for Toxic Substances and Disease Registry, Hazardous Substances Data Bank, "1,2-Dichlorobenzene," as of January 22, 1992.

197. National Library of Medicine's Toxicology Information Program, Agency for Toxic Substances and Disease Registry, Hazardous Substances Data Bank, "2-Aminotoluene," as of January 22, 1992.

198. National Library of Medicine's Toxicology Information Program, Agency for Toxic Substances and Disease Registry, Hazardous Substances Data Bank, "Octachloro-naphthalene," as of January 22, 1992.

199. National Library of Medicine's Toxicology Information Program, Agency for Toxic Substances and Disease Registry, Hazardous Substances Data Bank, "n-Octane," as of January 22, 1992.

200. National Library of Medicine's Toxicology Information Program, Agency for Toxic Substances and Disease Registry, Hazardous Substances Data Bank, "Oxalic Acid," as of January 22, 1992.

201. National Library of Medicine's Toxicology Information Program, Agency for Toxic Substances and Disease Registry, Hazardous Substances Data Bank, "1,4-Benzenediamine," as of January 22, 1992.

202. National Library of Medicine's Toxicology Information Program, Agency for Toxic Substances and Disease Registry, Hazardous Substances Data Bank, "Paraldehyde," as of January 22, 1992.

203. National Library of Medicine's Toxicology Information Program, Agency for Toxic Substances and Disease Registry, Hazardous Substances Data Bank, "Pentaborane," as of January 22, 1992.

204. National Library of Medicine's Toxicology Information Program, Agency for Toxic Substances and Disease Registry, Hazardous Substances Data Bank, "Pentachloro-naphthalene," as of January 22, 1992.

205. National Library of Medicine's Toxicology Information Program, Agency for Toxic Substances and Disease Registry, Hazardous Substances Data Bank, "Pentachlorophenol," as of January 22, 1992.

206. National Library of Medicine's Toxicology Information Program, Agency for Toxic Substances and Disease Registry, Hazardous Substances Data Bank, "Phenylhydrazine," as of January 22, 1992.

207. National Library of Medicine's Toxicology Information Program, Agency for Toxic Substances and Disease Registry, Hazardous Substances Data Bank, "Phenol" as of January 22, 1992.

208. National Library of Medicine's Toxicology Information Program, Agency for Toxic Substances and Disease Registry, Hazardous Substances Data Bank, "Diphenyl Ether," as of January 22, 1992.

209. National Library of Medicine's Toxicology Information Program, Agency for Toxic Substances and Disease Registry, Hazardous Substances Data Bank, "Phenyl Glycidyl Ether," as of January 22, 1992.

210. National Library of Medicine's Toxicology Information Program, Agency for Toxic Substances and Disease Registry, Hazardous Substances Data Bank, "Phosgene," as of January 24, 1992.

211. National Library of Medicine's Toxicology Information Program, Agency for Toxic Substances and Disease Registry, Hazardous Substances Data Bank, "Phosphine," as of January 24, 1992.

212. National Library of Medicine's Toxicology Information Program, Agency for Toxic Substances and Disease Registry, Hazardous Substances Data Bank, "Orthophosphoric Acid," as of January 24, 1992.

213. National Library of Medicine's Toxicology Information Program, Agency for Toxic Substances and Disease Registry, Hazardous Substances Data Bank, "Phosphorus Sulfide," as of January 24, 1992.

214. National Library of Medicine's Toxicology Information Program, Agency for Toxic Substances and Disease Registry, Hazardous Substances Data Bank, "Phosphorus," as of January 24, 1992.

215. National Library of Medicine's Toxicology Information Program, Agency for Toxic Substances and Disease Registry, Hazardous Substances Data Bank, "Phthalic Anhydride," as of January 24, 1992.

216. National Library of Medicine's Toxicology Information Program, Agency for Toxic Substances and Disease Registry, Hazardous Substances Data Bank, "Picric Acid," as of January 24, 1992.

217. National Library of Medicine's Toxicology Information Program, Agency for Toxic Substances and Disease Registry, Hazardous Substances Data Bank, "Pindone," as of January 24, 1992.

218. National Library of Medicine's Toxicology Information Program, Agency for Toxic Substances and Disease Registry, Hazardous Substances Data Bank, "Propane," as of January 24, 1992.

219. National Library of Medicine's Toxicology Information Program, Agency for Toxic Substances and Disease Registry, Hazardous Substances Data Bank, "Propyleneimine," as of January 24, 1992.

220. National Library of Medicine's Toxicology Information Program, Agency for Toxic Substances and Disease Registry, Hazardous Substances Data Bank, "1,2-Dichloropropane" as of January 24, 1992.

221. National Library of Medicine's Toxicology Information Program, Agency for Toxic Substances and Disease Registry, Hazardous Substances Data Bank, "1,2-Propylene Oxide," as of January 24, 1992.

222. National Library of Medicine's Toxicology Information Program, Agency for Toxic Substances and Disease Registry, Hazardous Substances Data Bank, "Pyrethrum," as of January 24, 1992.

223. National Library of Medicine's Toxicology Information Program, Agency for Toxic Substances and Disease Registry, Hazardous Substances Data Bank, "1,4-Benzoquinone," as of January 24, 1992.

224. National Library of Medicine's Toxicology Information Program, Agency for Toxic Substances and Disease Registry, Hazardous Substances Data Bank, "2-Pentyl Acetate," as of January 24, 1992.

225. National Library of Medicine's Toxicology Information Program, Agency for Toxic Substances and Disease Registry, Hazardous Substances Data Bank, "sec-Butyl Acetate," as of January 24, 1992.

226. National Library of Medicine's Toxicology Information Program, Agency for Toxic Substances and Disease Registry, Hazardous Substances Data Bank, "sec-Butyl Alcohol," as of January 24, 1992.

227. National Library of Medicine's Toxicology Information Program, Agency for Toxic Substances and Disease Registry, Hazardous Substances Data Bank, "Selenium," as of January 24, 1992.

228. National Library of Medicine's Toxicology Information Program, Agency for Toxic Substances and Disease Registry, Hazardous Substances Data Bank, "Sodium Fluoroacetate," as of January 24, 1992.

229. National Library of Medicine's Toxicology Information Program, Agency for Toxic Substances and Disease Registry, Hazardous Substances Data Bank, "Sodium Hydroxide," as of January 24, 1992.

230. National Library of Medicine's Toxicology Information Program, Agency for Toxic Substances and Disease Registry, Hazardous Substances Data Bank, "Stibine," as of January 24, 1992.

231. National Library of Medicine's Toxicology Information Program, Agency for Toxic Substances and Disease Registry, Hazardous Substances Data Bank, "Methyl Propyl Ketone," as of January 24, 1992.

232. National Library of Medicine's Toxicology Information Program, Agency for Toxic Substances and Disease Registry, Hazardous Substances Data Bank, "Sulfur Dioxide," as of January 24, 1992.

233. National Library of Medicine's Toxicology Information Program, Agency for Toxic Substances and Disease Registry, Hazardous Substances Data Bank, "Sulfur Monochloride," as of January 24, 1992.

234. National Library of Medicine's Toxicology Information Program, Agency for Toxic Substances and Disease Registry, Hazardous Substances Data Bank, "Sulfuryl Fluoride," as of January 24, 1992.

235. National Library of Medicine's Toxicology Information Program, Agency for Toxic Substances and Disease Registry, Hazardous Substances Data Bank, "Dithion," as of January 24, 1992.

236. National Library of Medicine's Toxicology Information Program, Agency for Toxic Substances and Disease Registry, Hazardous Substances Data Bank, "Tellurium," as of January 24, 1992.

237. National Library of Medicine's Toxicology Information Program, Agency for Toxic Substances and Disease Registry, Hazardous Substances Data Bank, "tert-Butyl Acetate," as of January 24, 1992.

238. National Library of Medicine's Toxicology Information Program, Agency for Toxic Substances and Disease Registry, Hazardous Substances Data Bank, "Tetrachloronaphthalene," as of January 24, 1992.
239. National Library of Medicine's Toxicology Information Program, Agency for Toxic Substances and Disease Registry, Hazardous Substances Data Bank, "Tetraethyl Lead," as of January 24, 1992.
240. National Library of Medicine's Toxicology Information Program, Agency for Toxic Substances and Disease Registry, Hazardous Substances Data Bank, "Tetrahydrofuran," as of January 24, 1992.
241. National Library of Medicine's Toxicology Information Program, Agency for Toxic Substances and Disease Registry, Hazardous Substances Data Bank, "Tetramethyl Lead," as of January 24, 1992.
242. National Library of Medicine's Toxicology Information Program, Agency for Toxic Substances and Disease Registry, Hazardous Substances Data Bank, "Thiram," as of January 24, 1992.
243. National Library of Medicine's Toxicology Information Program, Agency for Toxic Substances and Disease Registry, Hazardous Substances Data Bank, "Titanium Dioxide," as of January 24, 1992.
244. National Library of Medicine's Toxicology Information Program, Agency for Toxic Substances and Disease Registry, Hazardous Substances Data Bank, "Tributyl Phosphate," as of January 24, 1992.
245. National Library of Medicine's Toxicology Information Program, Agency for Toxic Substances and Disease Registry, Hazardous Substances Data Bank, "Triethylamine," as of January 24, 1992.
246. National Library of Medicine's Toxicology Information Program, Agency for Toxic Substances and Disease Registry, Hazardous Substances Data Bank, "Freon 13B1," as of January 24, 1992.
247. National Library of Medicine's Toxicology Information Program, Agency for Toxic Substances and Disease Registry, Hazardous Substances Data Bank, "Triphenyl Phosphate," as of January 24, 1992.
248. National Library of Medicine's Toxicology Information Program, Agency for Toxic Substances and Disease Registry, Hazardous Substances Data Bank, "Turpentine," as of January 24, 1992.
249. National Library of Medicine's Toxicology Information Program, Agency for Toxic Substances and Disease Registry, Hazardous Substances Data Bank, "Vinyl Chloride," as of January 24, 1992.
250. National Library of Medicine's Toxicology Information Program, Agency for Toxic Substances and Disease Registry, Hazardous Substances Data Bank, "Vinyl Toluene," as of January 24, 1992.
251. National Library of Medicine's Toxicology Information Program, Agency for Toxic Substances and Disease Registry, Hazardous Substances Data Bank, "Warfarin," as of January 24, 1992.
252. National Library of Medicine's Toxicology Information Program, Agency for Toxic Substances and Disease Registry, Hazardous Substances Data Bank, "Zinc Chloride," as of January 24, 1992.
253. National Library of Medicine's Toxicology Information Program, Agency for Toxic Substances and Disease Registry, Hazardous Substances Data Bank, "Zinc Oxide," as of January 24, 1992.
254. National Library of Medicine's Toxicology Information Program, Agency for Toxic Substances and Disease Registry, Hazardous Substances Data Bank, 1,1,2,2,-Tetrachloroethane," as of January 24, 1992.
255. National Library of Medicine's Toxicology Information Program, Agency for Toxic Substances and Disease Registry, Hazardous Substances Data Bank, "1,1,2-Trichloroethane," as of January 24, 1992.
256. National Library of Medicine's Toxicology Information Program, Agency for Toxic Substances and Disease Registry, Hazardous Substances Data Bank, "1,2,3-Trichloropropane," as of January 24, 1992.

257. National Library of Medicine's Toxicology Information Program, Agency for Toxic Substances and Disease Registry, Hazardous Substances Data Bank, "2,4,6-Trinitrotoluene," as of January 24, 1992.

258. National Library of Medicine's Toxicology Information Program, Agency for Toxic Substances and Disease Registry, Hazardous Substances Data Bank, "Methylhydrazine," as of February 9, 1992.

259. National Library of Medicine's Toxicology Information Program, Agency for Toxic Substances and Disease Registry, Hazardous Substances Data Bank, "Ethylene Glycol," as of February 9, 1992.

260. National Library of Medicine's Toxicology Information Program, Agency for Toxic Substances and Disease Registry, Hazardous Substances Data Bank, "1,2-Dinitrobenzene," as of February 9, 1992.

261. National Library of Medicine's Toxicology Information Program, Agency for Toxic Substances and Disease Registry, Hazardous Substances Data Bank, "4-Nitroaniline," as of February 9, 1992.

262. National Library of Medicine's Toxicology Information Program, Agency for Toxic Substances and Disease Registry, Hazardous Substances Data Bank, "1-Chloro-4-Nitrobenzene," as of February 9, 1992.

263. National Library of Medicine's Toxicology Information Program, Agency for Toxic Substances and Disease Registry, Hazardous Substances Data Bank, "Dowtherm A," as of February 9, 1992.

264. National Library of Medicine's Toxicology Information Program, Agency for Toxic Substances and Disease Registry, Hazardous Substances Data Bank, "Paraquat," as of January 24, 1992.

265. National Library of Medicine's Toxicology Information Program, Agency for Toxic Substances and Disease Registry, Hazardous Substances Data Bank, "Tetraethyl Pyrophosphate," as of January 24, 1992.

266. National Library of Medicine's Toxicology Information Program, Agency for Toxic Substances and Disease Registry, Hazardous Substances Data Bank, "Tri-O-Cresyl Phosphate," as of January 24, 1992.

267. National Library of Medicine's Toxicology Information Program, Agency for Toxic Substances and Disease Registry, Hazardous Substances Data Bank, "Diborane," as of January 14, 1992.

268. National Library of Medicine's Toxicology Information Program, Agency for Toxic Substances and Disease Registry, Hazardous Substances Data Bank, "1,1-Dimethylhydrazine," as of January 11, 1992.

269. National Library of Medicine's Toxicology Information Program, Agency for Toxic Substances and Disease Registry, Hazardous Substances Data Bank, "1,3-Dintrobenzene," as of January 14, 1992.

270. National Library of Medicine's Toxicology Information Program, Agency for Toxic Substances and Disease Registry, Hazardous Substances Data Bank, "Isopropylamine," as of January 18, 1992.

271. National Library of Medicine's Toxicology Information Program, Agency for Toxic Substances and Disease Registry, Hazardous Substances Data Bank, "Naphtha," as of January 19, 1992.

272. National Library of Medicine's Toxicology Information Program, Agency for Toxic Substances and Disease Registry, Hazardous Substances Data Bank, "alpha-Chloroactephenone," as of January 24, 1992.

273. National Library of Medicine's Toxicology Information Program, Agency for Toxic Substances and Disease Registry, Hazardous Substances Data Bank, "sec-Hexyl Acetate," as of January 24, 1992.

274. National Library of Medicine's Toxicology Information Program, Agency for Toxic Substances and Disease Registry, Hazardous Substances Data Bank, "Hydrogen Chloride," as of January 24, 1992.

275. National Library of Medicine's Toxicology Information Program, Agency for Toxic Substances and Disease Registry, Hazardous Substances Data Bank, "Methyl Cellosolve," as of January 24, 1992.

276. National Library of Medicine's Toxicology Information Program, Agency for Toxic Substances and Disease Registry, Hazardous Substances Data Bank, "Ethyl Amyl Ketone," as of January 24, 1992.

277. National Library of Medicine's Toxicology Information Program, Agency for Toxic Substances and Disease Registry, Hazardous Substances Data Bank, "Methyl Amyl Alcohol," as of January 24, 1992.

278. National Research Council, *Indoor Pollutants,* Washington, DC: National Academy Press, 1981.

279. National Research Council, Assembly of Life Sciences, Committee on Aldehydes, Based on Toxicology and Environmental Health Hazards, *Formaldehyde and Other Aldehydes,* Washington, DC: National Academy Press, 1981.

280. National Research Council, Assembly of Life Sciences, Subcommittee on Immunotoxicology, Based in Toxicology and Environmental Health Hazards, *Biologic Markers in Immunotoxicology,* Washington, DC: National Academy Press, 1992.

281. National Research Council, Board of Environmental Studies and Toxicology, Published proceedings from the *Workshop on Health Risks from Exposure to Common Indoor Household Products in Allergic or Chemically Diseased Persons,* Washington, DC: National Academy Press, 1987.

282. New Jersey Department of Health, "Hazardous Substance Fact Sheet 'Chlorpyrifos,'" 1986.

283. New Jersey Department of Health, "Hazardous Substance Fact Sheet 'Antimony,'" 1986.

284. New Jersey Department of Health, "Hazardous Substance Fact Sheet 'Arsenic,'" 1986.

285. New Jersey Department of Health, "Hazardous Substance Fact Sheet 'Formaldehyde,'" 1986.

286. New York Department of Law; Robert Abrams, attorney general, "The Secret Hazards of Pesticides," June 1991.

286a. "99.9 Percent?" *Concrete Facts* 1(1) (March 1991).

287. Pacific Toxicology Laboratories, "Human Toxic Chemical Exposure and Directory of Services," Los Angeles, CA.

287a. Perfecto, I.; Baldemar, V., "Farm Workers: Among The Least Protected," EPA Journal, 18(1), March/April 1992.

288. Procter & Gamble Co., label for Ivory Free Conditioner, U.S. patent pending, 1982.

289. Raloff, J., "Arsenic in water: Bigger cancer threat," *Science News,* April 18, 1992.

290. Redmond Products, product label for Aussie Mega Shampoo with Papaya, 1986.

291. Roach, S.A., and S.M. Rappaport, "But They Are Not Thresholds: A Critical Analysis of the Documentation of Threshold Limit Values," *American Journal of Industrial Medicine* 17 (1990): 727–753.

292. Rossol, M., editor, "NTP Lists New Carcinogens," *Acts Facts* 6(4) (April 1992).

293. Russell, B., "Zero Just Keeps Getting Smaller," *Pest Control,* Jan. 1992.

294. Russell, D., "Incineration Battle Flares in Arkansas," *Toxic Times,* The National Toxic Campaign Fund, April 1991.

295. Sax, N., and R.J. Sewis, *Hazardous Chemicals Desk Reference* New York: Van Norts and Reinhold, 1987.

296. Schnare, D.W., et al., "Evaluation of a Detoxification Regimen for Fat Stored Xenobiotics," *Medical Hypotheses* 9 (1982): 265–282.

297. Swanson, J.R., "Formaldehyde: The Psychological and Educational Implications of Formaldehyde Toxicology," Seattle, WA: University of Washington, College of Education, 1984.

298. Terr, A.I., "Clinical Ecology in the Workplace," *Journal of Occupational Medicine,* 31(3): (March 1989) 257–261.

299. Thomas, C.L., editor, *Taber's Cyclopedic Medical Dictionary,* 16th edition Philadelphia, PA: F.A. Davis Company, 1989.

300. Thrasher, J.D. and A. Broughton. *The Truth About the Indoor Formaldehyde Crisis: The Poisoning of Our Homes and Workplaces,* Santa Ana, CA: Ceadora, 1989.

301. U.S. Congress, "Neurotoxicity: Identifying and Controlling Poisons of the Nervous System," Office of Technology Assessment, April 1990, U.S. Government Printing Office, Washington, DC, GPO Stock No. #052-003-01184-1.

302. U.S. Congress, "Neurotoxins: At Home and the Workplace," 99th Congress, 2nd Session, April 24, 1987, Senate Hearing 100-70, printed for use of the Committee on Environment and Public Works, U.S. Government Printing Office, Washington, DC.

303. U.S. Department of Health and Human Services, Public Health Service, National Cancer Institute, "Everything Doesn't Cause Cancer," March 1990.

304. U.S. Department of Health and Human Services, Public Health Service, Centers for Disease Control, National Institute for Occupational Safety and Health, "NIOSH Pocket Guide to Chemical Hazards," June 1990, U.S. Government Printing Office, Washington, DC.

305. U.S. Department of Health and Human Services, Public Health Services, Centers for Disease Control, National Institute for Occupational Safety and Health, Division of Standards Development and Technology Transfer, "Occupational Safety and Health Guidelines for Chemical Hazards," 1988, U.S. Government Printing Office, Washington, DC, Publication No. 89-104.

306. U.S. Department of Health and Human Services, Public Health Services, Centers for Disease Control, National Institute for Occupational Safety and Health, Division of Standards Development and Technology Transfer, "Occupational Safety and Health Guidelines for Chemical Hazards," 1988, U.S. Government Printing Office, Washington, DC, Publication No. 88-118.

307. U.S. Department of Health and Human Services, Public Health Service, Centers for Disease Control, National Institute for Occupational Safety and Health, "NIOSH Mini-Alert – Request for Assistance in Controlling Carbon Monoxide Hazard in Aircraft Refueling Operations," Feb. 1984.

308. U.S. Department of Health and Human Services, Public Health Service, Centers for Disease Control, National Institute for Occupational Safety and Health, "NIOSH Current Intelligence Bulletin 32 – Arsine (Arsenic Hydride) Poisoning in the Workplace," Aug. 3, 1979.

309. U.S. Department of Health and Human Services, Public Health Service, Centers for Disease Control, National Insitute for Occupational Safety and Health," "NIOSH Current Intelligence Bulletin 34 – Formaldehyde: Evidence of Carcinogenicity," April 15, 1981.

310. U.S. Department of Health and Human Services, Public Health Service, Centers for Disease Control, National Institute for Occupational Safety and Health," NIOSH Current Intelligence Bulletin 35 – Ethylene Oxide (EtO)," May 22, 1981.

311. U.S. Department of Health and Human Services, Public Health Service, Centers for Disease Control, National Institute for Occupational Safety and Health, "NIOSH Current Intelligence Bulletin 36 – Silica Flour: Silicosis (Crystalline Silica)," June 30, 1981.

312. U.S. Department of Health and Human Services, Public Health Service, Centers for Disease Control, National Institute for Occupational Safety and Health, "NIOSH Current Intelligence Bulletin 37 – Ethylene Dibromide (EDB) (Revised)," Oct. 26, 1981.

313. U.S. Department of Health and Human Services, Public Health Service, Centers for Disease Control, National Institute for Occupational Safety and Health, "NIOSH Current Intelligence Bulletin 39 – Glycol Ethers: 2-Methoxyethanol and 2-Ethoxyethanol," May 2, 1983.

314. U.S. Department of Health and Human Services, Public Health Service, Centers for Disease Control, National Institute for Occupational Safety and Health, "NIOSH Current Intelligence Bulletin 41 – 1,3-Butadiene," Feb. 9, 1984.

315. U.S. Department of Health and Human Services, Public Health Service, Centers for Disease Control, Natinal Institute for Occupational Safety and Health, "NIOSH Current Intelligence Bulletin 42 – Cadmium (Cd)," Sept. 27, 1984.

316. U.S. Department of Health and Human Services, Public Health Service, Centers for Disease Control, National Institute for Occupational Safety and Health, "NIOSH Current Intelligence Bulletin 43 – Monohalomethanes: Methyl Chloride, Methyl Bromide, Methyl Iodide," Sept. 27, 1984.

317. U.S. Department of Health and Human Services, Public Health Service, Centers for Disease Control, National Institute for Occupational Safety and Health, "NIOSH Current Intelligence Bulletin 44 – Dinitrotoluenes (DNT)," July 5, 1986.

318. U.S. Department of Health and Human Services, Public Health Service, Centers for Disease Control, National Institute for Occupational Safety and Health, "NIOSH Current

Intelligence Bulletin 45 — Polychlorinated Biphenyls (PCBs): Potential Health Hazards from Electrical Equipment Fires or Failures," Feb. 24, 1986.

319. U.S. Department of Health and Human Services, Public Health Service, Agency for Toxic Substances and Disease Registry, "Toxicology Profile for Acrolein," Dec. 1990, Syracuse Research Corporation.

320. U.S. Department of Health and Human Services, Public Health Service, Agency for Toxic Substances and Disease Registry, "Toxicology Profile for Silver," Dec. 1990, Clement International Corporation.

321. U.S. Department of Health and Human Services, Public Health Service, Agency for Toxic Substances and Disease Registry, "Toxicology Profile for Di-n-Butylphthalate," Dec. 1990, Life Systems, Inc.

322. U.S. Department of Health and Human Services, Public Health Service, Agency for Toxic Substances and Disease Registry, "Toxicology Profile for Asbestos," Dec. 1990, Life Systems, Inc.

323. U.S. Department of Health and Human Services, Public Health Service, Agency for Toxic Substances and Disease Registry, "Toxicology Profile for Ammonia," Dec. 1990, Syracuse Research Corporation.

324. U.S. Department of Health and Human Services, Public Health Service, Agency for Toxic Substances and Disease Registry, "Toxicology Profile for Copper," Dec. 1990, Syracuse Research Corporation.

325. U.S. Department of Health and Human Services, Public Health Service, Agency for Toxic Substances and Disease Registry, "Toxicology Profile for Ethylene Oxide," Dec. 1990, Life Systems, Inc.

326. U.S. Department of Health and Human Services, Public Health Service, Agency for Toxic Substances and Disease Registry, "Toxicology Profile for Nitrobenzene," Dec. 1990, Life Systems, Inc.

327. U.S. Department of Health and Human Services, Public Health Service, Agency for Toxic Substances and Disease Registry, "Toxicology Profile for Toxaphene," Dec. 1990, Clement Associates.

328. U.S. Department of Health and Human Services, Public Health Service, Agency for Toxic Substances and Disease Registry, "Toxicology Profile for 1,1,1-Trichloroethane," Dec. 1990, Syracuse Research Corporation.

329. U.S. Department of Health and Human Services, Public Health Service, Agency for Toxic Substances and Disease Registry, "Toxicology Profile for Acrylonitrile," Dec. 1990, Life System, Inc.

330. U.S. Department of Health and Human Services, Public Health Service, Agency for Toxic Substances and Disease Registry, "Toxicology Profile for Chlorobenzene," Dec. 1990, Life Systems, Inc.

331. U.S. Department of Health and Human Services, Public Health Service, Agency for Toxic Substances and Disease Registry, "Toxicology Profile for Chloromethane," Dec. 1990, Syracuse Research Corporation.

332. U.S. Department of Health and Human Services, Public Health Service, Agency for Toxic Substances and Disease Registry, "Toxicology Profile for Creosote," Dec. 1990, Clement International Corporation.

333. U.S. Department of Health and Human Services, Public Health Service, Agency for Toxic Substances and Disease Registry, "Toxicology Profile for cis, trans 1,2-Dichloroethane," Dec. 1990, Syracuse Research Corporation.

334. U.S. Department of Health and Human Services, Public Health Service, Agency for Toxic Substances and Disease Registry, "Toxicology Profile for 1,1-Dichloroethane," Dec. 1990, Clement International Corporation.

335. U.S. Department of Health and Human Services, Public Health Service, Agency for Toxic Substances and Disease Registry, "Toxicology Profile for Ethylbenzene," Dec. 1990, Clement International Corporation.

336. U.S. Department of Health and Human Services, Public Health Service, Agency for Toxic Substances and Disease Registry, "Toxicology Profile for Naphthalene, 2-Methylnaphthalene," Dec. 1990, Life Systems, Inc.

337. U.S. Department of Health and Human Services, Public Health Service, Agency for

Toxic Substances and Disease Registry, "Toxicology Profile for Polycyclic Aromatic Hydrocarbons," Dec. 1990, Clement International Corporation.

338. U.S. Department of Health and Human Services, Public Health Service, Agency for Toxic Substances and Disease Registry, "Toxicology Profile for 2,4,6-Trichlorophenol," Dec. 1990, Clement International Corporation.

339. U.S. Department of Health and Human Services, Public Health Service, Agency for Toxic Substances and Disease Registry, "Toxicology Profile for Total Xylenes," Dec. 1990, Clement Associates, Inc.

340. U.S. Department of Health and Human Services, Public Health Service, Agency for Toxic Substances and Disease Registry, "Toxicology Profile for Aluminum," July 1992, Clement Associates, Inc.

341. U.S. Department of Health and Human Services, Public Health Service, Agency for Toxic Substances and Disease Registry, "Draft for Public Comment: Toxicology Profile for Trichloroethylene," Oct. 1991, Clement International Corporation.

342. U.S. Department of Health and Human Services, Public Health Service, Agency for Toxic Substances and Disease Registry, "Draft for Public Comment: Toxicology Profile for Tetrachloroethylene," Oct. 1991, Clement International Corporation.

343. U.S. Department of Health and Human Services, Public Health Service, Agency for Toxic Substances and Disease Registry, "Draft for Public Comment: Toxicology Profile for Selected PCBs (Arcoclor-1260, -1254, -1248, -1242, -1232, -1221, and -1016)," Oct. 1991, Syracuse Research Corporation.

344. U.S. Department of Health and Human Services, Public Health Service, Agency for Toxic Substances and Disease Registry, "Draft for Public Comment: Toxicology Profile for Nickel," Oct. 1991, Syracuse Research Corporation.

345. U.S. Department of Health and Human Services, Public Health Service, Agency for Toxic Substances and Disease Registry, "Draft for Public Comment: Toxicology Profile for Methylene Chloride," Oct. 1991, Life Systems, Inc.

346. U.S. Department of Health and Human Services, Public Health Service, Agency for Toxic Substances and Disease Registry, "Draft for Public Comment: Toxicology Profile for Lead," Oct. 1991, Clement International Corporation.

347. U.S. Department of Health and Human Services, Public Health Service, Agency for Toxic Substances and Disease Registry, "Draft for Public Comment: Toxicology Profile for 1,4-Dichlorobenzene," Oct. 1991, Life Systems, Inc.

348. U.S. Department of Health and Human Services, Public Health Service, Agency for Toxic Substances and Disease Registry, "Draft for Public Comment: Toxicology Profile for Cyanide," Oct. 1991, Syracuse Research Corporation.

349. U.S. Department of Health and Human Services, Public Health Service, Agency for Toxic Substances and Disease Registry, "Draft for Public Comment: Toxicology Profile for Chromium," Oct. 1991, Syracuse Research Corporation.

350. U.S. Department of Health and Human Services, Public Health Service, Agency for Toxic Substances and Disease Registry, "Draft for Public Comment: Toxicology Profile for Chloroform," Oct. 1991, Syracuse Research Corporation.

351. U.S. Department of Health and Human Services, Public Health Service, Agency for Toxic Substances and Disease Registry, "Toxicology Profile for Cadmium," July 1992, Life Systems, Inc.

352. U.S. Department of Health and Human Services, Public Health Service, Agency for Toxic Substances and Disease Registry, "Draft for Public Comment: Toxicology Profile for 1,3-Butadiene," Oct. 1990, Syracuse Research Corporation.

353. U.S. Department of Health and Human Services, Public Health Service, Agency for Toxic Substances and Disease Registry, "Toxicology Profile for Boron," July 1992, Life Systems, Inc.

354. U.S. Department of Health and Human Services, Public Health Service, Agency for Toxic Substances and Disease Registry, "Draft for Public Comment: Toxicology Profile for Beryllium," Oct. 1991, Syracuse Research Corporation.

355. U.S. Department of Health and Human Services, Public Health Service, Agency for Toxic Substances and Disease Registry, "Draft for Public Comment: Toxicology Profile for 2,3-Benzofuran," Oct. 1990, Life Systems, Inc.

356. U.S. Department of Health and Human Services, Public Health Service, Agency for Toxic Substances and Disease Registry, "Draft for Public Comment: Toxicology Profile for Benzene," Oct. 1991, Clement Associates, Inc.

357. U.S. Department of Health and Human Services, Public Health Service, Agency for Toxic Substances and Disease Registry, "Draft for Public Comment: Toxicology Profile for Arsenic," Oct. 1991, Life Systems, Inc.

358. U.S. Department of Health and Human Services, Public Health Service, Agency for Toxic Substances and Disease Registry, "Toxicology Profile for Barium," July 1992, Clement Associates, Inc.

359. U.S. Department of Health and Human Services, Public Health Service, Agency for Toxic Substances and Disease Registry, "Draft for Public Comment: Toxicology Profile for Carbon Disulfide," Oct. 1990, Clement Associates, Inc.

360. U.S. Department of Health and Human Services, Public Health Service, Agency for Toxic Substances and Disease Registry, "Toxicology Profile for 1,2-Dibromoethane," July 1992, Clement Associates, Inc.

361. U.S. Department of Health and Human Services, Public Health Service, Agency for Toxic Substances and Disease Registry, "Draft for Public Comment: Toxicology Profile for cis-, trans- 1,3-Dichloropropene," Oct. 1990, Syracuse Research Corporation.

362. U.S. Department of Health and Human Services, Public Health Service, Agency for Toxic Substances and Disease Registry, "Draft for Public Comment: Toxicology Profile for Di(2-ethylhexyl)phthalate," Oct. 1991, Life Systems, Inc.

363. U.S. Department of Health and Human Services, Public Health Service, Agency for Toxic Substances and Disease Registry, "Draft for Public Comment: Toxicology Profile for Fluorides, Hydrogen Fluorine, and Fluorine (F)," July 1991, Clement Associates, Inc.

364. U.S. Department of Health and Human Services, Public Health Service, Agency for Toxic Substances and Disease Registry, "Toxicology Profile for Manganese," July 1992, Life Systems, Inc.

365. U.S. Department of Health and Human Services, Public Health Service, Agency for Toxic Substances and Disease Registry, "Draft for Public Comment: Toxicology Profile for Methyl Parathion," Oct. 1990, Clement Associates, Inc.

366. U.S. Department of Health and Human Services, Public Health Service, Agency for Toxic Substances and Disease Registry, "Toxicology Profile for Nitrophenols: 2-Nitrophenol, 4-Nitrophenol," July 1992, Syracuse Research Corporation.

367. U.S. Department of Health and Human Services, Public Health Service, Agency for Toxic Substances and Disease Registry, "Draft for Public Comment: Toxicology Profile for Styrene," Oct. 1990, Life Systems, Inc.

368. U.S. Department of Health and Human Services, Public Health Service, Agency for Toxic Substances and Disease Registry, "Draft for Public Comment: Toxicology Profile for Tin," Oct. 1990, Life Systems, Inc.

369. U.S. Department of Health and Human Services, Public Health Service, Agency for Toxic Substances and Disease Registry, "Toxicology Profile for Vanadium," July 1992, Clement Associates, Inc.

370. U.S. Department of Health and Human Services, Public Health Service, Agency for Toxic Substances and Disease Registry, "Draft for Public Comment: Toxicology Profile for Antimony," Oct. 1990, Syracuse Research Corporation.

371. U.S. Department of Health and Human Services, Public Health Service, Agency for Toxic Substances and Disease Registry, "Draft for Public Comment: Toxicology Profile for Bromomethane," Oct. 1990, Life Systems, Inc.

372. U.S. Department of Health and Human Services, Public Health Service, Agency for Toxic Substances and Disease Registry, "Toxicology Profile for 2-Butanone," July 1992, Syracuse Research Corporation.

373. U.S. Department of Health and Human Services, Public Health Service, Agency for Toxic Substances and Disease Registry, "Toxicology Profile for Cobalt," July 1992, Syracuse Research Corporation.

374. U.S. Department of Health and Human Services, Public Health Service, Agency for Toxic Substances and Disease Registry, "Toxicology Profile for 2,4-Dichlorophenol," July 1992, Syracuse Research Corporation.

375. U.S. Department of Health and Human Services, Public Health Service, Agency for Toxic Substances and Disease Registry, "Draft for Public Comment: Toxicology Profile for Endosulfan, Endosulfan Alpha, Endosulfan Beta, Endosulfan Sulfate," Oct. 1990, Clement Associates, Inc.

376. U.S. Department of Health and Human Services, Public Health Service, Agency for Toxic Substances and Disease Registry, "Draft for Public Comment: Toxicology Profile for Methyl Mercaptan," Oct. 1990, Life Systems, Inc.

377. U.S. Department of Health and Human Services, Public Health Service, Agency for Toxic Substances and Disease Registry, "Draft for Public Comment: Toxicology Profile for Pyridine," Oct. 1990, Life Systems, Inc.

378. U.S. Department of Health and Human Services, Public Health Service, Agency for Toxic Substances and Disease Registry, "Toxicology Profile for Thallium," July 1992, Life Systems, Inc.

379. U.S. Department of Health and Human Services, Public Health Service, Agency for Toxic Substances and Disease Registry, "Draft for Public Comment: Toxicology Profile for 1,2,3-Trichloropropane," Oct. 1990, Syracuse Research Corporation.

380. U.S. Department of Health and Human Services, Public Health Service, Agency for Toxic Substances and Disease Registry, "Toxicology Profile for Vinyl Acetate," July 1992, Clement Associates, Inc.

381. U.S. Department of Health and Human Services, Public Health Service, Agency for Toxic Substances and Disease Registry, "Draft for Public Comment: Toxicology Profile for Vinyl Chloride," Oct. 1991, Clement International Corporation.

382. U.S. Department of Health and Human Services, Public Health Service, Agency for Toxic Substances and Disease Registry, "Toxicology Profile for Cresols," July 1992, Syracuse Research Corporation.

383. U.S. Department of Health and Human Services, Public Health Service, Centers for Disease Control, National Institute for Occupational Safety and Health, "NIOSH Current Intelligence Bulletin 48 — Organic Solvent Neurotoxicity," March 31, 1987.

384. U.S. Department of Health and Human Services, Public Health Service, Centers for Disease Control, National Institute for Occupational Safety and Health, "NIOSH Alert — Request for Assistance in Preventing Deaths of Farm Workers in Manure Pits," May 1990.

385. U.S. Department of Health and Human Services, Public Health Service, Centers for Disease Control, National Institute for Occupational Safety and Health, "NIOSH Alert — Request for Assistance in Preventing Bladder Cancer from Exposure to o-Toluidine and Aniline," Dec. 1990.

386. U.S. Department of Health and Human Services, Public Health and Human Services, Public Health Service, Centers for Disease Control National Institute of Occupational Safety and Health, "NIOSH Alert — Request for Assistance in Preventing Adverse Health Effects from Exposure to Dimethylformamide (DMF)," Sept. 1990.

387. U.S. Department of Health and Human Services, Public Health Service, Centers for Disease Control, National Institute for Occupational Safety and Health, "NIOSH Alert — Request for Assistance in Preventing Lead Poisoning in Construction Workers," Aug. 1991.

388. U.S. Department of Health and Human Services, Public Health Service, Centers for Disease Control, National Institute for Occupational Safety and Health, "Regulations, Recommendations and Assessments Extracted from RTECS: A Subfile of the Registry of Toxic Effects of Chemical Substances," Sept. 1986, U.S. Government Printing Office.

389. U.S. Department of Health and Human Services, Public Health Service, Centers for Disease Control, National Institute for Occupational Safety and Health, "NIOSH Current Intelligence Bulletin 54 — Environmental Tobacco Smoke in the Workplace: Lung Cancer and Other Health Effects," June 1991, U.S. Government Printing Office, Washington, DC.

390. U.S. Department of Health and Human Services, Public Health Service, Centers for Disease Control, National Institute for Occupational Safety and Health, "NIOSH Current Intelligence Bulletin 52 — Ethylene Oxide Sterilizers in Health Care Facilities: Engineering Controls and Work Practices," July 13, 1989, U.S. Government Printing Office, Washington, DC.

391. U.S. Department of Health and Human Services, Public Health Service, Centers for Disease Control, National Institute for Occupational Safety and Health, "NIOSH Current

Intelligence Bulletin 53 – Toluene Diisocyanate (TDI) and Toluenediamine: Evidence of Carcinogenicity," Dec. 1989, U.S. Government Printing Office, Washington, DC.

392. U.S. Department of Health and Human Services, Public Health Service, Centers for Disease Control, National Institute for Occupational Safety and Health, "NIOSH Current Intelligence Bulletin 55 – Carcinogenicity of Acetaldehyde and Malonaldehyde, and Mutagenicity of Related Low-Molecular-Weight Aldehydes," Sept. 1991, U.S. Government Printing Office, Washington, DC.

393. U.S. Department of Health and Human Services, Public Health Service, Centers for Disease Control, National Institute for Occupational Safety and Health, "NIOSH Current Intelligence Bulletin 51 – Carcinogenic Effects of Exposure to Propylene Oxide," July 13, 1989, U.S. Government Printing Office, Washington, DC.

394. U.S. Department of Health and Human Services, Public Health Service, Centers for Disease Control, National Institute for Occupational Safety and Health, "NIOSH Current Intelligence Bulletin 50 – Carcinogenic Effects of Exposure to Diesel Exhaust," Aug. 1988, U.S. Government Printing Office, Washington, DC.

395. U.S. Department of Health and Human Services, Public Health Service, Centers for Disease Control, National Institute for Occupational Safety and Health, "NIOSH Current Intelligence Bulletin 20 – Tetrachloroethylene (perchloroethylene)," Jan. 20, 1978, U.S. Government Printing Office, Washington, DC.

396. U.S. Department of Health and Human Services, Public Health Service, Centers for Disease Control, National Institute for Occupational Safety and Health, "NIOSH Current Intelligence Bulletin 23 – Ethylene Dibromide and Disulfiram Toxic Interaction," April 11, 1978, U.S. Government Printing Office, Washington, DC.

397. U.S. Department of Health and Human Services, Public Health Service, Centers for Disease Control, National Institute for Occupational Safety and Health, "NIOSH Current Intelligence Bulletin 24 – Direct Blue 6, Direct Black 38, Direct Brown 95: Benzidine Derived Dyes," April 17, 1978, U.S. Government Printing Office, Washington, DC.

398. U.S. Department of Health and Human Services, Public Health Service, Centers for Disease Control, National Institute for Occupational Safety and Health, "NIOSH Current Intelligence Bulletin 25 – Ethylene Dichloride (1,2-dichloroethane)," April 19, 1978, U.S. Government Printing Office, Washington, DC.

399. U.S. Department of Health and Human Services, Public Health Service, Centers for Disease Control, National Institute for Occupational Safety and Health, "NIOSH Current Intelligence Bulletin 27 – Chloroethanes: Review of Toxicity," Aug. 21, 1978, U.S. Government Printing Office, Washington, DC.

400. U.S. Department of Health and Human Services, Public Health Service, Centers for Disease Control, National Institute for Occupational Safety and Health, "NIOSH Current Intelligence Bulletin 28 – Vinyl Halides Carcinogenicity: Vinyl Bromide, Vinyl Chloride, Vinylidene," Sept. 21, 1978, U.S. Government Printing Office, Washington, DC.

401. U.S. Department of Health and Human Services, Public Health Service, Centers for Disease Control, National Institute for Occupational Safety and Health, "NIOSH Current Intelligence Bulletin 29 – Glycidyl ethers," Oct. 12, 1978, U.S. Government Printing Office, Washington, DC.

402. U.S. Department of Health and Human Services, Public Health Service, Centers for Disease Control, National Institute for Occupational Safety and Health, "NIOSH Current Intelligence Bulletin 30 – Epichlorohydrin," Oct. 12, 1978, U.S. Government Printing Office, Washington, DC.

403. U.S. Department of Health and Human Services, Public Health Service, Centers for Disease Control, National Institute for Occupational Safety and Health, "NIOSH Current Intelligence Bulletin 1 – Chloroprene," Jan. 20, 1975, U.S. Government Printing Office, Washington, DC.

404. U.S. Department of Health and Human Services, Public Health Service, Centers for Disease Control, National Institute for Occupational Safety and Health, "NIOSH Current Intelligence Bulletin 2 – Trichloroethylene (TCE)," June 6, 1975, U.S. Government Printing Office, Washington, DC.

405. U.S. Department of Health and Human Services, Public Health Service, Centers for Disease Control, National Institute for Occupational Safety and Health, "NIOSH Current

Intelligence Bulletin 3 — Ethylene Dibromide (EDB)," July 7, 1975, U.S. Government Printing Office, Washington, DC.

406. U.S. Department of Health and Human Services, Public Health Service, Centers for Disease Control, National Institute for Occupational Safety and Health, "NIOSH Current Intelligence Bulletin 4 — Chrome Pigment," June 24 and Oct. 7, 1975, and Oct. 8, 1976, U.S. Government Printing Office, Washington, DC.

407. U.S. Department of Health and Human Services, Public Health Service, Centers for Disease Control, National Institute for Occupational Safety and Health, "NIOSH Current Intelligence Bulletin 5 — Asbestos: Asbestos Exposure During Servicing of Motor Vehicle Brake and Clutch Assemblies," Aug. 8, 1975, U.S. Government Printing Office, Washington, DC.

408. U.S. Department of Health and Human Services, Public Health Service, Centers for Disease Control, National Institute for Occupational Safety and Health, "NIOSH Current Intelligence Bulletin 7 — Polychlorinated Biphenyls (PCBs)," Nov. 3, 1975, U.S. Government Printing Office, Washington, DC.

409. U.S. Department of Health and Human Services, Public Health Service, Centers for Disease Control, National Institute for Occupational Safety and Health, "NIOSH Current Intelligence Bulletin 9 — Chloroform," March 15, 1976, U.S. Government Printing Office, Washington, DC.

410. U.S. Department of Health and Human Services, Public Health Service, Centers for Disease Control, National Institute for Occupational Safety and Health, "NIOSH Current Intelligence Bulletin 14 — Inorganic Arsenic — Respiratory Protection," Sept. 27, 1976, U.S. Government Printing Office, Washington, DC.

411. U.S. Department of Health and Human Services, Public Health Service, Centers for Disease Control, National Institute for Occupational Safety and Health, "NIOSH Current Intelligence Bulletin 17 — 2-Nitropropane," April 25, 1977, U.S. Government Printing Office, Washington, DC.

412. U.S. Department of Health and Human Services, Public Health Service, Centers for Disease Control, National Institute for Occupational Safety and Health, "NIOSH Current Intelligence Bulletin 18 — Acrylonitrile," July 1, 1977, U.S. Government Printing Office, Washington, DC.

413. U.S. Department of Health and Human Services, Public Health Service, Centers for Disease Control, National Institute for Occupational Safety and Health, "Proposed National Strategies for the Prevention of Leading Work-Related Disease and Injuries: Neurotoxic Disorders," 1988, Government Printing Office, Washington, DC.

414. U.S. Department of Health and Human Services, Public Health Service, National Library of Medicine, "Toxicology Data Network: Fact Sheet," March 1991.

415. U.S. Department of Health, Education, and Welfare; Public Health Service; Centers for Disease Control; National Institute for Occupational Safety and Health, "NIOSH Current Intelligence Bulletin 21: Trimellitic Anhydride (TMA)," Feb. 3, 1978.

416. U.S. Department of Housing and Urban Development, "Manufactured Home Construction and Safety Standards; Final Rule," Federal Register, 24 CFR Part 3280, Aug. 9, 1984.

416a. U.S. Department of Labor and Occupational Safety and Health Administration, "Labor Department Asks Court for 30-Day Stay, Forms Task Force on Court's Air Contaminants Decision," USDL 92-463, July 17, 1992.

416b. U.S. Department of Labor and Occupational Safety and Health Administration, "Labor Department Seeks 11th Circuit Rehearing on Air Contaminants," USDL 92-554, August 27, 1992.

416c. U.S. Department of Labor and Occupational Safety and Health Administration, "OSHA Reduces Permissible Exposure Limits for Cadmium by 95 Per Cent," USDL 92-561, August 31, 1992.

417. U.S. Department of Labor and Occupational Safety and Health Administration, U.S. Department of Health and Human Services, Public Health Service, Centers for Disease Control, National Institute of Occupational Safety and Health, "Health Hazard Alert — 2-Nitropropane," Oct. 1, 1980.

417a. U.S. Department of Labor and Occupational Safety and Health Administration, May 27, 1992, Federal Register, Vol. 57, pp. 22289-22328.

418. U.S. Department of Labor and Occupational Safety and Health Administration, U.S. Department of Health and Human Services, Public Health Service, Centers for Disease Control, National Institute of Occupational Safety and Health, "Health Hazard Alert — Benzidine-, o-Toluidine-, and o-Dianisidine–Based Dyes," Dec. 1980.

419. U.S. Department of Labor, Office of Information, Occupational Safety and Health, New release, "Osha Proposes 20-Fold Reduction in Methylene Chloride Exposure to Cut Cancer Risk," Nov. 6, 1991, usdl 91-573.

420. U.S. Environmental Protection Agency, "Cyclohexnone: Response to the Interagency Testing Committee," Federal Registry, Jan. 3, 1984; 49(1): 136–142.

421. U.S. Environmental Protection Agency, "Evaluation of Emission Factors for Formaldehyde from Certain Wood Processing Operations, Final Report," May-Aug. 1989.

422. U.S. Environmental Protection Agency, "Guidelines for Development Toxicity Risk Assessment: Notice," Federal Register, Oct. 5, 1991.

423. U.S. Environmental Protection Agency, "List of Pesticide Product Inert Ingredients," July 25, 1986, and updated on Jan. 15, 1992.

424. U.S. Environmental Protection Agency, "Memorandum: Further Developmental Toxicity Testing on Cyclohexanone," May 4, 1988.

424a. U.S. Environmental Protection Agency, "Tsca Carpet Policy Dialogue Information Package," March 1992.

425. U.S. Environmental Protection Agency, "Tsca Section 4 Profile of Isobutyl Alcohol," Nov. 14, 1991.

426. U.S. Environmental Protection Agency, "Tsca Section 4 Profile of 1-Butanol," Nov. 14, 1991.

427. U.S. Environmental Protection Agency, "Tsca Section 4 Profile of Acetone," Nov. 14, 1991.

428. U.S. Environmental Protection Agency, Air and Radiation, Research and Development, "Indoor Air Facts No. 4 (revised), Sick Building Syndrome," April 1991.

429. U.S. Environmental Protection Agency, Air Quality Planning and Substances, "Natich Data Base Report on State, Local, and epa Air Toxics Activities," July 1990.

430. U.S. Environmental Protection Agency, Office of Air Quality Planning and Standards, "Locating and Estimating Air Emissions from Source of Styrene, Interim Report," Oct. 1991.

431. U.S. Environmental Protection Agency, Office of Pesticides and Toxic Substances, "Memorandum: Request for Assistance on Cyclohexanone," Aug. 23, 1984.

432. U.S. Environmental Protection Agency, Office of Toxic Substances, Economic and Technology Division, "Toxics in the Community, National and Local Perspectives: The 1989 Toxics Release Inventory National Report," Sept. 1991, Government Printing Office.

433. U.S. Environmental Protection Agency, Office of Toxic Substances, "Risk Management Level II, Pollution Prevention Scoping Document for Acrylontrile, cas# 107-13-1," Nov. 21, 1991.

434. U.S. Environmental Protection Agency, Office of Toxic Substances, "RM1 Meeting Summary: 1,2-Dibromoethane (ebd)," May 17, 1990.

435. U.S. Environmental Protection Agency, Office of Toxic Substances, "RM1 Meeting Summary: Hydroquinone," May 17, 1990.

436. U.S. Environmental Protection Agency, Office of Toxic Substances, "RM1 Meeting Summary: Vinyl Acetate Status Report," Feb. 1, 1991.

437. U.S. Environmental Protection Agency, Office of Toxic Substances, "RM1 Meeting Summary: Mesityl Oxide," June 7, 1990.

438. U.S. Environmental Protection Agency, Office of Toxic Substances, "Rab RM-1 Presentation for Cyclohexanone," Nov. 15, 1990.

439. U.S. Environmental Protection Agency, Office of Toxic Substances, "RM1 Meeting Summary: Cyclohexanone," November 15, 1990.

440. U.S. Environmental Protection Agency, Office of Toxic Substances, "RM1 Meeting Summary: Isophorone," Jan. 16, 1991.

441. U.S. Environmental Protection Agency, Office of Toxic Substances, "RM1 Meeting Summary: Cumene," Jan. 10, 1991.

442. U.S. Environmental Protection Agency, Office of Toxic Substances, "RM1 Meeting Summary: 1,2-Dichloropropane," June 5, 1991.

443. U.S. Environmental Protection Agency, Office of Toxic Substances, "RM1 Meeting Summary: 2-Nitropropane," May 29, 1991.

444. U.S. Environmental Protection Agency, Office of Toxic Substances, "RM1 Meeting Summary: Hydrogen Cyanide (HCN)," May 17, 1990.

445. U.S. Environmental Protection Agency, Office of Toxic Substances, "Revised RAD RM1 Document for Isocyanates," October 1, 1991 (revised), RAB/ECAD TS-778.

446. U.S. General Accounting Office, "Indoor Air Pollution: Federal Efforts Are Not Effectively Addressing a Growing Problem," October, 1991, GAO/RCED-92-8.

447. U.S. General Accounting Office, "Lawn Care Pesticides: Risks Remain Uncertain While Prohibited Safety Claims Continue," March 1990.

448. U.S. General Accounting Office, "Pesticides: Food Consumption Data of Little Value to Estimate Some Exposures," 1991, Report No. GAO/RCED-91-125.

449. U.S. General Accounting Office, "Reproductive and Developmental Toxicants: Regulatory Actions Provide Uncertain Protection," October 1991. (GAO/PEMD-92-3).

450. U.S. General Accounting Office, "Disinfectants: EPA Lacks Assurance They Work," August 1990.

451. U.S. Public Health Service, Agency for Toxic Substances and Disease Registry, U.S. Environmental Protection Agency, "Toxicological Profile for Toluene," December 1989.

452. Wallace, L.A., W.C. Nelson, E. Pellizzari, J.H. Raymer, and K.W. Thomas, U.S. Environmental Protection Agency, Research Triangle Institute, "Identification of Polar Volatile Organic Compounds in Consumer Products and Common Microenvironments," presented at the 84th Annual Meeting & Exhibition, Air & Waste Management, Vancouver, B.C., June 16–21, 1991.

453. Warner, B., "Coping with Toxic Chemicals in the Interiorscape," *The New Leaf Press,* July 1988, Vol. 3., No. 7.

454. Washington Institute of Neurosciences, Inc., "Halstad-Reitan Neuropsychological Testing," patient information package (undated), Seattle, WA.

455. Washington Institute of Neurosciences, Inc., "About the Brainmap," patient information package (undated), Seattle, WA.

456. Western Family, product label for Hydrogen Peroxide 3% Solution U.S.P., ca. 1992.

457. Williams, M.L., et al, "Environmental Health Center – Dallas Outpatient Information Booklet," 1984.

458. Working Notes on Community Right-to-Know, "Hazardous Waste Recycling: A Risky Business," Feb./March 1991.

459. Xerox Corporation, Material Safety Data Sheet No. A-0024 for 1040/1045/1050/5045/5052 Dry Ink Plus, Jan. 17 1983.

460. Xerox Corporation, Material Safety Data Sheet No. B-0223 for 1040/1045/1050/5052/5052 Developer, Jan. 18, 1983.

Index

A

AA 122, 125
a,a-Butadiene 138
Abdominal effects 11, 124, 127, 131, 132, 136, 137, 138, 139, 142, 143, 145, 147, 151, 152, 155, 157, 158, 163, 164, 171, 173, 175, 177, 181, 188–191, 194, 195, 196, 198, 201–203, 207, 210–213, 215, 216, 219, 220, 222–225, 228, 229, 233, 234, 236–239, 240–242, 248, 250–252; *see also* stomach (gastric)
Abortion, spontaneous 11, 125, 130, 131, 133, 150, 153, 159, 162, 169, 178, 196, 199, 221, 234, 238, 250, 252
Absolute ethanol 122, 172
Absorbant materials 79, 125
Acaricides 79, 132, 143, 151, 158, 162, 170, 210, 236
Acetaldehyde 19, 21, 23, 25–29, 31, 32, 50, 52, 57–60, 65, 66, 68, 70, 74, 76, 77, 80, 82, 84, 86, 90, 94, 95, 100, 103, 106–109, 112, 113, 115, 122, 172, 174, 205
p-Acetaldehyde 122, 217
Acetaminophen 79, 123, 214
Acetanilide 123
Acetic acid 16, 17, 19, 23, 25, 27, 30–32, 35, 38, 45–46, 49–50, 55–56, 58–60, 63–66, 69–71, 73, 76–79, 83–85, 90–97, 99, 101–102, 104, 106, 108–109, 111–113, 115, 118–120, 122, 123, 145, 161, 172, 185, 200
Acetic acid anhydride 122
Acetic acid, ethenyl ester 122, 249
Acetic acid, vinyl ester 122, 249
Acetic aldehyde 122
Acetic anhydride 13, 16, 19, 21, 23–25, 27, 30–32, 35, 38, 41, 48, 50, 54–57, 59, 60, 61, 62, 63–65, 70, 73, 76, 77, 79, 82, 85, 86, 91, 92, 94, 95, 97, 102, 104–109, 112, 115, 120, 122–124, 172
Acetic ester 123, 173

Acetic ether 123, 173
Acetic oxide 122, 123
Acetone 14, 16, 17, 19, 21–25, 27–29, 31, 33, 36, 37, 39, 40, 42, 43, 50, 51, 55, 56, 58, 59, 60, 62–64, 69–71, 73, 76, 77, 79–81, 85–87, 89, 91–94, 100, 104–106, 108, 109, 111–115, 117–120, 123, 148, 155, 167, 195, 206, 227
Acetonitrile 12, 14, 17, 19–26, 31, 35, 36, 38, 39, 40, 47, 48, 50, 53–57, 59, 63, 64, 66, 67, 69–71, 73–75, 77, 81, 86, 88, 92, 93, 104–110, 112, 113, 115, 116, 118, 123, 156, 180, 204
3-(alpha-Acetonyl)-benzyl-4-hydroxycoumarin 124, 251
1-Acetoxyethylene 124, 249
alpha-Acetoxytoluene 124, 135
Acetylene dichloride 124, 161
Acetylene tetrabromide 11, 13, 15, 36, 40, 41, 45, 50, 51, 52, 60, 69, 70, 73, 75, 77, 84, 92–93, 96, 103, 104, 110, 111, 114, 115, 118, 120, 124, 236, 237
Acetylene tetrachloride 124, 237
Acetylene trichloride 126, 244
Acetyl oxide 122, 124
Acidosis 11, 127, 139, 152, 157, 168, 179, 182, 183, 195, 201, 217, 218, 234
Acintene DP 124, 196
Acquinite (tn) 124, 150
Acraldehyde 124
Acritet 124, 125
Acrolein 11, 13, 14, 19, 25, 29, 31, 45, 48, 58, 61, 62, 65, 66, 67, 73, 76, 77, 79–82, 84, 86, 90, 95, 97, 98, 101, 103, 105–111, 115, 117, 124–126, 130, 216, 277
Acroosteolysis, occupational 11, 249, 250
Acrylaldehyde 124, 125
Acrylamide 12, 18, 19, 24, 26, 30, 31, 33, 34, 36, 42, 49, 52, 53, 59, 61, 62, 65, 67, 73, 75–77, 79, 80, 85, 87, 89, 92, 106–109, 114, 116, 119, 125, 227
Acrylamide monomer 125
Acrylic acids 125, 145, 195

G

REFERENCE